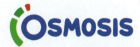

HIGH-YIELD PHYSIOLOGY NOTES

1st Edition

The Osmosis Team

2019

Copyright © 2017–2019 by Osmosis
ALL RIGHTS RESERVED

This book or any portion thereof may not be reproduced or used in any manner whatsoever without the express written permission of the publisher except for the use of brief quotations in a book review. For permission requests, email us with the subject "Attention: Permissions Coordinator," at the address below.

hi@osmosis.org

ISBN 978-1-947769-11-3

Osmosis
37 S. Ellwood Avenue
Baltimore, MD 21224
www.osmosis.org

Printed in Canada

Designed by Fergus Baird, Lauren DiVito, Heidi Hildebrandt, Tanner Marshall, & Kyle Slinn
Copyedited by Fergus Baird, Thomas Bush, Damien Caissie, Elizabeth Krupa, & Jessica MacEachern
Cover design by Robyn Hughes, Aileen Lin, Brittany Norton, & Vince Waldman

Fonts:
Nunito by Vernon Adams., Open Font License;
STIX2Math & STIX2Text, by STI Pub Companies, Open Font License

Written by writers all around the globe.
TC 10 9 8 7 6 5 4 3 2 1

1st Edition

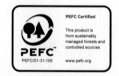

We'd like to thank our Osmosis Prime members, our supporters, the hundreds of volunteers who double check our facts and translate our videos, and of course, our viewers on YouTube. You all have played a huge part in helping us make the best learning experiences possible.

If you find any mistakes, let us know here:
osms.it/feedback-physio

Osmosis Team

Hillary Acer, BA
Alex Aranda, AA
Amin Azzam, MD, MA
Fergus Baird, MA
Damien Caissie, BA
Kaia Chessen, MScBMC
Evan Debevec-McKenney, BA
Harry Delaney, MBChB
Rishi Desai, MD, MPH
Allison Dollar, BFA
Ursula Florjanczyk, MScBMC
Caleb Furnas, MA
Shiv Gaglani, MBA
Guillermo Galizzi
Sam Gillespie, BSc

Meagan Harcastle, BS
M. Ryan Haynes, PhD
Heidi Hildebrandt, MA
Michael Holewinski
Robyn Hughes, MScBMC
Aileen Lin, MScBMC
Justin Ling, MD, MS
Kara Lukasiewicz, PhD, MScBMC
John Maloney MFA
Tanner Marshall, MS
Samantha McBundy, MFA
B. Gil McIntire
Ashwin Menon, MS, MSEd, BE
Sam Miller, BA
Katie Murphy, BA

Brandon Newton, BBA
Elizabeth Nixon-Shapiro, MSMI, CMI
Brittany Norton, MFA
Che Nxusani, BSc
Marisa Pedron, BA
Viviana Popa, MD candidate
Pauline Rowsome, BSc
Kyle Slinn, BScN, RN, MEd
Diana Stanley, MBA
Sean Tackett, MD, MPH
Vincent Waldman, PhD
Will Wei
Sidney Williams
Owen Willis, MEd
Yifan Xiao, MD

EDITORS

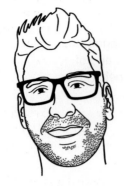

Harry Delaney
BSc. (Hons), MBChB

Harry is a content editor and erstwhile script writer for Osmosis. He completed his medical degree at The University of Warwick and is a registrar in anatomical pathology at University College London Hospital. Harry has taught and examined undergraduate medical students at all stages and is never happier than when teaching first years anatomy in the dissecting lab! He just spent a year living in Munich, Germany.

In his free time there he skied the Alps in the winter and walked them in the summer. When he's not sliding down the piste in a heap, he enjoys live comedy, gaming, and riding his motorcycle.

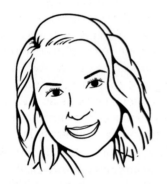

Elizabeth Krupa
MD

Elizabeth is an editor and reviewer with Osmosis. She is originally from Winnipeg, Canada and completed medical school in Krakow, Poland at the Jagiellonian University Medical College. Her interests in medicine lie in pediatrics and pet therapy which she hopes to integrate into her future practice. Elizabeth enjoys painting, the outdoors, and trying new recipes inspired by her travels in Europe!

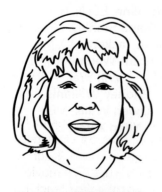

Lisa Miklush
PhD, RNC, CNS

Lisa writes and reviews content for Osmosis. At the University of San Diego, she completed her PhD with a focus on health outcomes of high-risk infants. Lisa loves contributing to online education. She has created educational content for Khan Academy Medicine and has over 15 years of experience teaching graduate and undergraduate nursing students.

When she isn't teaching or working for Osmosis, Lisa spends time in her garden, feeding birds, and walking the local trails with her husband.

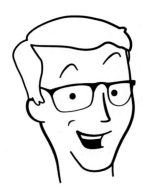

Kyle Slinn
BScN, MEd, RN

Kyle is a project manager and instructional designer at Osmosis. He wears many hats, such as leading collaboration efforts with the YouTube community, prototyping future projects, producing videos, leading internationalization efforts, and designing Osmosis's textbooks and high-yield notes. A jack-of-all-trades. Before Osmosis, he worked as a project coordinator for Khan Academy Medicine, where he managed the creation of videos, questions, and text-based articles for MCAT and NCLEX-RN students.

Kyle also worked in the pediatric intensive care unit as a nurse at the Children's Hospital of Eastern Ontario, in Ottawa, Canada. He received his Bachelor of Science in nursing from the University of Ottawa and holds a Master of Education in distance education from Athabasca University.

With his free time, Kyle loves to go on adventures, rock climb, ski, play board games, and play musical instruments.

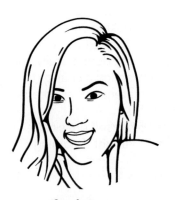

Ashley Thompson
BS, MD

Ashley is a content writer and editor for Osmosis. Originally from Vancouver, Canada, she completed her Bachelor of Science degree in biology at the University of Victoria, and is a lover of all things nature, even the Vancouver rain! Her enthusiasm for traveling led her to Europe where she completed her MD degree at Jagiellonian University in Krakow, Poland. Here, she cultivated her passions for teaching and medical education, developing interactive workshops and leading interest groups as a way to engage medical students outside of the traditional classroom setting. Ashley is currently a resident at SUNY Upstate Medical University in Syracuse, New York and is awaiting all the four beautiful seasons the east coast has to offer.

When she does have the occasional time off, she loves to hike, snowboard, surf, or hang out with her super cool cat, Nugget.

CONTRIBUTORS

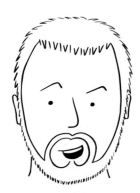

Fergus Baird
MA

Fergus is a copywriter, copy editor and textbook designer at Osmosis, and he dabbles in a little scriptwriting for the YouTube channel as well.

Before moving to Canada, Fergus lived in a small village in Scotland. He earned his master's degree in English literature at Concordia University in Montréal, writing his thesis on history and the graphic novel. Prior to joining the Osmosis team, Fergus worked as a GIF curator, a movie subtitler, a meme master, and a ghost writer, and spent a year teaching elementary school kids in Japan.

When he's not eating or cooking elaborate meals for his friends, Fergus spends his spare time playing video games and the theremin, drawing strange pictures, and consuming horror media in all its gruesome forms.

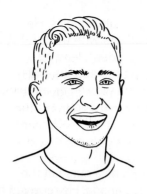

Thomas Bush

Thomas writes notes and scripts for Osmosis. With a background in the physical sciences, he loves creating short and sweet explanations for tough medical topics. From his office in not-so-sunny Poland, he also teaches others about linguistics and technology. Thomas is a firm believer that deep understanding is the key to effective learning, and he makes sure to incorporate that idea in all of his work!

When he's not looking for the answer to obscure and oddly specific medical questions, Thomas loves biking, cooking, and traveling the world.

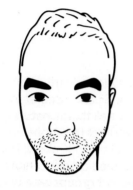

Damien Caissie
BA

Damien serves as a content editor with Osmosis. Having recently moved to Toronto following a stint living in South Korea, Damien spends his days renewing his passion for reality television and baking cookies. After studying English literature at the University of New Brunswick and Concordia, Damien has taught English and history domestically and abroad. Lending his talents to Osmosis has given Damien a chance to develop engaging and approachable educational material for our readers.

Being Canadian, Damien has excelled at preparing himself physically and mentally for long winters, though can often be caught dreaming of Floridian beaches in unguarded moments.

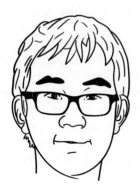

Kaien Gu
BSc

Kaien writes content for Osmosis. He completed his BSc in biochemistry at McGill University and is currently studying medicine at the University of Manitoba. Outside of that, he has a passion for research, having been involved in various projects for almost a decade. His current projects involve rheumatology and the long-term outcome of rheumatic diseases.

Outside of all of this, Kaien enjoys travelling, eating out, and playing squash in his free time.

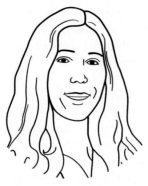

Robyn Hughes
MScBMC

Robyn is an illustrator with Osmosis who has also created layouts for print material. She completed her BSc in life sciences at Queen's University, where she discovered her love of anatomy and pathophysiology. She then completed her Master of Science in biomedical communications at the University of Toronto, where she learned how to effectively communicate scientific information through visual design. Robyn is grateful that she is able to use her skills to help develop quality educational resources.

She is passionate about the arts, and when she is not working, you will most likely find her at a musical theatre rehearsal or dance class!

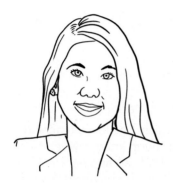

Jennifer Lee

Jennifer is currently a third-year med student and content writer for Osmosis. At the University of Florida, Jennifer considered a career in music and fashion merchandise before stumbling upon a volunteering opportunity for an underserved clinic and committing to medicine.

When she's not watching puppy videos on Instagram, Jennifer enjoys college football, margaritas on the beach, and exploring new eateries.

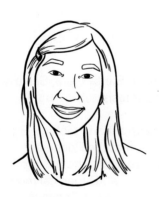

Aileen Lin
MScBMC

Aileen is a content illustrator and figure-caption writer for Osmosis. She loves taking complex ideas and making them approachable and easy to understand, especially thorugh visuals. Aileen grew up in Calgary, where she spent many weekends hiking in the Rocky Mountains. She completed a BSc in cognitive science at the University of Toronto. Recently, she completed her Master of Science in biomedical communications, also at the University of Toronto, where she was able to combine her enthusiasm for both science and art. Now, she is excited to be involved in creating great educational resources for students!

In her free time, she enjoys playing video games, playing board games, reading, and making things with her hands (such as crafts and desserts).

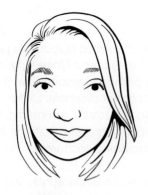

Jessica MacEachern, MA

Jessica MacEachern edits copy for Osmosis. She has an MA in creative writing from Concordia University in Montréal, Québec. She is a PhD candidate in English studies at the Université de Montréal, as well as a part-time professor in Concordia's English Department.

Jessica studies feminist poetry—and occasionally writes it, too. She began her secondary education in psychology at the University of New Brunswick, where she received a student research grant to study sex differences in spatial cognition. As with her hero Gertrude Stein (the modernist poet who studied under the psychologist William James) these early pursuits in the scientific study of the mind continue to inform her creative explorations.

When she's not reading or writing, Jessica is likely pinned underneath her darling cat, Kitty—though this is generally true even if she has a book in hand.

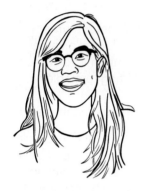

Patricia Nguyen, BScKin, MScBMC

Patty has two great passions: science and comics. She loves teaching people about interesting scientific concepts through images (even better if they can be cartoons!). During her spare time, you can find her munching on french pastries and drawing comics about life, mental health and relationships.

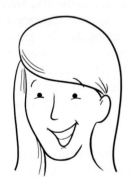

Brittany Norton, MFA

Brittany is a medical illustrator currently based in Santa Clara, California, who creates illustrations and animations for Osmosis.

Unable to choose between her passions for both art and biology, Brittany decided to pursue a degree in medical illustration at the Rochester Institute of Technology. Since graduating with an MFA, she has worked as a video illustrator for Khan Academy as well as a 3D medical modeler/animator for a patient education startup in Silicon Valley. She loves drawing all things anatomical and helping others understand complex concepts through the universal language of art.

When she's not working, Brittany can be found jamming out to Disney music, planning her next traveling adventure, or chasing down neighborhood dogs to pet.

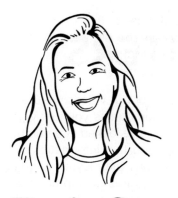

Jennifer Ring
M.H.Sc., S-LP(C) Reg.
CASLPO

Jennifer is a content editor for Osmosis. She completed her B.Sc in life sciences at Queen's University, with a minor in psychology. Once finished, she moved to Toronto to complete her Master of Health Sciences in speech–language pathology. She has a background in alternative and augmentative communication, autism, and supportive communication. Jennifer is committed to improving access to easily understood and evidence-based medical information for everyone who may want it.

In her free time, Jennifer loves to travel, explore the great outdoors, and spend time lakeside with friends and family.

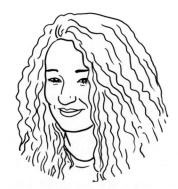

Gordana Sendić

Gordana is a note writer and reviewer for Osmosis. She is excited to provide thorough, comprehensive, and enjoyable notes that make med students' lives much easier! Since she is a med student herself, she understands the struggle! She studies at the University of Belgrade's Faculty of Medicine in Serbia. Gordana also has experience as an undergraduate student demonstrator at her university. She is interested in internal medicine and surgical specialties.

In her free time she enjoys philosophy, traveling, classical music, painting, singing, dancing, and the occasional Netflix binge (she is one of those people who wants to do everything at once in life). But she remains committed to one goal, however: to learn as much as she can about everything!

WORDS FROM THE WRITERS

The High-Yield Notes project started back in March of 2017. When writing scripts for our videos we use a lot of different resources during our initial research period. Textbooks are great, but sometimes you just want to quickly learn the key points of a disease without wading through paragraphs of text. We looked at a number of resources that try to do this, but they all had issues. Some of them were missing important information or had numerous factual inaccuracies (frightening!). Some of them were hard to use: simply, their layout and visual aesthetic needed some work. Some of them neglected to include memory aids or pictures to help tie together what the text was saying. None of them let us make notes easily on the pages themselves. Most of them didn't actually cover all the content you need to know on a particular exam. All of them were geared exclusively for the medical profession.

We couldn't find what we wanted, and it occurred to us that we had an opportunity to make the product we were searching for. So we did. It also gave us a chance to expand beyond the scope of our many videos. As such, these notes have more fleshed-out symptoms, diagnoses, and treatment sections than our videos.

This proved to be a massive effort. This was the longest project we had ever done and one of the most complex. This book was assembled by an army of people. We had over 25 writers write the book, and several reviewers, designers, and copyeditors carefully comb through it. Harry, our pathologist, single-handedly sourced all of the images over the better part of a year, curating an impressive library for us. Every single person involved cared deeply about making this the best learning experience possible and I think their passion shines through on every page.

Our Osmosis users' involvement provided essential insights as well. We interviewed dozens of you over video chat and received hundreds of responses from the surveys we sent out asking you how our prototypes for this book could improve. Your comments were incredibly helpful. You valued more images, tables, and clean, thoughtful design even if it heightened our page-count. You wanted mnemonics to help you remember information and you wanted us to signal important information to remember. So, we delayed our book's release and ensured that those suggestions were included.

And here we are! The first edition of this book is complete. Thank you so much for getting us this far. We all hope you like what we've built, not only using it while in school, but continue to draw knowledge from it long after as an invaluable resource.

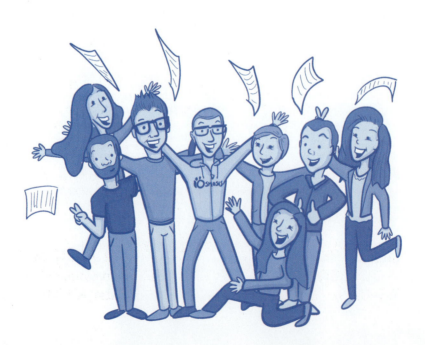

WORDS FROM THE FOUNDERS

Welcome to Osmosis High-Yield Physiology Notes, our third volume in a series of high-yield notes covering pathology and physiology. We are very proud of how our growing library of physiology videos is helping learners in the health professions, and are thrilled to offer these high-yield notes as an essential companion to the Osmosis learning platform.

Our six core company values, modeled after the human body, guide our approach to everything we create for our learners. The first of these values is "Start with the Heart" because we care deeply about your success. Our passionate and dedicated writers, editors, and illustrators refined every page to deliver concise notes that won't just help you memorize essential facts, but also strengthen your conceptual understanding of each and every topic. Whether through these notes, our popular videos, or unique features on the Osmosis platform, we want to ensure that Osmosis is a comprehensive and trustworthy partner in your education.

We've listened to countless Osmosis learners as we developed these notes and would welcome your feedback as well. Indeed, one of our other core values is to "Open Your Arms," signifying our team's approachability. Thus, please feel free to share any suggestions, concerns, feedback, and new ideas.

Osmosis's high-yield notes have received a tremendous amount of positive feedback from our community and we're thrilled to finally offer them in print. High-Yield Physiology Notes is packed with illustrations, diagrams, and other visual resources to help strengthen your knowledge. Rather than dryly scanning through and memorizing facts, we want to ensure that you are building a strong conceptual understanding of health science topics. Overall, we believe that learning should be joyful. Let Osmosis give you a hand with these notes!

While you may not be able to sleep with your head on these notes and "learn by Osmosis," you can use the powerful and comprehensive Osmosis learning platform to watch the corresponding pathology and physiology videos, actively quiz yourself with tens of thousands of associated practice questions and flashcards, and set up a personalized study schedule. We encourage you to visit www.osmosis.org to learn more.

Best wishes Osmosing!

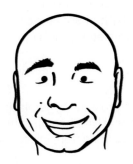

Shiv Gaglani
MBA
Co-founder & CEO

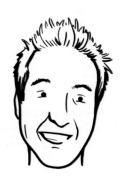

M. Ryan Haynes
PhD (Neuroscience)
Co-founder & CTO

HOW TO USE THIS BOOK

This book has a few unique features to help you get the most out of it:

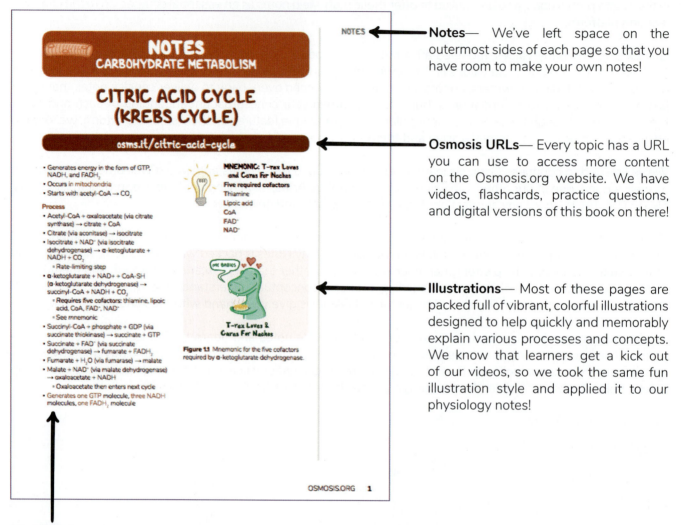

Notes— We've left space on the outermost sides of each page so that you have room to make your own notes!

Osmosis URLs— Every topic has a URL you can use to access more content on the Osmosis.org website. We have videos, flashcards, practice questions, and digital versions of this book on there!

Illustrations— Most of these pages are packed full of vibrant, colorful illustrations designed to help quickly and memorably explain various processes and concepts. We know that learners get a kick out of our videos, so we took the same fun illustration style and applied it to our physiology notes!

Highlighting— We spent a lot of time editing this book so that only the most essential, important information on each topic is included, but even then, some topics still have a ton of information to remember. To help you determine what information is absolutely important, we've highlighted some words and phrases for you. One caveat: if the first word in a list (complications, signs and symptoms etc) is highlighted, assume the whole list is important. For example,

- Adults:
    - *Acquired disease:* kidney stones (most common cause), benign prostatic hyperplasia, blood clot, contiguous malignant diseases (prostate/bladder/cervix cancer, retroperitoneal lymphoma), contiguous inflammation (prostatitis, ureteritis, urethritis, retroperitoneal fibrosis), tissue scarring from injury/surgery, uterus enlargement during pregnancy

That's silly, why don't we highlight all of the words? We did in earlier drafts. Large blocks of colored text looks gross. We spent many days trying to nail down a system that looks nice, but also allows you to make your own highlights. This was what we settled on. Our recommendation? Keep your own highlighter nearby!

CONTENTS

SUBJECT: BIOCHEMISTRY

	PAGE
Carbohydrate metabolism	
Citric acid cycle (Krebs cycle)	1
Electron transport chain & oxidative phosphorylation	2
Gluconeogenesis	4
Glycogen metabolism	6
Glycolysis	9
Pentose phosphate pathway	10
Fat & cholesterol metabolism	
Cholesterol metabolism	13
Fatty acid synthesis	15
Fatty acid oxidation	18
Ketone body metabolism	21
Nucleic acid metabolism	
Nucleotide metabolism	23
Protein metabolism	
Amino acids & protein folding	29
Enzyme function	31
Amino acid metabolism	32
Nitrogen & the urea cycle	33
Protein structure & synthesis	38

SUBJECT: BIOSTATISTICS & EPIDEMIOLOGY

	PAGE
Introductory biostatistics	
Introduction to biostatistics	41
Mean, median, & mode	43
Probability	44
Range, variance, & standard deviation	46
Types of data	47
Causation & validity	
Causality	48
Bias	49
Confounding	50
Interaction	50
Community health	
Modes of infectious disease transmission	52
Outbreak investigations	52

SUBJECT: BIOSTATISTICS & EPIDEMIOLOGY

	PAGE
Disease surveillance	53
Vaccination & herd immunity	54
Epidemiology measures	
Direct standardization	55
Indirect standardization	55
Incidence & prevalence	58
Measures of risk	58
Odds ratio	59
Attributable risk (AR)	60
Mortality rates & case-fatality	60
DALY & QALY	61
Non-parametric tests	
Chi-squared test	62
Fisher's exact test	62
Kaplan–Meier survival analysis	63
Kappa coefficient	63
Mann–Whitney U test	63
Spearman's rank correlation coefficient	64
Parametric tests	
ANOVA	65
Correlation	67
Hypothesis testing	68
Linear regression	68
Logistic regression	69
Type I & type II errors	69
Statistical probability distributions	
Normal distribution & z-scores	71
Standard error of the mean	72
Paired t-tests	72
One-tailed & two-tailed tests	72
Study design	
Sampling	74
Placebo effect & masking	74
Case-control (retrospective) study	74
Cohort study	75
Cross-sectional (prevalence) study	76
Ecologic study	77
Randomized control trial (RCT)	78
Testing	
Sensitivity (SN) & specificity (SF)	79
Positive & negative predictive value	81
Test precision & accuracy	82

SUBJECT
CARDIOVASCULAR PHYSIOLOGY | PAGE

Cardiovascular anatomy & physiology
- Cardiovascular anatomy & physiology — 83
- Lymphatic anatomy & physiology — 90
- Normal heart sounds — 94
- Abnormal heart sounds — 95

Blood pressure regulation
- Baroreceptors — 105
- Chemoreceptors — 107
- Renin-angiotensin aldosterone system — 109

Cardiac cycle
- Measuring cardiac output - Fick principle — 111
- Cardiac & vascular function curves — 111
- Altering cardiac & vascular function curves — 112
- Pressure-volume loops — 113
- Changes in pressure-volume loops — 115
- Cardiac work — 116
- Cardiac preload — 117
- Cardiac afterload — 118
- Law of Laplace — 118
- Frank–Starling relationship — 119
- Stroke volume, ejection fraction, & cardiac output — 120

Cardiac electrophysiology
- Action potentials in pacemaker cells — 121
- Action potentials in myocytes — 122
- Electrical conduction in the heart — 123
- Cardiac conduction velocity — 123
- Excitability & refractory periods — 124
- Cardiac excitation-contraction coupling — 125
- Cardiac length tension — 126
- Cardiac contractility — 126

Electrocardiography
- ECG basics — 128
- ECG normal sinus rhythm — 129
- ECG rate & rhythm — 129
- ECG intervals — 130
- ECG axis — 131
- ECG transition — 131
- ECG cardiac hypertrophy & enlargement — 133
- ECG myocardial infarction & ischemia — 134

SUBJECT
CARDIOVASCULAR PHYSIOLOGY | PAGE

Hemodynamics
- Blood pressure, blood flow, & resistance — 136
- Pressures in the cardiovascular system — 137
- Resistance to blood flow — 141
- Laminar flow & Reynolds number — 143
- Compliance of blood vessels — 144

Normal variations of the cardiovascular system
- Cardiovascular changes during exercise — 146
- Cardiovascular changes during hemorrhage — 147
- Cardiovascular changes during postural change — 149

Specific circulations
- Cerebral circulation — 152
- Coronary circulation — 153
- Control of blood flow circulation — 154
- Microcirculation & Starling forces — 155

Thermoregulation
- Cardiovascular temperature homeostasis — 157

SUBJECT
CELLULAR PHYSIOLOGY | PAGE

Cellular structure & processes
- Cellular structure & function — 160
- Cell membrane — 162
- Selective permeability of the cell membrane — 163
- Extracellular matrix — 164
- Cell-cell junctions — 166
- Endocytosis & exocytosis — 167
- Osmosis — 168
- Resting membrane potential — 169
- Cell signaling pathways — 170
- Cytoskeleton & intracellular motility — 177
- Nuclear structure — 179

SUBJECT	
CELLULAR PHYSIOLOGY	**PAGE**
Cellular pathology	
Necrosis & apoptosis	181
Oncogenes & tumor suppressor genes	184
Hyperplasia & hypertrophy	185
Metaplasia & dysplasia	186
Atrophy, aplasia, & hypoplasia	186
Free radicals & cellular injury	187
Ischemia	188
Inflammation	188

SUBJECT	
DERMATOLOGY	**PAGE**
Skin structures	
Skin anatomy & physiology	190
Hair, skin, & nails	192
Wound healing	194

SUBJECT	
EMBRYOLOGY	**PAGE**
Early weeks	
Human development days 1–4	196
Human development days 4–7	199
Human development week 2	200
Human development week 3	201
Germ layers	
Ectoderm	204
Mesoderm	205
Endoderm	206
Early structures	
Development of the digestive system & body cavities	209
The hedgeog signalling pathway	212
Development of the placenta	214
Development of the umbilical cord	216
Development of the fetal membranes	218
Development of twins	219

SUBJECT	
EMBRYOLOGY	**PAGE**
Body system structures	
Development of the skeletal system	221
Development of the muscular system	225
Development of the limbs	227
Development of the cardiovascular system	228
Fetal circulation	232
Development of the respiratory system	235
Development of the gastrointestinal system	238
Development of the renal system	243
Development of the integumentary system	247
Head & neck structure	
Pharyngeal arches, pouches, & clefts	249
Development of teeth	252
Development of the brain	253
Development of cranial nerves & autonomic nervous system	256
Development of the spinal cord	257
Development of the ear	258
Development of the eye	260

SUBJECT	
ENDOCRINE PHYSIOLOGY	**PAGE**
Anatomy & physiology	
Endocrine anatomy & physiology	262
Pituitary hormones	
Adrenocorticotropic hormone	269
Growth hormone	271
Thyroid hormone	273
Adrenal hormones	
Synthesis of adrenocortical hormones	276
Cortisol	278
Pancreatic hormones	
Glucagon	280
Insulin	281
Somatostatin	283

SUBJECT	
ENDOCRINE PHYSIOLOGY	**PAGE**
Calcium & phosphate hormonal regulation	
Calcitonin	284
Parathyroid hormone	286
Vitamin D	289

SUBJECT	
GASTROINTESTINAL PHYSIOLOGY	**PAGE**
Anatomy & physiology	
Gastrointestinal anatomy & physiology	293
Gastrointestinal function	
Enteric nervous system	302
Gastrointestinal hormones	305
Satiety	308
Upper gastrointestinal tract	
Chewing & swallowing	309
Salivary secretion	311
Slow waves	313
Esophageal motility	316
Gastric motility	319
Gastric secretion	321
Digestion & absorption	
Hydration	326
Carbohydrates & sugars	326
Proteins	327
Fats	328
Vitamins	330
Intestinal fluid balance	331
Liver, gall bladder, and pancreas	
Bile secretion & enterohepatic circulation	332
Liver anatomy & physiology	333
Pancreatic secretion	337

SUBJECT	
GENETICS	**PAGE**
Population genetics	
Mendelian genetics & Punnett squares	338
Independent assortment of genes & linkage	339
Inheritance patterns	341
Evolution & natural selection	344
Hardy–Weinberg equilibrium	344
Epigenetics	345
Lac operon	345
Gene regulation	346
Gel electrophoresis & genetic testing	347
Polymerase chain reaction	348
Transcription, translation, & replication	
DNA structure	349
DNA replication	351
Transcription	354
Translation	355
Cell cycle	357
Mitosis & meiosis	358
Genetic mutations & repair	360

SUBJECT	
HEMATOLOGY	**PAGE**
Blood components & function	
Blood components	364
Platelet plug formation (primary hemostasis)	365
Coagulation (secondary hemostasis)	367
Role of vitamin K in coagulation	367
Anticoagulation, clot retraction, & fibrinolysis	369
Blood groups & transfusions	370

SUBJECT	
IMMUNOLOGY	**PAGE**
Immune system	
Introduction to the immune system	372
Vaccines	375
B & T cells	
Antibody classes	377
B cell activation & differentiation	378
B cell development	381
Cell mediated immunity of CD4 cells	383
Cell mediated immunity of natural killer & CD8 cells	384
Cytokines	385
MHC class I & MHC class II molecules	386
Somatic hypermutation & affinity maturation	389
T cell activation	390
T cell development	391
VDJ rearrangement	393
Contraction of the immune response	
Anergy, exhaustion, & clonal deletion	395
B & T cell memory	396
Contracting the immune response	399
Innate immunity	
Innate immune system	400
Complement system	402

SUBJECT	
MUSCULOSKELETAL PHYSIOLOGY	**PAGE**
Bones, joints, & cartilage	
Skeletal system anatomy & physiology	405
Cartilage	407
Bone remodeling & repair	410
Fibrous, cartilage, & synoial joints	411
Muscles	
Muscular system anatomy & physiology	414
Slow twitch & fast twitch muscle fibers	418
Sliding filament model of muscle contraction	419
ATP & muscle contraction	420
Neuromuscular junction & motor unit	421

SUBJECT	
NEUROLOGY	**PAGE**
Anatomy & physiology	
Nervous system anatomy & physiology	423
Neuron action potential	433
Anatomy & physiology of the eye	434
Anatomy & physiology of the ear	440
Autonomic nervous system	
Sympathetic nervous system	445
Parasympathetic nervous system	447
Adrenergic receptors	450
Cholinergic receptors	452
Blood brain barrier & CSF	
Blood brain barrier	455
Cerebrospinal fluid	456
Brain functions	
Sleep	459
Consciousness	460
Learning	460
Attention	460
Memory	461
Language	461
Emotion	462
Stress	462
Motor nervous system	
Motor cortex	464
Motor neurons & muscle spindles	465
Pyramidal & extrapyramidal tracts	468
Cerebellum	474
Basal ganglia: direct & indirect pathway of movement	477
Spinal cord reflexes	480
Sensory nervous system	
Sensory receptor function	481
Somatosensory pathways	482
Somatosensory receptors	484
Photoreception	486
Optic pathways	487
Auditory transduction & pathways	489
Vestibular transduction	491
Vestibulo-ocular reflex & nystagmus	494
Olfactory transduction & pathways	494
Taste & the tongue	497
Spinal cord & nerves	
Brachial plexus	500
Cranial nerves	503

SUBJECT	
RENAL PHYSIOLOGY	**PAGE**
Anatomy & physiology	
Renal anatomy & physiology	510
Acid-base physiology	
Acid-base map & compensatory mechanisms	515
Buffering & Henderson–Hasselbalch equation	516
Physiologic pH & buffers	517
Plasma anion gap	518
The role of the kidney in acid-base balance	518
Metabolic acidosis	519
Metabolic alkalosis	520
Respiratory acidosis	521
Respiratory alkalosis	522
Fluids in the body	
Body fluid compartments	523
Water shifts between body fluid compartments	525
Renal clearance	528
Renal blood flow regulation	
Renal blood flow regulation	530
Measuring renal plasma flow & renal blood flow	532
Renal electrolyte regulation	
Glomerular filtration	533
Proximal convoluted tubule	535
Loop of Henle	536
Distal convoluted tubule	537
TF/Px ratio & TF/Pinlin	538
Calcium homeostasis	539
Magnesium homeostasis	539
Phosphate homeostasis	540
Potassium homeostasis	540
Sodium homeostasis	541
Renal reabsorption & secretion	
Tubular reabsorption & secretion	543
Tubular reabsorption of glucose	543
Tubular secretion of para-animohippuric acid (PAH)	545
Urea recycling	547
Weak acids & bases - non-ionic diffusion	547

SUBJECT	
RENAL PHYSIOLOGY	**PAGE**
Water regulation	
Osmoregulation	548
Kidney countercurrent multiplication	549
Antidiuretic hormone	552
Free water clearance	554

SUBJECT	
REPRODUCTIVE PHYSIOLOGY	**PAGE**
Female reproductive system	
Anatomy & physiology of the female reproductive system	555
Oxytocin & prolactin	559
Menstrual cycle	561
Pregnancy	562
Labor	565
Breastfeeding	570
Menopause	572
Estrogen & progesterone	573
Male reproductive system	
Anatomy & physiology of the male reproductive system	576
Testosterone	579
Sexual development	
Development of the reproductive system	581
Puberty & Tanner staging	586

SUBJECT	
RESPIRATORY PHYSIOLOGY	**PAGE**
Anatomy & physiology	
Respiratory system	588
Breathing mechanics	
Lung volumes & capacities	594
Anatomic & physiologic dead space	595
Ventiliation	596
Alveolar gas equation	597
Compliance of lungs & chest wall	597
Combined pressure-volume curves for the lung & chest wall	598
Alveolar surface tension & surfactant	598
Airflow, pressure, & resistance	599
Breathing cycle	600
Breathing regulation	
Breathing control	601
Pulmonary chemoreceptors & mechanoreceptors	602
Gas exchange	
Ideal (general) gas law	603
Boyle's law	604
Dalton's law	604
Henry's law	605
Fick's laws of diffusion	605
Graham's law	606
Gas exchange in the lungs	607
Diffusion-limited & perfusion-limited gas exchange	609
Gas transport	
Oxygen binding capacity & oxygen content	611
Oxygen-hemoglobin dissociation curve	612
Erythropoietin (EPO)	615
Carbon dioxide transport in blood	615
Regulation of pulmonary blood flow	617
Zones of pulmonary blood flow	618
Pulmonary shunts	619
Ventilation perfusion ratios & V Q mismatch	621
Hypoxemia & hypoxia	622
Normal variations	
Pulmonary changes during exercise	625
Pulmonary changes at high altitude & altitude sickness	627

NOTES
CARBOHYDRATE METABOLISM

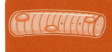

CITRIC ACID CYCLE (KREBS CYCLE)

osms.it/citric-acid-cycle

- Generates energy in the form of GTP, NADH, and $FADH_2$
- Occurs in mitochondria
- Starts with acetyl-CoA → CO_2

Process
- Acetyl-CoA + oxaloacetate (via citrate synthase) → citrate + CoA
- Citrate (via aconitase) → isocitrate
- Isocitrate + NAD^+ (via isocitrate dehydrogenase) → α-ketoglutarate + NADH + CO_2
  - Rate-limiting step
- α-ketoglutarate + NAD^+ + CoA-SH (α-ketoglutarate dehydrogenase) → succinyl-CoA + NADH + CO_2
  - Requires five cofactors: thiamine, lipoic acid, CoA, FAD^+, NAD^+
  - See mnemonic
- Succinyl-CoA + phosphate + GDP (via succinate thiokinase) → succinate + GTP
- Succinate + FAD^+ (via succinate dehydrogenase) → fumarate + $FADH_2$
- Fumarate + H_2O (via fumarase) → malate
- Malate + NAD^+ (via malate dehydrogenase) → oxaloacetate + NADH
  - Oxaloacetate then enters next cycle
- Generates one GTP molecule, three NADH molecules, one $FADH_2$ molecule

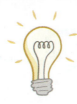

MNEMONIC: T-rex Loves and Cares For Nachos
Five required cofactors
Thiamine
Lipoic **a**cid
CoA
FAD⁺
NAD⁺

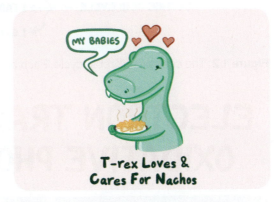

Figure 1.1 Mnemonic for the five cofactors required by α-ketoglutarate dehydrogenase.

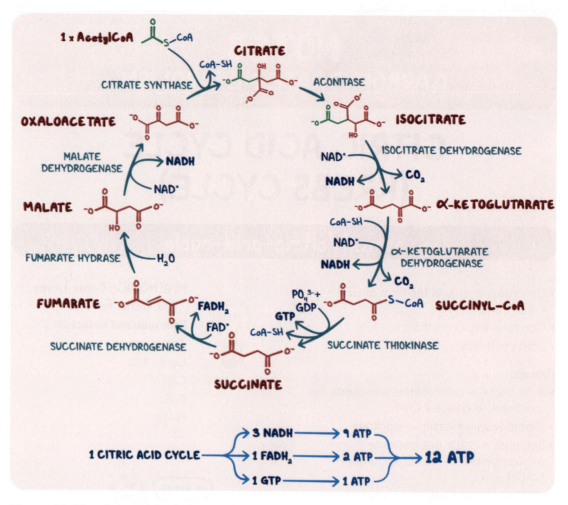

Figure 1.2 The citric acid (Krebs) cycle. Each acetyl-CoA molecule generates 12 ATP.

ELECTRON TRANSPORT CHAIN & OXIDATIVE PHOSPHORYLATION

osms.it/etc-and-oxidative-phosphorylation

Oxidative phosphorylation
- Generates energy as ATP
- Occurs in inner mitochondrial membrane

Electron transport chain
- Series of proteins, lipids, metals that facilitates electron movement → proton gradient used to create ATP
- Starts with electron donors NADH, $FADH_2$
  - NADH from cytoplasm comes through malate-aspartate shuttle
- $FADH_2$ from cytoplasm comes through glycerol-3-phosphate shuttle
- NADH donates electron to complex I (contains flavin mononucleotide, iron-sulfur centers) → NAD^+
- $FADH_2$ donates electron to complex II (i.e. succinate dehydrogenase) → FAD
- Electrons from either complex flow into coenzyme Q (ubiquinone)
- Coenzyme Q passes electrons to cytochromes (proteins with heme

groups — $Fe^{3+} + e^- \leftrightarrow Fe^{2+}$): complex III (cytochromes b and c1) → cytochrome c → complex IV (cytochrome oxidase: cytochromes a, a3) → oxygen
- Movement of electrons → electrical current → complexes I, III, IV use this energy to pump protons across inner mitochondrial membrane
- Protons can move back into mitochondria through F_0 → proton gradient forms, powering F_1: ADP → ATP
  - Collectively called complex V
- An ADP/ATP antiport pumps ATP into cytoplasm of the cell, supplies complex V with new ADP

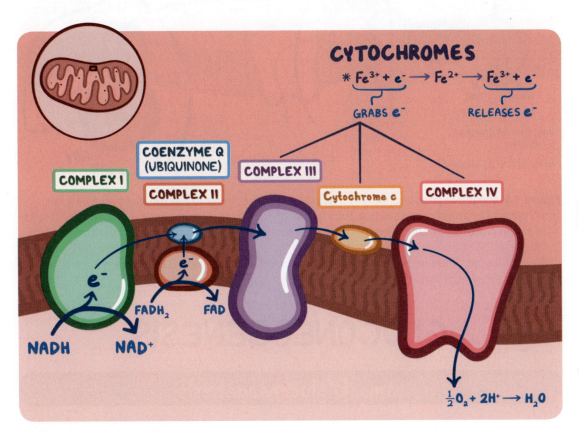

Figure 1.3 The flow of electrons through the electron transport chain, which takes place in the inner mitochondrial membrane.

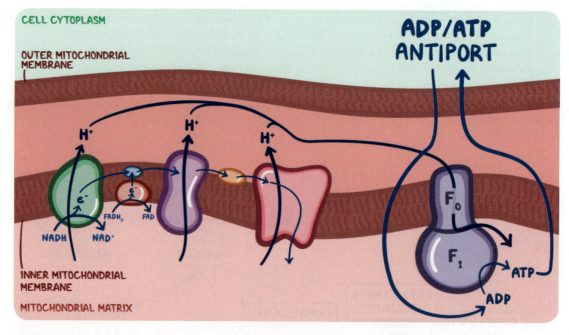

Figure 1.4 Oxidative phosphorylation. The passing of electrons along the electron transport chain generates an electrical current, which provides the energy that allows complexes I, III, and IV to pump protons into the space between the inner and outer mitochondrial membranes. This creates a gradient across the inner mitochondrial membrane. The protons use proton channel F_0 to flow down the gradient, back into the mitochondrial matrix. F_0 is attached to enzyme F_1, an ATP synthase, which uses the proton gradient to phosphorylate ADP → ATP.

GLUCONEOGENESIS

osms.it/gluconeogenesis

- Synthesis of glucose from non-carbohydrate substrates
    - E.g. amino acids, lactate, glycerol
- Occurs primarily in liver cells; also in epithelial cells of kidney, intestine
    - Inside cytoplasm, mitochondria, endoplasmic reticulum
- Starts with glycogenolysis after glucose depletion

Process
- Like backwards glycolysis, with three exceptions
- Obtaining pyruvate
    - Lactate (via lactate dehydrogenase) → pyruvate
    - Amino acids (not leucine, lysine); e.g. alanine (via alanine transaminase) → pyruvate
- Obtaining ATP, glycerol
    - Triacylglyceride breakdown → fatty acids and glycerol → acetyl CoA + ATP (β-oxidation)
- Pyruvate (via pyruvate carboxylase) → oxaloacetate
- Oxaloacetate (malate dehydrogenase) → malate
- Malate leaves mitochondria; malate (via malate dehydrogenase) → oxaloacetate
- Oxaloacetate (via PEPCK) → phosphoenolpyruvate (PEP)
- PEP undergoes reversed glycolysis reactions until dihydroacetone-phosphate (DHAP)
    - Alternatively, glycerol (via glycerol kinase) → glycerol-3-phosphate;

glycerol-3-phosphate (via glycerol-3-phosphate dehydrogenase) → DHAP
- DHAP (via aldolase) → fructose-1,6-bisphosphate
- Fructose-1,6-bisphosphatase → fructose-6-phosphate
  - Rate-limiting step
- Fructose-6-phosphate (via isomerase) → glucose-6-phosphate
- Glucose-6-phosphate (via glucose-6-phosphatase) → glucose

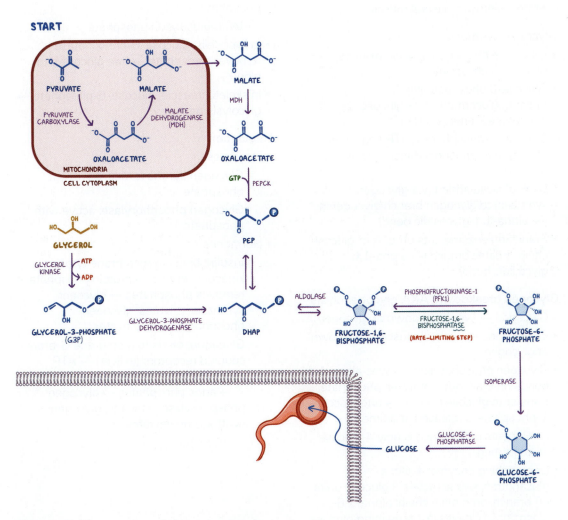

Figure 1.5 The process of gluconeogenesis.

GLYCOGEN METABOLISM

osms.it/glycogen-metabolism

- Polymer of glucose molecules linked by glycosidic bonds
- Stores energy in skeletal muscle, liver

Glycogen synthesis
- Glucose + phosphate (via hexokinase) → glucose-6 phosphate
- Glucose-6 phosphate (via phosphoglucomutase) → glucose-1-phosphate + energy (UTP)
- Glucose-1-phosphate + UTP (via UDP-glucose pyrophosphorylase) → UDP-glucose
- UDP-glucose added (via glycogen synthase) to glycogen branch/glycogenin (→ alpha-1,4-glycosidic bond)
- Branching enzyme cuts off part of glucose chain, creates branch (→ alpha-1,6-glycosidic bond)

Glycogen breakdown, AKA glycogenolysis
- Glucagon → liver breakdown of glycogen
- Epinephrine → skeletal muscle breakdown of glycogen
- Glycogen phosphorylase cleaves alpha-1,4 bonds on branches; catalyzes phosphate transfer to glucose residue → one glucose-1-phosphate is released at a time
    - Repeats until branch is only 4 glucose units long
- Debranching enzyme: 4-alpha-glucanotransferase moves 3 glucose units off branch, onto main chain; alpha-1,6-glucosidase cleaves last remaining glucose
- Cleaved glucose-1-phosphate (via phosphoglucomutase) → glucose-6-phosphate
    - With glucose-6-phosphate
- In liver cells, glucose-6-phosphatase removes phosphate → free glucose into blood
- In skeletal muscle, glucose-6-phosphate → glycolysis pathway

Regulation
- Principles
    - *Glycogen synthase:* active without phosphate
    - *Glycogen phosphorylase:* active with phosphate
- Hormones
    - *Insulin:* binds to membrane tyrosine kinase receptors → protein phosphatase removes phosphates → glycogen synthase activates, glycogen phosphorylase deactivates
    - *Glucagon:* binds to membrane G-protein coupled receptors (in liver) → ATP (adenylyl cyclase) → cAMP → kinase A → adds phosphates → glycogen phosphorylase activates, glycogen synthase deactivates

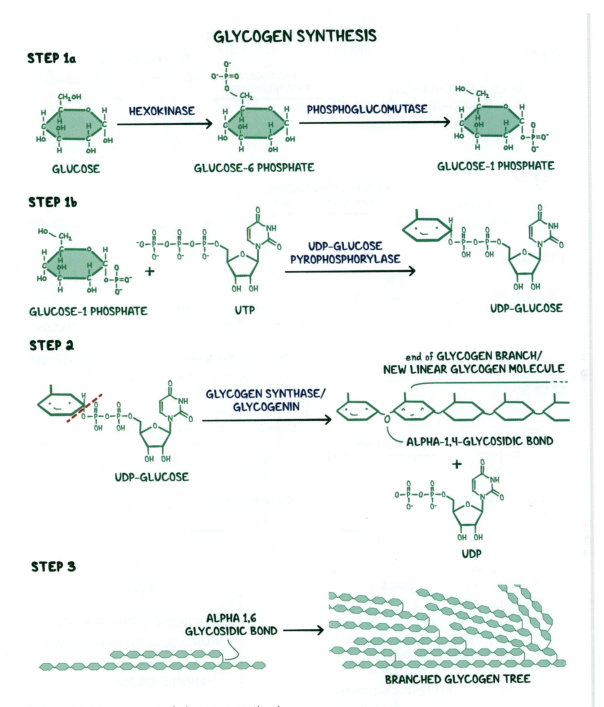

Figure 1.6 The process of glycogen synthesis.

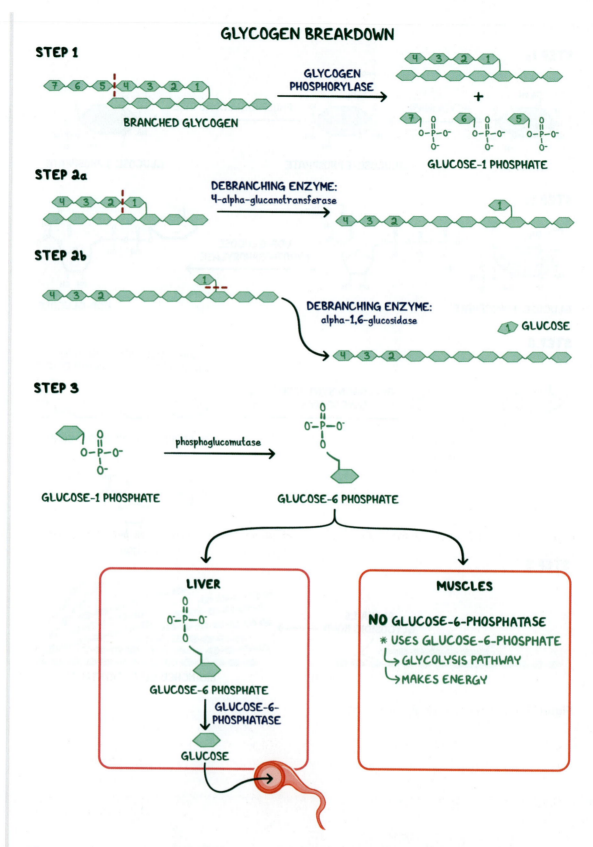

Figure 1.7 Glycogen breakdown. The process is completed differently in the liver and skeletal muscles due to the respective presence and absence of glucose-6-phosphatase in each.

Chapter 1 Biochemistry: Carbohydrate Metabolism

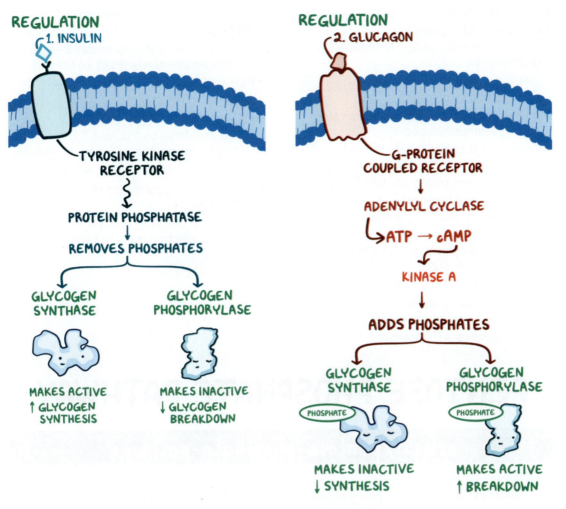

Figure 1.8 The role of insulin in the regulation of glycogen levels.

Figure 1.9 The role of glucagon in the regulation of glycogen levels.

GLYCOLYSIS

osms.it/glycolysis

- Energy-producing breakdown of glucose into pyruvate
- Occurs in cytoplasm of all cells

PROCESS
- Glucose transporter (GLUT) carries glucose into cell
- Kinases (hexokinase, glucokinase) phosphorylate glucose → conformational change, i.e. glucose can't diffuse out) →
glucose-6-phosphate
  - Uses one ATP molecule
- Glucose-6-phosphate (via phosphoglucoisomerase) → fructose-6-phosphate
- Fructose-6-phosphate (via phosphofructokinase-1) → fructose-1,6-bisphosphate
  - Rate-limiting step
  - Uses one ATP molecule

OSMOSIS.ORG 9

Enzyme activation
- Fructose-6-phosphate (via phosphofructokinase-2) → fructose-2,6-bisphosphate
  - Up-regulated by insulin; down-regulated by glucagon
  - Fructose-2,6-bisphosphate activates phosphofructokinase-1
- Fructose-1,6-bisphosphate (via aldolase) → glyceraldehyde 3-phosphate (G3P) + dihydroacetone-phosphate (DHAP)
  - DHAP (via isomerase) → G3P → 2x G3P molecules per glucose
- G3P (via G3P-dehydrogenase) → 1,3-diphosphoglycerate (1,3-BPG); H^+ + NAD^+ → NADH (x2)
  - 2x NADH enter electron transport chain
- 1,3-BPG + ADP (via phosphoglycerate kinase) → 3-phosphoglycerate + ATP (x2)
  - Creates two ATP molecules
- 3-phosphoglycerate (via mutase) → 2-phosphoglycerate (x2)
- 2-phosphoglycerate (via enolase) → phosphoenolpyruvate (PEP) + H_2O (x2)
- PEP + ADP (via pyruvate kinase) → pyruvate + ATP (x2)
  - Creates two ATP molecules
  - Up-regulated by fructose-1,6-bisphosphate (feed-forward regulation)
  - Down-regulated by ATP, alanine
- In total, process generates two ATP molecules
- In cells with oxygen, pyruvate enters citric acid cycle, electron transport chain to make more ATP
  - 30–32 in total

PENTOSE PHOSPHATE PATHWAY

osms.it/pentose-phosphate-pathway

- Synthesis of ribose, NADPH from unused glucose
- Occurs in cytoplasm of all cells

Irreversible oxidative phase
- Glucose-6-phosphate + $NADP^+$ (via glucose-6-phosphate dehydrogenase) → 6-phosphogluconate + NADPH
  - Rate-limiting step
- 6-phosphogluconate + $NADP^+$ (6-phosphogluconate dehydrogenase) → ribulose-5-phosphate + NADPH + CO_2

Reversible non-oxidative phase
- Two options:
  - Ribulose-5-phosphate (via isomerase) → ribose-5-phosphate
  - Ribulose-5-phosphate (via epimerase) → xylulose-5-phosphate

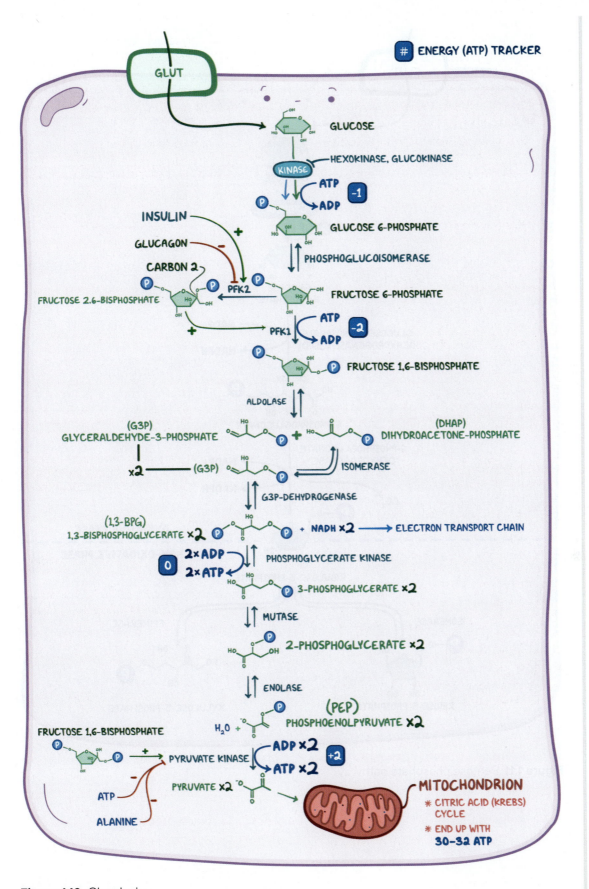

Figure 1.10 Glycolysis.

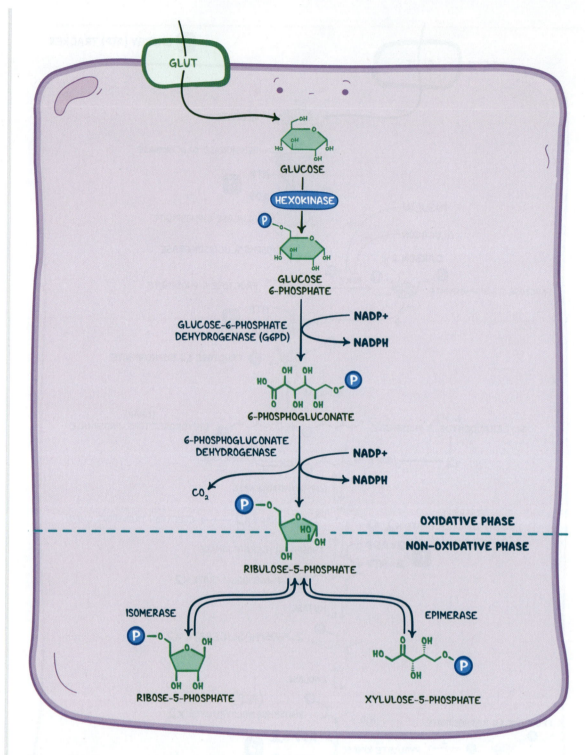

Figure 1.11 Pentose phosphate pathway.

NOTES
FAT & CHOLESTEROL METABOLISM

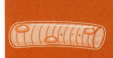

CHOLESTEROL METABOLISM

osms.it/cholesterol-metabolism

- Cholesterol insoluble in water → moves through blood stream with lipoproteins
- Cholesterol used in cell membrane for flexibility, durability
  - At ↓ temperature, cholesterol squeezed between phospholipid molecules, keeps membrane fluid
  - At ↑ temperature, cholesterol pulls phospholipid molecules together
- Cholesterol used by adrenal glands, gonads; makes steroid hormones
  - Adrenal glands form corticosteroids (e.g. cortisol, aldosterone); testes (testosterone); ovaries (estradiol, progesterone)

CHOLESTEROL SYNTHESIS

- Mevalonate pathway; occurs in smooth endoplasmic reticulum

Pathway

- Two acetyl-CoA molecules joined by acetyl-CoA acyltransferase → acetoacetyl-CoA, CoA
- HMG-CoA synthase combines acetoacetyl-CoA, acetyl-CoA → 3-hydroxy-3-methylglutaryl-CoA (HMG-CoA), CoA
- HMG-CoA reductase reduces HMG-CoA into mevalonate, removes CoA-SH, water
  - Rate limiting cholesterol synthesis step
- Mevalonate-5-kinase uses ATP to phosphorylate mevalonate → mevalonate-5-phosphate
- Phosphomevalonate kinase uses ATP to phosphorylate mevalonate-5-phosphate → mevalonate pyrophosphate
- Mevalonate pyrophosphate decarboxylase removes carboxyl group → isopentenyl pyrophosphate
- Geranyl transferase condenses three isopentenyl pyrophosphate molecules → farnesyl pyrophosphate
- Squalene synthase condenses two farnesyl pyrophosphate molecules → squalene
- Oxidosqualene cyclase converts squalene into lanosterol (cyclization)
- Lanosterol converted into 7-dehydrocholesterol, eventually cholesterol

Cholesterol synthesis regulation

- SREBP, INSIG1, SCAP (collection of proteins)
  - ↓ cholesterol → INSIG1 falls off of SCAP-SREBP → SREBP cleaving → binds sterol regulatory element → ↑ HMG-CoA reductase gene expression

CHOLESTEROL USE & STORAGE

- Majority of cholesterol used by liver, ends up as bile acids
- Include cholic acids, chenodeoxycholic acids
  - Conjugation with taurine forms taurocholic acid, taurochenodeoxycholic acid respectively
  - Conjugation with glycine forms glycocholic acid, glycochenodeoxycholic acid respectively
- Stored in gallbladder
- Released into intestines after meals, aids fat digestion
- Most reabsorbed by intestine; some eliminated through feces
  - *Enterohepatic circulation*: reabsorbed bile acids enter portal bloodstream, return to liver cells

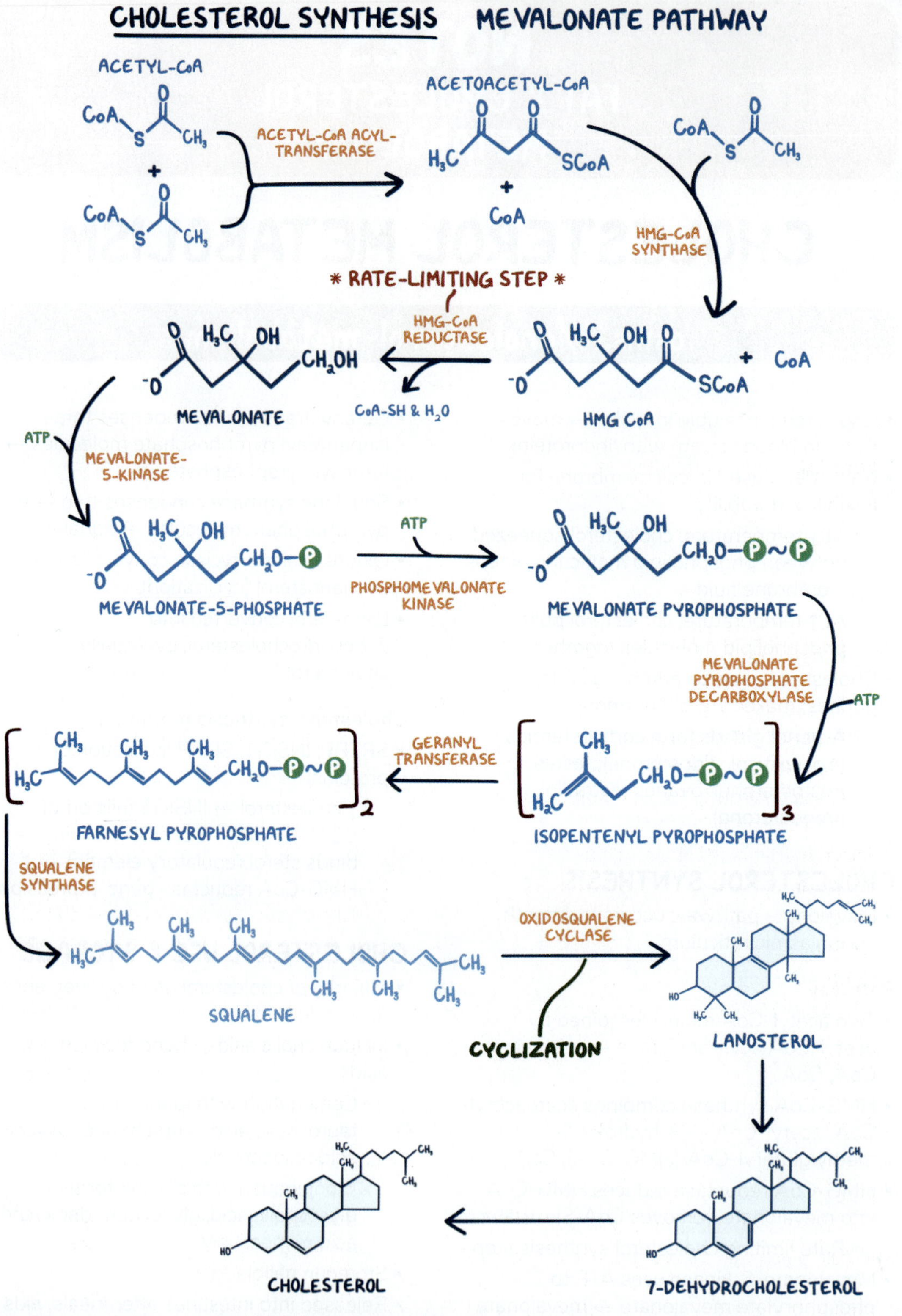

Figure 2.1 Cholesterol synthesis via the mevalonate pathway.

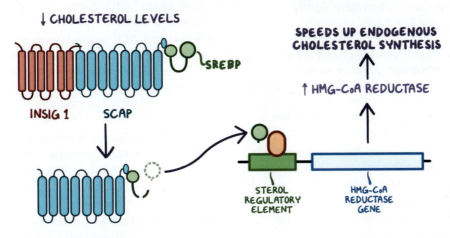

Figure 2.2 Cholesterol synthesis regulation.

FATTY ACID SYNTHESIS

osms.it/fatty-acid-synthesis

- **Fatty acids:** simplest lipid form
  - Long carbon, hydrogen chain atoms
  - **Classification:** short, medium, long, very long chain fatty acids
- Short, medium chain fatty acids
  - Primarily obtained from diet
- Long, very long chain fatty acids
  - Synthesized by liver, fat cells
- **Synthesis:** combine acetyl-CoA molecules into palmitoyl-CoA
  - 16 carbon chain fatty acid; precursor to longer chain fatty acids

BEFORE FATTY ACID SYNTHESIS

- Acetyl-CoA must be obtained
- In response to insulin, cells take in glucose
  - Consumed as carbohydrates
- In cell, glycolysis breaks glucose down into pyruvate molecules
- Mitochondria convert pyruvate into acetyl-CoA using pyruvate dehydrogenase
- Typically, acetyl-CoA combines with oxaloacetate, enters citric acid cycle → forms citrate → forms electron carriers (join electron transport chain in oxidative phosphorylation) → creates adenosine triphosphate (ATP)

FATTY ACID SYNTHESIS

- ATP inhibits enzymes needed for citric acid cycle
  - Allows additional acetyl-CoA to be funneled toward pathways involving fatty acid synthesis

Stages

- Acetyl-CoA combines with oxaloacetate → forms citrate → crosses mitochondrial membrane into cytoplasm
- In cytoplasm, citrate lyase cleaves citrate into acetyl-CoA, oxaloacetate
  - Malic enzyme converts oxaloacetate into pyruvate ($NADP^+$ → NADPH in process), which can cross back into membrane
  - Then converted back into oxaloacetate by pyruvate carboxylase
- Acetyl-CoA carboxylase adds carboxyl group to acetyl-CoA → forms malonyl-CoA
  - Rate limiting fatty acid synthesis step
  - Requires ATP, biotin, carbon dioxide (A-

- B-C) as cofactors
  - **Acetyl-CoA carboxylase:** tightly regulated (hormonal, allosteric regulation); hormonal regulation uses insulin, glucagon to remove/add phosphate group on acetyl-CoA carboxylase; insulin ↑ activity/vice versa; allosteric regulation uses citrate, fatty acids to ↑/↓ acetyl-CoA carboxylase activity by allosteric binding
- Multiple enzymes form fatty acid synthase complex (acyl carrier protein (ACP) on one end, cysteine amino acid on other)
- Acetyl-CoA ACP transacylase removes CoA group from acetyl-CoA, attaching resulting acetate to ACP → moves to cysteine residue
- Malonyl-CoA ACP transacylase removes CoA group from malonyl-CoA, attaching resulting malonate to ACP
- 3-ketoacyl-ACP synthase cuts off carbon (was added to malonate earlier), released as CO_2 (leaving behind acetate) → condenses it with acetate on cysteine residue → forms four carbon chain (using one NADPH molecule for each process)
- Malonyl-CoA added across seven cycles forming 16 carbon chain fatty acid polymer
  - Each cycle uses one acetyl-CoA (converted into malonyl-CoA), two NADPH molecules
- In total, eight acetyl-CoA molecules (including initial molecule) used along with 14 NADPH molecules

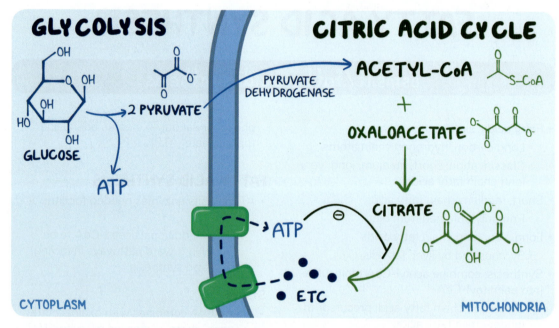

Figure 2.3 Acetyl-CoA is produced by mitochondria using pyruvate molecules (made during glycolysis). ATP inhibits citric acid cycle enzymes so that acetyl-CoA can be used in fatty acid synthesis pathways.

Chapter 2 Biochemistry: Fat & Cholesterol Metabolism

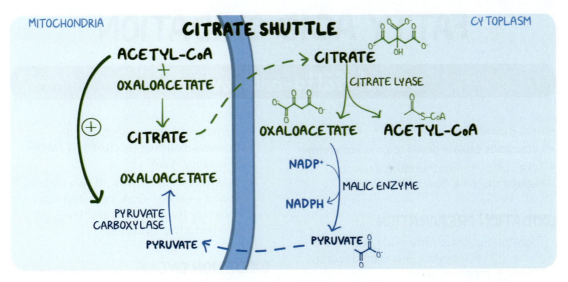

Figure 2.4 The citrate shuttle transports acetyl-CoA out of the mitochondria by combining it with oxaloacetate to form citrate. Once citrate is in the cytoplasm, it is converted back to oxaloacetate and acetyl-CoA, allowing acetyl-CoA to be used in fatty acid synthesis.

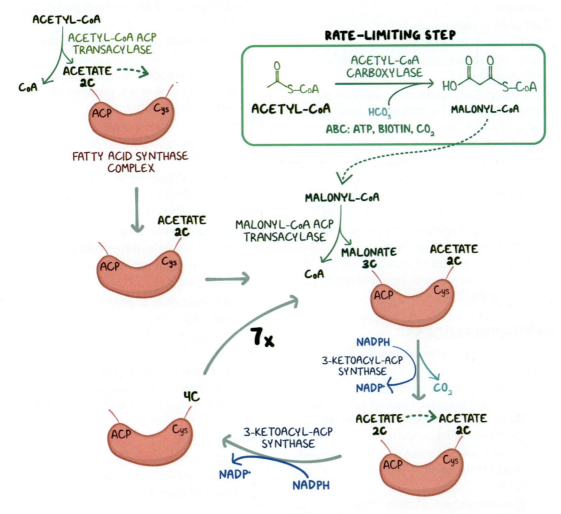

Figure 2.5 Fatty acid synthesis. Malonyl-CoA added across seven cycles → 16 carbon chain fatty acid polymer called palmitoyl-CoA.

OSMOSIS.ORG 17

FATTY ACID OXIDATION

osms.it/fatty-acid-oxidation

- AKA β-oxidation
- Fatty acids broken down to produce energy
- Takes place in mitochondria of heart, skeletal muscles, liver cells

OXIDATION PREPARATION

- Triglycerides (three fatty acids attached to glycerol) in adipocytes → broken down by hormone sensitive lipase
    - ↓ blood glucose → ↑ glucagon → ↑ hormone sensitive lipase → ↑ fatty acid breakdown
- Fatty acids leave fat cells → enter bloodstream
- Albumin in blood binds to fatty acids → carries them to target cells
- Fatty acid dissociates from albumin → diffuses into cell
- Fatty acyl-CoA synthetase adds CoA to end of fatty acid (→ fatty acyl-CoA), using up two ATP molecules
- Fatty acyl-CoA cannot cross cell membrane, carnitine shuttle used
    - Carnitine acyltransferase 1 (outer membrane) replaces CoA on fatty acid with carnitine (→ fatty acyl-carnitine)
    - Fatty acyl-carnitine, CoA cross inner mitochondrial membrane
    - Carnitine acyltransferase 2 (inner membrane) replaces carnitine on fatty acid with CoA (→ fatty acyl-CoA)

OXIDATION PROCESS

- Occurs on α, β carbon atoms of fatty acyl-CoA
    - Acyl-CoA dehydrogenase moves one hydrogen from each carbon to nearby flavin adenine dinucleotide molecule (FAD) → $FADH_2$, enoyl-CoA
    - Enoyl-CoA hydratase transfers hydroxyl group to β carbon → β-hydroxyacyl-CoA
    - β-hydroxyacyl-CoA dehydrogenase removes two hydrogens from β carbon transferring one to nicotinamide adenine dinucleotide (NAD) → NADH, β-ketoacyl-CoA
    - β-ketothiolase cleaves off two carbon atoms → acetyl-CoA, fatty acyl-CoA molecule (two carbons shorter—which can be further oxidized)

OXIDATION CYCLE

- **One oxidation cycle:** 1 NADH, 1 $FADH_2$, 1 acetyl-CoA
- Fatty acids with even number of carbon atoms
    - Oxidation repeats until just acetyl-CoA remains
- Fatty acids with odd number of carbon atoms
    - Oxidation repeats until three carbon propionyl-CoA is left; propionyl-CoA is broken down differently
- Propionyl-CoA carboxylase
    - Adds carboxyl group to propionyl-CoA → methylmalonyl-CoA
    - **Cofactors required:** ATP, biotin, carbon dioxide (A-B-C)
- Methylmalonyl-CoA mutase
    - Rearranges carbon atoms on methylmalonyl-CoA → succinyl-CoA
    - **Cofactor required:** Vitamin B_{12}
- Succinyl-CoA
    - Can enter citric acid cycle/used for heme synthesis
- Very long fatty acids (22 carbons atom/longer)
    - Peroxisomes may be needed
    - Peroxisomal oxidation uses different enzymes until fatty acid is smaller than 22 carbon atoms
- NADH, $FADH_2$
    - Can enter electron transport chain
    - Creates ATP → approximately three + two ATP molecules

- Acetyl-CoA
  - Can enter citric acid cycle
  - Creates more NADH, FADH$_2$ → approximate total of 12 ATP molecules

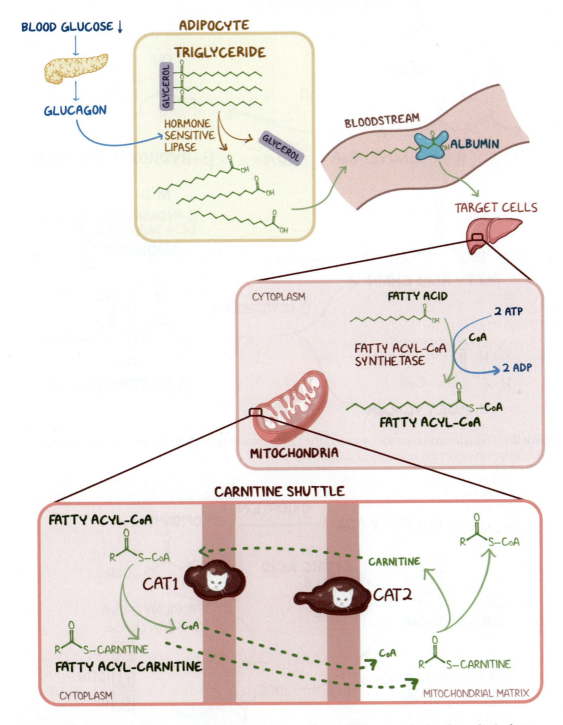

Figure 2.6 Oxidation preparation requires the use of two ATP molecules and results in fatty acyl-CoA being present in the mitochondrial matrix.

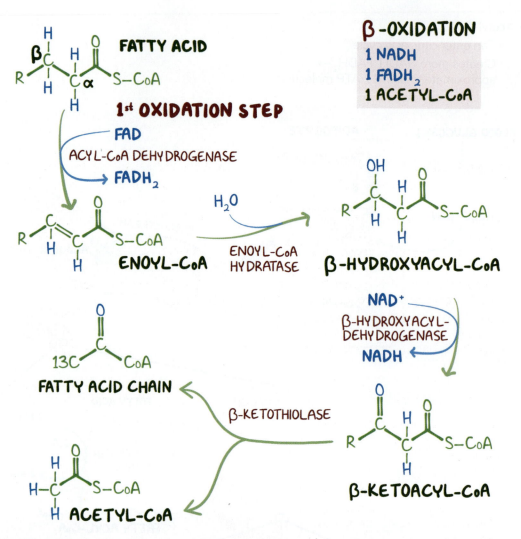

Figure 2.7 Oxidation preparation requires the use of two ATP molecules and results in fatty acyl-CoA being present in the mitochondrial matrix.

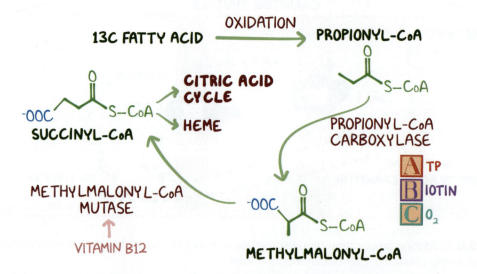

Figure 2.8 Fatty acid oxidation when the fatty acid has an odd number of carbon atoms.

KETONE BODY METABOLISM

osms.it/ketone-body-metabolism

KETONE BODIES

- Acetoacetate, β-hydroxybutyrate, acetone (all contain ketone C=O group)
- Produced by liver mitochondria using acetyl-CoA
  - During physiological states such as fasting, carbohydrate-restrictive diets (e.g Atkins, ketogenic diet), intense exercise, pathological states such as Type 1 diabetes mellitus, alcoholism (lack of glucose to power cells)
- Released into bloodstream → picked up by majority of cells → re-converted into acetyl-CoA → enter mitochondria, produce ATP

KETONE BODY SYNTHESIS

- Two acetyl-CoA molecules are joined (acetyl-CoA acyltransferase) → acetoacetyl-CoA + CoA
- HMG-CoA synthase
  - Acetoacetyl-CoA + acetyl-CoA → 3-hydroxy-3-methylglutaryl-CoA (HMG-CoA) + CoA (rate-limiting ketone body synthesis step)
- HMG-CoA lyase removes acetyl-CoA from HMG-CoA → acetoacetate
- Remaining ketone bodies formed
  - β-hydroxybutyrate dehydrogenase adds hydrogen from NADPH to acetoacetate → β-hydroxybutyrate
  - Acetoacetate in blood spontaneously loses a carbon → acetone (exhaled through lungs)

KETONE BODY BREAKDOWN

- β-hydroxybutyrate, acetoacetate in blood diffuses into peripheral tissue mitochondria
  - β-hydroxybutyrate dehydrogenase converts β-hydroxybutyrate back into acetoacetate
- Thiophorase can add CoA from succinyl-CoA to acetoacetate → form acetoacetyl-CoA, succinate
- β-ketothiolase cleaves acetoacetyl-CoA with CoA → forms two acetyl-CoA molecules
  - Can enter citric acid cycle to make ATP

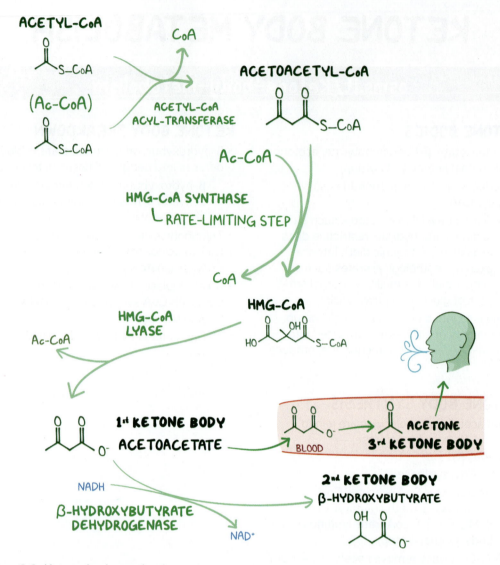

Figure 2.9 Ketone body synthesis.

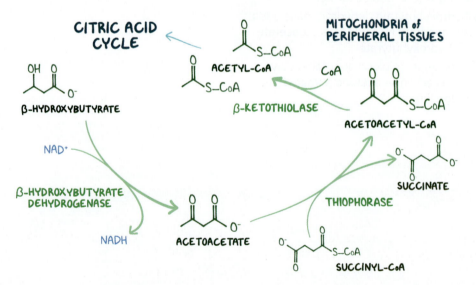

Figure 2.10 Ketone body breakdown.

NOTES
NUCLEIC ACID METABOLISM

NUCLEOTIDE METABOLISM
osms.it/nucleotide-metabolism

Nucleotides
- Building blocks of DNA, RNA
- Consist of 5 carbon sugar, phosphate group, nitrogenous base/nucleobase
  - *5 carbon sugar:* deoxyribose (→ DNA) or ribose (→ RNA)
  - *Nucleobase:* pyrimidine (cytosine, thymine for DNA, uracil for RNA) or purine (adenine, guanine)
  - Sugar + nucleobase = nucleoside

- RNA nucleosides (resulting nucleotide)
  - Adenine + ribose = adenosine (monophosphate → AMP)
  - Guanine + ribose = guanosine (monophosphate → GMP)
  - Cytosine + ribose = cytidine (monophosphate → CMP)
  - Uracil + ribose = uridine (monophosphate → UMP)

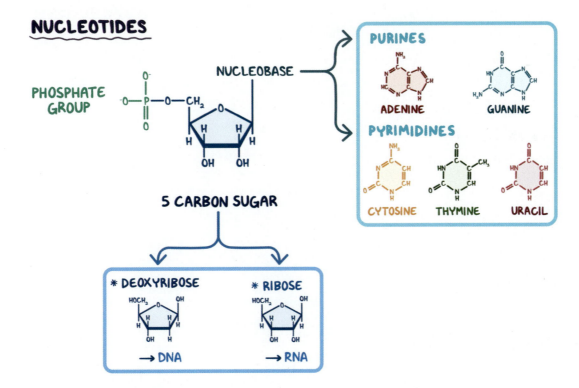

Figure 3.1 Nucleotide components: a phosphate group, a sugar (deoxyribose or ribose), and a nucleobase (adenine, guanine, cytosine, thymine, and uracil).

- DNA nucleosides (resulting nucleotide)
  - Adenine + deoxyribose = deoxyadenosine (monophosphate → dAMP)
  - Guanine + deoxyribose = deoxyguanosine (monophosphate → dGMP)
  - Cytosine + deoxyribose = deoxycytidine (monophosphate → dCMP)
  - Thymine + deoxyribose = deoxythymidine (monophosphate → dTMP)

De novo nucleotide synthesis
- RNA nucleotides start with ribose-5-phosphate
  - Then for pyrimidine nucleotides (UMP and CMP)
  - Then for purine nucleotides (AMP and GMP)
- DNA nucleotides start with diphosphates of RNA nucleotides
  - Ribonucleotide diphosphate reductase reduces ribose to deoxyribose
  - Molecules then lose phosphate groups → dCMP, dUMP, dAMP, dGMP
  - Thymidylate synthetase converts dUMP into dTMP

Nucleotide breakdown
- Pyrimidine rings C,T,U broken down into CO_2 + NH_3, excreted through exhalation/urine
- Purine rings G,A degraded into uric acid, excreted through urine

Salvage pathway
- Guanine, hypoxanthine from purine breakdown can be restored into GMP, AMP

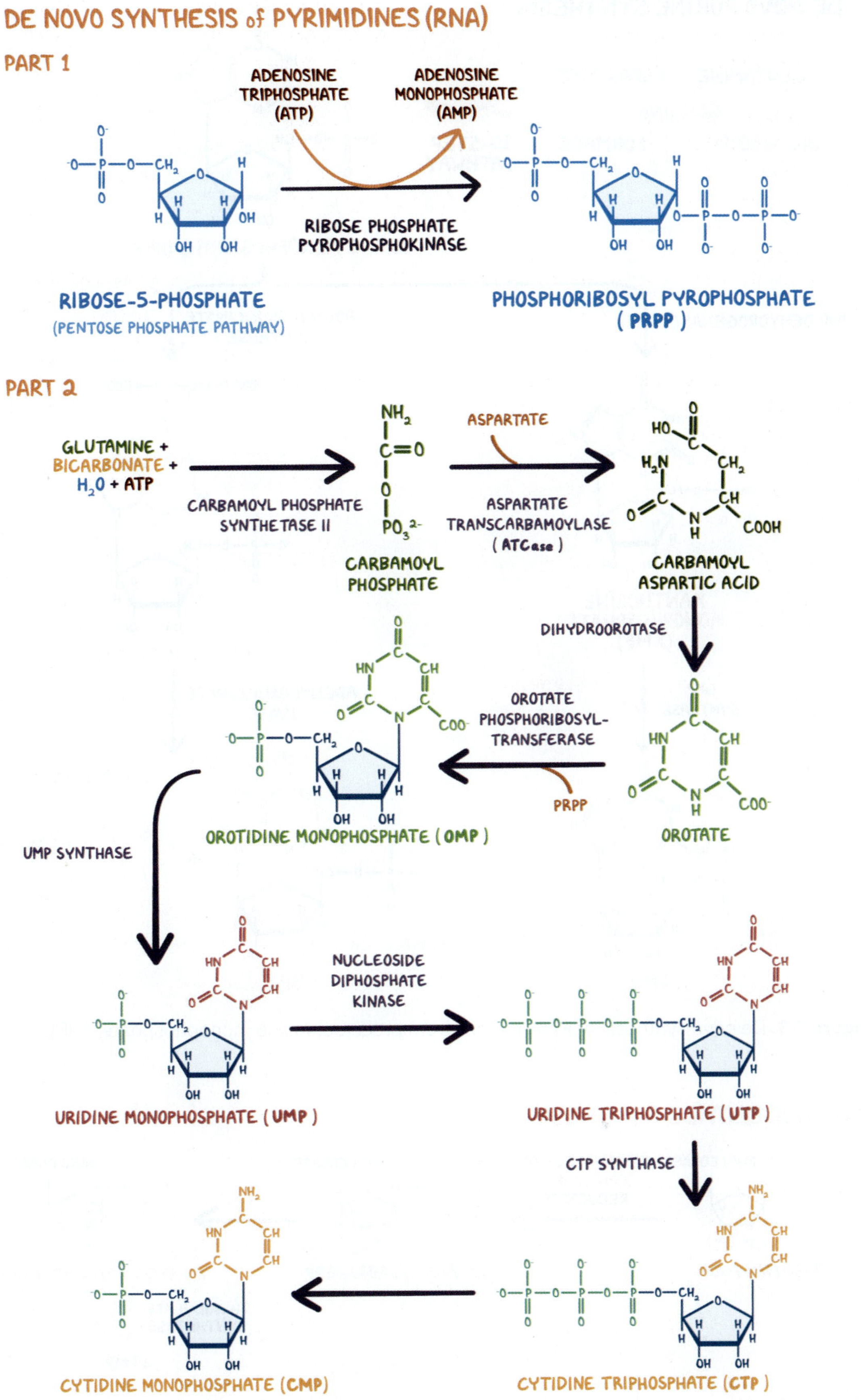

Chapter 3 Biochemistry: Nucleic Acid Metabolism

DE NOVO SYNTHESIS of PYRIMIDINES (RNA)

PART 1

RIBOSE-5-PHOSPHATE (PENTOSE PHOSPHATE PATHWAY) → [Ribose phosphate pyrophosphokinase, ATP → AMP] → PHOSPHORIBOSYL PYROPHOSPHATE (PRPP)

PART 2

GLUTAMINE + BICARBONATE + H_2O + ATP → [Carbamoyl phosphate synthetase II] → CARBAMOYL PHOSPHATE → [Aspartate transcarbamoylase (ATCase), Aspartate] → CARBAMOYL ASPARTIC ACID → [Dihydroorotase] → OROTATE → [Orotate phosphoribosyl-transferase, PRPP] → OROTIDINE MONOPHOSPHATE (OMP) → [UMP synthase] → URIDINE MONOPHOSPHATE (UMP) → [Nucleoside diphosphate kinase] → URIDINE TRIPHOSPHATE (UTP) → [CTP synthase] → CYTIDINE TRIPHOSPHATE (CTP) → CYTIDINE MONOPHOSPHATE (CMP)

Figure 3.2 De novo synthesis of RNA pyrimidines. CTP naturally loses phosphate groups → CMP.

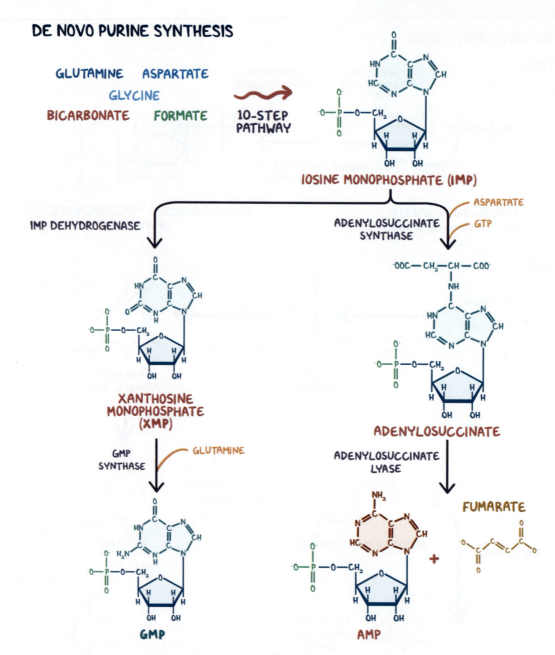

Figure 3.3 De novo synthesis of RNA purines from precursor iosine monophosphate (IMP).

Figure 3.4 DNA nucleotide synthesis from diphosphates of RNA nucleotides.

Chapter 3 Biochemistry: Nucleic Acid Metabolism

PURINE BREAKDOWN

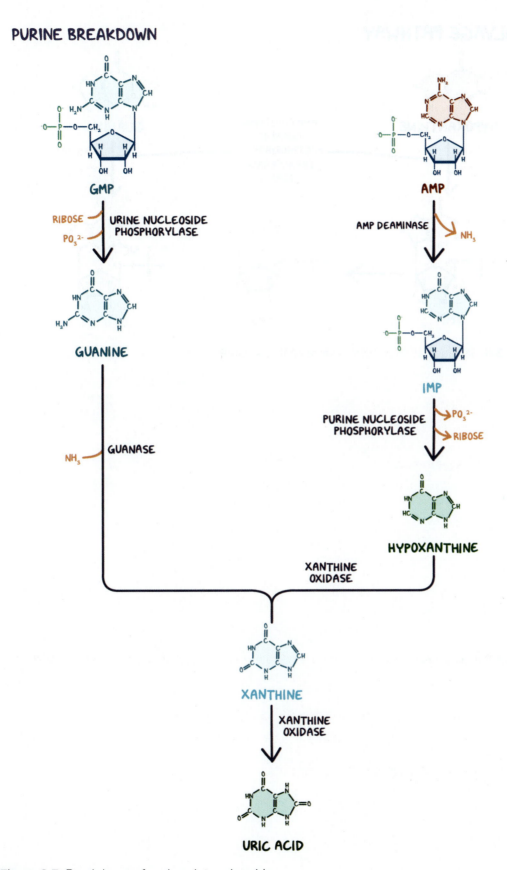

Figure 3.5 Breakdown of purines into uric acid.

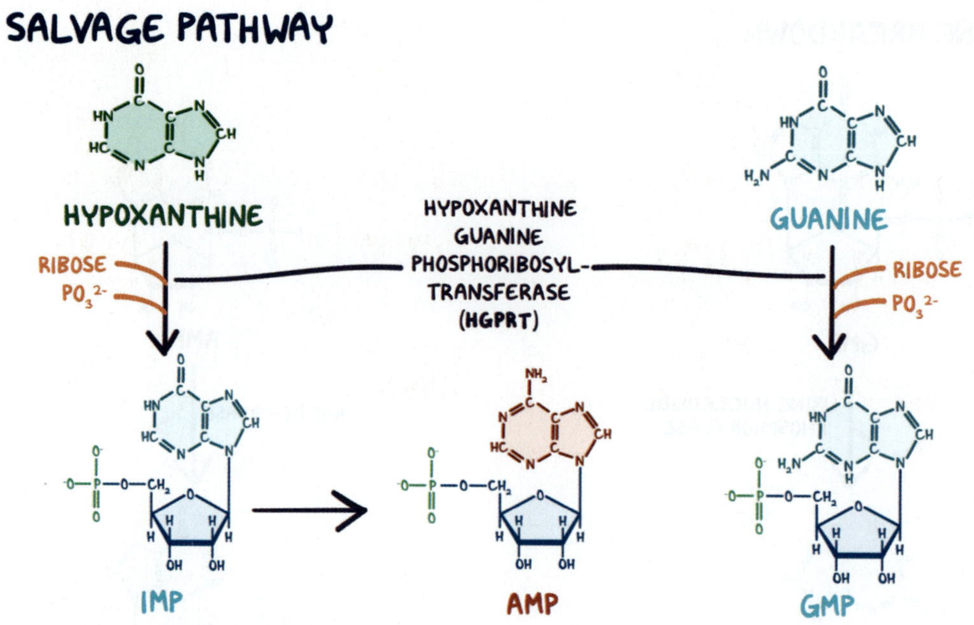

Figure 3.6 Salvage pathways that restore AMP and GMP.

NOTES
PROTEIN METABOLISM

AMINO ACIDS & PROTEIN FOLDING

osms.it/amino-acids-protein-folding

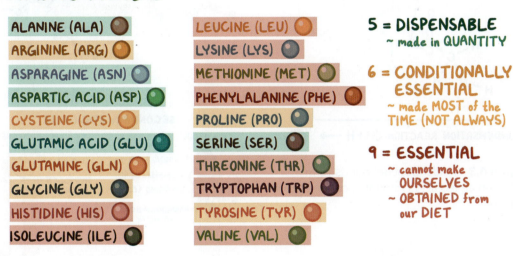

Figure 4.1 The 20 amino acids used by humans.

- **Amino acids:** organic compounds with -NH$_2$, -COOH groups
- Side chain gives specific properties
    - **Hydrophilic:** polar side chains → acidic (e.g. carboxyl); basic (e.g. amine)
    - **Hydrophobic:** non-polar side chains → alkyl, aromatic
- Molecular charge depends on pH
    - **Low pH:** + amine, 0 carboxyl
    - **High pH:** - carboxyl, 0 amine
    - **Neutral:** + amine, - carboxyl → zwitterion
- **Zwitterion:** compound with both positive, negative charges
    - Occurs in each amino acid at specific pH (AKA pI/isoelectric point)

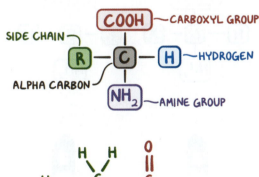
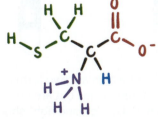

Figure 4.2 Amino acid structure.

OSMOSIS.ORG 29

- **Proteins:** amino acid chains connected by peptide bonds
  - **Peptide bond:** amide bond formed between amino acids by condensation of -NH_2 with -COOH → releases H_2O
  - **Resonance:** electrons shared across bond → partial double-bond character → improved strength
- **Amino acids:** chiral molecules
  - Enantiomers/mirror images are distinct
  - Proteins only made of L-amino acids
- Protein production occurs in ribosomes

Primary, secondary, tertiary, quaternary protein structures

- **Primary:** linear amino acid sequence connected by peptide bonds
- **Secondary:** α-helix, β-pleated sheet
- **Tertiary:** overall shape, including secondary structures, with other features (e.g. disulfide bridge, hydrophobic bonds)
- **Quaternary:** final level; combination of multiple amino acid chains (e.g. hemoglobin)

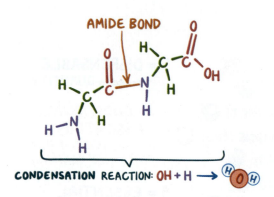

Figure 4.3 Amide (peptide) bonds form between amino acids through a condensation reaction.

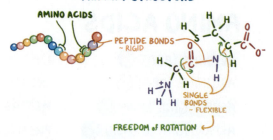

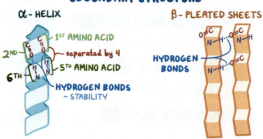

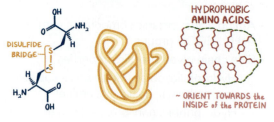

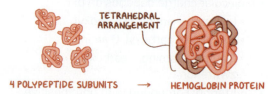

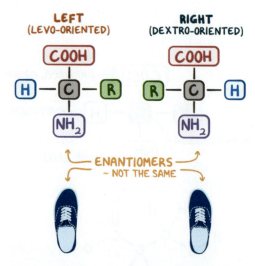

Figure 4.4 Enantiomers are two forms that look like mirror images but are not interchangeable, like a left and right shoe. Proteins are only made out of levo-oriented amino acids.

Figure 4.5 The four levels of structure for proteins.

ENZYME FUNCTION

osms.it/enzyme-function

- **Enzymes:** biochemical reaction catalysts
- Substrates bind to active site → enzyme-substrate complex
- Not used up in reactions
- Highly specific (e.g. amylase in saliva → large carbohydrate breakdown)

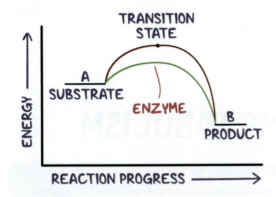

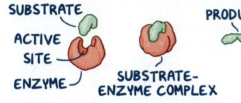

Figure 4.6 Transition state: intermediate step in reaction with high energy. Enzymes speed up reactions by binding substrate (enzyme-substrate complex), which stabilizes the transition state and decreases the amount of extra energy required for the reaction to proceed.

- **Enzyme kinetics:** catalysis rate
- V_{max}: maximum reaction velocity with fixed enzyme quantity
    - ↑ substrate → ↑ velocity, until all enzymes bind
    - ↑ enzymes → ↑ V_{max}
    - ↓ enzymes → ↓ V_{max}
    - Non-competitive inhibition (inhibitory molecule binds to active/allosteric site → prevents substrate binding) → ↓ V_{max}

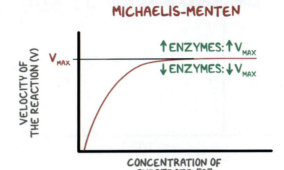

Figure 4.7 Michaelis–Menten graph: used to visualize enzyme kinetics. With a fixed amount of enzyme, the reaction velocity ↑ as substrate is added, until the active sites on all of the enzymes become saturated. At this point, the reaction speed plateaus → V_{max}.

- K_m: substrate concentration when reaction velocity is half of maximum
    - ↑ enzyme affinity (e.g. activator molecules) → ↓ K_m
    - ↓ enzyme affinity (e.g. competitive inhibition) → ↑ K_m

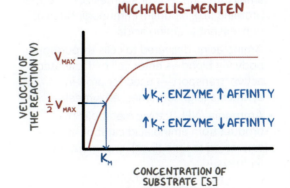

Figure 4.8 K_m is found using a Michaelis–Menten diagram by identifying ½ V_{max} on the y-axis, then finding the corresponding substrate concentration value on the x-axis.

- Lineweaver–Burk plot
  - Based on Michaelis–Menten equation
  $$V_0 = \frac{V_{max}[S]}{K_m+[S]} \rightarrow \frac{1}{V_0} = \frac{K_m+[S]}{V_{max}[S]}$$

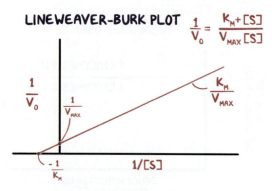

Figure 4.9 The Lineweaver–Burk plot shows K_m and V_{max} as functions of the x, y intercepts.

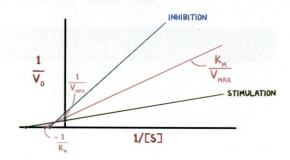

Figure 4.10 Processes that ↑ V_{max} ↓ $1/V_{max}$ → the line slopes lower on the graph than the control. Processes that ↓ V_{max} ↑ $1/V_{max}$ → the line slopes higher on the graph than the control.

AMINO ACID METABOLISM

osms.it/amino-acid-metabolism

- Dietary protein broken down into amino acids → used to synthesize other proteins
  - Excess amino acids used for energy/stored as fat/glycogen
- Portal vein delivers absorbed amino acids (and other nutrients) to liver after uptake by small intestine → liver synthesizes needed proteins (e.g. albumin, immunoglobulins), non-essential amino acids
- Amino acids delivered to cells throughout body via blood → enter cell by facilitated/active transport → used for protein synthesis (e.g. hormones, enzymes)
- Ammonia (NH_4^+): toxic metabolic by-product from amino acid catabolism → converted to urea (liver) → eliminated (kidneys)

Transamination
- Reversible reaction
  - Transfers nitrogen-containing amine group to another molecule
- Amino group transferred (via aminotransferase + vitamin B_6 cofactor) ⇌ alpha ketoglutarate (acceptor molecule) → alpha-keto acid + glutamate
  - Glutamate oxidatively deaminated in liver mitochondria → ammonia byproduct converted to urea (via urea cycle) → eliminated (kidneys)

Deamination
- Nitrogen-containing amine group removal (via deaminase) → amino acid utilized for energy
- Produces ammonia → converted to urea → renal excretion

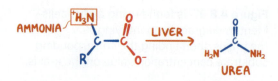

Figure 4.11 Ammonia → urea in the liver.

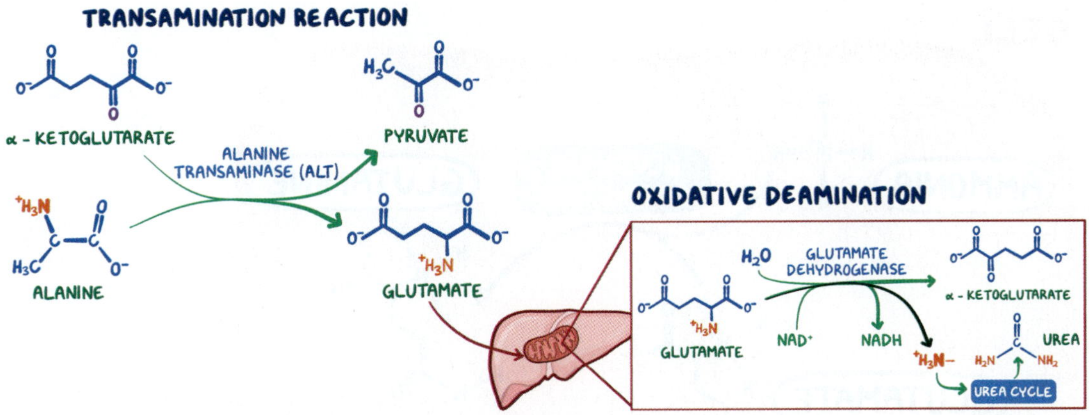

Figure 4.12 Example of a transamination reaction with amino acid alanine. ALT switches the amino group on alanine with the oxygen group on α-ketoglutarate, resulting in ketoacid pyruvate and amino acid glutamate, which has the amino group. Glutamate is the only amino acid that doesn't have to transfer its amine group to another molecule. It undergoes oxidative deamination, a process that removes hydrogens and an amino group.

NITROGEN & THE UREA CYCLE

osms.it/nitrogen-and-urea-cycle

- **Ammonia (NH_3):** toxic protein catabolism byproduct; detoxification by liver (forming non-toxic urea)

AMMONIA

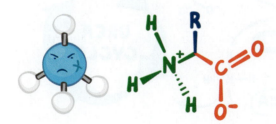

Figure 4.13 Ammonia is composed of a nitrogen-containing amino group, an acidic carboxyl group, and a side chain.

- NH_3 reaches liver in two ways, sometimes as glutamate

Glutamine synthetase system
- From all tissues
- **Glutamine synthetase:** NH_3 + glutamate → glutamine
- Glutamine transported through blood
- **Glutaminase:** glutamine → NH_3 + glutamate
- In liver mitochondria

Glucose-alanine cycle
- Only from muscle
- **Glutamate dehydrogenase:** NH_3 + alpha-ketoglutarate → glutamate
- **Alanine transaminase:** glutamate + pyruvate → alpha-ketoglutarate + alanine
- Alanine transported through blood
- **Alanine transaminase:** alpha-ketoglutarate + alanine → glutamate + pyruvate

Glutamate–NH_3 conversion: two ways
- **Glutamate dehydrogenase:** glutamate → NH_3 + alpha-ketoglutarate
  - Free NH_3 enters urea cycle
- **Aspartate transaminase:** glutamate + oxaloacetate → aspartate + alpha-ketoglutarate
  - Aspartate carries NH_3 into urea cycle

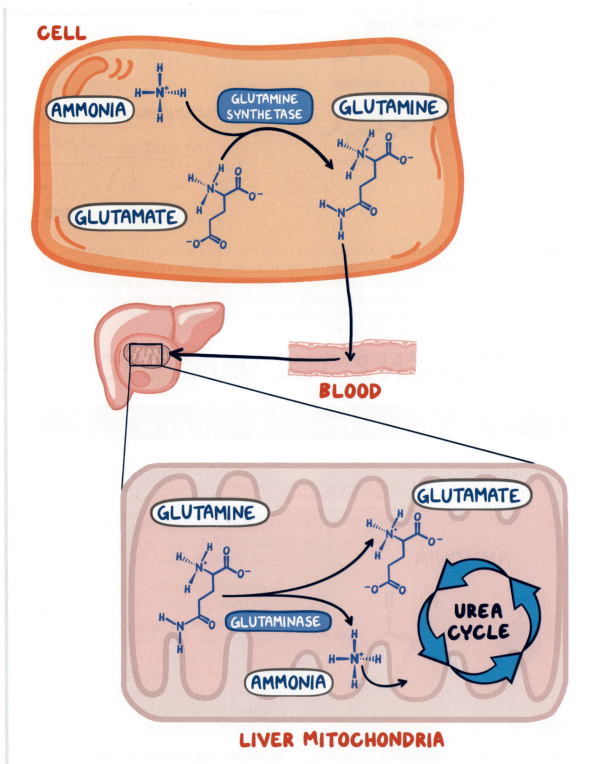

Figure 4.14 The glutamine synthetase system of ammonia reaching the liver.

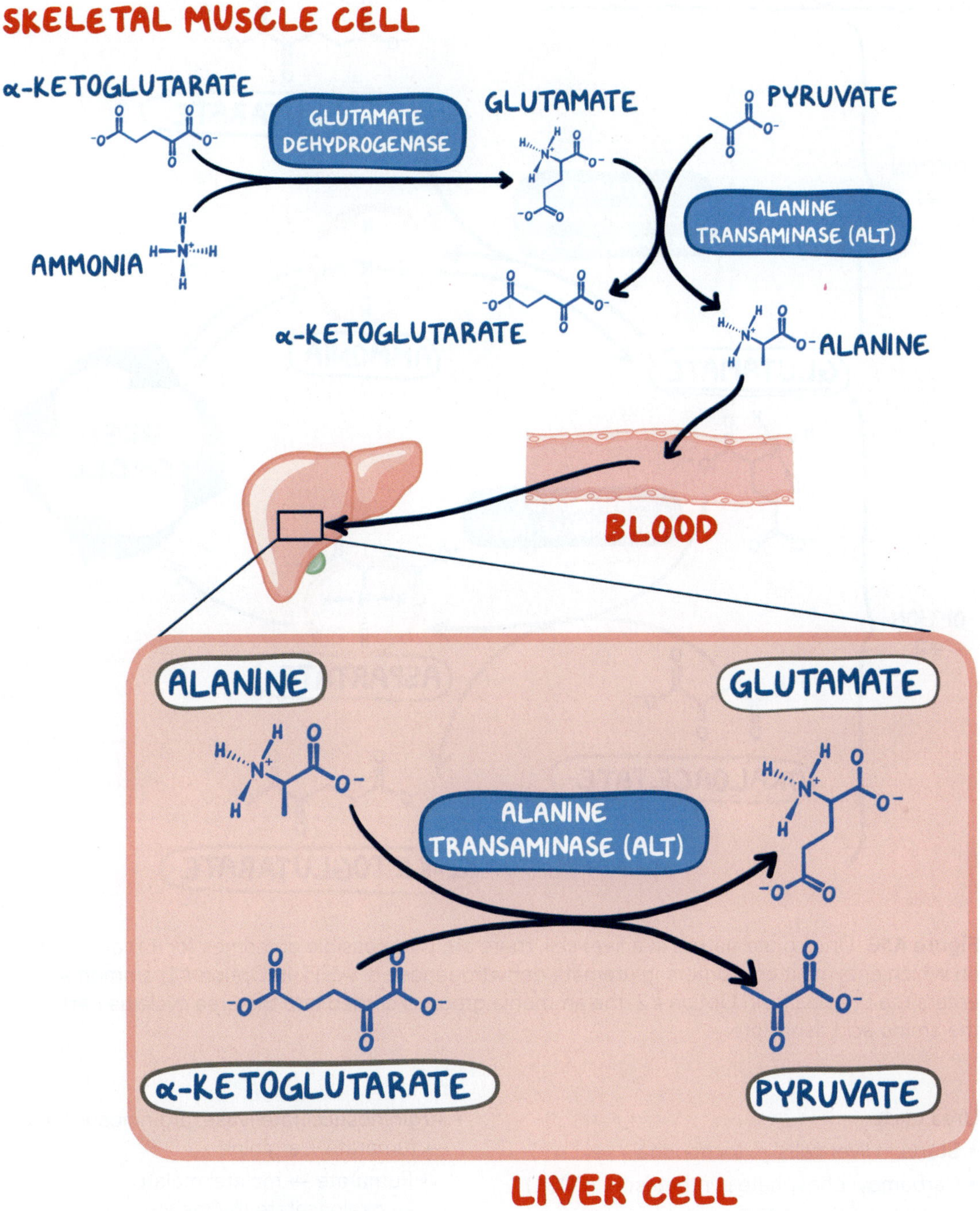

Chapter 4 Biochemistry: Protein Metabolism

Figure 4.15 The glucose-alanine cycle of ammonia reaching the liver.

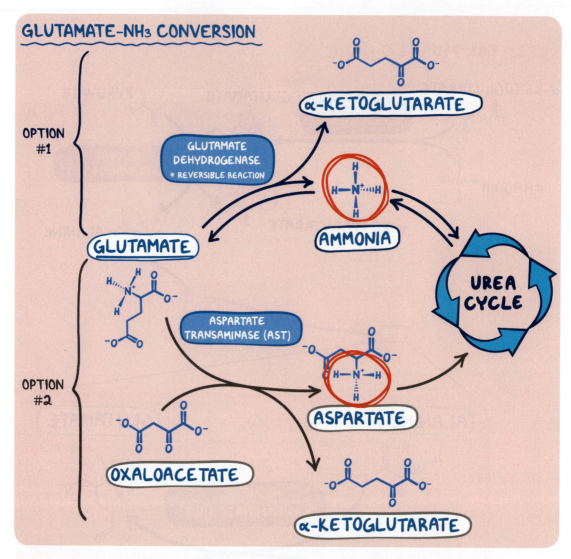

Figure 4.16 Once glutamate is in a liver cell, there are two possible outcomes for it that depend on which enzyme it encounters (glutamate dehydrogenase or AST). In Option #1, ammonia enters the urea cycle; in Option #2, the ammonia group is carried into the urea cycle as part of the amino acid aspartate.

Urea cycle

- Starts in liver cells' mitochondria
- Carbamoyl phosphate synthetase 1 (CPS1)
  - $NH_3 + CO_2 + 2ATP \rightarrow$ carbamoyl phosphate
  - N-acetylglutamate → ↑ CPS1 affinity for ammonia (by allosteric binding)
- **Ornithine transcarbamylase:** ornithine + carbamoyl phosphate → citrulline + phosphate
- Citrulline moves to cytoplasm
- **Argininosuccinate synthetase:** citrulline + aspartate + ATP → argininosuccinate
- **Argininosuccinate lyase:** argininosuccinate → fumarate + arginine
  - Fumarate → malate; malate → oxaloacetate (by malate dehydrogenase); oxaloacetate + glutamate → aspartate + alpha-ketoglutarate (by aspartate transaminase) → aspartate can enter next cycle
  - Arginine → urea + ornithine (by arginase) → ornithine can enter next cycle
- Resulting urea then enters blood, excreted by kidneys

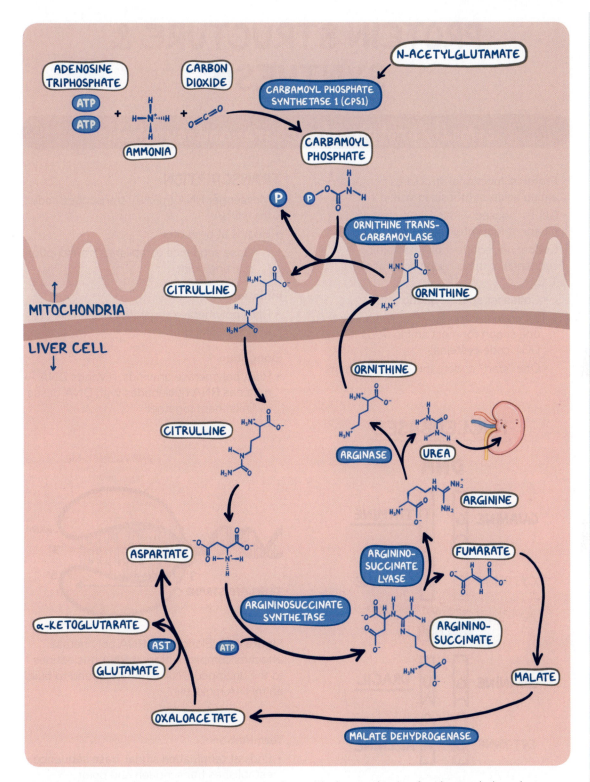

Figure 4.17 Illustration of the urea cycle, starting with the synthesis of carbamoyl phosphate from ATP, ammonia, and carbon dioxide, with the help of enzyme CPS1.

PROTEIN STRUCTURE & SYNTHESIS

osms.it/protein-structure-and-synthesis

- **Proteins:** functional structures composed of amino acids; synthesized within cells
- **Genes,** housed within DNA, provide blueprint for protein synthesis
- **Codon:** nucleotide triplet containing sequence of three nucleotide bases (A, G, T, C)
  - Codes for specific amino acid
  - 64 codons code for 20 amino acids; > one codon for most amino acids (UUU, UGC code cysteine)
  - One "start" codon; three "stop" codons

TRANSCRIPTION

- Messenger RNA (mRNA) transcribes code from DNA
- Begins at promoter
  - Base sequence establishes transcription starting point

Initiation
- RNA polymerase separates DNA helix at promoter site

Elongation
- RNA polymerase unwinds, rewinds DNA → matches RNA nucleotides with DNA bases → links them together

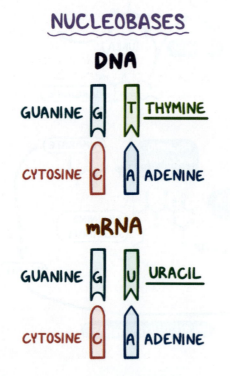

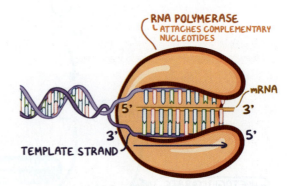

Figure 4.19 Elongation: RNA polymerase attaches complementary mRNA nucleotides to the unzipped DNA template strand to build an mRNA molecule.

Figure 4.18 The four nucleobases used in DNA are guanine, cytosine, thymine, and adenine. In mRNA, uracil (U) is used rather than thymine.

Termination
- Ends at termination signal; base sequence establishes transcription end point

Pre-mRNA formed
- Contains non-coding areas (introns)
  - Spliceosomes snip out introns → functional mRNA
  - mRNA complex proteins added → guide mRNA out of nucleus

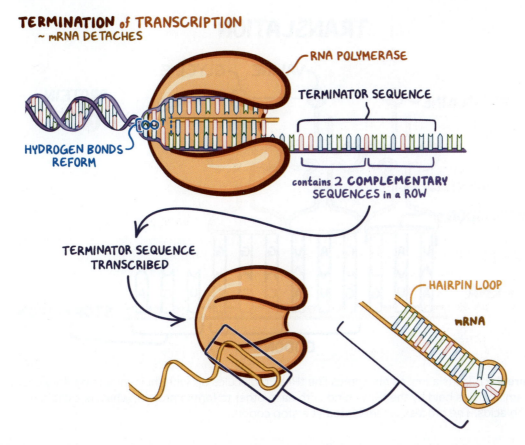

Figure 4.20 Termination: when the two complementary sequences in the terminator sequence get transcribed into mRNA, they bond with each other, creating a hairpin loop that causes the RNA polymerase to detach from the DNA strand.

TRANSLATION
- Base sequence contained in mRNA translated into assembled polypeptide

Three RNA types required
- *mRNA:* carries coded message out of nucleus to ribosome in cytoplasm
- *Ribosomal RNA (rRNA):* "workbench" for protein synthesis
- *Transfer RNA (tRNA):* brings amino acids to workbench assembly site at ribosome
  - Folded into "cloverleaf" shape
  - *Acceptor stem:* attaches to amino acid
  - *Anticodon:* complementary to mRNA codon (tRNA binds with mRNA through complementary base pairing)

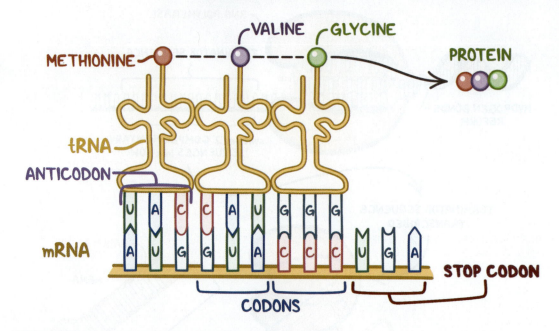

Figure 4.21 Translation: as ribosomes line tRNA molecules up with their complementary codons, the amino acids held by the tRNA bind with each other to form a protein, which is a chain of amino acids. The process is terminated at a stop codon.

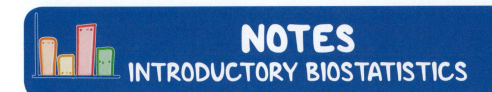

NOTES
INTRODUCTORY BIOSTATISTICS

INTRODUCTION TO BIOSTATISTICS

osms.it/intro-biostatistics

- *Statistics:* process of collecting, organizing, analyzing data set variables
- *Biostatistics:* focus on data related to living things
- *Descriptive statistics:* summarizes, describes population information
- *Inferential statistics:* examines relationships between two/more variables → applies results of sample population to target population

POPULATION & SAMPLE

Population
- Group (people, specimens, events) with defined criteria (e.g. October–March emergency room visits)
- *Parameter:* numerical population description (e.g. range, mean, standard deviation)
  - μ = population mean
  - σ = population standard deviation

Sample
- Subset drawn from population (e.g. influenza-related October–March emergency room visits)
- Represents population → inferences can be made about population
- *Statistic:* numerical sample description (e.g. range, mean, standard deviation)
- $\bar{X}$ = sample mean
- SD = sample standard deviation
- *Sampling error:* sample does not accurately reflect population
  - Usually due to wide variation within sample
  - ↑ sample size helps avoid sampling error

- *Selection bias:* sample does not accurately reflect population
  - Occurs when precautions to obtain representative sample are not used
  - Randomization helps eliminate bias

Case (data point)
- Single observation (e.g. one individual visiting emergency room for influenza symptoms)

TYPES OF HYPOTHESES

Null hypothesis (H_0)
- States that there is no relationship between variables
- Any observed relationship due to chance (e.g. no relationship between body mass index (BMI), hypertension)

Alternative hypothesis (research hypothesis)
- States expected relationship between variables (e.g. relationship between BMI, hypertension)

Hypothesis testing
- Statistical methods used to determine relationship strength between variables, how much of observed relationship is due to chance, significance of observations
- *Statistical significance:* relationship between variables is caused by something other than chance
- Usually defined by a p-value of < 0.05 (5%); "p" stands for "probability"
  - *Type 1 error:* probability of incorrectly rejecting null hypothesis (i.e. concluding significant relationship between

variables when there is not)
- Type 2 error: incorrectly accepting null hypothesis (i.e. concluding there is no significant relationship between variables, missing present association)
• Clinical significance: practical importance of study results that may not be statistically significant

RELIABILITY & VALIDITY
• Measurement characteristics used to collect data

Validity: accuracy
• Instrument actually measures variable (concept, construct) it is supposed to measure (e.g. urine dipstick accurately detects proteinuria)
• Valid instrument must be reliable

Reliability: repeatability
• Instrument consistently yields same results with repeated measurements (e.g. urine dipstick reliably detects proteinuria with each measurement)
• Reliable instrument may/may not be valid

TYPES OF VARIABLES
• Variable: defined characteristic being studied; can assume different values
• Independent variable: manipulated (treatment) variable
• Dependent variable: outcome variable; influenced by independent variable
  - What is effect of X (independent variable) on Y (dependent variable); how is X related to Y?
  - E.g. what is the effect of lipid-lowering drug (X) on individual's cholesterol level (Y)?

GRAPHIC DESCRIPTION OF DATA
• When values are plotted on graph → variety of frequency distributions (curves) result
• Properties of distributions: central tendency, dispersion

Normal (Gaussian) curve
• Symmetrical distribution of scores around mean
  - Forms classic bell shape
  - Values lie within two standard deviations of mean
  - Most natural phenomena show this type of distribution
  - Parametric tests utilized in research

Non-Gaussian curve
• Asymmetrical distribution of scores around mean
  - Skewed (negatively/positively) curve
  - Kurtotic (flat/peaked) curve (leptokurtic—thin, positive kurtosis; platykurtic—flat negative kurtosis)
  - Nonparametric tests utilized in research

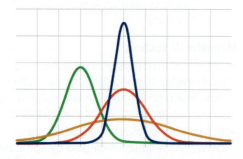
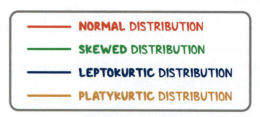

Figure 5.1 Visualization of normal (red), skewed (green) and kurtotic (blue and yellow) distributions.

MEAN, MEDIAN, MODE

osms.it/mean-median-mode

- Central tendency measures
- More curve symmetry → more alike mean, median, mode

Mean ($\bar{X}$)
- Central value calculated by adding each value in data set → dividing by total number of data points
- *Expressed as formula*: total sum of individual data points $X_1, X_2, ..., X_n$, divided by n (number of data points)

$$\bar{X} = \frac{(X_1 + X_2, ..., +X_n)}{n}$$

$$\frac{17+19+20+20+21+21+22}{7} = \frac{140}{7} = 20$$

- Can be influenced by an extreme value (outlier) → skewed data

Median
- Calculates central value when possible outliers present
- Divides set of data into two halves
  - Half of values > median, half < median
- Most commonly used expression of central tendency
- Arrange data in order of magnitude → find midpoint

17 19 20 20 21 21 22 100

- Odd number of values → one "middle" number
- Even number of values → two middle-values values (20, 21)
  - Calculate median by averaging two values: (20+21)/2 = 20.5

Mode
- Central value appearing most often in data sequence
  - Bimodal (two modal), trimodal (three modes), amodal

17 19 20 20 21 21 22 100

  - Bimodal dataset with two mode values of 20, 21
- Not affected by outliers

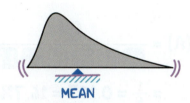

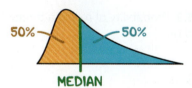

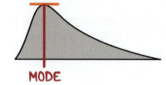

Figure 5.2 Mean, median, and mode in a skewed curve.

PROBABILITY

osms.it/probability

- Relative likelihood that event will/will not occur
- To calculate chance that event/outcome will occur → divide number of times event happened by number of times event could have happened
  - E.g. event A is rolling a die and getting a three
  - Since a die has six sides, there are six possible numbers, so the probability (P) of rolling a three is 1/6, or 0.167 (16.7%)

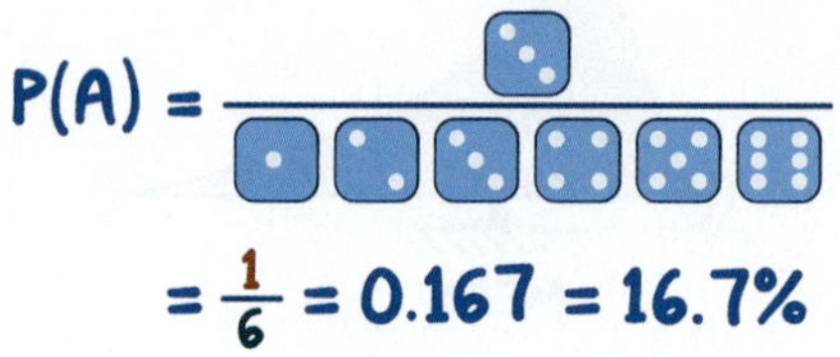

$$P(A) = \frac{1}{6} = 0.167 = 16.7\%$$

Figure 5.3 Probability of rolling a three on a six-sided die.

RULES

Rule 1
- Probability of event A can range anywhere from 0% to 100%
  - $0 \leq P(A) \leq 1$

Rule 2
- Sum of probabilities of all possible outcomes = 1

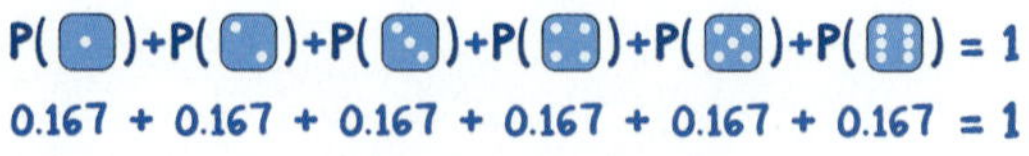

$$P(⚀)+P(⚁)+P(⚂)+P(⚃)+P(⚄)+P(⚅) = 1$$
$$0.167 + 0.167 + 0.167 + 0.167 + 0.167 + 0.167 = 1$$

Figure 5.4 Visualization of Rule 2.

Rule 3 (complement rule)
- Probability that event will not occur = 1 minus probability that it does occur
  - $P = 1 - P(A)$

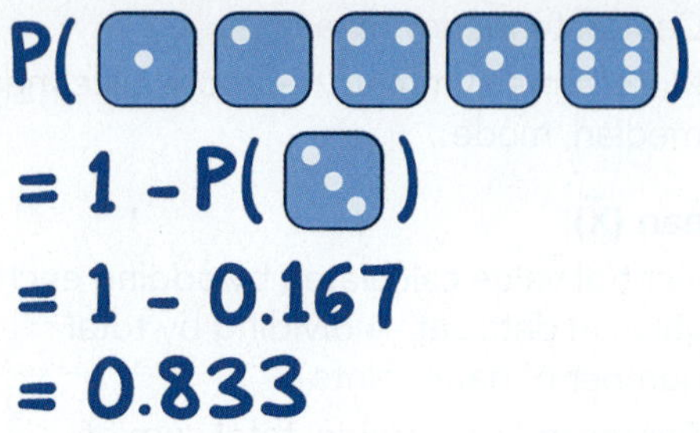

$$P(⚀⚁⚂⚃⚅)$$
$$= 1 - P(⚂)$$
$$= 1 - 0.167$$
$$= 0.833$$

Figure 5.5 Probability of not rolling a three = 1 - P(rolling a three).

Rule 4
- Probability of two disjoint (mutually exclusive) events = the sum of the first event plus the second event
  - $P(A \text{ or } B) = P(A) + P(B)$

Rule 5
- Probability for two not disjoint (not mutually exclusive) events = sum of the probability of event A and the probability of event B, minus the probability of event A and B together
  - $P(A \text{ or } B) = P(A) + P(B) - P(A \text{ and } B)$

Rule 6
- Probability of two independent events = probability of the first event multiplied by the probability of the second event
  - $P(A \text{ and } B) = P(A) \times P(B)$

Rule 7
- Conditional probability (probability of event A, given what happens in event B) = probability of event A and event B divided by probability of event B

Rule 8
- Probability of events A, B = probability of event A multiplied by conditional probability of event B given event A occurred

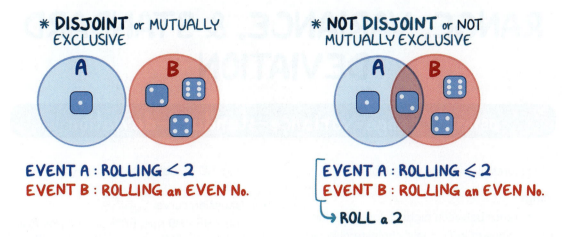

Figure 5.6 A visualization of the difference between mutually exclusive and not mutually exclusive events.

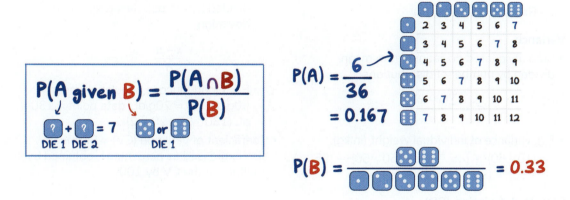

Figure 5.7 Rule 7, conditional probability: determining P(A) and P(B) when event A depends on event B. In this case, we are finding the probability that the roll of two dice adds up to seven (event A) given that the first die is either a five or a six (event B). Once P(A) and P(B) are known, they are used to solve for P(A given B).

RANGE, VARIANCE, & STANDARD DEVIATION

osms.it/range-variance-standard-deviation

- Measures distribution of variables

Range
- Difference between highest, lowest value
- E.g. Range of individuals' cholesterol levels
  - 130, 150, 152, 158, 165, 289, 354
  - Range 354 - 130 = 224mg/dL
- E.g. individual weight (in kg)
  - 10 + 45 + 50 + 55 + 90
  - Range = 90 - 10 = 80

Variance
- Sum of squared deviations from mean, divided by number of distributions

$$\sigma^2 = \frac{\Sigma(x - \bar{x})^2}{n}$$

- E.g. variance of individual weight (in kg)
  - $(10 - 50)^2 + (45 - 50)^2 + (50 - 50)^2 + (55 - 50)^2 + (90 - 50)^2 / (5) = 650 \text{ kg}^2$

Standard deviation (SD)
- Square root of variance

$$\sigma = \sqrt{\frac{\Sigma(x - \bar{x})^2}{n}}$$

- E.g. SD of individual weight: $\sqrt{650}$ = 25.5kg
- In Gaussian curve
  - **68 - 95 - 99 rule:** 68% of data points lie within 1 SD from mean; 95% lie within 2 SD, 99% lie within 3 SD
- Z-score = number of SD data point is away from mean
  - Data point minus the population mean, divided by the population standard deviation

$$\frac{x - \mu}{\sigma}$$

  - E.g. blood glucose population mean = 90g/dL, SD = 20g/dL, data point = 130g/dL (130 - 90 / 20 = 2)
- Coefficient of variation (CV) = SD/mean; also expressed as percentage, obtained by multiplying the CV by 100

TYPES OF DATA

osms.it/types-of-data

- Determining type of data to be collected helps establish which sort of distributions can logically be used to describe variable

Nominal data
- Can assume one of a limited number of possible values (e.g. ABO blood types)
  - No meaningful rank order; no median, mean, standard deviation; mode used for analysis
  - Includes dichotomous variables (e.g. normal, abnormal)

Ordinal data
- Ordered in meaningful way (e.g. systolic murmur ranking from 1–6)
  - Follows order, but quantitative differences not clear (do not indicate degree of difference between observations)
  - Median, mode can be used; mean usually not suitable to describe sample/population

Discrete data
- Measured in whole numbers (no decimal values)
  - E.g. number of pregnancies

Continuous data
- Can take on infinite number of value (e.g. weight, height, blood glucose)
  - Mean, median, mode, standard deviation can be calculated

Interval data
- Indicates meaningful quantitative difference between two values; values can be placed in clear, logical order
  - E.g. temperature on Celsius/Fahrenheit scale; difference between 90° and 60° measured as 30°
  - Arbitrary zero point
  - Mean, median, mode, standard deviation can be calculated

Ratio data
- Has absolute, meaningful zero point
- Can use multiplication, addition, subtraction to calculate ratios
- Mean, median, mode using ratio data

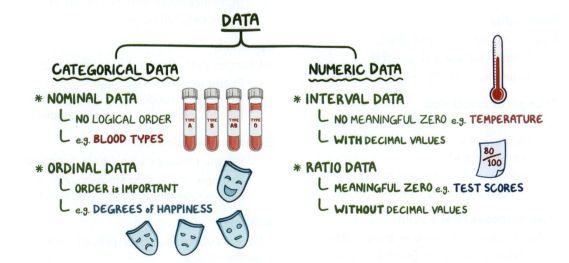

Figure 5.8 Types of data.

NOTES
CAUSATION & VALIDITY

CAUSALITY

osms.it/causality

- Consequential relationship between two events (e.g. A caused B)
  - *Contrast with correlation:* association between two events
- Consequential relationship may be direct/indirect
  - *Direct:* event caused direct consequence which → effect (A → B)
  - *Indirect:* initial event → another event → final effect (A → x → y → B)
- Correlation is not equal to causation
  - Two correlated events may seem to have consequential relationship; sometimes due to random chance/external factors/confounding (noncausal) variables

ESTABLISHING CAUSALITY
- To establish causality between set of events, relationship must meet following criteria

Temporality
- Cause happened before effect
  - Event A followed by Event B
  - *Example:* smoking → lung cancer

Strength of association
- Relational closeness between two events
  - Measured by relative risk, odds ratio, correlations, etc.
  - *Example:* how closely is smoking related to developing lung cancer?

Dose-response relationship
- More exposure to cause → greater effect
  - Longer exposure to Event A → more risk of Event B
  - *Example:* the longer you smoke, the higher your risk of developing lung cancer

Biologic coherence
- Causal mechanism for effect agrees with current knowledge
  - *Example:* factually known that cigarettes contain carcinogenic agents

Biologic plausibility
- Proposed mechanism of effect makes sense according to current knowledge
  - *Example:* because we know cigarettes contain carcinogenic agents, it makes sense that cigarette-smoke exposure → higher probability of developing lung cancer

Consistency with other knowledge
- Association has been shown repeatedly
  - *Example:* it has been repeatedly proven that smoking confers higher risk of developing lung cancer

Specificity
- Chances that effect is due to other causes
  - *Example:* can there be another explanation for developing lung cancer besides exposure to cigarette smoke?

Experimental evidence
- When you remove cause, effect disappears
  - *Example:* if you stop smoking, your risk of developing lung cancer decreases

Analogy
- Similar events have been proven to cause similar effects
  - *Example:* smoking other substances has

been known to cause lung pathology

CAUSAL RELATIONSHIP TYPES

Necessary and sufficient
- Presence of A required, present in adequate amounts to cause B
    - *Example:* autosomal dominant mutation with complete penetrance both necessary, sufficient for disease to develop

Necessary but not sufficient
- Presence of A required, not present in adequate amounts to cause B
    - *Example:* heat required to cause burn, however, low heat will not cause burn; it is necessary but not sufficient

Not necessary but sufficient
- Presence of A not required, but is enough to cause B
    - *Example:* gunshot to head sufficient to cause death, however, not necessary, as there are many other causes of death

Not necessary and not sufficient
- Presence of A not needed nor enough to cause B
    - *Example:* urinary infection not necessary nor sufficient to cause pelvic inflammatory disease; urinary infection can be present without pelvic inflammatory disease, individual can have pelvic inflammatory disease without having urinary tract infection

BIAS

osms.it/bias

- Error in one step of study design/conduction/analysis → results interpretation that is different from truth
    - Many types of biases, no common classification

SELECTION BIAS
- Errors made when choosing/following population to be studied
    - Can occur at different stages of study
    - Most commonly occurs when chosen sample is not representative of population

MEASUREMENT BIAS
- AKA information bias
- Errors made when measuring data/results of interest
    - Most commonly results in results misclassification which can be differential/non-differential

Differential misclassification
- Error in measurement more likely to occur in one group than another
    - Results of one group will be inherently different to other group's results
    - *Example:* blood glucose levels of groups measured by different machines; one gave accurate results, other reported inaccurate results

Non-differential misclassification
- Measurement error likely to have occurred in both groups
    - Results among two groups will not differ greatly
    - *Example:* machine used to determine blood glucose levels for both groups was inaccurate

OTHER BIAS TYPES
- Information gathering, management can → other bias types
- AKA information bias

Procedure bias
- People allocated to different groups not treated identically
    - Usually due to lack of blinding

- *Example:* people in one group spend more time in hospital than other group

Recall bias
- Awareness of event/effect influences individual's recall of cause
  - Most common in retrospective studies
  - *Example:* after a person with cancer knows that radiation exposure is a cancer development risk factor, the person may place more emphasis on exposure to radiation than someone without cancer

Lead-time bias
- Early diagnosis extends follow-up period, making it seem as if event being studied took longer to progress
  - *Example:* early cervical cancer detection may make it seem as if cancer is less aggressive because of more time spent living with diagnosis

Observer-expectancy bias
- When belief in intervention's effectiveness interferes with reported treatment outcome
  - *Example:* researcher's belief in drug efficacy may interfere with reported results

CONFOUNDING

osms.it/confounding

- Occurs when external event is related to possible cause, outcome of interest but is not on causal pathway
- Example: study exploring relationship between exercising, overall health, we know that
  - Exercising known to improve overall health
  - Exercising associated with healthy lifestyle, but is not result of healthy lifestyle

INTERACTION

osms.it/interaction

- Combination of two/more factors changes disease incidence compared to influence they would have had individually
  - Describes way multiple factors interact to produce event

Synergism
- Refers to potentiation effect multiple factors may have on one another
- Example: 2 + 2 = 5

Antagonism
- Refers to inhibition effect multiple factors may have on one another
- Example: 2 + 2 = 3

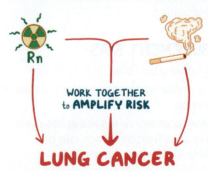

Figure 6.1 Biological interaction is when two exposures, like radon gas and cigarette toxins, work together to influence an outcome, like lung cancer.

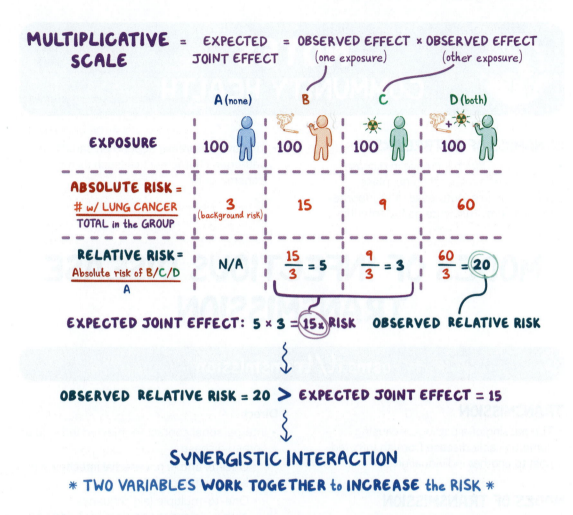

Figure 6.2 A graph representing data collected from four groups with 100 people per group: those with no exposure to radon or cigarette toxins (A), those with exposure to only cigarette toxins (B), those with exposure to only radon (C), and those with exposure to both radon and cigarette toxins (D). The multiplicative scale was used to calculate the expected joint effect of radon and cigarette toxins based on their independent effects (columns B and C). These two exposures are said to have a synergistic interaction because observed relative risk > expected joint effect. If observed relative risk had been < expected joint effect, the interaction would have been antagonistic.

NOTES
COMMUNITY HEALTH

DYNAMICS OF OUTBREAKS
- Outbreak: sudden increase in disease occurrence in a specific time, place, population (e.g. outbreaks of foodborne-related norovirus acute gastroenteritis)
- Infective outbreaks depend on causative pathogen characteristics (such as mode of transmission)

MODES OF INFECTIOUS DISEASE TRANSMISSION

osms.it/transmission

TRANSMISSION
- The passing of a pathogen-causing communicable disease from an infected host to another individual/group

MODES OF TRANSMISSION
- Depends on responsible organism's characteristics

Direct
- Interpersonal contact → infected individuals spread disease
  - One-to-one (e.g. venereal infection with sexual intercourse)
  - One-to-multiple (e.g. influenza with a violent sneeze in a crowded environment)

Indirect
- Common vehicle (e.g. contaminated air, water/food supply, needle-sharing)
- Vectors (e.g. mosquito/tick)

OUTBREAK INVESTIGATIONS

osms.it/outbreak-investigations

CHARACTERISTICS OF AN OUTBREAK
- *Explosive*: in epidemic curve, there is a fast, abrupt rise in number of cases, followed by fast, abrupt fall
- *Indirect transmission*: infection limited to individuals who share common exposure
- *Direct transmission*: often impossible to associate new cases to primary case (first symptomatic case occurring in defined setting)

STEPS TO INVESTIGATE AN OUTBREAK

Validate outbreak's existence in a population
- Define number of cases (numerator)
- Define the extent of the population susceptible to disease (denominator)
- Determine whether number of observed cases is more than expected number of cases
- Calculate the attack rate: proportion of an initially disease-free population that develops disease
    - Proportion is used because the individuals in the numerator (those who have the disease) are included in the denominator (the total population)

Investigate cases by looking for interactions of time, person, place
- Are there interactions between variables?

Develop hypotheses
- Consider existing knowledge about the disease, findings from current investigation

Test hypotheses
- Analyze data (e.g. case-control study, laboratory tests such as chemical/immunological fingerprinting)

Recommend measures for disease control, prevention
- E.g. remove infection source, establish environmental controls (interrupt disease transmission), improve sanitation, immunize susceptible individuals

DISEASE SURVEILLANCE

osms.it/disease-surveillance

- Essential public health tool, aimed at predicting, observing, minimizing outbreaks
- Based on systematic collection, analysis, interpretation of epidemiologic data
- Monitored parameters examples
    - Changes in disease incidence/mortality
    - Changes in quantity of risk factors for a disease in environment
    - Completeness of vaccination coverage
    - Prevalence of drug-resistant organisms

MODALITIES OF SURVEILLANCE

Passive
- Using existing data on reportable diseases such as anthrax, cholera, gonorrhea
- Pros
    - Comparatively inexpensive, easy to develop
    - Areas that require urgent intervention are quickly identified by international comparisons
- Cons
    - Surveillance is not the primary responsibility of case-reporting individuals
    - Local outbreaks may be missed

Active
- Implementing surveillance program (e.g. field visits to clinics, hospitals, communities)
- Pros
    - Reporting more accurate; individuals recruited specifically for surveillance program
    - Local outbreaks are more likely to be identified
- Cons
    - More expensive to develop, maintain

DIFFICULTIES
- Obtaining reliable data in low-income countries → underreporting risk
    - Areas may be difficult to reach
    - Communication with central authorities can be challenging
    - Resources such as diagnostic laboratories not always available

VACCINATION & HERD IMMUNITY

osms.it/vaccination-herd-immunity

HERD IMMUNITY BASICS
- *Herd immunity*: phenomenon in which entire population is indirectly protected against disease when critical percentage of members are immune
  - Immunity can be innate/acquired through vaccination/by naturally recovering from infection
  - The higher the proportion of immune people in a population, the less likely the encounter between a susceptible person and an infected one → chain of infection is disrupted

Conditions
- Host is a single species
- Transmission of the organism must be spread by direct contact
- No reservoir outside the human host
- Infections must induce solid immunity

HERD IMMUNITY & COMMUNITY HEALTH
- The critical percentage of immune individuals needed to achieve herd immunity varies according to disease contagiousness (e.g. 94% in measles [highly communicable] → increased number of individuals need to be immune)
- Because of herd immunity, vaccination programs do not necessitate yield 100% immunization rates, yet can achieve highly effective protection by immunizing critical percentage of a population
- Herd immunity is important for public health because individuals who cannot develop immunity or cannot be vaccinated depend on herd immunity (e.g. newborn infants, individuals with immunodeficiency due to HIV/AIDS, cancer, cancer treatments)

NOTES: EPIDEMIOLOGY MEASURES

DIRECT STANDARDIZATION

osms.it/direct-standardization

STANDARDIZATION
- Methods used to compare health event rates of two/more populations (e.g. mortality rates) by standardizing characteristics responsible for inter-population differences
- E.g. remove confounding variables (age) when comparing two groups' crude mortality rate (CMR) to get age-adjusted mortality rate
  - CMR: number of people who died in one group, divided by the group population (100,000 or 1,000)

DIRECT STANDARDIZATION
- Compares differences in health events among two/more populations by calculating age-adjusted rate
- Used when event distribution in each age group within population is known
- Process for calculating direct standardization for age-adjusted mortality rate
  - Choose reference (standard) population (e.g. separate population such as a national-level population)
  - Multiply other population of interest's age-specific mortality rates to number of people in each age group of reference population
  - Add up number of expected deaths from all age groups
  - Calculate age-adjusted mortality rate
  - Compare two age-adjusted mortality rates

INDIRECT STANDARDIZATION

osms.it/indirect-standardization

- Used when number of events/mortality rates in each age group within population is not known
- Process for calculating indirect standardization for age-adjusted mortality rate
  - Choose reference population with known mortality rates
  - Multiply other population of interest's age-specific mortality rates to number of people in each age group of reference population
  - Add up number of expected deaths from all age groups
  - Calculate standardized mortality ratio (SMR)

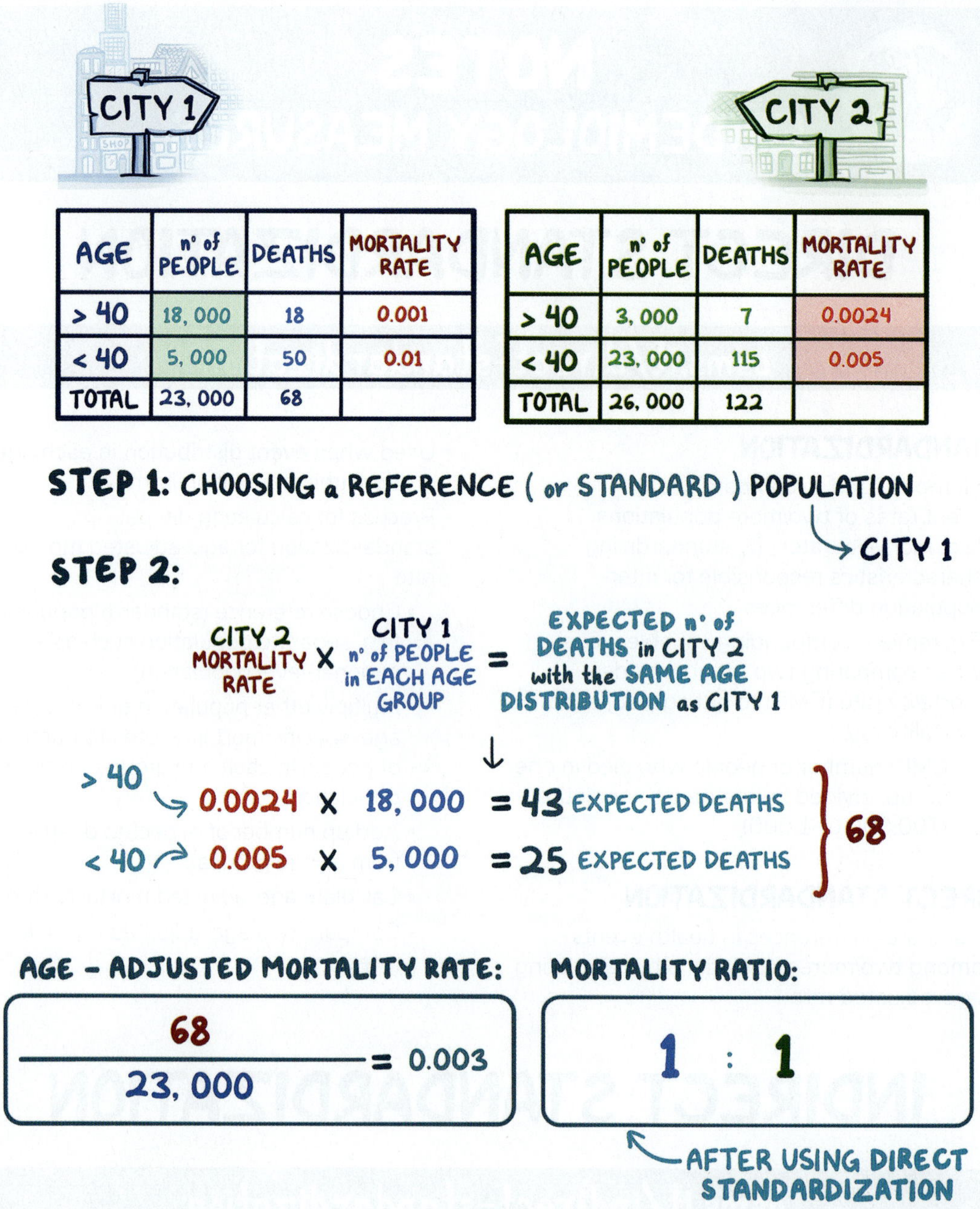

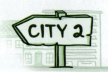

Figure 8.1 Using direct standardization to find the age-adjusted mortality rate for City 2, using City 1 as the reference population.

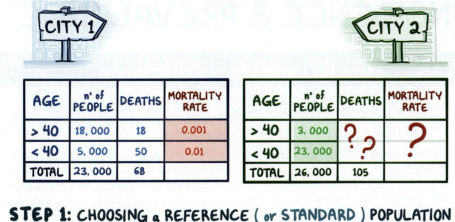

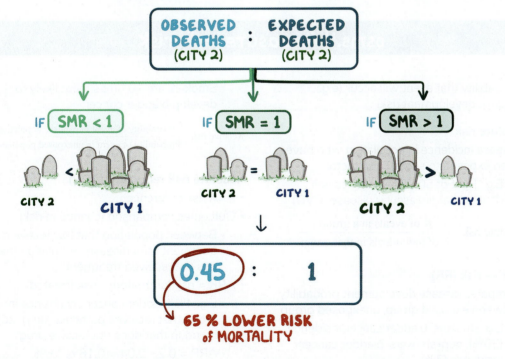

Figure 8.2 Using indirect standardization to find the standardized mortality ratio for City 2, using City 1 as the reference population.

INCIDENCE & PREVALENCE

osms.it/incidence-prevalence

- Measures number of people who have disease
- Reported as population percentage/ratio (e.g cases per 1000)

Incidence
- Number of new disease cases in population over time period (usually one year)
  - Affected by preventive measures (vaccination, diagnostic techniques)

Prevalence
- Number of total (old, new) disease cases in population in particular time point (point prevalence)
  - Shows disease commonness in group of people
  - Affected by cure rate, survival rate, death rate, recurrence

Relationship between incidence and prevalence
- New disease cases (incidence) added to amount of disease present in population (baseline prevalence) → ↑ prevalence
- ↑ death rate, cure rate → ↓ prevalence (↓ total disease cases)
- If incidence > death/cure rate → net ↑ prevalence; if incidence < death/cure rate → net ↓ prevalence

$$\text{prevALence} = \frac{\text{ALL cases}}{\text{population at risk}}$$

$$\text{iNcidence} = \frac{\text{New cases}}{\text{population at risk}}$$

MEASURES OF RISK

osms.it/measures-of-risk

- Probability that event will occur (e.g. disease development risk)

Absolute risk
- Disease incidence in population who have been exposed to specific risk factor
  - E.g. 1 out of 50 (2%) diabetics will develop cardiovascular disease (CVD)

$$\text{Absolute risk} = \frac{\text{\# of events in a group}}{\text{\# of individuals in that group}}$$

Relative risk (RR)
- Compares disease development probability between exposed group, unexposed group
  - E.g. smokers' bladder cancer incidence (30%), non-smokers' bladder cancer incidence (3%)
  - RR = 0.3/0.03 = 10
  - Smokers are 10 times more likely to develop bladder cancer

$$\text{Relative risk} = \frac{\text{Probability of event in exposed population}}{\text{Probability of event in unexposed population}}$$

Absolute risk reduction (ARR)
- AKA risk difference
- Outcomes comparison (change in risk)
  - Between population that has received treatment for a disease, population that has not received treatment
- ARR = risk (untreated) - risk (treated)
  - E.g. 4% bladder cancer occurrence in group that receives particular drug, 20% in group that does not receive drug
  - ARR = 0.2 - 0.04 = 0.16 or 16%
  - For every 100 individuals receiving drug, 16 bad outcomes would be avoided

Number needed to treat
- Determines how many individuals should be treated with medication to prevent one person from developing bladder cancer
  - Number needed to treat: 1/0.16 = 6.25
  - About six people should be treated

$$\text{\# needed to treat} = \frac{1}{\text{Absolute risk reduction}}$$

ODDS RATIO

osms.it/odds-ratio

- Measures association between exposure (e.g. risk factor, health characteristic), outcome (e.g. disease, mortality)
  - E.g. Which group is at higher risk of experiencing an adverse outcome? Does an intervention change risk degree for a group?
- *Used in case-control studies:* case group with identified outcome, control group without identified outcome
- Calculated using 2X2 frequency table
  - Divide odds of disease in exposed individuals by odds of disease in unexposed individuals

$$OR = \frac{a/c}{b/d} = \frac{ad}{bc}$$

$$OR = \frac{40/20}{60/80} = \frac{2}{0.75} = 2.66$$

- OR = 1 → exposure does not affect odds of outcome
- OR > 1 → exposure associated with higher odds of outcome
- OR < 1 → exposure associated with lower odds of outcome

2 x 2 FREQUENCY TABLE

	+ (DISEASE)	– (NO DISEASE)
+ (EXPOSED)	a: # of exposed individuals (smokers) w/bladder cancer = 40	b: # of exposed individuals (smokers) w/o bladder cancer = 60
– (UNEXPOSED)	c: # of unexposed cases w/bladder cancer = 20	d: # of unexposed cases w/o bladder cancer = 80

ATTRIBUTABLE RISK (AR)

osms.it/attributable-risk

- AKA risk difference/excess risk
- Measures difference in disease risk between exposed population, unexposed population
    - Often used in cohort studies

AR for exposed individuals

$$AR = \frac{A}{A+B} - \frac{C}{C+D}$$

2 x 2 FREQUENCY TABLE

	+ (DISEASE)	− (NO DISEASE)	TOTALS
+ (EXPOSED)	a: # of exposed individuals (smokers) w/bladder cancer = 40	b: # of exposed individuals (smokers) w/o bladder cancer = 60	100
− (UNEXPOSED)	c: # of unexposed cases w/bladder cancer = 20	d: # of unexposed cases w/o bladder cancer = 80	100
	60	140	200

$$AR = \frac{40}{100} - \frac{20}{100} = 0.4 - 0.2 = \frac{20}{100}$$

$$\frac{AR}{\text{incidence in exposed}} \times 100$$

$$\frac{20}{40} \times 100 = 50\%$$

- 50% of bladder cancer incidence → attributable to smoking in exposed population

AR for population (PAR)

PAR = incidence in population − incidence in unexposed

$$PAR = \frac{60}{200} - \frac{20}{100} = 0.3 - 0.2 = \frac{10}{100}$$

$$\frac{10}{20} \times 100 = 50\%$$

MORTALITY RATES & CASE-FATALITY

osms.it/mortality_rates_case-fatality

- **Mortality rate**: death incidence in population over period of time

Annual mortality rate

- Mortality rate from all causes (crude death rate)
    - Calculated by taking total number of deaths from all causes in one year divided by total number of people at risk in population at mid-year
- Annual mortality = total number of deaths (850) ÷ total number of people at risk in population at mid-year (500,000) = 0.0017

- Percent: 0.0017 × 100 = 0.17%
- Per 100,000: 0.0017 × 100,000 = 170 (170 death per 100,000 people during year)

Population-specific mortality rate
- Mortality rate for specific sub-population (e.g. biologically-female individuals; cancer-related deaths, neonatal mortality)
    - E.g. neonatal mortality rate = number of deaths among children < 28 days old (during given time interval) ÷ number of live births (during same time interval) × 1,000

Case-fatality rate
- Percent of people that die within certain period of time post-diagnosis
    - Calculated by dividing number of post-diagnosis deaths by total number of diagnosed individuals, multiplied by 100
- Measures disease severity

$$\text{Case mortality rate from disease A} = \frac{40}{250} = 0.16 = 16\%$$

DALY & QALY

osms.it/DALY-QALY

- *Disease burden measurement*: impact of health problem on individual/population

Disability-Adjusted Life Years (DALY)
- Determines disease burden according to years of life, or to compare specific intervention's effect (e.g. new medication reducing diabetes risk)
    - Morbidity, mortality combined into single metric
- DALY: years of lost life due to premature death (YLL) + years lived disability (YLD)
    - YLL: number of deaths (N) × standard life expectancy at age of death in years (L)
    - YLD: number of incident cases (I) × disability weight (DW) × average duration of disability in years (L)
    - DW: reflects disease severity on 0 (perfect health) to 1 (dead) scale

Quality-Adjusted Life Years (QALY)
- Determines disease burden according to quality of years of life, relative value of interventions (e.g. cost-utility analysis); guides healthcare-resource prioritization
- Measures years of life with illness/disability (considered less than year of healthy life)
- QALY = number of years lived × utility weight
    - One healthy year of life = 1 QALY (1 year of life × 1 utility weight)
    - One year of life lived in situation with illness/disability (e.g. chronic pain) = 1 year × 0.5 (utility weight) = 0.5 QALYs
    - Death: assigned value of 0 QALYs

NOTES
NON-PARAMETRIC TESTS

NON-PARAMETRIC TESTS
- For data that is assumed to not be distributed normally
- For nominal/ordinal level variables

CHI-SQUARED TEST

osms.it/chi-squared_test

- Chi-square (X^2) goodness-of-fit test
- Test compares categorical variables
  - Assesses for significant association
- Examines whether collected data is significantly different than theoretical model
  - How "good is the fit" between data, what is expected
- Null hypothesis: no significant difference between theorized/expected, observed ratios
  - $X^2 =$ sum of [(observed − expected)^2/expected]
- Use X^2 table to find critical X^2
  - Adjusted for degrees of freedom [n − 1], at selected p-value
- Accept null hypothesis if X^2 < critical X^2

CHI-SQUARE TEST OF INDEPENDENCE
- For analysis of contingency tables (or crosstabs tables)
- Investigates whether two/more categorical variables are statistically significant
- Used for multiple variables
- Degrees of freedom = (# of rows − 1) x (# of columns − 1)
- Requires > 5 data points in all cells of table; whole numbers
- Higher X^2 results in lower p-value

FISHER'S EXACT TEST

osms.it/Fisher_exact_test

- Variant of chi-square test
  - Used with small sample size
- Used to determine exact probability of association between two categorical variables (i.e. significance of association [contingency] between classifications)
  - Use for 2 x 2 contingency tables (< 5 in a cell)
  - p-values calculated exactly
  - $p < 0.05$, unlikely to be random association

KAPLAN-MEIER SURVIVAL ANALYSIS

osms.it/Kaplan-Meier_survival_analysis

- Estimates survival from lifetime data; measures fraction of survivors over treatment time; simplest method of computing survival over time
    - Plot of percent survival versus time; generated from status at last observation, time to event
    - Large sample size → approaches population effect
- Accounts for censored data; withdrawn from study, lost to follow-up; alive at last follow-up (i.e. right-censoring—data above a certain value, but otherwise unknown)
- Limited capacity to estimate survival adjusted for covariates

KAPPA COEFFICIENT

osms.it/kappa-coefficient

- AKA Cohen's kappa coefficient
- Measure of inter-rater agreement
- Compares ability of different raters to classify categorical variables
- **Interobserver agreement**: accounts for agreement that occurs by chance, when raters measure same thing, using same observation method
- Calculated from observed, expected frequencies from diagonal of contingency table
- If kappa = 1
    - Agreement is perfect
- If kappa = 0
    - Agreement is no better than if agreement happened by chance
- Example for interpreting agreement based on kappa coefficient
    - **None**: < 0
    - **Fair**: 0.20–0.40
    - **Moderate**: 0.40–0.60
    - **Good**: 0.60–0.80
    - **Very good**: 0.80–1.00

MANN-WHITNEY U TEST

osms.it/Mann-Whitney_u_test

- Nonparametric test equivalent to unpaired t-test
- Compares differences between two unpaired groups that are not normally distributed
- Uses number ranks rather than raw data
- Provides p-value indicating whether or not groups are significantly different from each other ($p < 0.05$; unlikely to happen by chance)

SPEARMAN'S RANK CORRELATION COEFFICIENT

osms.it/Spearmans-rank-correlation-coefficient

- Spearman's rho (ρ)
- Non-parametric equivalent of Pearson's correlation coefficient
- Measure strength, direction of monotonic association between two ranked variables
  - Monotonic association means variables increase together (i.e. as value of one variable increases value of other variable increases also/as value of one variable increases, other variable value will decrease)
  - Does not have to be linear, but must be entirely increasing/entirely decreasing (may include plateaus)
  - Use for continuous/discrete ordinal, interval, ratio variables
- Sign indicates direction of association
  - x and y increasing → +ve ρ; x and y decreasing → –ve ρ
- ρ increases as correlation approaches perfect monotone relationship between variables
- Two formulas
  - One for when there are no tied ranks
  - One for tied ranks
- Use critical values (r_s) from Spearman's rank coefficient tables to determine significance of r (Spearman's coefficient of sample)

NOTES
PARAMETRIC TESTS

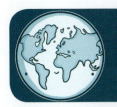

PARAMETRIC TESTS
- ANOVA, t-tests
- Use for following data
  - Randomly selected samples
  - Independent observations
  - Population standard deviations (SDs) are same
  - Data distributed normally/approximately normally

ANOVA

osms.it/one-way_ANOVA
osms.it/two-way_ANOVA
osms.it/repeated-measures_ANOVA

- AKA analysis of variance
- Determines differences between > two samples
  - Measures differences among means
- F-ratio (F statistic)
  - F = (variance between groups) / (variance within each group)
- Computer program calculates p-value from F; use F to accept/reject null hypothesis
  - F approx. = 1; p large; accept null hypothesis
  - F large → p small (alpha set at 0.05 significant → reject null hypothesis)
- Assumptions
  - Samples drawn randomly; sample groups have homogeneity of variance (i.e. from same population; interval, ratio data)

1-way ANOVA
- Between groups design
- One independent variable
  - May have multiple levels (e.g. drug A effect vs. drug B vs. placebo on specified outcome)

Factorial ANOVAs
- Factorial designs
- Two-way, three-way, four-way ANOVA, more (two, three, four, etc. independent variables)

Single-factor repeated measures ANOVA
- ANOVAs involving repeated measures/ within groups/subjects
- One independent variable with multiple levels tested within one subject group (e.g. drug A vs. drug B vs. placebo tested within same individuals at different times)
- ↓ variation effect between sample groups

LOWERING SYSTOLIC BLOOD PRESSURE

ONE-WAY ANOVA

MEDICATION A — MEDICATION B — MEDICATION C
GROUP A — GROUP B — GROUP C

TWO-WAY ANOVA

MEDICATION A SIX WEEKS — MEDICATION B SIX WEEKS — MEDICATION C SIX WEEKS
YOUNGER OLDER — YOUNGER OLDER — YOUNGER OLDER

REPEATED MEASURES ANOVA

MEDICATION A ONE MONTH — MEDICATION A THREE MONTHS — MEDICATION A SIX MONTHS
GROUP A — GROUP A — GROUP A

Figure 10.1 Examples demonstrating a one-way, two-way, and repeated measures ANOVA. The one-way ANOVA has one independent variable (medication type) with multiple levels (medications A, B, and C). The two-way ANOVA looks at two independent variables (medication type and age category) that each have multiple groups (medications A, B, and C; younger and older). The repeated measures ANOVA follows the same group of people over a period of time to measure the effects of the same medication over time. In this case, the independent variable is time, divided into three groups (one month, three months, and six months), and the dependent variable is systolic blood pressure.

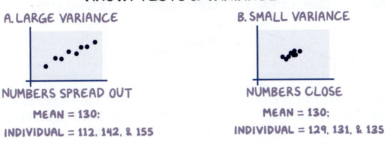

Figure 10.2 All ANOVA tests assume that the groups have equal variance. A large variance means that the numbers are very spread out from the mean; a small variance means that the numbers are very close to the mean. Variances between groups are considered unequal when the variance of one group is greater than twice the variance of the other group.

CORRELATION

osms.it/correlation

- Investigates relationships between variables; determines strength, type (positive/negative) relationship
- Correlation coefficient: r ($-1 > r < +1$)
  - Perfect positive correlation: $r = +1$
  - Perfect negative correlation: $r = -1$
  - No correlation: $r = 0$
  - Strong correlation: $r > 0.5 < -0.5$
  - Weak correlation: $0 < r < 0.5$, or $0 > r > -0.5$
- Pearson product-moment coefficient: interval/ratio data; calculates linear relationship degree between two variables
- Confidence interval (CI): population based on correlation coefficient
  - Indicates range within population correlation coefficient lies
- P-value for correlation coefficient based on null hypothesis
  - I.e. if true ($p > 0.05$), no correlation between variables
- Coefficient of determination: r^2 or R^2 ($0 < R^2 < 1$)
  - Fraction of variation of variable of interest (x axis) due to another variable of interest (y axis)
  - Remaining proportion due to natural variability
  - Low R^2 may indicate poor linear relationship, may be strong nonlinear relationship
- Eta-squared (η^2): analogous to R^2 for ANOVA
- Correlation ≠ causation, consider
  - How strong is association?
  - Does effect always follow cause?
  - Is there a dose response?
  - Relationship biologically plausible, coherent?
  - Consistent finding?
  - Other factors involved?
  - Good experimental evidence?
  - Analogous examples?

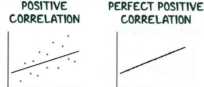
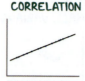

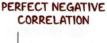
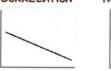
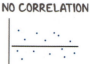

Figure 10.3 Scatterplots are used to plot measurements, with one measured variable on each axis. Each data point represents one individual. A trend line is drawn to best represent the collection of data points on the plot, with roughly half the points above the line and the other half below the line. A perfect positive or negative correlation means that the trend line passes through every single data point.

HYPOTHESIS TESTING

osms.it/hypothesis-testing

- Calculating sample size required to test hypothesis
- Equations used for calculating power can also be used to calculate sample size for a predefined alpha (0.05)
- Requires knowledge of
  - Clinically important effect size (larger sample size needed to detect smaller effects)
  - Surrogate endpoint use rather than direct outcome
  - Desired power; alpha (if not 0.05); confidence interval
  - Statistical tests to be used
  - Data lost to follow-up
  - Test group SD; population of interest expected frequency within test group
- Statistician's advice
  - Optimize sample size, avoid underpowered studies, enable valid data interpretation

LINEAR REGRESSION

osms.it/linear-regression

- *Simple linear regression*: assumes linear relationship; slope ≠ 0; data points close to line
- Examine weight of two variables' (x, y) effects; predict effects of x on y
- Fit best straight line to x, y plot of data
  - Equation: y = bx + a (x and y are independent variables; b = slope of line (regression coefficient); a = intercept)
- 95% CI for slope range; larger sample → narrower CI; if range does not include zero → real correlation suggested
- p-value for null hypothesis
  - No linear correlation (i.e. slope = 0; $p < 0.05$ → real correlation suggested)

OTHER REGRESSION ANALYSES

- Multiple linear regression
  - Examines effects of more than one variable on y
- Multiple nonlinear regression
  - Examines correlations among nonlinear data, more than one independent variable

- Logistic regression
  - Predicts likelihood of categorical event in presence of multiple independent variables

LOGISTIC REGRESSION

osms.it/logistic-regression

- **Predictive analysis**: describes relationship between binary dependent variable (i.e. takes one of two values), multiple independent variables
- Assumptions
  - **Dichotomous outcome** (e.g. yes/no; present/absent; dead/alive)
  - **No outliers**: assess using z scores
  - **No intercorrelations**: assess using correlation matrix
- May use logit (assumes log distribution of event's probability)/probit (model assumes normal distribution)

- **Rule of 10**: stable values if based on minimum of 10 observations per independent variable
- **Regression coefficients**: indicate contribution of individual independent variables; odds ratios
- Tests to assess significance of independent variable
  - Likelihood ratio test; Wald test
- **Bayesian inference**: prior (known) distributions for regression coefficients; conjugate prior; automatic software (e.g. OpenBUGS, JAGS to simulate priors)

TYPE I & TYPE II ERRORS

osms.it/type-I-and-type-II-errors

POWER
- Refers to test probability correctly rejecting false null hypothesis
- Power: (1 – beta)
  - Likelihood that statistically non-significant result is correct (i.e. not false negative—type II error)
- Medical research
  - Power typically set at 0.80
- Increasing power
  - ↓ type II error chance; ↑ type I error chance
- Power increases when ↑ sample size, ↓ SD, ↑ effect size

EFFECT SIZE
- Relationship strength between variables
- Statistical significance does not necessarily indicate clinical significance
- Random variation (SD) may ↓ differences between outcomes of interest between hypothesis' test groups

$$ES = \frac{\overline{X_1} - \overline{X_2}}{SD}$$

  - ES is effect size
  - X_1 is the mean for Group 1
  - X_2 is the mean for Group 2
  - SD is the standard deviation from either group

- Adjust for variation in test groups with Cohen's d (assumes each group's SD is same)
    - Cohen's d = (mean 1 − mean 2)/SD
    - 0.2 = small effect size
    - 0.5 = medium effect size
    - ≥ 0.8 = large effect size

SAMPLE SIZE
- Smaller sample size
    - ↑ sampling error chance
    - Lower power
    - ↑ type II error chance (false negative)

BAYESIAN THINKING
- Relates p-value to context
    - Can involve complex mathematics
- Measures event probability given incomplete information
- Joint distribution between given information (usually probability density), experimental results

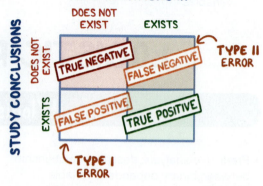

Figure 10.4 A Type I error occurs when no true relationship exists between two variables, but the study concludes there is one; a type II error occurs when there is a true relationship between two variables, but the study concludes there is no relationship.

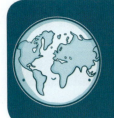

NOTES
STATISTICAL PROBABILITY DISTRIBUTIONS

NORMAL DISTRIBUTION & Z-SCORES

osms.it/normal-distributions-z_scores

NORMAL DISTRIBUTION
- Data grouped around central value, no left/right bias, in "bell curve" shape
- Probability distribution for normal random variable x
- $f(x) = \dfrac{1}{\sigma\sqrt{2\pi}} e^{-(\frac{1}{2})[(x-\mu)/\sigma]^2}$
- μ = mean of normal random variable x
- σ = standard deviation
- π = 3.1416 ...
- e = 2.71828 ...
- Normal distribution: μ = 0, σ = 1

Z-SCORES
- Standardized score
- Uses data set mean, standard deviation to determine measurement location
    - Represents deviation from mean
- Expressed in standard deviations
- Sample z-score for measurement x
- $z = \dfrac{x - \bar{u}}{\sigma}$
- μ = population mean
- σ = standard deviation

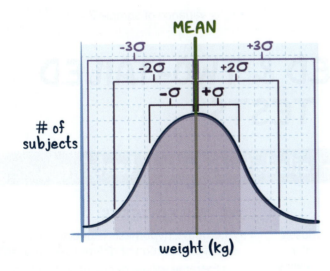

BELL CURVE

1 standard deviation:
68% = +/- σ

2 standard deviations:
95% = +/- 2σ

3 standard deviations:
99% = +/- 3σ

STANDARD ERROR OF THE MEAN

osms.it/standard-error-of-mean

- AKA SEM, standard deviation
- $\sigma_{\bar{x}} = \dfrac{\sigma}{\sqrt{n}}$

- σ = standard deviation
- n = sample size

PAIRED T-TESTS

osms.it/paired-t-test

- Statistical hypothesis test (parametric)
- Determines if two groups are statistically different (compares two groups' means)
- Groups can occur naturally (e.g. smokers compared to non-smokers)/groups can be created experimentally (e.g. control group compared to treatment group)
- t = $\dfrac{\text{difference between means}}{\text{variance/sample size}}$
- = $\dfrac{\text{sample mean - population mean}}{\text{sample standard error of the mean}}$

- $\dfrac{\bar{x}_1 - \bar{x}_2}{\sqrt{\dfrac{s_1^2}{n_1} + \dfrac{s_2^2}{n_2}}}$

- x_1 = mean of sample 1
- x_2 = mean of sample 2
- n_1 = sample size of sample 1
- n_2 = sample size of sample 2
- s_1^2 = variance of sample 1 = $\dfrac{\sum(x_1 - \bar{x}_1)^2}{n_1 - 1}$
- s_2^2 = variance of sample 2 = $\dfrac{\sum(x_2 - \bar{x}_2)^2}{n_1 - 1}$

ONE-TAILED & TWO-TAILED TESTS

osms.it/one-tailed-two-tailed-tests

- **Tails**: ends of probability curve
- Alternative (research) hypothesis proposes groups under investigation are different in some way/relationship between them exists

ONE-TAILED TESTS

- Alternative hypothesis is directional (i.e. specifies direction of difference/relationship)
  - Extreme values of one of distribution tails are of interest given difference type/expected relationship (solid theoretical

basis required for one-tailed test)
- Alternative hypothesis predicts relationship between groups either positive/negative (e.g. Group A will score higher on particular test than Group B)

TWO-TAILED TESTS

- Alternative hypothesis is non-directional (i.e. non-specified direction of difference/relationship)
  - Extreme values on either tail of sampling distribution support null hypothesis rejection (e.g. Group A scores will be different than Group B)

NOTES
STUDY DESIGN

SAMPLING

osms.it/sampling

- Selection of individuals for study from specific population
- Aims to represent, estimate characteristics of that population

PLACEBO EFFECT & MASKING

osms.it/placebo-effect-and-masking

WHAT IS THE PLACEBO EFFECT?
- Refers to situation where study participant's belief in treatment brings about positive effect
    - E.g. individuals given placebo drug tend to report improvements even when treatment has no real effect
- Placebos can be affected by study participant's psychological responses to context in which treatment is taking place
- Placebo can be drug/pharmacologically inactive substance indistinguishable from an active treatment/can be based on any expectation the person may have about intervention under study
- Useful in studying rate of side effects, reactions to drug

WHAT IS MASKING?
- Subjects and/or investigators are unaware of treatment assignment
    - *Single blind:* subjects are unaware of treatment assignment
    - *Double blind:* subjects, investigators are unaware of treatment assignment
    - *Triple blind:* treatment administrator unaware of treatment assignment

CASE-CONTROL STUDY

osms.it/case-control_study

- Study that determines potential risk factors in individuals with condition
- May rely on individual recall, past medical history, autopsy
- *Example:* Percentage of people who gave birth to child with condition A who had previously taken drug B during pregnancy
    - All children either do or do not have condition A
    - We assess whether they did/did not

take drug B during pregnancy

Pros
- More easily examines rare diseases than prospective studies; less expensive and time-consuming
- Individuals not exposed to possible risk factors
- Past medical history used to determine potential multiple risk factors

Cons
- Potential problems matching cases and controls
  - E.g. study may be influenced by characteristics not being studied (confounding variables)
- Potentially biased (relies on individual recall)
  - E.g. study candidates may emphasize potential risk factors rather than controls

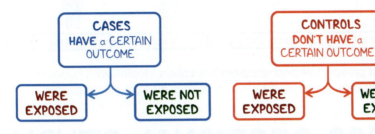

Figure 12.1 Case-control study design.

COHORT STUDY

osms.it/cohort-study

- Measures disease within group of individuals (cohort) over period of time
- Focuses on disease development
- **Two types:** prospective cohort, retrospective cohort

PROSPECTIVE COHORT STUDY
- AKA longitudinal, concurrent cohort study
- Results not known until after intervention
- Used to follow up on people who received treatment/were exposed to risk factors
- Laboratory tests often used as surrogate markers – for example, increase in hemoglobin immediately after blood transfusion assumed to mean that transfusion was effective
- **Example:** RSV rates of premature birth cohorts

Pros
- Easier to conduct than randomized controlled studies
- Useful information on risk
- Matching decreases influence of confounding variables

Cons
- Expensive, time-consuming
- Follow-up with people over time can be difficult; subjects may be lost

RETROSPECTIVE COHORT (HISTORICAL COHORT, NONCONCURRENT PROSPECTIVE) STUDY
- Same prospective cohort study design but uses past data to determine future time frame; study and obtention of results faster
- Use pre-existing population to decrease study duration
- Can be conducted relatively quickly, inexpensively
  - E.g. mortality rates according to duration of smoking

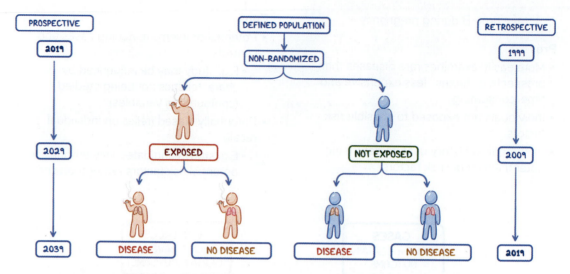

Figure 12.2 Design of prospective and retrospective cohort studies with hypothetical time frames. Exposed = smokers, not exposed = non-smokers, disease = lung cancer.

CROSS-SECTIONAL STUDY

osms.it/cross-sectional_study

- Study that observes a group of people at one point in time
- Examines relationship between an exposure (variable), disease being investigated
- *Example:* the relationship between endometrial cancer, hormone replacement therapy (HRT)

Pros
- Less time-consuming, expensive than longitudinal studies, as individual follow-up not necessary
- Good for establishing overall association between exposure and disease
- Can establish disease prevalence (number of individuals with particular disease in their lifetime)

Cons
- Establishes disease prevalence but not incidence (percentage of individuals who may develop a particular disease within a year)
- Does not establish temporal relationship between exposure and disease
- Potentially biased if surveys used
- *Retrospective studies:* data quality may be compromised due to poor recall/"recall bias," where people are more likely to recall certain events

Chapter 12 Epidemiology: Study Design

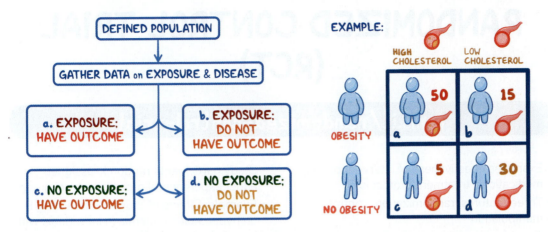

Figure 12.3 Design of a cross-sectional (prevalence) study. *Example:* obesity is the exposure, and high cholesterol is the outcome.

ECOLOGIC STUDY

osms.it/ecologic-study

- Observes at least one variable
  - Exposure/outcome
- Measured at group level
- At least one comparison group, disease occurrence compared between groups
- Often used to make large-scale comparisons

- Examples
  - Rate of cancer occurrence in one population
  - Average sunlight exposure at different geographical locations
  - Comparing per capita dietary fat consumption, cardiovascular disease mortality
  - Disease occurrence compared between groups

RANDOMIZED CONTROL TRIAL (RCT)

osms.it/randomized-control-trial

- Examines effectiveness of intervention (e.g. medications, treatment protocols)
- *Three features:* randomization, control, manipulation
- Considered gold standard of experimental research, identifying cause-and-effect relationships
- Study participants randomly assigned either experimental group or control group
- *Example:* Effects of drug A versus drug B on hypercholesterolemia in individuals with type 2 diabetes mellitus

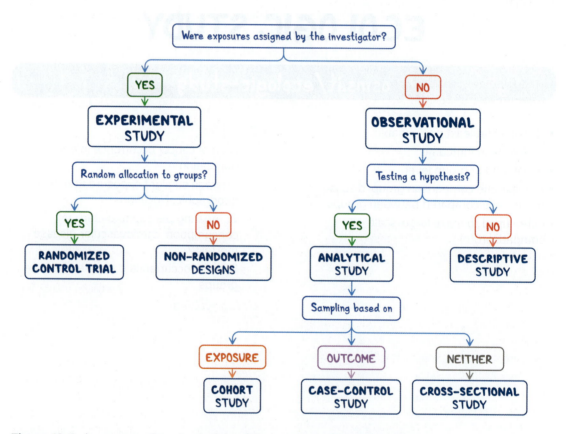

Figure 12.4 A summary flowchart of the different types of study designs.

NOTES: TESTING

SENSITIVITY (SN) & SPECIFICITY (SF)

osms.it/sensitivity-specificity

- Validity measure; concerned with how close test's result is to truth (i.e. did test/instrument measure what it is intended to measure?)
  - No perfect test → some miscalculation degree inevitable (i.e. healthy individual tests positive for disease → false positive; sick individual tests negative → false negative)
  - Sn, Sp: complementary test characteristic measures must be used together

SENSITIVITY

- Population proportion who test positive for disease, have disease
- AKA true positive rate
- Highly sensitive test with positive result identifies people who are truly diseased (true positives), some healthy people (false positives)
- *Sensitivity:* proportion containing all truly positive, false positives
- Can assume two things
  - Test with high sensitivity is negative, individual must be healthy → rule out disease
  - Test with high sensitivity is positive, individual may/may not have disease (ensure lack of false positive; further testing required)
  - High sensitivity negative test → useful for ruling-out disease

SPECIFICITY

- Population proportion tests negative for disease, free of disease
  - AKA true negative rate
- Highly specific test with negative result
- Identifies all people who are truly free of disease (true negatives), some sick people (false negatives)
- *Specificity:* proportion containing all truly negative, false negatives; two things assumed
  - Test with high specificity positive → confirm disease
  - Test with high specificity negative → individual may/may not have disease (ensure not false negative; further testing required)
- Positive test with high specificity → useful disease confirmation

CUTOFF POINT

- *For continuous variables:* sensitivity, specificity may overlap → midpoint usually sought (avoids misclassification)
- Cutoff point needed to distinguish between normal/healthy, abnormal/unhealthy results

High cutoff point
- *Highly specific:* low false positives
  - Everyone categorized as abnormal has disease
- *Poorly sensible:* high false negatives
  - Not everyone categorized as normal is free of disease

- I.e. previous hypertension definition stated 140/90mmHg as cutoff point
  - *Highly specific:* everyone categorized as abnormal has disease
  - *Poorly sensitive:* not everyone categorized as normal is free of disease

Low cutoff point
- *Poorly specific:* high false positives
  - Not everyone categorized as abnormal has disease
- *Highly sensitive:* low false negatives
  - Everyone categorized as normal is free of disease
- I.e. new hypertension definition states 120/80mmHg as cutoff point
  - *Poorly specific:* not everyone categorized as abnormal has diseases
  - *Highly sensitive:* everyone categorized as normal is free of disease

Cutoff point determined by test's purpose
- Screening test
  - Needs to detect all possible diseased → low cutoff point → highly sensitive → low false negatives
- Confirmatory test
  - Need to be sure of disease presence → high cutoff point → highly specific → low false positives

SEQUENTIAL & SIMULTANEOUS TESTING

Sequential testing
- AKA two-stage testing
- Consecutive tests performed with different characteristics → obtain more specific results
  - Perform first test → positive → perform second test → positive → disease likely present
  - Perform first test → negative → disease not likely present
- Similar to "double checking" results
- First test often easier/cheaper/less invasive than second test
- Sensitivity, specificity calculations must include both tests' characteristics
- *Net sensitivity:* proportion of true cases that test positive on both first, second test
  - First test sensitivity x second test sensitivity
- *Net specificity:* proportion of healthy people that test negative on either first, second test
  - (First test specificity + second test specificity) - (first test specificity * second test specificity)

Simultaneous testing
- Two tests with different characteristics performed at same time → more sensitive results
  - Simultaneous testing: three groups of people
  - People detected only by Test A
  - People detected only by Test B
  - People detected by both Test A and Test B
  - Pools all possibly relevant information → more sensitive results
- Sensitivity, specificity calculations must include both tests' characteristics
- *Net sensitivity:* proportion of true cases that test positive on either test A or B
  - (Test A sensitivity + Test B sensitivity) - (Test A sensitivity x Test B sensitivity)
- *Net specificity:* proportion of healthy people that test negative on both tests A and B
  - Test A specificity x Test B specificity

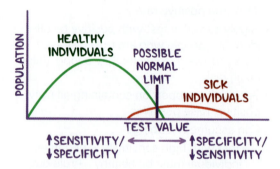

Figure 13.1 Illustration showing how sensitivity and specificity are affected by moving the cut-off point.

SENSITIVITY & SPECIFICITY

		DISEASE		TESTING TOTAL	MEASURES
		PRESENT	ABSENT		
TEST	POSITIVE	True positives (TP)	False positives (FP)	Total positive test (TP + FP)	Positive Predictive Value (PPV) = <u>true positives</u> / total positives
	NEGATIVE	False negatives (FN)	True negatives (TN)	Total negative test (FN + TN)	Negative Predictive Value (NPV) = <u>true negatives</u> / total negatives
TOTAL DISEASE		Total disease (TP + FN)	Total no disease (FP + TN)	Total population (TP + FP + TN + FN)	Muscles, liver
MEASURES		Sensitivity = <u>true positives</u> / total disease	Specificity = <u>true negatives</u> / total no disease	Prevalence = <u>Total disease</u> / total population	

POSITIVE & NEGATIVE PREDICTIVE VALUE

osms.it/positive-negative-predictive-value

- **PPV**: probability that if test is positive, person has disease
  - Divide true positives, total positive test number
- **NPV**: probability that if test is negative, person is free of disease
  - Divide true negatives, total negative test number

- Both measures directly influenced by prevalence, test specificity
  - **High prevalence**: more likely that person has disease → ↑ PPV
  - **Low prevalence**: less likely that person has disease → ↑ NPV
  - **Low prevalence**: need a good test in confirming disease (high specificity) → ↑ PPV

TEST PRECISION & ACCURACY

osms.it/test-precision-accuracy

- Both concerned with how likely test to be reproduced → return results close to truth
    - Neither measuring devices nor people perfect → affects test precision, accuracy
- **Test precision:** how repeatable test results are over time, regardless of result accuracy
    - **High precision test:** consistently deliver similar results, regardless of whether true/not
- **Test accuracy:** how true test results are, regardless of test repeatability
    - **High accuracy test:** gives correct results; cannot always be reproduced

- Comparing test precision, accuracy
    - Oximeter consistently (precisely) reports true pO_2 (accurately)
    - Oximeter consistently (precisely) reports pO_2 20% lower than truth (not accurate)
    - Oximeter inconsistently (not precise) reports true pO_2 (accurate)
    - Oximeter inconsistently (not precise) reports pO_2 20% lower than truth (not accurate)

CARDIOVASCULAR ANATOMY & PHYSIOLOGY

osms.it/cardiovascular-anatomy-physiology

CARDIOVASCULAR SYSTEM
- Cardia-, cardi-, cardio-
  - Heart, which pumps blood
- **Vascular:** blood vessels (carry blood to body, return it to heart)
- Delivers oxygen, nutrients to organs, tissues
- Removes waste (carbon dioxide, other cellular respiration by-products) from organs, tissues

MORPHOLOGY
- **Size:** about size of person's first (correlated with person's size)
- **Shape:** blunt cone-shaped
- **Position:** slightly shifted to left side
- **Location**
  - Lies in mediastinum in thoracic cavity
  - Sits on top of diaphragm (main breathing muscle)
  - Behind sternum (breast bone)
  - In front of vertebral column
  - Between lungs
  - Enclosed, protected by ribs
  - Right, left sides separated by muscular septum

Heart wall layers
- **Epicardium:** covers surface of heart, great vessels (AKA visceral pericardium)
- **Myocardium:** muscular middle layer
  - **Cardiac muscle cells:** striated branching cells with many mitochondria, intercalated disks for synchronous contraction
  - **Cardiac myocytes:** striated, branching cells with fibrous cardiac skeleton

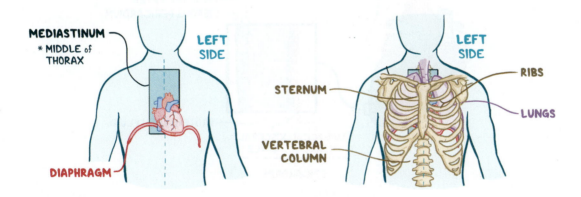

Figure 14.1 Heart location relative to other thoracic structures.

(supports muscle tissue, crisscrossing connective tissue collagen fibers); coronary vessels (lie on outside of heart, penetrate into myocardium to bring blood to that layer)
- **Endocardium**: innermost layer
    - Made of thin epithelial layer, underlying connective tissue
    - Lines heart chamber, valve
- **Pericardium**: double-layered sac surrounding heart
    - *Fibrous pericardium*: outer layer; tough fibrous connective tissue anchors heart within mediastinum
    - *Serous pericardium*: simple squamous epithelium layer
    - *Parietal pericardium*: lines fibrous pericardium
    - *Visceral pericardium (epicardium)*: covers outer surface of heart
    - Cells of parietal, visceral pericardium secrete protein-rich fluid (pericardial fluid) → fills space between layers (lubricant for heart, prevents friction)

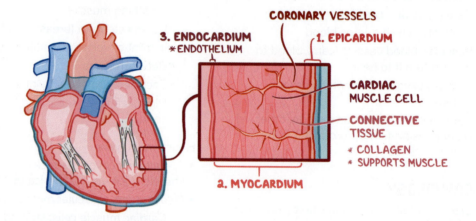

Figure 14.2 Heart wall layers, from superficial to deep.

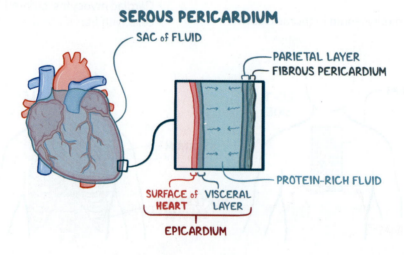

Figure 14.3 Layers of the pericardium (the double-layered sac surrounding the heart.)

Atrioventricular valves
- Separate atria from ventricles
- Tricuspid valve
  - Three cusps with chordae tendinae (tether valve to papillary muscle)
  - Prevents blood backflow into right atrium (right ventricle contracts → papillary muscles contract, keep chordae tendineae taut)
- Bicuspid / mitral valve
  - **Two cusps:** anterior, posterior leaflet
  - Both have chordae tendineae tethered to papillary muscles in left ventricle
  - Prevents blood backflow back into left atrium

Semilunar valves
- Located where two major arteries leave ventricles
- Pulmonary valve
  - Three half-moon shaped cusps
  - Prevents blood backflow into right ventricle
- Aortic valve
  - Three cusps
  - Prevents blood backflow into left ventricle

Blood flow physiology
- Deoxygenated blood enters right side of heart via superior, inferior vena cava (veins)
- Coronary sinus (tiny right atrium opening) collects blood from coronary vessels → right atrium → tricuspid valve → right ventricle → pulmonary valve → pulmonary trunk → pulmonary arteries → pulmonary arterioles → pulmonary capillaries → alveoli
- Blood collects oxygen from alveoli, removes carbon dioxide
- Oxygenated blood travels through pulmonary venules → pulmonary veins → left atrium → bicuspid/mitral valve → left ventricle → aortic valve → aorta → organs, tissues
- Deoxygenated blood returns to heart

SYSTEMIC VS. PULMONARY CIRCULATION
- Pulmonary, systemic circulation both pump same amount of blood

Pulmonary circulation
- Low pressure system
- Right side of heart pumps deoxygenated blood through pulmonary circulation to collect oxygen
  - Right atrium → right ventricle → pulmonary arteries → lungs

Systemic circulation
- High pressure system
- Left side of heart pumps oxygenated blood to systemic circulation
  - Pulmonary veins → left atrium → left ventricle → aorta → body
  - Left ventricle three times thicker than right ventricle (↑ systemic circulation resistance)

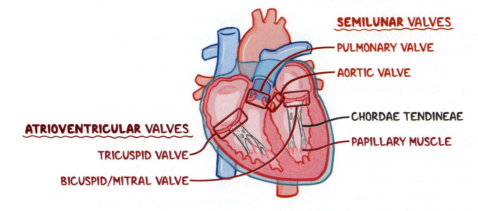

Figure 14.4 The four heart valves. The chordae tendineae and papillary muscles attached to the atrioventricular valves prevent blood backflow into the atria.

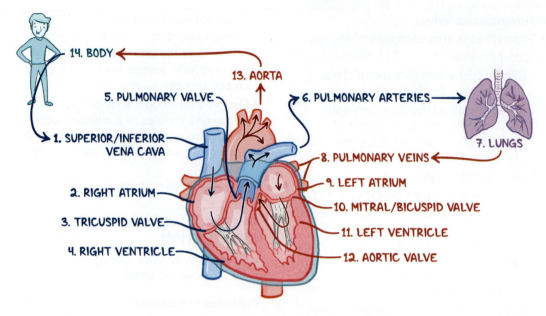

Figure 14.5 Blood flow physiology starting with the superior and inferior vena cavae bringing deoxygenated blood from the body to the right atrium of the heart.

VENTRICULAR SYSTOLE VS. DIASTOLE

Systole
- Ventricular contraction/atrial relaxation
- Occurs during S1 sound
    - Aortic, pulmonic valves open → blood pushed into aorta, pulmonary arteries
- Systolic blood pressure
    - Arterial pressure when ventricles squeeze out blood under high pressure
    - Peripheral pulse felt

Diastole
- Ventricular relaxation/atrial contraction
- Occurs during S2 sound
    - Tricuspid, mitral valves open → blood fills ventricles
- Diastolic blood pressure
    - Ventricles fill with more blood (lower pressure)

BLOOD DISTRIBUTION
- **Average adult:** 5L/1.32gal total blood volume (not cardiac output)
- 10% of total volume (approx. 500ml/0.13gal) in pulmonary arteries, capillaries, pulmonic circulatory veins
- 5% of total volume (250ml/0.07gal) in one of four heart chambers
- 15% (750ml/0.2gal) in systemic arteries
    - 15% to brain
    - 5% nourishes heart
    - 25% to kidneys
    - 25% to GI organs
    - 25% to skeletal muscles
    - 5% to skin
- 5% (250ml/0.07gal) in systemic capillaries
- 65% (3.25L/0.86gal) in systemic veins
- Numbers can change (e.g. exercise)

BLOOD FLOW TERMINOLOGY

Preload
- Amount of blood in left ventricle before contraction
- Determined by filling pressure (end diastolic pressure)
- "Volume work" of heart

Afterload
- Resistance (load) left ventricle needs to push against to eject blood during contraction
- "Tension work" of heart
- Components include
    - Amount of blood in systemic circulation

Chapter 14 Cardiovascular Physiology: Cardiovascular Anatomy & Physiology

- Degree of arterial vessel wall constriction (for left side of heart, main afterload source is systemic arterial resistance; for right side of heart, main afterload source is pulmonary arterial pressure)

Stroke volume (SV)
- Blood volume (in liters) pumped by heart per contraction
- Determined by amount of blood filling ventricle, compliance of ventricular myocardium

Cardiac output (CO)
- Blood volume pumped by heart per minute (L/min)
- CO = SV * heart rate
- Example
  - SV = 70mL ejected per contraction
  - HR = 70bpm
  - CO = 70 * 70 = 4900mL/min = 4.9L/min

Venous return
- Blood-flow from veins back to atria

Ejection fraction (EF)
- Percentage of blood leaving heart during each contraction
- EF = (stroke volume/end diastolic volume) * 100

Frank–Starling Mechanism
- Ventricular contraction strength related to amount of ventricular myocardial stretch
- Maximum contraction force achieved when myocardial actin, myosin fibers are stretched about 2–2.5 times normal resting length

BLOOD VESSEL LAYERS ("TUNICS")

Tunica intima (interna)
- Innermost layer

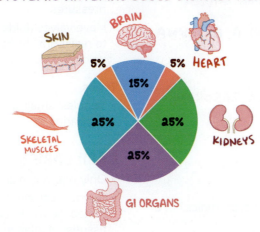

Figure 14.6 A: Total blood volume distribution in an average adult. B: Systemic arterial blood distribution.

- Endothelial cells create slick surface for smooth blood flow
- Receives nutrients from blood in lumen
- Only one cell thick
    - Larger vessels may have subendothelial basement membrane layer (supports endothelial cells)

Tunica media
- Middle layer
- Mostly made of smooth muscle cells, elastin protein sheets
- Receives nutrients from blood in lumen

Tunica externa
- Outermost layer
- Made of loosely woven fibers of collagen, elastic
    - Protects, reinforces blood vessel; anchors it in place
- Vaso vasorum ("vessels of the vessels")
    - Tunica externa blood vessels are very large, need own blood supply

ARTERIES

Key features
- High pressure, thicker than veins, no valves

Types
- "Elastic" arteries (conducting arteries)
    - Lots of elastin in tunica externa, media
    - Stretchy; allows arteries to expand, recoil during systole, diastole
    - Absorbs pressure
    - Largest arteries closest to heart (aorta, main branches of aorta, pulmonary arteries) have most elastic in walls
- Muscular arteries (distributing arteries)
    - Carry blood to organs, distant body parts
    - Thick muscular layer
- Arterioles (smallest arteries)
    - Artery branches when they reach organs, tissues
    - Major systemic vascular resistance regulators
    - Bulky tunica media (thick smooth muscle layer)
    - Regulate blood flow to organs, tissues
    - Contract (vasoconstriction) in response to hormones/autonomic nervous system, ↓ blood/↑ systemic resistance
    - Vasodilate (relax) ↑ blood flow to organs/tissues, ↓ systemic resistance
    - Ability to contract/dilate provides thermoregulation

VEINS

Key features
- Low pressure
- Cannot tolerate high pressure but are distensible → adapts to different volumes, pressures
- Have valves (folds in tunica interna) to resist gravity, keep blood flowing unidirectionally heart

Types
- **Venules**: small veins that connect to capillaries

CAPILLARIES
- Only one cell thick (flat endothelial cells)
- Oxygen, carbon dioxide, nutrients, metabolic waste easily exchanged between tissues; circulation through capillary wall by diffusion

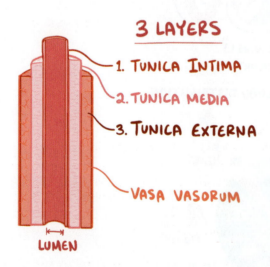

Figure 14.7 The three layers, or "tunics," of a blood vessel.

Chapter 14 Cardiovascular Physiology: Cardiovascular Anatomy & Physiology

- Fluid moves out of vessel, into interstitial space (space between blood vessels, cells)
  - Water-soluble substances (ions) cross capillary wall through clefts, between endothelial cells, through large pores in fenestrated capillary walls
  - Lipid-soluble molecules (oxygen, carbon dioxide) dissolve, diffuse across endothelial cell membranes

BULK FLOW
- Passive water, nutrient movement across capillary wall down concentration gradient

Key features
- Moves large amounts of water, substances in same direction through fenestrated capillaries
- Material movement
- Faster transport method
- Regulates blood, interstitial volume
- Filtration, reabsorption
- Continuous fluid mixing between plasma, interstitial fluid

Types
- *Filtration*: bulk flow when moving from blood to interstitium
- *Reabsorption*: bulk flow when moving from interstitium to blood

Other characteristics
- *Kidney*: major site of bulk flow where waste products are filtered out, nutrients reabsorbed
- Fluid filters out of capillaries into interstitial space (net filtration) at arteriolar end, reabsorbed (net reabsorption) at venous end
  - Hydrostatic interstitial fluid pressure draws fluid into capillary
  - Hydrostatic capillary pressure pushes fluid out of capillary
  - Colloid interstitial fluid pressure pushes fluid out of capillary
  - Colloid capillary pressure draws fluid into capillary

MICROCIRCULATION
- *Microcirculation*: arterioles + capillaries + venules
- Arteriole blood flow through capillary bed, to venule (nutrient, waste, fluid exchange)
  - Capillary beds composed of vascular shunt (vessel connects arteriole, venule to capillaries), actual capillaries
  - Terminal arteriole → metarteriole → thoroughfare channel → postcapillary venule
  - *Precapillary sphincter*: valve regulates blood flow into capillary
  - Various chemicals, hormones, vasomotor nerve fibers regulate amount of blood entering capillary bed

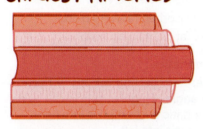
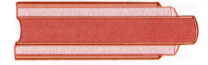
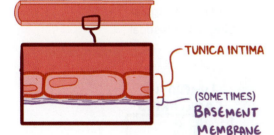
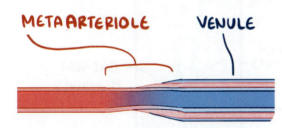

Figure 14.8 Key features of different blood vessel types.

LYMPHATIC ANATOMY & PHYSIOLOGY

osms.it/lymphatic-anatomy-physiology

LYMPHATIC SYSTEM

Function
- Fluid balance
  - Returns leaked interstitial fluid, plasma proteins to blood, heart via lymphatic vessels
  - *Lymph*: name of interstitial fluid when in lymph vessels
  - *Lymphedema*: lymph dysfunctional/absent (lymph node removal in cancer) → edema forms
- Immunity
- Fat absorption

Lymphatic capillaries
- Collect interstitial fluid leaked by capillaries
- Found in all tissues (except bone, teeth, marrow)
  - Microscopic dead-ended vessels unlike blood capillaries, helps fluid remain inside
  - Usually found next to blood capillaries
- Lymph moves via breathing, muscle contractions, arterial pulsation in tight tissues
- Carries particles away from inflammation sites/injury towards bloodstream, stopping first through lymph nodes that filter out harmful substances
- Overlapping endothelial cells create valves; prevent backflow, infectious spread
- *Lacteals*: specialized lymphatic capillaries found in small intestine villi
  - Carry absorbed fats into blood
  - *Chyle*: fat-containing lymph

Larger lymphatics
- Capillaries → collecting vessels → trunks → ducts → angle of jugular, subclavian veins; right lymphatic duct empties into right angle, thoracic into left
- Collecting vessels have more valves, more anastomoses than veins
  - Superficial collecting vessels follow veins
  - Deep collecting vessels follow arteries
- Lymphatic trunks
  - *Paired*: lumbar, bronchomediastinal, subclavian, jugular
  - *Singular*: intestinal

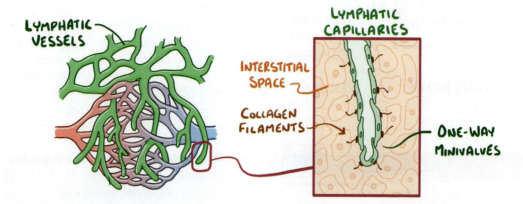

Figure 14.9 Lymphatic vessels collect interstitial fluid (which is then called lymph) and return it to the veins. Lymphatic capillaries have minivalves that open when pressure in the interstitial space is higher than in the capillary and shut when pressure in the interstitial space is lower.

Chapter 14 Cardiovascular Physiology: Cardiovascular Anatomy & Physiology

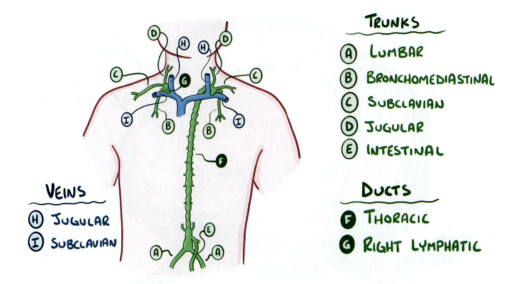

Figure 14.10 Lymphatic system structures and their locations in the body.

- Ducts
  - Upper right lymphatic drains right arm; right thorax; right side of head, neck
  - Thoracic duct drains into cisterna chyli (a dilation created to gather all lymph drained from body area that's not covered by upper right lymphatic duct)

LYMPHOID CELLS

- **Lymphocytes:** T subtype activate immune response; B subtype → plasma cells, produce antibodies
- **Macrophages:** important in T cell activation, phagocytosis
- **Dendrocytes:** return to nodes from inflammation sites to present antigens
- **Reticular cells:** similar to fibroblasts; create mesh to contain other immune cells

LYMPHOID TISSUES

- Reticular connective tissue
- **Composition:** macrophage-embedded reticular fibers
- Loose
  - Diffuse lymphoid tissue
  - Venules enter, filters blood
  - Found in all organs
- Dense
  - Follicles/nodules
  - Mostly contain germinal centers
  - Found in larger organs (lymph nodes)/ individually (mucosa)

LYMPHOID ORGANS

Spleen
- Largest lymphoid tissue in body
- Located below left side of diaphragm
- Blood supplied by splenic artery; blood leaves spleen via splenic vein
  - Capsules with projections into organ, form splenic trabeculae
- Function
  - Macrophages remove foreign particles, pathogens from blood
  - Red blood cell turnover
  - Compound storage (e.g. iron)
  - Platelet/monocyte storage
  - **Blood reservoir:** stores about 300mL/0.08gal
  - Fetal erythrocyte production
- Histology
  - *White pulp:* lymphocyte, macrophage islands that surround central arteries
  - *Red pulp:* composed mostly of red blood cells, macrophages; macrophages remove old red blood cells, platelets; splenic cords (reticular tissues running between venous sinusoids)

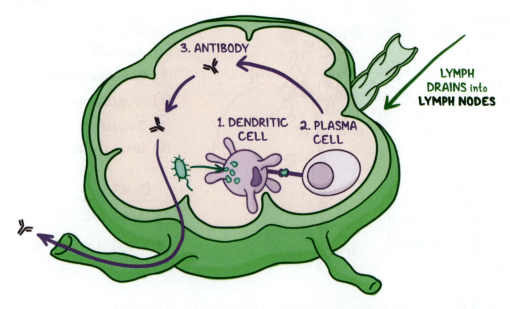

Figure 14.11 In lymph nodes, dendritic cells present pieces of pathogens they come across to B cells. If a dendritic cell presents something foreign to a B cell, the B cell turns into a plasma cell and starts secreting antibodies, which flow into the lymph and exit the lymph node.

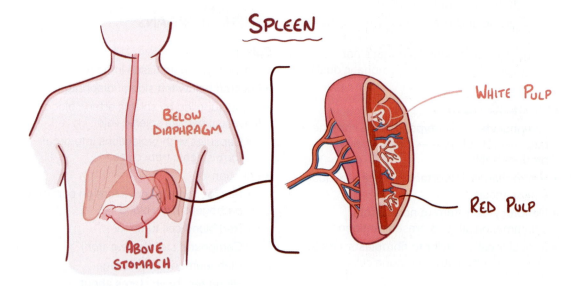

Figure 14.12 Spleen location, histology.

Lymph nodes
- Hundreds scattered throughout body, often grouped along lymphatic vessels
  - Superficial, deep
  - Many found in inguinal, axillary, cervical regions
- Function
  - Lymph filtration, immune system activation
- Kidney-shaped formations
  - Built like tiny spleens, 1–25cm/0.4–9.8in long
  - Covered by capsule with trabeculae, extend inward; trabeculae divide nodes sectionally
- Cortex
  - Subcapsular sinus, lymphoid follicle, germinal center

- Medulla
  - Medullary cord, medullary sinus
- Lymph flows through afferent lymphatic vessels → enters node through hilum → subcapsular sinus → cortex → medullary sinus → exiting via efferent lymphatic vessels in hilum
  - Fewer efferent vessels than afferent vessels, slows traffic down → allows node to filter lymphatic fluid
- Swollen painful nodes indicate inflammation, painless nodes may indicate cancer

Thymus
- Located between sternum, aorta in mediastinum
- Two lobes, many lobules composed of cortex, medulla
  - *Cortex:* T lymphocyte maturation site (immature T lymphocytes move from bone marrow to thymus for maturation)
  - *Medulla:* contains some mature T lymphocytes, macrophages, cell-clusters called thymic corpuscles (corpuscles contain special T lymphocytes thought to be involved in preventing autoimmune disease)
- Lymphocyte production site in fetal life
  - Active in neonatal, early life; atrophies with age

Bone marrow
- *B cells:* made, mature in bone marrow
- *T cells:* made in bone marrow, mature in thymus

Mucosa-associated lymphoid tissue (MALT)
- Lymphoid tissue that is associated with mucosal membranes
- *Tonsils:* lymphoid-tissue ring around pharynx
  - Have crypts (epithelial invaginations) which trap bacteria
  - *Palatine:* paired tonsils on each side of pharynx (largest tonsils, most often inflamed)
  - *Lingual:* near base of tongue
  - *Pharyngeal:* near nasal cavity (called adenoid when inflamed)
  - *Tubal:* near Eustachian tube
- *Peyer's patches:* small bowel MALT

Appendix
- Worm-like large bowel extension
- Contains numerous lymphoid follicles
- Fights intestinal infections

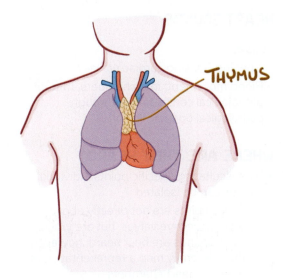

Figure 14.13 Thymus location.

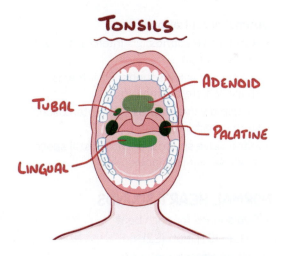

Figure 14.14 Tubal, pharyngeal (adenoid), palatine, and lingual tonsils create a lymphoid-tissue ring around pharynx.

NORMAL HEART SOUNDS

osms.it/normal-heart-sounds

HEART SOUNDS

Causes
- Opening / closing cardiac valves
- *Blood movement*: into chambers, through pathological constrictions, through pathological openings

WHERE ARE THEY HEARD?
- By auscultating specific points individual sounds can be isolated
  - These points are not directly above their respective valves, but are where valve sounds are best heard; however, they generally map a representation of different heart chambers
- Knowing normal heart size, auscultation locations allows for enlarged (diseased) heart detection

Optimal auscultation sites
- *Aortic valve sounds*: 2nd intercostal, right sternal margin
- *Pulmonary valve sounds*: 2nd intercostal space, left sternal margin
- *Tricuspid valve sounds*: $4/5^{th}$ intercostal, left sternal margin
- *Mitral valve sounds*: 5th intercostal space, midclavicular line (apex)

NORMAL HEART SOUNDS
- Two sounds for each beat
  - Lub (S1), dub (S2)
- Factors affecting intensity
  - Intervening tissue, fluid presence, quantity
  - Mitral valve closure speed (mitral valve contraction strength)

S1 heart sound
- "*Lub*": low-pitched sound
- Marks beginning of systole/end of diastole
- Early ventricular contraction (systole) → ventricular pressure rises above atrial pressure → atrioventricular valves close → S1
- *S1*: mitral, tricuspid closure
  - Intensity predominantly determined by mitral valve component, loudest at apex
- S1 (lub) louder, more resonant than S2 (dub)
- S1 displays negligible variation during breathing

S2 heart sound
- "*Dub*": higher-pitched sound
- Marks end of systole/beginning of diastole
- *S2*: semilunar valves (aortic, pulmonic) snap shut at beginning of ventricular relaxation (diastole) → short, sharp sound
- Best heard at Erb's point, 3rd intercostal space on left, medial to midclavicular line
- Splits on expiration
  - During expiration S2 split into earlier aortic component; later, softer pulmonic component (A2 P2). Lower intrathoracic pressure during inspiration → ↑ right ventricular preload → ↑ right ventricular systole duration → delays P2
  - ↓ left ventricular preload during inspiration → shorter ventricular systole, earlier A2
  - A2, P2 splitting during inspiration usually about 40ms
  - A2, P2 intensity roughly proportional to respective systemic. pulmonary circulation pressures
  - P2 best heard over pulmonic area

Chapter 14 Cardiovascular Physiology: Cardiovascular Anatomy & Physiology

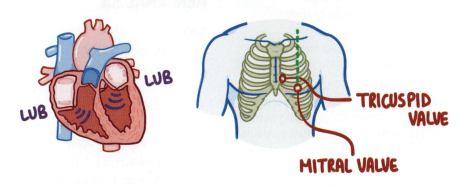

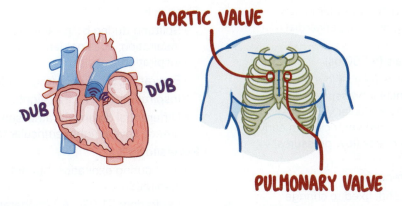

Figure 14.15 Valves that close to produce S1 and S2 sounds and optimal auscultation sites.

ABNORMAL HEART SOUNDS

osms.it/abnormal-heart-sounds

ABNORMAL S1

Loud S1
- As left ventricle fills, pressure increases
- As left atrium empties, pressure increases as it empties against increasingly pressure-loaded ventricle; as atrium approaches empty, pressure begins to decrease
- *Differential diagnosis*: short PR interval, mild mitral stenosis, hyperdynamic states
- Short PR interval (< 120ms)
  - Normally atrioventricular valve leaflets drift towards each other before onset of systole
  - Shorter PR interval → less time to drift closure → wider closure distance → louder S1
  - Short PR interval → incomplete ventricular emptying → higher ventricular filling pressure → ventricular pressure crosses critical atrioventricular valve closing threshold while atrial pressures are still high → load snap

- Mild mitral stenosis
  - Significant force required to close stenotic mitral valve → large atrioventricular pressure gradient required
  - Slam shut with increased force, producing loud sound
- Hyperdynamic states
  - Shortened diastole → large amount of ongoing flow across valve during systole → leaflets wide apart, pressure remains high
  - Results in forceful atrioventricular valve closure

Soft S1
- *Differential diagnosis*: long PR intervals, severe mitral stenosis, left bundle branch block, chronic obstructive pulmonary disease (COPD), obesity, pericardial effusion
- Long PR intervals (> 200ms)
  - Atrium empties fully → low pressure → low ventricular pressure required to close atrioventricular valves → valves close when ventricle is in early acceleration phase (low pressures) → soft sound
- Severe mitral stenosis
  - Leaflets too stiff, fixed to change position

Variable S1
- Auscultatory alternans
  - When observed with severe left ventricular dysfunction, correlate of pulsus alternans
- *Differential diagnosis*: atrioventricular dissociation, atrial fibrillation, large pericardial effusion, severe left ventricular dysfunction

Split S1
- S1 usually a single sound
  - Near-simultaneous mitral, tricuspid valve closures; soft intensity of tricuspid valve closure
- Splitting usually from tricuspid valve closure being delayed relative to mitral valve closure
- *Differential diagnosis*: right bundle branch block, left-sided preexcitation, idioventricular rhythm arising from left ventricle

ABNORMAL S2

Split S2
- Physiological S2 splitting
  - *Expiration*: S1 A2P2 (no split)
  - *Inspiration*: S1 A2....P2 (40ms split)
- Wide split
  - *Detection*: splitting during expiration
  - *Expiration*: S1 A2..P2 (slight split)
  - *Inspiration*: S1 A2.......P2 (wide split)
  - *Differential diagnosis*: right bundle branch block, left ventricle preexcitation, pulmonary hypertension, massive pulmonary embolism, severe mitral regurgitation, constrictive pericarditis
- Fixed split
  - Splitting during both expiration, inspiration; does not lengthen during inspiration
  - *Expiration*: S1 A2..P2 (slight split)
  - *Inspiration*: S1 A2..P2 (slight split)
  - *Differential diagnosis*: atrial septal defect, severe right ventricular failure
- Reversed split
  - Split during expiration, but not inspiration
  - *Expiration*: S1 P2....A2 (moderate split)
  - *Inspiration*: S1 P2A2
  - *Differential diagnosis*: left bundle branch block, right ventricle preexcitation, aortic stenosis/AR

Abnormal single S2 variants
- Loud P2
  - *Expiration*: S1 A2P2
  - *Inspiration*: S1 A2....P2!
  - *Diagnosis*: pulmonary hypertension
- Left ventricular outflow obstruction
  - Absent A2
  - *Expiration*: S1 P2
  - *Inspiration*: S1 P2
  - *Diagnosis*: severe aortic valve disease
- Fused A2/P2
  - *Expiration*: S1 A2P2
  - *Inspiration*: S1 A2P2
  - *Differential diagnosis*: ventricular septal defect with Eisenmenger's syndrome, single ventricle

Chapter 14 Cardiovascular Physiology: Cardiovascular Anatomy & Physiology

ADDED HEART SOUNDS

S3 heart sound
- S3 (ventricular gallop)
  - Low-pitched early diastolic sound
  - Best heard in mitral/apex region
  - Left lateral decubitus position
- Associated with volume overload conditions
- Early diastolic sound, produced in rapid filling phase → excessive volume filling ventricle in short period → rapid filling → chordae tendineae tensing → S3 sound
- *Children/adolescents:* may be normal
- *Middle aged/elderly person:* usually pathological
  - Over 40 years old: indicative of left ventricular failure
- Auscultatory summary: S1... S2.S3... S1

S4 heart sound
- S4 *(atrial gallop):* low pitched late diastolic (pre-systolic) sound, best heard in mitral/apex region, left lateral decubitus position
- Associated with hypertension, left ventricular hypertrophy, ischaemic cardiomyopathy
- *Pressure overload:* thought to be caused by atrial contraction into stiff / non-compliant ventricle
- Chronic heart contraction effort against increased pressure → hypertrophy → stiff ventricle (concentric hypertrophy)
- Always pathological
- Auscultatory summary: S4.S1...S2...S4.S1

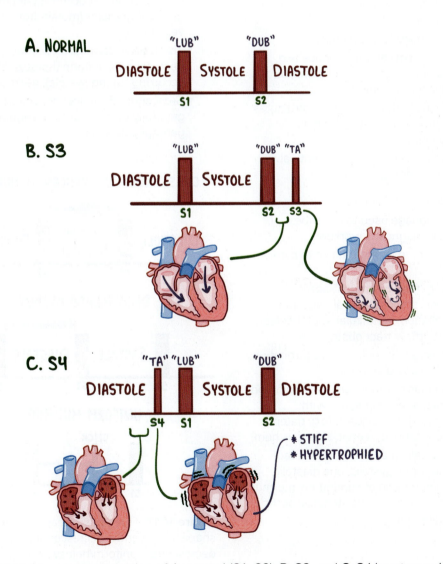

Figure 14.16 Linear representation of **A:** normal (S1, S2), **B:** S3, and **C:** S4 heart sounds.

Summation gallop
- Superimposition of atrial, ventricular gallops during tachycardia
- Heart rate ↑ → diastole shortens more than systole → S3, S4 brought closer together until they merge

HEART MURMURS

Key features
- Blood flow silent when laminar, uninterrupted
- Turbulent flow may generate abnormal sounds (AKA "heart murmurs")
- Murmurs can be auscultated with stethoscope

Causes
- May be normal in young children, some elderly individuals
- ↓ blood viscosity (e.g. anaemia)
- ↓ diameter of vessel, valve, orifice (e.g. valvular stenosis, coarctation of aorta, ventricular septal defect)
- ↑ blood velocity through normal structures (e.g. hyperdynamic states—sepsis, hyperthyroid)
- Regurgitation across incompetent valve (e.g. valvular regurgitation)

Describing heart murmurs
- Specific language used to describe murmurs in diagnostic workup
- *Timing*: refers to timing relative to cardiac cycle
    - *Systolic "flow murmurs"*: aortic, pulmonic stenosis; mitral, tricuspid regurgitation; ventricular septal defect; aortic outflow tract obstruction
    - *Diastolic*: aortic, pulmonic regurgitation; mitral, tricuspid stenosis
    - Continuous murmurs are least common, generally seen in children with congenital heart disease (e.g. patent ductus arteriosus, cervical venous hum)
    - Occasionally may have two related murmurs, one systolic, one diastolic; gives impression of continuous murmur (e.g. concurrent aortic stenosis, aortic regurgitation)
- Location
    - Location on chest wall where murmur is best heard
- Radiation
    - Location where murmur is audible despite not lying directly over heart
    - Generally radiate in same direction as turbulent blood is flowing
    - *Aortic stenosis*: carotid arteries
    - *Tricuspid regurgitation*: anterior right thorax
    - *Mitral regurgitation*: left axilla
- Shape
    - How sound intensity changes from onset to completion
    - Shape determined by pattern of pressure gradient driving turbulent flow, loudest segment occurring at time of greatest gradient (moment of highest velocity)
    - *Three basic shapes*: crescendo-decrescendo, uniform (holosystolic when occurring during systole), decrescendo
    - Crescendo-decrescendo, uniform generally systolic; decrescendo murmurs generally diastolic

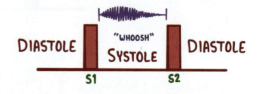

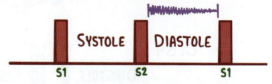

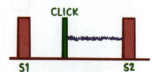

Figure 14.17 Three basic heart murmur shapes: crescendo-decrescendo, decrescendo, uniform/holosystolic.

- Pitch
  - High pressure gradients → high pitched murmurs (e.g. mitral regurgitation, ventricular septal defect)
  - Large volume of blood-flow across low pressure gradients → low pitched murmurs (e.g. mitral stenosis)
  - If both high pressure, high flow (severe aortic stenosis), both high, low pitches are produced simultaneously → subjectively unpleasant/"harsh" sounding murmur
- Intensity
  - Murmur loudness graded on scale from I–VI
  - Dependent on blood velocity generating murmur; acoustic properties of intervening tissue; hearing; examiner experience; stethoscope used, ambient noise presence
  - I: barely audible
  - II: faint, but certainly present
  - III: easily, immediately heard
  - IV: associated with thrill (palpable vibration over involved heart valve)
  - V: heard with only edge of stethoscope touching chest wall
  - VI: heard without stethoscope (or without it making direct contact with chest wall)
- Quality
  - Subjective, attempt to describe timbre, depends on how many different base frequencies of sound are generated, relative amplitude of various harmonics
  - Mitral regurgitation: blowing/musical
  - Mitral stenosis: rumbling
  - Aortic stenosis: harsh
  - Aortic regurgitation: blowing
  - Still's murmur (benign childhood): musical
  - Patent ductus arteriosus: machine-like

Diagnostic maneuvers (dynamic auscultation)

- Some maneuvers may elicit characteristic intensity/timing changes (changes in hemodynamics during maneuvers)
- Dynamic auscultation: listening for subtle changes during physical maneuvers
- Inspiration
  - ↓ intrathoracic pressure → ↑ pulmonary venous return to right heart → ↑ right heart stroke volume → right sided murmurs → ↑ intensity
  - Dilation of pulmonary vascular system → ↓ pulmonary venous return to left side of heart → ↓ left heart stroke volume → left side murmurs → ↓ intensity
- Expiration
  - ↑ intrathoracic pressure → ↓ venous return to right heart → ↓ right ventricle stroke volume → ↓ intensity of right sided murmurs
  - ↑ pulmonary venous return to left side → ↑ left ventricle stroke volume → left sided murmur → ↑ intensity
- Valsalva maneuver
  - Forceful exhalation against closed glottis
  - ↓ venous return to heart → ↓ left ventricular volume → ↓ cardiac output
  - Murmurs of hypertrophic obstructive cardiomyopathy, occasionally mitral valve prolapse → ↑ intensity
  - All other systolic murmurs → ↓ intensity
- Isometric handgrip
  - Squeeze two objects (such as rolled towels) with both hands
  - Do not simultaneously Valsalva
  - If unconscious, simulate by transient arterial occlusion (BP cuffs applied to both upper arms, inflated to 20–40mmHg above systolic blood pressure for 20 seconds)
  - ↑ venous return, ↑ sympathetic tone → ↑ heart rate, systemic venous return → ↑ cardiac output → murmurs from mitral regurgitation, aortic regurgitation, ventricular septal defect → ↑ intensity
  - Murmur from hypertrophic obstructive cardiomyopathy → ↓ intensity
  - Murmur from aortic stenosis → most commonly unchanged
- Leg elevation
  - Lying supine, both legs raised 45°
  - ↑ venous return → ↑ left ventricular volume
  - Murmur from hypertrophic obstructive cardiomyopathy → ↓ intensity
  - Murmurs from aortic stenosis, mitral regurgitation may → ↑ intensity

- Müller's maneuver
  - Nares closed, forcibly suck on incentive spirometer/air-filled syringe for 10 seconds (conceptual opposite of Valsalva)
    - ↓ venous return → ↓ left ventricular volume → ↓ systemic venous resistance murmur from hypertrophic obstructive myopathy → ↑ intensity
    - Murmur from aortic stenosis may → ↓ intensity
- Squatting to standing
  - Abruptly stand up after 30 seconds of squatting
    - ↓ venous return → ↓ left ventricular volume
    - Murmur from hypertrophic obstructive cardiomyopathy → ↑ intensity
    - Murmur from aortic stenosis may → ↓ intensity
- Standing to squatting
  - From standing upright, squat down
  - If unable to squat, examiner can passively bend knees up towards abdomen to mimic maneuver
    - ↑ venous return → ↑ left ventricular volume
    - Murmur from hypertrophic obstructive cardiomyopathy → ↓ intensity
    - Murmur from aortic stenosis may → ↑ intensity
    - Murmur from aortic regurgitation → ↑ intensity

Systolic murmurs

- Aortic stenosis
  - **Aortic valve auscultation site:** 2nd intercostal, right sternal margin
  - S1, closing of mitral valve, during systole → heart contracts against closed stenotic aortic valve → pressure must rise during systole to force open stenotic aortic valve → valve pops open → produces ejection click
  - Followed by ↑ flow as heart contracts more forcefully to empty left ventricle → murmur intensity ↑ as flow across partially open valve ↑
  - Chamber begins to empty → pressure, flow diminish → ↓ murmur intensity
  - Radiates to neck/carotids (murmur occurs in aorta, these are its first branches)
  - **Auscultatory summary:** S1. Ejection click. Crescendo-decrescendo murmur. S2
- Pulmonic stenosis
  - **Pulmonary valve auscultation site:** 2nd intercostal space, left sternal margin
  - S1, closing of tricuspid valve, during systole
  - Heart contracts against closed pulmonic valve → pressure builds during systole, forcing open stenotic pulmonic valve → valve pops open → ejection click
  - Flow rate increases as heart contracts more forcefully to empty right ventricle → murmur gets louder as flow across partially open valve increases → chamber empties → pressure, flow diminishing → ↓ murmur intensity
  - Radiates to neck/carotids, back
  - **Auscultatory summary:** S1. Ejection click. Crescendo-decrescendo murmur. S2
- Mitral regurgitation
  - **Mitral valve auscultation site:** 5th intercostal space, midclavicular line/apex
  - Holo-/pansystolic murmur (occurs for systole duration)
  - Normal S1 as mitral valve closes → in mitral regurgitation, valve cannot completely close → pressure builds in left ventricle (with closed aortic valve) → blood forced back through partially closed mitral valve → murmur occurs along with S1 as long as pressures remain high enough
  - Aortic valve will open to redirect majority of blood → left ventricle continues contracting → continuously raised pressures → blood continuously flowing through partially closed mitral valve (whole of systole)
  - As heart continues to contract, pressure ↑, but atrium becomes more compliant. Even though blood-flow across partially closed valve may ↑, pressure in atrium does not significantly increase
  - Left ventricle pressure notably higher than left atrium → sound does not

Chapter 14 Cardiovascular Physiology: Cardiovascular Anatomy & Physiology

change throughout murmur
- Referred to as "flat" murmur because intensity does not change
- Radiates to axilla due to direction of regurgitant jet
- *Auscultatory summary:* S1. Flat murmur. S2

- Tricuspid regurgitation
  - *Tricuspid valve auscultation site:* 4/5th intercostal, left sternal margin
  - Holo-/pansystolic murmur
  - Normal S1 occurs due to tricuspid valve closure → pulmonic valve closed, pressure rises in right ventricle
  - In tricuspid regurgitation, valve cannot completely close → pressure builds in right ventricle → blood forced back out through partially closed tricuspid valve → murmur is continuous as long as pressures remain high enough
  - Pulmonic valve opens to redirect blood → left ventricle maintains contraction (thus raises pressure) → blood continues flowing through partially closed tricuspid valve (through whole systole)
  - Arium becomes more compliant as it fills → atrium pressure does not significantly increase
  - Right ventricle pressure notably higher than that of right atrium → murmur sound does not change throughout murmur
  - Referred to as "flat" murmur (intensity does not change)
  - *Auscultatory summary:* S1. flat murmur. S2

- Mitral valve prolapse
  - *Mitral valve auscultation site:* 5th intercostal space, midclavicular line/apex
  - Mitral valve billows into left atrium → clicking sound (unlike aortic stenosis, not associated with ejection of blood, non-ejection click, mid-late systolic)
  - Ventricle contracts → mitral valve closure → S1 → pressure rises → mitral valve accelerates into left atrium → stops abruptly (chordae tendineae restraint) → rapid tensing → click
  - Often associated with mitral regurgitation → after click murmur of mitral regurgitation may follow
  - *Auscultatory summary:* S1. Mid systolic click with late systolic murmur. S2

Diastolic murmurs
- Aortic regurgitation
  - *Aortic regurgitation auscultation site:* left parasternal border
  - Blood flows back through incompletely closed aortic valve
  - Occurs between S2, S1
  - S2, aortic valve closure → mitral valve opens, heart in diastole → blood enters left ventricle through regurgitant valve, through normal filling via mitral valve
  - Initially, low pressure in ventricle (compared to systemic blood pressure forcing blood through regurgitant valve) → ventricle fills → as pressure mounts, less flow through regurgitant valve → decrescendo murmur
  - Early diastolic decrescendo murmur
  - *Auscultatory summary:* S1. S2. Early diastolic decrescendo murmur. S1

- Pulmonic regurgitation
  - *Pulmonic regurgitation auscultation site:* upper left parasternal border
  - Blood flows back through incompletely closed pulmonic valve
  - Occurs between S2, S1
  - S2 aortic valve closure → tricuspid valve opens, heart in diastole → incomplete pulmonic valve closure → right ventricle fills via incompletely closed pulmonic valve as well as tricuspid valve
  - Initially → low ventricle pressure allows for high flow through regurgitant valve → pressure rises, ↓ flow through regurgitant valve → decrescendo murmur
  - Early diastolic decrescendo murmur
  - *Auscultatory summary:* S1. S2. Early diastolic decrescendo murmur. S1

- Mitral stenosis
  - *Mitral valve auscultation site:* 5th intercostal space, midclavicular line/apex
  - Mitral valve can't open efficiently
  - S2 → aortic valve closure → milliseconds later, mitral valve should open (fill ventricle during diastole), only small opening occurs

Systolic Murmurs

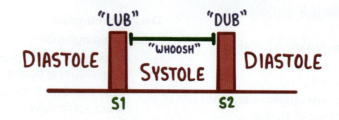

Stenosis
└ Aortic or Pulmonic Valve

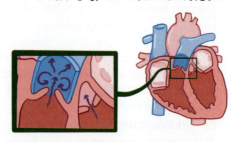 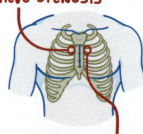

- Aortic Valve Stenosis
- Pulmonary Valve Stenosis

Regurgitation
└ Mitral or Tricuspid Valve

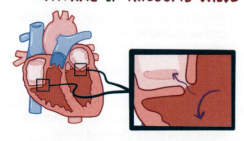 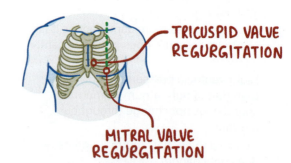

- Tricuspid Valve Regurgitation
- Mitral Valve Regurgitation

Mitral Valve Prolapse
~ if severe enough → Mitral Regurgitation

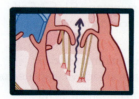

Ventral Septal Defect
* Holosystolic Murmur

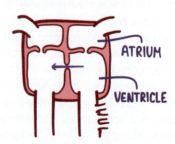

- Atrium
- Ventricle

Figure 14.18 Causes of systolic murmurs.

- Beginning of diastole, highest flow of blood comes from left atrium to left ventricle (rapid filling), fills more blood at beginning of diastole (beginning due to highest pressure difference) → most intense phase of murmur
- Aortic valve closure → mitral valve opens, due to stenotic leaflets, they can only open slightly → chordae tendineae snap as limit is reached (similar to ejection snap) → opening snap from stenotic leaflets shooting open (milliseconds after S2) → highest intensity of murmur thereafter → murmur diminishes as pressure equalises
- End of diastole atrium contracts to force remaining blood into left ventricle → atrial kick sound (presystolic accentuation at end of murmur)
- *Auscultatory summary:* S1. S2. Opening snap. Decrescendo mid diastolic rumble. Atrial kick. S1

- Tricuspid stenosis
  - *Tricuspid valve auscultation site:* 4/5th intercostal space, left sternal margin
  - Tricuspid valve can't open efficiently
  - S2 → pulmonic valve closure → milliseconds later, tricuspid valve should open (fill ventricle during diastole), only small opening occurs
  - Beginning of diastole, high flow of blood comes from right atrium to right ventricle (rapid filling), fills more blood at beginning of diastole (due to highest pressure difference) → most intense murmur phase
  - Pulmonic valve closure → tricuspid valve opens (due to stenotic leaflets, they can only open slightly) → chordae tendineae snap as limit is reached (similar to ejection snap) → opening snap from stenotic leaflets shooting open (milliseconds after S2) → highest murmur intensity thereafter → murmur diminishes as pressures equalise
  - End of diastole atrium contracts to force remaining blood into left ventricle → atrial kick sound (presystolic accentuation at end of murmur)
  - *Auscultatory summary:* S1. S2. Opening snap. Decrescendo mid diastolic rumble. Atrial kick. S1

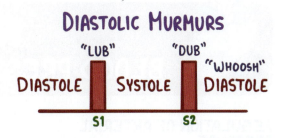

Figure 14.19 Diastolic murmurs are heard as a "whoosh" after S2.

Murmur Identification
- Detect murmur?
  - Yes/no
- Identify phase?
  - *Systolic/diastolic:* S1 -systole- S2 -diastole- S1 (in tachycardia, feel pulse → tapping → ejection phase, therefore S1)
- Which valves normally open/which valves normally closed
  - Systole, aortic and pulmonic, open (mitral and tricuspid, closed)
  - If systolic murmur, either open valves stenotic/closed valves regurgitant (1/4 choice)
  - Diastole, mitral and tricuspid, open (aortic and pulmonic, closed) (1/4 choice)
- To choose between four resultant options auscultate over respective areas, employ maneuvers as required

MISCELLANEOUS HEART SOUNDS
- Mechanical valve clicks
  - Distinctly audible, harsh, metallic sound
- Pericardial knock
  - Sound occasionally heard in constrictive pericarditis; similar in acoustics, timing to S3
- Tumor plop
  - Rare low-pitched early diastolic sound, occasionally heard in atrial myxoma presence
  - Occurs when relatively mobile tumour moves in front of mitral valve during diastole → functional mitral stenosis along with low pitched diastolic rumbling murmur

NOTES
BLOOD PRESSURE REGULATION

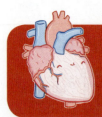

REGULATION OF ARTERIAL PRESSURE

- Must be maintained at a constant level of ~100mmHg
- Changes in blood pressure activate baroreceptors and/or chemoreceptors (fast response) and renin-angiotensin-aldosterone system (slow response), causing a series of events that eventually bring blood pressure back to normal (discussed later)
- Central mechanisms regulating blood pressure are cardiac output, peripheral resistance, and blood volume

Cardiac output and peripheral resistance relate to blood pressure

- P_a = cardiac output x TPR
    - P_a = mean arterial pressure
    - Cardiac output = cardiac output (mL/min)
    - TPR = total peripheral resistance (mmHg/mL/min)
- Mean arterial pressure varies directly with cardiac output and total peripheral pressure, can be changed by altering one or both
- Blood pressure varies directly with blood volume because cardiac output depends on blood volume
    - Cardiac output is equal to stroke volume (ml/min) times heart rate (beats/min)
    - Normal is 5–5.5L/min
- P_a is regulated by two mechanisms
    - *Baroreceptor reflex*: neurally mediated (short-term, fast response)
    - *Renin-angiotensin-aldosterone system*: hormonally mediated (long-term, slow response)

MEASURING BLOOD PRESSURE

- *Auscultatory method*: an indirect method of measuring pressure by listening to Korotkoff sounds in the brachial artery using a sphygmomanometer
1. Wrap blood pressure cuff around upper arm just above elbow
2. Rapidly inflate cuff until pressure in it exceeds systolic pressure (up to around 180mmHg) to stop blood flow
3. Press lightly with the stethoscope bell over the brachial artery just below edge of cuff
4. Reduce cuff pressure slowly and listen with stethoscope for sounds in the brachial artery while simultaneously observing the mercury gauge
    - The first tapping sound (Korotkoff sound) represents systolic pressure
    - When the tapping sound disappears, it represents diastolic pressure

HOMEOSTATIC IMBALANCES IN BLOOD PRESSURE

Normal blood pressure in adults

- Affected by age, weight, sex and race
- *Systolic pressure*: 90–120mmHg
- *Diastolic pressure*: 60–80mmHg

Hypertension

- Chronically elevated blood pressure
    - *Systolic pressure*: > 140mmHg
    - *Diastolic pressure*: > 90mmHg

Hypotension

- Low blood pressure
    - *Systolic pressure*: <90mmHg
    - *Diastolic pressure*: <60mmHg
- Often normal variation
- Acute hypotension
    - Can be a sign of circulatory shock
- Orthostatic hypotension
    - Temporary drop in blood pressure caused by rapidly standing up from a sitting or lying position
    - Common in the elderly
- Chronic hypotension
    - Often a sign of an underlying condition

Chapter 15 Cardiovascular Physiology: Blood Pressure Regulation

BARORECEPTORS
osms.it/baroreceptors

BARORECEPTOR REFLEX

- Short term, fast neural response to change in blood pressure
- Alters peripheral resistance and cardiac output
- Mediated by baroreceptor cells
  - Specialized nerve endings called mechanoreceptors, located in aortic arch and carotid sinus; sensitive to pressure or stretching
  - Most sensitive to rapid pressure changes
- **Carotid sinus baroreceptors**: responsive to both decreases and increases in pressure
- **Aortic arch baroreceptors**: predominantly responsive to increases in pressure
- Change in blood pressure activates reflex arc
  - Baroreceptors → afferent neurons → brain stem centers → processing information and generating response → efferent neurons → changes in the heart and blood vessels
  - Increase of blood pressure → stretching of baroreceptors → depolarizing receptor potential (higher rate action potential)
  - Decrease of blood pressure → decreased stretch of baroreceptors → hyperpolarizing potential (lower rate action potential)
- Sensitivity can be altered as a result of some diseases
- **Chronic hypertension**: result is adaptation of baroreceptors
  - Baroreceptors are adjusted to monitor pressure changes at higher setpoint
- **Atherosclerosis**: carotid sinus syndrome
  - Baroreceptors are more sensitive; even light pressure on the carotid sinus can cause extreme bradycardia

INTEGRATED FUNCTION OF BARORECEPTORS

Response to increased P_a

- ↑ *firing rate*: carotid sinus nerve (glossopharyngeal nerve, CN IX), aortic arch nerve afferent fibers (vagus nerve, CN X)
- Glossopharyngeal, vagus nerve fibers synapse in nucleus tractus solitarius of medulla, (transmits blood pressure information)
- Nucleus tractus solitarius governs coordinated response series; returns P_a down to normal levels
  - ↑ parasympathetic outflow to heart
  - ↓ sympathetic outflow to heart, blood vessels
- Decrease in sympathetic activity
  - Complements increase in parasympathetic activity → decrease in heart rate
  - Decrease in cardiac contractility
  - Decreased heart rate + decreased cardiac contractility → decrease in cardiac output → decrease of P_a (P_a = cardiac output × TPR)
  - Arteriolar vasodilation → decrease in TPR → decrease of P_a (P_a = cardiac output × TPR)
  - Vasodilation of veins → increased compliance of veins → increased unstressed volume → decreased stressed volume → reduction in P_a
- Once P_a reduced back to the set-point pressure (i.e., 100 mmHg), activity of the baroreceptors and the cardiovascular brainstem centers return to baseline level

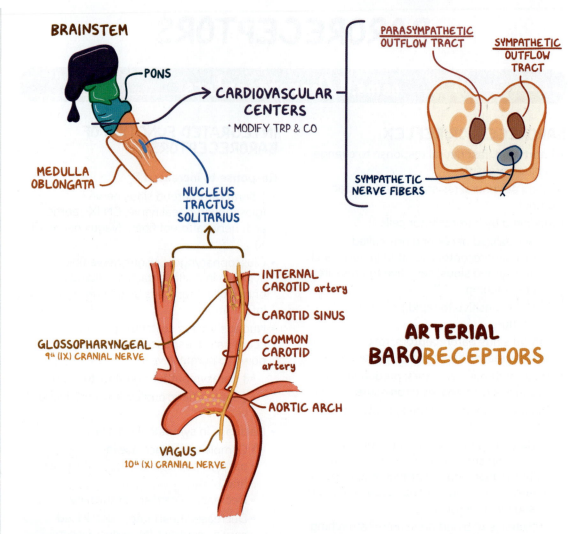

Figure 15.1 Locations of arterial baroreceptors and pathways that transmit their signals.

CARDIOPULMONARY (LOW PRESSURE) BARORECEPTORS

- Located in the vena cava, pulmonary arteries and atria
- These baroreceptors are volume receptors - they detect changes in blood volume
- Increased blood volume and subsequent increases in venous and atrial pressure are detected by cardiopulmonary baroreceptors which generates several responses

Cardiopulmonary baroreceptors responses

- Secretion of atrial natriuretic peptide (ANP), a polypeptide hormone secreted by the myocytes in the atrial wall
  - ANP causes generalized vasodilation
  - This vasodilatation in the kidney increases glomerular filtration rate which results in increased Na^{2+} and H_2O filtration and excretion → decreased blood volume
- Decreased secretion in ADH
  - Decreased water reabsorption in the collecting ducts → decreased blood volume
- Increase of heart rate (Bainbridge reflex)
  - Increased cardiac output → increased renal perfusion → increased Na^+ and H_2O excretion

Chapter 15 Cardiovascular Physiology: Blood Pressure Regulation

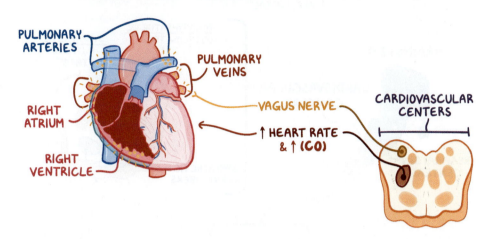

Figure 15.2 Locations of cardiopulmonary baroreceptors and pathway that transmits their signals.

CHEMORECEPTORS

osms.it/chemoreceptors

CHEMORECEPTOR REFLEX
- Blood pressure regulation pathway that involves chemoreceptors for O_2 in the aortic and carotid bodies
- Central and peripheral chemoreceptors

PERIPHERAL CHEMORECEPTORS
- Located in carotid bodies (near common carotid artery bifurcation, in aortic bodies along aortic arch)
- Very sensitive partial pressure of O_2 decreases
  - Also sensitive to partial pressure of CO_2 increases (pCO_2), pH decreases
- Reflex arc
  - Decreased pO_2 → chemoreceptors (afferent neurons) increase firing of action potential (hyperpolarization potential) → efferent neurons → increased sympathetic outflow → arterial vasoconstriction in skeletal muscle, renal and splanchnic circulation → increased total peripheral pressure
- These chemoreceptors are also involved in control of breathing

- Decrease of pO_2 causes an increase in ventilation which decreases the parasympathetic outflow to heart → ↑ heart rate → ↑ cardiac output

CENTRAL CHEMORECEPTORS
- Located in the medulla
- Most sensitive: CO_2, pH
- Less sensitive: O_2
- Reflex arc
  - Decrease in brain blood flow → increased pCO_2, decreased pH → chemoreceptors (afferent neurons) increase firing of action potential (hyperpolarization potential) → efferent neurons → increased sympathetic outflow → arterial vasoconstriction in skeletal muscle, renal and splanchnic circulation → increased total peripheral pressure

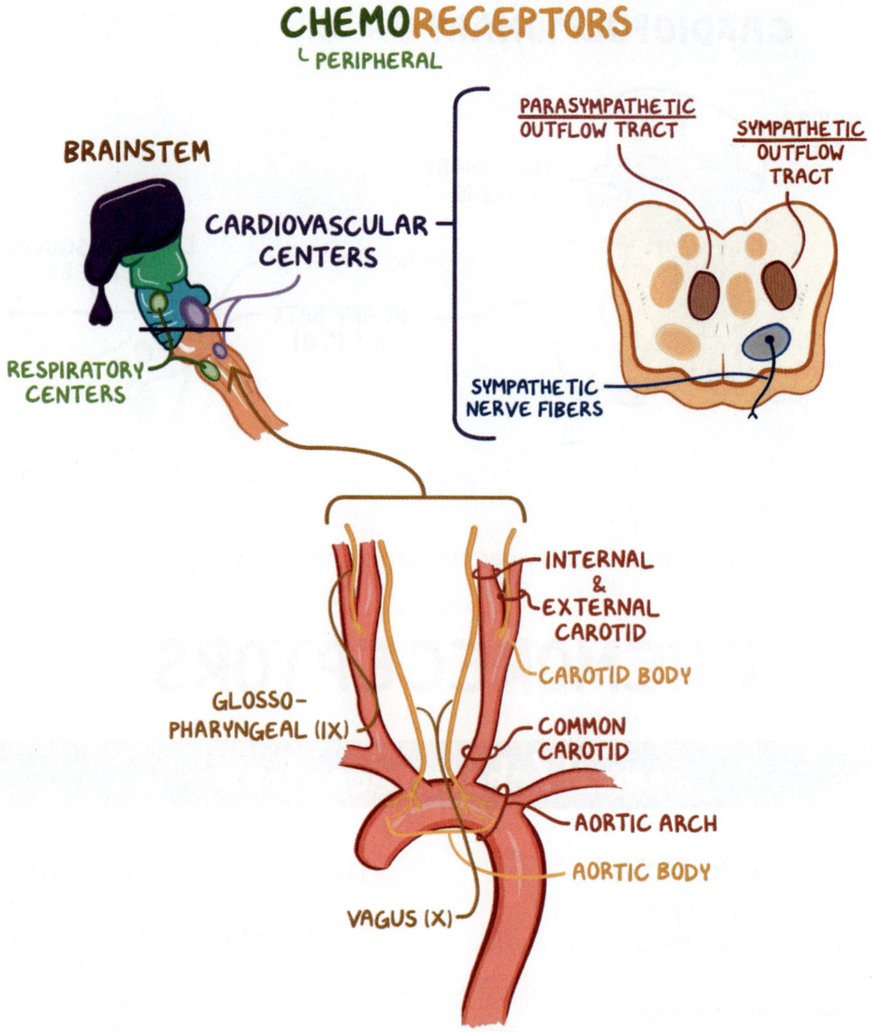

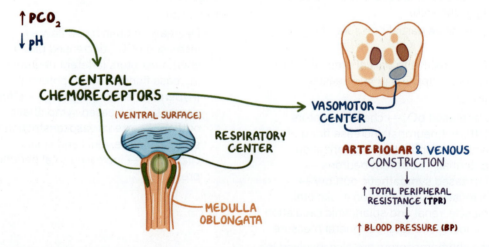

Figure 15.3 Locations of peripheral chemoreceptors and locations in the brainstem to which they transmit their signals.

Figure 15.4 Central chemoreceptors are located in the medulla of the brainstem and are most sensitive to changes in CO_2 and pH levels.

RENIN-ANGIOTENSIN ALDOSTERONE SYSTEM

osms.it/renin-angiotensin_aldosterone_system

- Hormonally mediated, slow regulation of blood pressure
- Regulates P_a by regulating blood volume

Direct renal mechanism
- Increase of P_a causes increased filtration rate in the tubules
- In this situation, the kidney cannot reabsorb filtrate fast enough → more fluid leaves the body in urine → blood volume and blood pressure drops

Indirect renal mechanism
- Renin-angiotensin aldosterone system
- Decrease of P_a and/or decrease of Na^+ concentration causes decrease in kidney perfusion which in turn causes a series of events
- Cells of the macula densa sense the change in blood volume/osmolarity and in turn stimulate renin production
  - Renin is an enzyme secreted by juxtaglomerular cells of the juxtaglomerular apparatus of the nephron
  - Renal sympathetic nerves and beta-1 agonists also cause renin production
- Renin converts angiotensinogen to angiotensin I
- Angiotensin-converting enzyme (ACE) in the lungs and kidneys converts angiotensin I to angiotensin II
  - Stimulates the synthesis and secretion of aldosterone in the glomerulosa cells of the adrenal gland
  - Aldosterone causes Na^+ reabsorption to increase in principal cells of renal distal tubule, collecting duct
  - Increased Na^+ concentration → increased osmolarity → increased ECF and blood volume
- Angiotensin II
  - Stimulates Na^+- H^+ exchange → increased Na^+ reabsorption
  - Stimulates antidiuretic hormone (ADH) secretion
  - Acts on hypothalamus (stimulates thirst, water intake)
  - Causes vasoconstriction of the arterioles → increased total peripheral resistance (TPR)

Antidiuretic hormone (ADH)
- Hormone produced in hypothalamus, secreted by pituitary gland's posterior lobe
- Stimulated by low blood volume, increase of serum osmolarity and angiotensin II
- Receptors for ADH
- **V1 receptors:** vasoconstriction of arterioles
- **V2 receptors:** increase water reabsorption by principal cells of the renal collecting duct

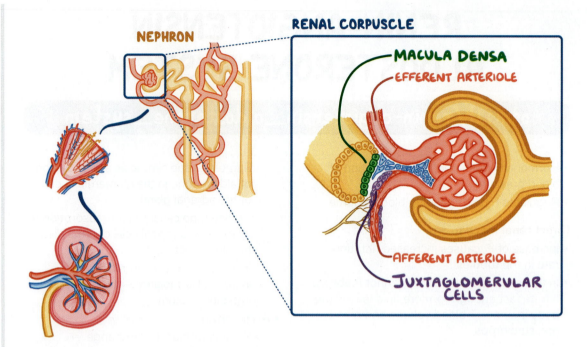

Figure 15.5 Macula densa cells are chemoreceptors located in the distal convoluted tubule. When they sense a ↓ in P_a and/or Na⁺, Cl⁻, they stimulate renin production by nearby juxtaglomerular cells. Renin initiates angiotensin II activation, which acts in multiple areas to increase blood pressure.

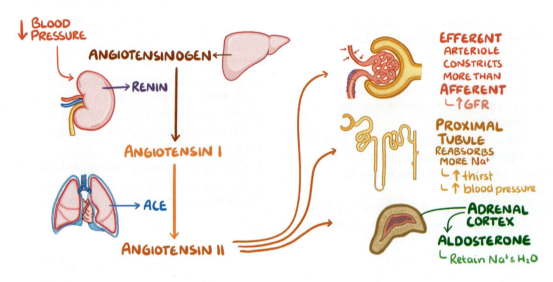

Figure 15.6 RAAS system summary.

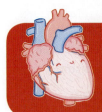

NOTES
CARDIAC CYCLE

MEASURING CARDIAC OUTPUT - FICK PRINCIPLE

osms.it/Fick-principle

- Model used to measure cardiac output (CO)
  - Output of left, right ventricles equal during normal cardiac function
- **Steady state**: rate of O_2 consumption = amount of O_2 leaving lungs via pulmonary vein - amount of O_2 returning via pulmonary arteries × CO
- Pulmonary blood flow of right heart = CO of left heart: used to calculate CO

Cardiac Output =
$$\frac{O_2 \text{ consumption}}{[O_2] \text{ pulmonary vein} - [O_2] \text{ pulmonary artery}}$$

- 250mL/minute = total O_2 consumption (70kg, biologically-male individual); pulmonary venous O_2 content = 0.20/mL; pulmonary arterial O_2 content = 0.15/mL

Cardiac Output =
$$\frac{250\text{mL/min}}{0.20\text{mL} - 0.15\text{mL}} = 5000\text{mL/min}$$

- Also measures blood flow to individual organs
  - Renal blood flow = renal O_2 consumption / renal arterial O_2 - renal venous O_2

CARDIAC & VASCULAR FUNCTION CURVES

osms.it/cardiac-and-vascular-function-curves

- Curves depicting functional connections between vascular system, right atrial pressure, and CO

CARDIAC FUNCTION CURVE (CO CURVE)
- Plot of relationship between left ventricle (LV) CO, right atrial (RA) pressure
- Based on Frank–Starling relationship describing CO dependence on preload
  - Preload (determined by RA pressure), independent variable; CO, dependent variable
  - ↑ venous return → ↑ RA pressure → ↑ LV end-diastolic volume (EDV)/preload, myocardial fiber stretch → ↑ CO
  - LV CO (L/min) = LV venous return/preload (RA pressure in mmHg)
  - Relationship remains intact with steady state of venous return
  - RA pressure 4mmHg → curve levels off at maximum 9L/min

VASCULAR FUNCTION CURVE

- Plot of relationship between venous return, RA pressure
- Independent of Frank–Starling relationship
  - Venous return independent variable; RA pressure dependent variable
  - Venous return, RA pressure: inverse relationship
- ↑ RA pressure → ↓ pressure gradient between systemic arteries, RA → ↓ venous return to RA; CO

Mean systemic pressure (MSP)
- Pressure equal throughout vasculature
- Influenced by blood volume, distribution

Total peripheral resistance (TPR)
- Primarily determined by pressure in arterioles; determines slope of curve
- ↓ TPR (↓ arteriolar resistance) → ↑ flow from arterial to venous circulation → ↑ venous return → clockwise rotation of curve
- ↑ TPR (↑ arteriolar resistance) → ↓ flow from arterial to venous circulation → ↓ venous return → counterclockwise rotation of curve

ALTERING CARDIAC & VASCULAR FUNCTION CURVES

osms.it/altering-cardiac-vascular-function-curves

- Curves combined → changes in CO visualized, cardiovascular parameters altered
- Curves can be displaced by changes in blood volume, inotropy, TPR

INOTROPIC AGENTS
- Alters cardiac curve
- Positive inotropic agents (e.g. digoxin) at any level of RA pressure
  - ↑ contractility, stroke volume (SV), CO → (1) cardiac curve shifts upward, (2) vascular function curve not affected, (3) x-intercept (steady state) shifts upward, to left
- Negative inotropic agents (e.g. beta-blockers)
  - Opposite effect

BLOOD VOLUME
- Alters vascular curve
- ↑ circulating volume (e.g. blood transfusion)
  - ↑ MSP → (1) curves intersect at ↑ CO, RA pressure, (2) parallel shift of x-intercept (steady state), vascular curve to right, (3) no change in TPR
- ↓ circulating volume (e.g. hemorrhage)
  - Opposite effect
- Changes in venous compliance are similar to blood volume changes
  - ↓ venous compliance → changes similar to ↑ circulating volume
  - ↑ venous compliance → changes similar to ↓ circulating volume

TOTAL PERIPHERAL RESISTANCE
- Alters both curves due to changes in afterload (cardiac curve), venous return (vascular curve)
- ↑ TPR → ↑ arterial pressure → ↑ afterload → ↓ CO → (1) downward shift of cardiac curve, (2) counterclockwise rotation of vascular curve, (3) ↓ venous return, (4) RA pressure unchanged, ↓/↑ (depending on cardiac, venous curve alteration), (5) curves intersect at altered steady state
- ↓ TPR (arteriolar dilation)
  - Opposite effect

PRESSURE-VOLUME LOOPS

osms.it/pressure-volume_loops

- Graphs represent pressure, volume changes in LV during one heartbeat (one cardiac cycle/"stroke work")
- Pressure in left ventricle on y axis, volume of left ventricle on x axis

FOUR PHASES

Ventricular filling during diastole
- At end of this phase:
  - Mitral valve closed
  - Left ventricle filled (EDV); relaxed, distended
  - EDV = 140mL

Isovolumic contraction
- Systole begins (ventricular contraction)
- No changes to ventricular volume (mitral, aortic valve closed)
- Pressure builds

Ventricular ejection
- Pressure in left ventricle > aortic pressure → aortic valve opens → blood ejected

Isovolumic relaxation
- Ventricle starts relaxing → aortic pressure > LV pressure → aortic valve closes
- End of systole
- ESV = 70mL

STROKE VOLUME (SV)
- STROKE VOLUME (SV)
- Amount of blood pumped by ventricles in one contraction
- SV = EDV - ESV

STROKE WORK (SW)
- Work of ventricles to eject a volume of blood (i.e. to eject SV)
- Represented by area inside of loop

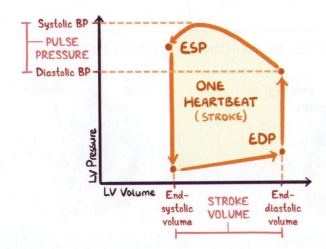

Figure 16.1 Measurements that can be obtained from the pressure-volume loop graph. Pulse pressure is measured in mmHg and reflects the throbbing pulsation felt in an artery during systole. Pulse pressure = systolic blood pressure - diastolic blood pressure. Stroke volume is measured in mL and is blood volume ejected by left ventricle during every heartbeat. Stroke volume = end-diastolic volume - end systolic volume.

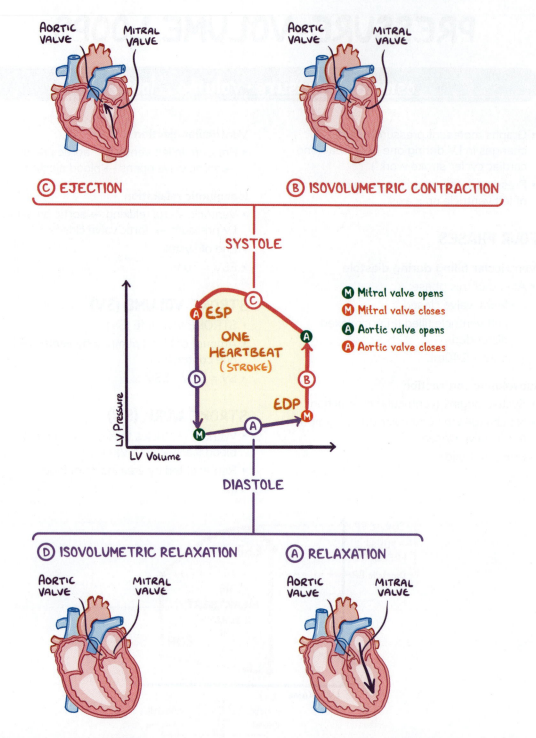

Figure 16.2 The four phases of the pressure-volume loop and the condition of the heart during each phase.

CHANGES IN PRESSURE-VOLUME LOOPS

osms.it/changes_in_pressure-volume_loops

- Cardiac parameters change → volume-pressure loops change
- ↑ preload (↑ EDV) → ↑ strength of contraction → ↑ stroke volume → larger loop
- ↑ afterload → ↑ ventricular pressure during isovolumetric contraction → ↑ less blood leaves ventricle → ↑ end-systolic volume

(ESV) → ↓ SV → loop narrower, taller (smaller SV, higher pressure; stroke work remains relatively stable)
- ↑ contractility → blood under ↑ pressure → longer ejection phase → left ventricular pressure = aortic pressure → ↑ SV, stroke work, ↓ ejection fraction (EF), EDV → loop widens

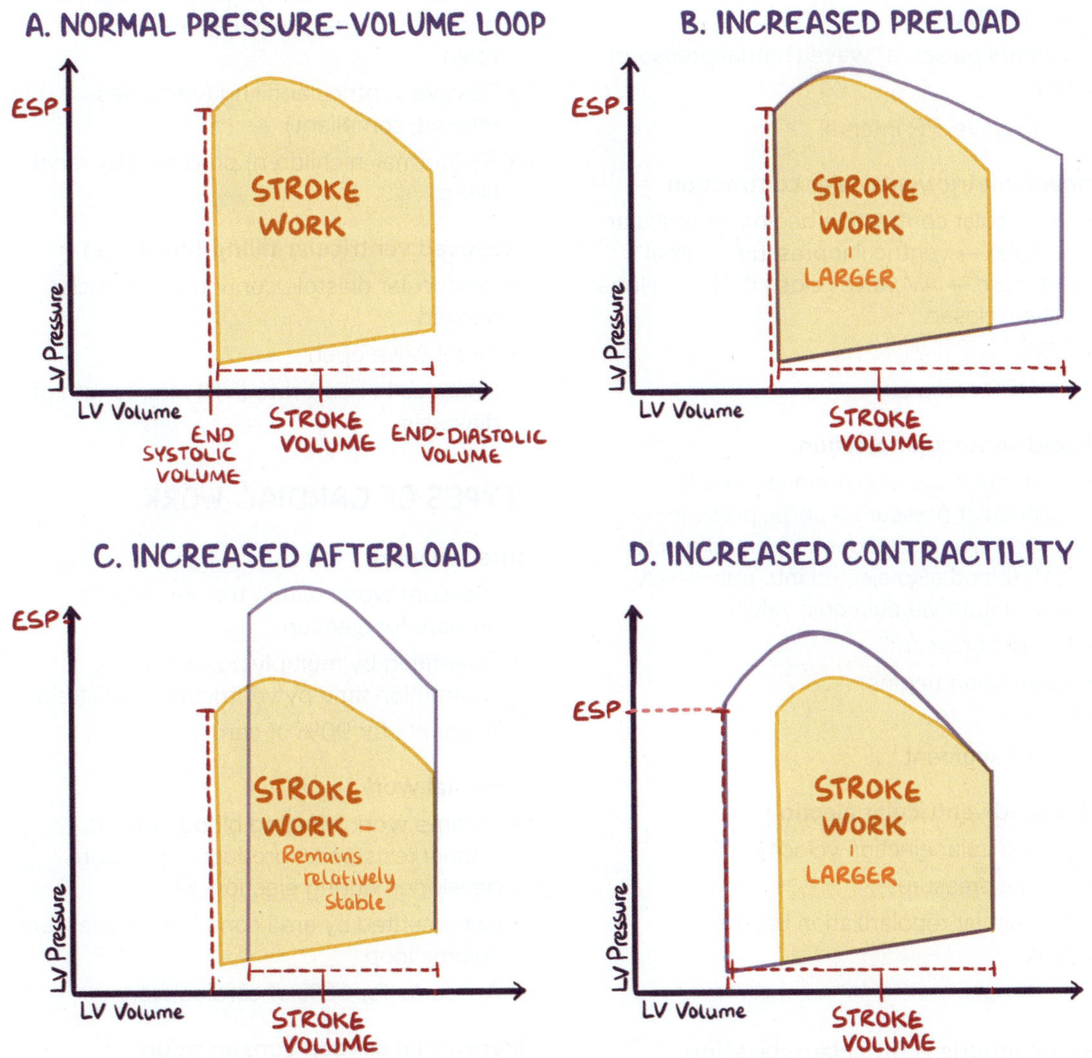

A. NORMAL PRESSURE-VOLUME LOOP
B. INCREASED PRELOAD
C. INCREASED AFTERLOAD
D. INCREASED CONTRACTILITY

Figure 16.3 Changes in stroke work as a result of increased preload (B), afterload (C), and contractility (D) represented on pressure-volume loop graphs.

CARDIAC WORK

osms.it/cardiac-work

- Work heart performs as blood moves from venous to arterial circulation during cardiac cycle

PHASES OF CARDIAC WORK

Atrial systole
- Begins when atria, ventricles in diastole
- Atrioventricular (AV) valves open → passive ventricular filling
- Atrial depolarization → atria contract (atrial kick during systole) → completes ventricular filling (EDV)
- **Venous pulse:** "a" wave (↑ atrial pressure)
- ECG
   - P wave, PR interval

Isovolumetric ventricular contraction
- Ventricular contraction begins (ventricular systole) → ventricular pressure > atrial pressure → AV valves close (S1); semilunar valves closed
- ECG
   - QRS complex

Rapid ventricular ejection
- Ventricular systole continues → left ventricular pressure > aortic pressure → aortic valve forced open → blood ejected (SV) (blood also ejected into pulmonary vasculature via pulmonic valve)
- ↑ aortic pressure
- Atrial filling begins
- ECG
   - ST segment

Reduced ventricular ejection
- ↓ ventricular ejection velocity
- ↑ atrial pressure
- Ventricular repolarization begins
- ECG
   - T wave

Isovolumetric ventricular relaxation
- Ventricles relaxed (ventricular diastole); ventricular pressure < aortic pressure → aortic valve closes (S2); causes dicrotic notch on aortic pressure curve
- All valves closed
- Ventricular volume
   - Constant
- Complete ventricular repolarization
- ECG
   - T wave ends

Rapid ventricular filling
- Ventricular diastole continues → ventricular pressure < atrial pressure → AV valves open
- Passive ventricular filling (ventricles relaxed, compliant)
- S3 (normal in children) produced by rapid filling

Reduced ventricular filling (diastasis)
- Ventricular diastole continues; ventricles relaxed
- Mitral valve open
- Changes in heart rate (HR) alter length of diastasis

TYPES OF CARDIAC WORK

Internal work
- **Pressure work:** within the ventricle to prepare for ejection
- Quantified by multiplying isovolumic contraction time by ventricular wall stress
- Accounts for 90% of cardiac work

External work
- **Volume work:** ejecting blood against arterial resistance; product of pressure developed during ejection, SV
- Represented by area contained in pressure-volume loop
- Accounts for 10% of cardiac work

Myocardial oxygen consumption
- Pressure work > volume work

- Aortic stenosis → ↑↑ pressure work → ↑↑ oxygen consumption, ↓ CO
- Strenuous exercise → ↑ volume work → ↑ oxygen consumption, ↑ CO

LV and right ventricle (RV)
- *Volume work*: CO LV = RV CO
- *Pressure work*: LV (aortic pressure 100mmHg) > RV (pulmonary pressure 15mmHg)
  - ↑ systemic pressure (e.g. hypertension) → ↑ LV pressure work → ventricular wall hypertrophy
  - Law of Laplace for sphere (e.g. heart): thickness of heart wall increases → greater pressure produced

CARDIAC PRELOAD

osms.it/cardiac-preload

- EDV: volume load created by blood entering ventricles at end of diastole before contraction
- Establishes sarcomere length, ventricular stretch as ventricles fill (length-tension relationship)

FACTORS AFFECTING PRELOAD

Venous pressure
- Includes blood volume, rate of venous return to RA
- ↑ blood volume, venous return → ↑ preload

Ventricular compliance
- *Flexibility*: ability to yield when pressure applied
- Compliant, "stretchy" ventricles → ↑ preload
- Noncompliant, stiff ventricles → ↓ preload

Atrial contraction
- Early ventricular diastole → ventricles relaxed, passively fill with blood from atria via open AV valves → late ventricular diastole atrial systole (atrial kick) → additional blood into ventricles
- Accounts for 20% of ventricular preload

Resistance from valves
- Stenotic mitral, tricuspid valves create inflow resistance → ↓ filling → ↓ preload
- Stenotic pulmonic, aortic valves create outflow resistance → ↓ emptying → ↑ preload

HR
- Normal heart rate allows adequate time for ventricles to fill
- Tachyarrhythmias → ↓ filling time → ↓ preload

CARDIAC AFTERLOAD

osms.it/cardiac-afterload

- Amount of resistance ventricles must overcome during systole
- Establishes degree, speed of sarcomere shortening, ventricular wall stress (force-velocity relationship)
- ↑ afterload → ↓ velocity of sarcomere shortening
- ↓ afterload → ↑ velocity of sarcomere shortening

FACTORS AFFECTING AFTERLOAD

LV
- Systemic vascular resistance (SVR)
- Aortic pressure

RV
- Pulmonary pressure

Resistance from valves
- Stenotic pulmonic, aortic valves create outflow resistance → ↑ afterload

LAW OF LAPLACE

osms.it/law-of-Laplace

- Describes pressure-volume relationships of spheres
- Blood vessels
    - \> radius of artery = > pressure on arterial wall
- Heart
    - Wall tension produced by myocardial fibers when ejecting blood depends on thickness of sphere (heart wall)
- Laplace's formula: tension on myocardial fibers in heart wall = pressure within ventricle x volume in ventricle (radius) / wall thickness

- $T = \dfrac{P \times r}{h}$
    - T = wall tension
    - P = pressure
    - r = radius of ventricle
    - h = ventricular wall thickness
- Dilation of heart muscle increases tension that must be developed within heart wall to eject same amount of blood per beat
- Myocytes of dilated left ventricle have greater load (tension)
    - Must produce greater tension to overcome aortic pressure, eject blood → ↓ CO

Chapter 16 Cardiovascular Physiology: Cardiac Cycle

FRANK–STARLING RELATIONSHIP

osms.it/Frank-Starling_relationship

- Loading ventricle with blood during diastole, stretching cardiac muscle → force of contraction during systole
- Length-tension relationship
  - Amount of tension (force of muscle contraction during systole) → depends on resting length of sarcomere → depends on amount of blood that fills ventricles during diastole (EDV)
  - Length of sarcomere determines amount of overlap between actin, myosin filaments, amount of myosin heads that bind to actin at cross-bridge formation
  - Low EDV → ↓ sarcomere stretching → ↓ myosin heads bind to actin → weak contraction during systole → ↓ SV
  - Too much sarcomere stretching prevents optimal overlap between actin, myosin → ↓ force of contraction → ↓ SV
- Allows intrinsic control of heart = venous return with SV
- Extrinsic control through sympathetic stimulation, hormones (e.g. epinephrine), medications (e.g. digoxin) → ↑ contractility (positive inotropy), SV
- Negative inotropic agents (e.g beta-blockers) → ↓ contractility → ↓ SV

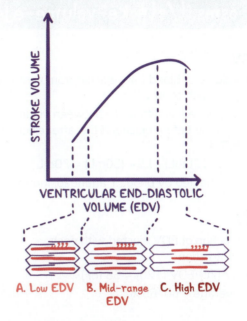

Figure 16.4 Graphical representation of the Frank–Starling relationship and sarcomere length at low, mid-range, and high EDVs. A mid-range EDV (B), where the volume of blood returning to the ventricles is increasing but is not too large (C), allows for best myosin-actin binding → ↑ strength of contractions → ↑ stroke volume.

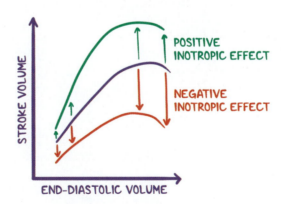

Figure 16.5 Graphical representation of positive and negative inotropic effects on the Frank–Starling relationship.

STROKE VOLUME, EJECTION FRACTION, & CARDIAC OUTPUT

osms.it/stroke-volume-ejection-fraction-cardiac-output

SV
- Volume of blood (mL) ejected from ventricle with each contraction
- Calculated as difference between volume of blood before ejection/EDV, after ejection (ESV)
- EDV (120mL) - ESV (50mL) = 70mL
- SV affected by preload, afterload, inotropy

EF
- Fraction of EDV ejected with each contraction
- SV (70)/EDV (120) = 58 (EF)
- Average = 50–65%

CO
- Volume of blood ejected by ventricles per minute
- SV (120) x HR (70) = 4900mL/min

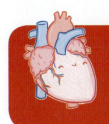

NOTES
CARDIAC ELECTROPHYSIOLOGY

ACTION POTENTIALS IN PACEMAKER CELLS

osms.it/pacemaker-cell-action-potentials

Pacemaker cells
- Groups of cardiac muscle cells with ability to spontaneously create action potential (automaticity) and comprise intrinsic conduction system
- Directly influenced by sympathetic and parasympathetic nervous systems
- Comprise about 1% of heart cells
- Differ in speed of spontaneous depolarization
- Cells with fastest rate of depolarization at any given time determine heart rhythm
  - Remaining/slower cells called latent pacemakers

SA node
- Primary pacemaker cells located in wall of right atrium
- Rate: 60–100bpm
  - Usually determines normal heart rhythm

Latent pacemaker cells
- AV node
  - Located at base of right atrium, near septum
  - Rate: 40–60bpm
- Bundle of His
  - Divides into right and left bundle branches, travels through septum between ventricles
  - Rate: 20–40bpm
- Purkinje fibers
  - Spread throughout ventricles
  - Rate: 20–40bpm

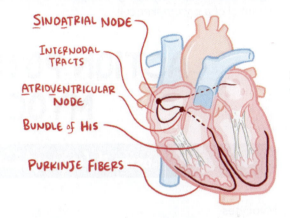

Figure 17.1 Locations of pacemaker cells within the heart.

Action potentials in pacemaker cells
- Rapid electrical changes across membrane of pacemaker cells
- Conducted to rest of heart

Action potential phases
- **Phase 4:** sodium moves into cell through funny channels (open in response to hyperpolarization); slowly depolarizes cell until threshold potential met
  - Responsible for instability of resting membrane potential
- **Phase 0:** strong inward calcium current; responsible for rapid depolarization
- **Phase 3:** strong potassium current moves out of cell; responsible for repolarization
  - Phases 1, 2 absent in pacemaker cells → no plateau

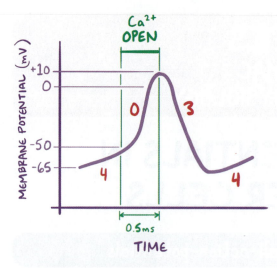

Figure 17.2 Graph depicting the action potential of a pacemaker cell.

ACTION POTENTIALS IN MYOCYTES

osms.it/myocyte-action-potentials

Myocytes
- Receive signal from from pacemaker cells causing them to contract
- Able to depolarize, spread action potentials
- Action potential phases:
  - **Phase 0 (depolarization phase):** rapid influx of sodium into cell (inward current); responsible for rapid depolarization
  - **Phase 1:** sodium current stops, potassium slowly flows out of cell; depolarization stops, re-polarization starts
  - **Phase 2:** calcium current moves into cell, balances potassium current moving out of cell; charge balance between inside, outside of cell creates plateau
  - **Phase 3:** calcium current moving into cell stops; potassium current moving out of cell continues; repolarization continues
  - **Phase 4:** potassium current moving out of cell approaches equilibrium between inside, outside of cell; sodium, calcium current moving into cell balance outward potassium current; resting membrane potential achieved

Chapter 17 Cardiovascular Physiology: Cardiac Electrophysiology

ELECTRICAL CONDUCTION IN THE HEART

osms.it/heart-electrical-conduction

- Transmission of electrical signals across heart cells leads to rhythmic myocardial contraction
- Intercalated discs connect cells and allow myocardium to act as syncytium
    - Contain desmosomes (holds cells together) and gap junctions (areas of low resistance to electrical flow)
- Cardiac action potential: sequential flow of electrons across ion channels in cardiac cell membranes, resulting in electrical activation of myocardial cells
    - Depolarization: cation movement into cell, producing positive cell charge relative to outside
    - Polarization: anion movement into cell, producing negative cell charge relative to outside
- Pathway of electrical conduction
    - Sinoatrial node (SA node) → atrial internodal fibers → atrioventricular node (AV node) → bundle of His → Purkinje fibers → ventricular myocytes
- These structures responsible for electrical conduction, spontaneous depolarization; do not generate contractile force

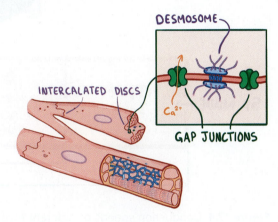

Figure 17.3 Desmosomes and gap junctions present at intercalated discs allow the myocardium to act as a syncytium.

CARDIAC CONDUCTION VELOCITY

osms.it/cardiac-conduction-velocity

- Speed at which depolarization wave spreads among myocardial cells
    - Measured in meters per second (m/s)
- Each myocardial structure has a different conduction speed related to its purpose
    - Slowest: AV node
    - Fastest: Purkinje fibers
- AV delay: slow conduction through AV node ensures adequate ventricular filling
    - Speed: 0.01–0.05m/s
    - Blood flows from atria to ventricles
- Rapid conduction through Purkinje fibers ensures adequate blood ejection
    - Speed: 2–4m/s

Velocity depends on two factors
- Amount of ions going into cell during action potential
    - More ions → faster depolarization → faster spread
    - Fewer ions → slower depolarization → slower spread

- **Interconnectedness** of myocardial conduction cells
  - More gap junctions → more interconnected cells → less resistance to ion flow between cells
  - Fewer gap junctions → fewer interconnected cells → increased resistance to ion flow between cells

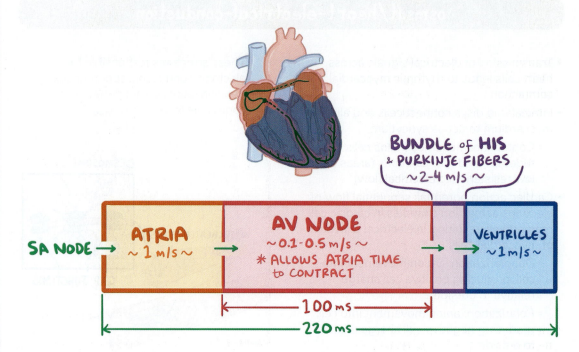

Figure 17.4 Conduction speeds of different myocardial structures.

EXCITABILITY & REFRACTORY PERIODS

osms.it/excitability-refractory-periods

Refractory period
- Time in which myocardial cell cannot be depolarized
- *Absolute refractory period*: no stimulus, no matter its size, can depolarize cell
  - Phases 0, 1; part of phase 2
- *Effective refractory period*: large stimulus can generate action potential
  - However, too weak to be conducted
- *Relative refractory period*: large stimulus can generate action potential
  - Big enough to be conducted

Excitability
- Ability of myocardial cells to depolarize in response to incoming depolarizing current
- *Supranormal period*: < normal stimulus may produce action potential large enough to be conducted
  - Resting membrane potential has not yet been achieved
  - Membrane potential closer to threshold than normal, refractory periods over

CARDIAC EXCITATION-CONTRACTION COUPLING

osms.it/cardiac_excitation-contraction_coupling

- Plateau in action potential of myocyte membrane allows influx of calcium, stimulating muscle contraction
    - Calcium enters cell via L-type voltage gated channels
    - Higher intracellular Ca^{2+} triggers release of more Ca^{2+} from sarcoplasmic reticulum through ryanodine receptors (AKA calcium-induced release)
    - Released Ca^{2+} attaches to troponin C → tropomyosin moves → actin-myosin cross bridges → contraction
- Cross bridges last as long as Ca^{2+} occupies troponin
    - Tension is proportional to intracellular Ca^{2+} concentration
- Intracellular Ca^{2+} removed by two mechanisms that induce relaxation, keep Ca^{2+} from damaging cell contents
    - Ca^{2+} ATPase uses ATP energy, Na^+/Ca^{2+} ATP exchanger uses Na^+ inward current to remove Ca^{2+} from cell through sarcolemmal membrane, remove Na^+ through Na^+/K^+ ATPase
    - Ca^{2+} ATPase removes Ca^{2+} into sarcoplasmic reticulum; calsequestrin 2 inside sarcoplasmic reticulum binds Ca^{2+}, keeping it inside

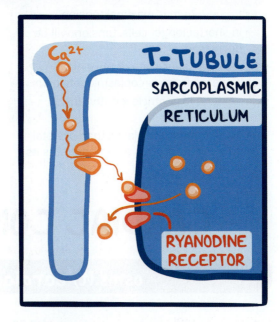

Figure 17.5 Depolarization of a cardiomyocyte by calcium-induced calcium release.

CARDIAC LENGTH TENSION

osms.it/cardiac-length-tension

- Degree filament overlap correlates to tension
  - L_{max} = 2.2 μm is maximal tension
  - In shorter/longer cells, tension will be decreased
- ↑ L → ↑ Ca^{2+} sensitivity of troponin C → ↑ Ca^{2+} release from sarcoplasmic reticulum
- Can extend to ventricle length/tension relationship curve
  - Cardiac muscle < elastic than skeletal; only ascending curve demonstrates its contraction
- ↑ **resting tension:** small changes produce ↑ tension
- Frank–Starling basis; ↑ fiber length → stronger contraction
  - Preload = LV end-diastolic volume (L), if ↑ means ventricular fiber length ↑
  - Afterload = aortic pressure; if preload ↑ → afterload tension and pressure ↑

CARDIAC CONTRACTILITY

osms.it/cardiac-contractility

- **Positive inotropes:** ↑ force of myocardial contraction
- **Negative inotropes:** ↓ force of myocardial contraction
- Proportional to Ca^{2+} concentration
  - Proportional to Ca^{2+} released
  - Depends on storage, current size

WHAT AFFECTS INOTROPISM? - AUTONOMIC NERVOUS SYSTEM

Sympathetic

- *Positive inotropic effects:* ↑ contractility
- Causes faster relaxation, faster refill, increased heart rate (HR)
- Increased tension development rate
  - ß1 receptor is G_s coupled, activates adenylyl cyclase → cAMP produced
  - pKA activated → phosphorylation → ↑ sarcolemmal Ca^{2+} channel activity → ↑ contraction
  - Phospholamban phosphorylation; stops sarcoplasmic Ca^{2+} ATPase inhibition, decreasing time of IC Ca^{2+}, making HR faster, systole shorter; Frank–Starling effective
  - Na^+/K^+ ATPase phosphorylation; increases relaxation due to secondary channel activations
  - Troponin I phosphorylation; Ca^{2+} binds less troponin C → effect on excitation contraction coupling, prolongs filling, higher ejection fraction

Parasympathetic

- **Negative inotropic effects:** ↓ contractility on atria via muscarinic receptors
- Acidosis also has negative inotropic effect → ↓ contractility
- G_k (type of G_i), adenylyl cyclase couple, resulting in
  - Decreased Ca^{2+} plateau current
  - ACh increases I_{kACh}
  - → ↓ action potential duration → ↓ Ca^{2+} current → ↓ AP width
- Phosphodiesterase metabolises cAMP, inhibit phosphodiesterase, increase contractility IP3 stimulates Ca release in SR, increases force of contraction

Chapter 17 Cardiovascular Physiology: Cardiac Electrophysiology

Heart rate (HR)
- HR increases contractility
- Diastole affected more than systole
- Ca can't be removed as quickly as it accumulates → new equilibrium
  - ↑ **action potentials/time:** increased total trigger Ca^{2+}, increased inward current
  - ↑ Ca^{2+} influx → ↑ stores; phospholamban phosphorylated, thus inhibited
- Positive staircase effect/Bowditch staircase/Treppe phenomenon
  - On first, beat still no extra Ca^{2+}
  - Afterward, Ca^{2+} accumulates until max Ca^{2+} storage achieved
- Postextrasystolic potentiation
  - Same effect as positive staircase
  - Extrasystole < powerful, but creates one more chance for calcium entry
  - Because the voltage channels are open more, postextrasystolic beat has higher tension than extrasystolic

WHAT AFFECTS INOTROPISM? – DRUGS

Cardiac glycosides
- Digoxin, digitoxin, ouabain; congestive heart failure treatment
  - Inhibit Na^+/K^+ ATPase; + inotropic, ↑ intracellular Na^+ changes Na/Ca → decreases exchange → intracellular calcium increases → increases tension
  - Nifedipine also acts on Ca^{2+} by blocking ryanodine receptors

Beta adrenergics
- Isoproterenol, norepinephrine, epinephrine, dopamine, dobutamine
  - ↑ cAMP → ↑ contractility

NOTES
ELECTROCARDIOGRAPHY (ECG)

ECG BASICS

osms.it/ECG-basics

- ECG traces provide information on heart's electrical activity, rate, rhythm
  - Depolarization waves moving towards electrode → positive deflection
  - Depolarization waves moving away from electrode → negative deflection
- 12 lead ECG (EKG) records heart electrical activity during heartbeat
  - Six limb leads (I, II, III, AVR, AVL, AVF)
  - Six chest leads (V1–V6)
- **P wave:** atrial depolarization
  - **PR interval:** beginning of atrial contraction to beginning of ventricular contraction (time for impulse to reach ventricles form sinus node)
- **PR segment:** end of P wave to beginning of QRS complex; signifies AV nodal delay
- **QRS complex:** ventricular depolarization
- **T wave:** ventricular repolarization
- **QT interval:** time from start of Q wave to end of T wave; represents time taken for ventricular depolarization, repolarization
- **U wave:** sometimes seen after T wave (not shown), represents purkinje fiber repolarization

RECORDING ECGs

- Recorded on 1mm graph paper (10mm = 1mV)

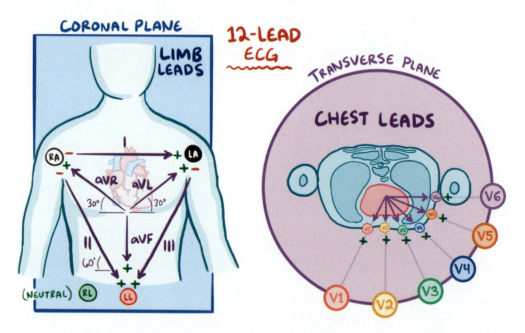

Figure 18.1 Lead placement in the coronal and transverse plane.

- x-axis = time (1mm = 0.04s)
- y-axis = voltage (10mm = 1mV)
- **Limb leads:** I, II, III, AVR, AVL, AVF
  - *Bipolar leads:* I, II, III
  - *Unipolar leads:* AVR, AVL, AVF (augmented voltage for right arm, left arm, left foot
  - *Lateral leads:* I, aVL, V5, V6
  - *Inferior leads:* II, III, AVF
  - Six limb leads provide six viewpoints of cardiac activity, in frontal plane
- Electrodes placed on shoulders, abdomen to record limb leads
- **Chest leads (precordial):** V1–V6
  - *Septal leads:* V1, V2
  - *Lateral leads:* V5, V6
  - *Anterior leads:* V3, V4
  - Six chest leads provide six viewpoints of cardiac activity, in horizontal plane

ECG NORMAL SINUS RHYTHM

osms.it/ECG-normal-sinus-rhythm

- P waves precede QRS complexes in 1:1 relationship
- SA node (sinus node), dominant centre of automaticity
  - Normal sinus rhythm 50–90bpm
- Constant RR interval
- Predictable recurring wave pattern (P-waves, QRS, T waves)
- P waves
  - Upright in leads I, II, AVF
  - Amplitude < 2.5mm in limb leads
  - *Sinus arrhythmia:* can be normal if sinus rate varies with respiratory cycle, relatively mild/abnormal if sinus rate varies unpredictably, very dramatic

ECG RATE & RHYTHM

osms.it/ECG-rate-rhythm

RATE DETERMINATION
- **Box method:** measure R-R interval by large boxes
  - *ECG grid:* thick lines 5mm apart (0.20s); thin lines 1mm (0.04s)
  - Locate R wave peak on thick line as "start"
  - *Label blocks (thick lines):* 300; 150; 100; 75; 60; 50
  - Locate next R wave peak to estimate heart rate
- **Fast heart rates:** use fine division within boxes for more accurate estimates
- **Slow heart rates:** use 2.5s marks at top of trace paper
- Locate R wave peak on large block line as "start"
- Count subsequent number of complete R waves in 10s strip (total strip)
- To calculate heart rate
  - Count number of QRS complexes across entire recording, multiply by six for heart rate; used to estimate heart rate during irregular rhythms

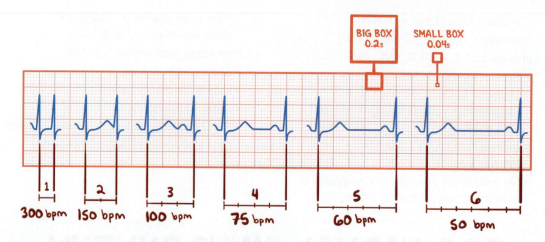

Figure 18.2 The Box method measures distance between R-R intervals to calculate the heart rate.

ECG INTERVALS

osms.it/ECG-intervals

PR INTERVAL & SEGMENT
- Normal interval 0.12–0.20s
  - Measure duration(s) from start of P to start of Q
- *Normal segment:* usually isoelectric, may be displaced

QRS INTERVAL
- *Normal QRS:* <0.10–0.12s (slight variation between references)
  - Measured from start of Q to end of S
- *QRS amplitude (voltage):* wide range of normal limits
  - *Low voltage:* < 5mm limb leads, < 10mm chest leads
  - Increased voltage can indicate left ventricular hypertrophy, right ventricular hypertrophy, may be normal
  - Narrow (< 0.12s) / wide (> 0.12s)

QT INTERVAL
- Normal QT < 50% RR interval, only for normal heart rates
- Measure QT from start of Q to end of T
- Measure RR interval as time between R-R

- QTc interval corrected for heart rate; 0.35–0.44s for normal heart rate (60–100bpm)
- Long QTc (> 500ms) → prone to rapid, potentially fatal ventricular rhythm

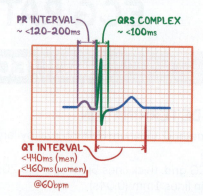

Figure 18.3 An ECG interval includes a segment and one or more waves and should be completed within a specific amount of time to be considered healthy.

ECG AXIS

osms.it/ECG-axis

- Mean direction (vector) of ventricular depolarization wavefront
  - Mean QRS vector normally downward from AV node through stronger left ventricle
- Normal axis range -30° to +90° of frontal plane
- Limb leads indicate vector deviation in frontal plane
  - Divided into four quadrants

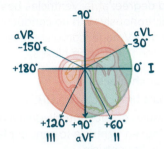

Figure 18.4 The green shows a normal range. The red bottom left quadrant would indicate right ventricular hypertrophy while the top right would indicate left ventricular hypertrophy.

ECG TRANSITION

osms.it/ECG-transition

- Chest leads provide information on vector rotation in horizontal plane
  - *Normal:* gradual transition of QRS through leads V1–V6
  - QRS complex switches from predominantly negative to positive either between V2, V3 or between V3, V4

R WAVE PROGRESSION

- *Early:* tall R wave in V1, V2
- *Delayed R:* transition point between V4, V5/between V5, V6
  - R amplitude > S; no progression through V5, V6
- *Reverse:* decreasing amplitude

ASSESSMENT FOR NORMAL REGULAR RHYTHM

- Is there a P before every QRS complex?
- Is there a QRS after every P?
- Are the P waves normal?

ABNORMAL RATES & RHYTHMS

- Conventionally defined, sinus bradycardia <60bpm
  - True normal adult resting heart rate is 50–90bpm
- Sinus tachycardia > 100bpm
- If SA node fails, other latent ectopic pacemakers capable of automaticity
  - Atria, AV junction, His bundle, bundle branches can set heart rate
  - Each foci has unique rate (atrial foci 60–80bpm; junctional foci 40–60bpm; ventricular foci 20–40bpm)
  - *Overdrive suppression:* mechanism by which only foci/node with highest firing frequency rate conducts impulses, suppresses other pacemaker sites

Heart blocks
- Sinus block
  - SA node temporarily ceases to conduct impulse; usually resumes, may cause escape rhythm

- AV block
  - *First degree:* prolonged PR interval > 0.2s
  - *Second degree:* some P waves conducted to ventricles, followed by QRS complex while some not
  - *Third degree:* atria, ventricles beat asynchronously with no conduction through AV node (complete dissociation between P, QRS complexes)

Bundle branch blocks
- Left bundle branch block (LBBB)
  - Activation of left ventricle delayed causing left ventricle to contract later than right ventricle
  - Broad QRS < 120ms
  - Secondary R wave (R') in leads V1-3
  - Slurred S wave in lateral leads (I, avL, V5–6)
  - Secondary repolarization abnormalities in right precordial leads (ST depression, T wave inversions)
- Right bundle branch block (RBBB)
  - Activation of right ventricle delayed causing right ventricle to contract later than left ventricle
  - Broad QRS < 120ms
  - Dominant S wave in V1
  - Absence of Q waves, broad monophasic R wave in lateral leads
- Left anterior fascicular block
  - Impulses conducted to left ventricle via left posterior fascicle
  - Left axis deviation
  - Increased R wave peak time in aVL
  - Small Q waves, tall R waves in leads 1, aVL
  - Small R waves, deep S waves in leads II, III, aVF
  - Increased QRS voltage in limb leads
  - Prolonged R wave peak time in aVL > 45ms
- Left posterior fascicular block
  - Impulses conducted to left ventricle via left anterior fascicle
  - Right axis deviation
  - Increased R wave peak time in aVF
  - Small R waves with deep S waves in leads I, aVL
  - Small Q waves with tall R waves in leads II, III, aVF
  - Increased QRS voltage in limb leads

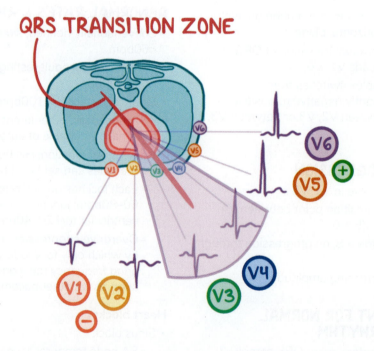

Figure 18.5 The QRS transition zone usually occurs in the V3 and V4 lead. V1 and V2 are mostly positive while V5 and V6 are mostly negative.

ECG CARDIAC HYPERTROPHY & ENLARGEMENT

osms.it/ECG-cardiac-hypertrophy-enlargement

ATRIAL DILATION/ENLARGEMENT
- Biphasic P waves > one small box in lead V1
- Initial component of wave larger
  - Right atrial enlargement
- Terminal component of wave larger
  - Left atrial enlargement
- Amplitude of P wave in any limb lead > 2.5mm
  - Probable right atrial enlargement

RIGHT VENTRICULAR HYPERTROPHY
- V1–V6 all consisting of small r waves, deep S waves (no R wave transition)
- Tall R wave in V1 that progressively shortens across to V6 (reverse R wave transition)
- Possible right axis deviation

LEFT VENTRICULAR HYPERTROPHY
- Deep S wave in lead V1
- Tall R wave in V5 and/or V6
- Sum of S wave depth in V1 + R wave height in either V5/V6 > 35mm
- Possible left axis deviation
- Left ventricular 'strain pattern'
  - Downsloping ST segments, T wave inversions in lateral leads

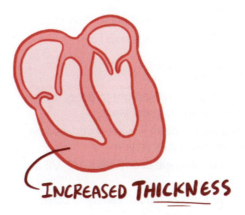

Figure 18.6 Hypertrophy is an enlargement of the muscle wall while an increase in volume is known as dilation.

CHARACTERISTICS of CARDIAC HYPERTROPHY

	LEFT	RIGHT
ATRIAL ENLARGEMENT	V1: Biphasic P; II: Double-Humped	II & V1: Big P
VENTRICULAR ENLARGEMENT	V1: Big R; V5: Big S	V1: Huge S; V5 & V6: Huge R

ECG MYOCARDIAL INFARCTION & ISCHEMIA

osms.it/ECG-cardiac-infarction-ischemia

MYOCARDIAL INFARCTION

- Complete/partial blockage in coronary artery causing myocardial damage
- *ST elevation MIs (STEMIs):* complete artery blockage
    - ST elevation present on ECG; emergency
- *Non-ST elevation MIs (NSTEMIs):* partial artery blockage
    - ST elevations not present on ECG
    - Less emergent than STEMI

ISCHEMIA

- Inverted T waves; slight to deep; most pronounced in chest leads
- *Angina:* transient T wave inversion; may occur without infarction
- Inverted T wave in any leads V2–V6 are abnormal
    - Suggest ischemia, variety of other pathologies
- *Acute or recent infarction:* elevated ST segment (slight to extensive)
    - One of the earliest ECG signs of infarction
    - Returns to baseline over time
- *Restricted coronary blood flow:* flat depressed ST segment
    - Suggests subendocardial infarction; any ST depression

NECROSIS

- Pathologic Q wave; > 0.04s, amplitude < ⅓ - ¼mm the R wave height
    - Non-pathological q waves < 0.04s considered normal
- Ignore AVR lead; record leads with Q (pathological), q (physiological) waves; ST depression/elevation; inverted T waves
- Anterior left ventricular infarction (q in V5, V6)
    - Chest leads anterior location; Q waves in leads V1, V2, V3 /V4
- Posterior infarction
    - Large R in leads V1, V2; possible Q in V6
    - *Mirror test:* invert, examine reflection for vQ, ST elevation in leads V1, V2
- *Lateral infarction:* Q in leads I, AVL
- *Inferior infarction:* Q in leads II, III, AVF

ECG CHARACTERISTICS of COMMON ARRHYTHMIAS

	ISCHEMIA	INFARCTION
SUBENDOCARDIAL	Stable angina; ST Depressions	Unstable angina; NSTEMI; ST Depresssions; T wave Inversion
TRANSMURAL	Unstable angina; NSTEMI; ST Depresssions; T wave Inversion	STEMI; T wave inversions; Hyperacute T waves; ST elevation; Pathologic Q waves

NOTES
HEMODYNAMICS

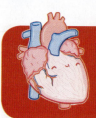

BLOOD PRESSURE, BLOOD FLOW, & RESISTANCE

osms.it/blood-pressure-blood-flow-resistance

PRESSURE (P)
- Force over area → blood pressure is force of blood over blood vessel surface area

BLOOD FLOW (Q)
- Volume (cm^3) blood flow through vessel over period of seconds (s)
- E.g. Q = 83cm^3/s

Determined by two factors
- ΔP = Pressure gradient (mmHg); difference in pressure between two blood vessel ends
- R = Resistance (mmHg/mL per min)
  - Q=ΔP/R
- Q directly proportional to pressure gradient
  - Increased pressure gradient → increased blood flow
- Q inversely proportional to resistance
  - Increased resistance → decreased blood flow

BLOOD FLOW VELOCITY (v)
- Major mechanism for changing blood flow is changing resistance
- Blood flow velocity (v) is distance (cm) traveled in certain amount of time (s)
- Using the equation for area (A) of a circle, $(d/2)^2 \times \pi$, we get $(2/2)^2 \times \pi = 3.14 cm^2$
- Since cardiac output = blood flow → convert L/min to cm^3/s → $1000 cm^3$ in a L, 60 seconds in a minute, multiplying those equals 83cm^3/sec
- Rearranging formula, velocity equals flow rate divided by area, equals about 26cm/s, about 1km/hr

TOTAL PERIPHERAL RESISTANCE (TPR)
- Resistance of entire systemic vasculature
  - Can be measured by substituting cardiac output for flow (Q), pressure difference between aorta, vena cava for ΔP
- Resistance within an organ
  - Can be measured by substituting organ blood flow for flow (Q), pressure difference in pressure between organ artery, vein for ΔP

PRESSURES IN THE CARDIOVASCULAR SYSTEM

osms.it/cardiovascular-system-pressures

- Blood pressure highest in large arteries (e.g. brachial artery), about 120/80mmHg

SYSTOLIC BLOOD PRESSURE
- First/top number
- Pressure in aorta caused by ventricular contraction
- During systole, heart contracts → transfers kinetic energy (140mmHg) to blood → aortic elastic walls stretched, where some kinetic energy stored as elastic energy of walls (form of potential energy) → blood pressure drops to 120mmHg (systolic pressure)

DIASTOLIC BLOOD PRESSURE
- Second/bottom number
- Pressure caused by recoil of arteries during diastole
- During diastole, heart relaxes, aortic valves close → kinetic energy drops to 50mmHg → potential energy of stretched aortic walls adds to kinetic energy again when walls recoil → pressure rises to 60mmHg (diastolic pressure) → allows blood to move forward
- **Pulse pressure**: difference between systolic, diastolic pressure

Mean arterial pressure (MAP/P_a)
- Average blood pressure during cardiac cycle including systolic, diastolic blood pressure
- MAP, pulse pressure decline with distance from heart

MAP measured in two ways
- Diastole lasts longer than systole, therefore MAP is equal to one third systolic pressure plus two thirds diastolic pressure
  - MAP = ⅓ systolic pressure + ⅔ diastolic pressure
- For person with normal blood pressure of 120/80mmHg
  - MAP = ⅓ 120 + ⅔ 80 = 93mmHg
- Diastole lasts longer than systole; roughly equal to diastolic pressure plus one-third pulse pressure

$$MAP = Diastolic\ pressure + \frac{pulse\ pressure}{3}$$

- For person with normal blood pressure of 120/80mmHg

$$MAP = 80 mmHg + \frac{120 mmHg}{3} = 93 mmHg$$

- MAP demonstrated using relationship of blood flow, blood pressure, resistance, applying the following equation
- $Q = \Delta P / R \rightarrow P_i - P_f = Q \times R$
  - P_i = mean arterial pressure (MAP)
  - P_f = central venous pressure (CVP)
  - Q = blood flow, equals cardiac output (CO)
  - R = resistance; combined resistance of all of blood vessels of systemic circulation equals systemic vascular resistance (SVR)
- Applying this equals the following
  - MAP - CVP = CO × SVR
- CVP is a small number, usually ignored; equation simplified
  - MAP = CO × SVR
- Based on this relationship → increased resistance will cause increased blood pressure

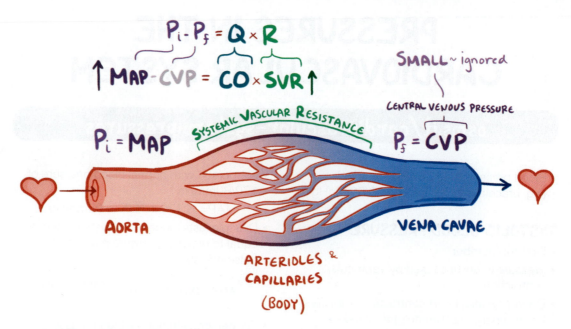

Figure 19.1 Visualization of MAP equation components.

PRESSURE GRADIENT

- Pressure gradient pressure difference between two ends of blood vessel
  - Gradient from aorta to arteriole ends
- Pressures in different parts of cardiovascular system not equal, keeps blood moving
- Blood flow generated by heart pumping action, moves along pressure gradient from high pressure areas (arteries) to low pressure areas (veins)
- Fluctuations on arterial side
  1. Blood ejected into aorta → pressure rises
  2. Small amount of blood backflows into ventricles
  3. Valves close → pressure drops
  4. Dicrotic notch/incisura pressure drop followed by small pressure increase as a result of valve recoiling
  5. Aorta settles, heart relaxes → pressure drops

- Pulse pressure lower in aorta than in large arteries → because pressure from blood travels faster than blood itself; pressure waves bounce off branch points in arteries which increases pressure even more
- Systolic pressure higher in large arteries than aorta, blood keeps moving forward
- Diastolic pressure is lower than in large arteries → mean arterial pressure mostly affected by diastolic pressure → mean arterial pressure is higher in aorta → driving force for blood flow
  - **For example:** aortic systolic pressure is 115mmHg; diastolic pressure is 85mmHg → Mean arterial pressure is 95mmHg; large artery systolic pressure is 120mmHg; diastolic pressure is 80mmHg → mean arterial pressure is 93mmHg

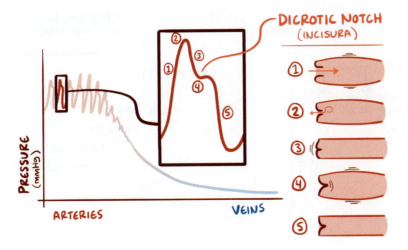

Figure 19.2 The five stages of fluctuation in arterial pulse pressure.

SYSTEMIC CIRCULATION
- Mean pressure in aorta results from two factors
  - Blood volume (cardiac output)
  - Compliance (low compliance → high pressure)
- Pressure remains high in large arteries because of high elastic recoil

Small arteries
- Pressure decreases; biggest pressure drop is in arterioles (30mmHg)
  - Occurs because arterioles develop high resistance to flow

Capillaries
- Pressure drops for 30mmHg to 10mmHg
- Two causes for pressure drop
  - Fluid filtration in capillaries
  - Increase frictional resistance
- Pressure drop is less than in arterioles
  - Many capillaries running in parallel → reduces total resistance (total resistance for vessels in parallel is less than resistance in any individual vessel)

Veins
- Systolic pressure drops even further → 4mmHg in vena cava, 2mmHg in right atrium
  - Venous pressure too low to promote venous return to heart
- Factors that facilitate venous return
  - **Muscular pump:** as muscles contract, relax they compress surrounding veins, force blood towards heart
  - **Respiratory pump:** during inhalation, abdominal pressure increases, forces blood in local veins forward
  - **Sympathetic vasoconstriction:** as smooth muscle in veins contracts, blood pushed towards heart

PULMONARY CIRCULATION
- Right ventricle → lungs → left atrium
- **Pulmonary arteries:** systolic pressure 25mmHg; diastolic pressure 8mmHg
  - Mean arterial pressure → 25 (⅓) + 8 (⅔) = 14mmHg
- **Capillaries:** pressure drops to 10mmHg
- **Pulmonary vein:** pressure drops to 8mmHg
- **Left atrium:** pressure drops to 2–5mmHg

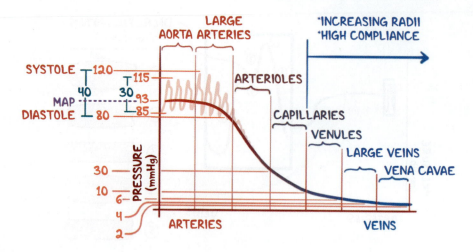

Figure 19.3 Visualizing pressures throughout the systemic cardiovascular system.

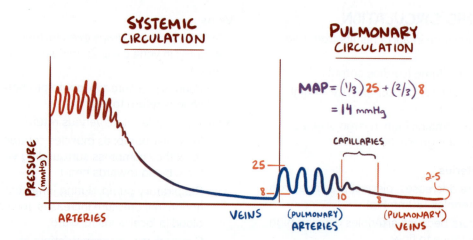

Figure 19.4 Visualizing pressures in the pulmonary circulation.

RESISTANCE TO BLOOD FLOW

osms.it/resistance-to-blood-flow

RESISTANCE

- Opposition to flow → amount friction as blood passes through blood vessels
- Determined by
  - Blood viscosity
  - Total length blood vessels
  - Diameter blood vessels

Poiseuille Equation

- Describes relationship between resistance, blood vessel diameter, blood viscosity

$$R = \frac{8\eta l}{\pi r^4}$$

- R = resistance
- η = blood viscosity
- l = length of blood vessel
- r^4 = radius (diameter) blood vessel raised to fourth power

Points expressed by Poiseuille equation

- Resistance to blood flow is directly proportional to blood viscosity, blood vessel length
- Resistance to flow is inversely proportional to radius to fourth power (r^4) → when radius decreases, resistance increases by fourth power → e.g radius decreases by one half, resistance increases 16-fold

SERIES & PARALLEL RESISTANCE

- Resistance also depends on blood vessel arrangement → series/parallel

Series resistance

- Sequential flow from one vessel to next
- Illustrated by arrangement of blood vessels within an organ
- Major artery → smaller arteries → arterioles → capillaries → venules → veins
- Total resistance of system arranged in series is equal to sum of individual resistances

$$R_{total} = R_{arteries} + R_{arterioles} + R_{capillaries} + R_{venules} + R_{veins}$$

- Blood flow at each part of system is identical but pressure decreases progressively (greatest decrease in arterioles)

Parallel resistance

- Simultaneous flow through each parallel vessel
- Illustrated by arrangement of arteries branching off aorta
- Cardiac output → aorta → branching → cerebral, coronary, renal system etc. → capillaries → venules → veins → vena cava → right atrium
- Total resistance less than any individual resistance

$$\frac{1}{R_{total}} = \frac{1}{R_1} + \frac{1}{R_2} + \frac{1}{R_3} + \frac{1}{R_4} + \frac{1}{R_5} + ...$$

- Numbered subscripts represent cerebral, renal, coronary, other systems
- Blood flow in each system is only small portion of total blood flow → no pressure lost in major arteries (remains same as in aorta)

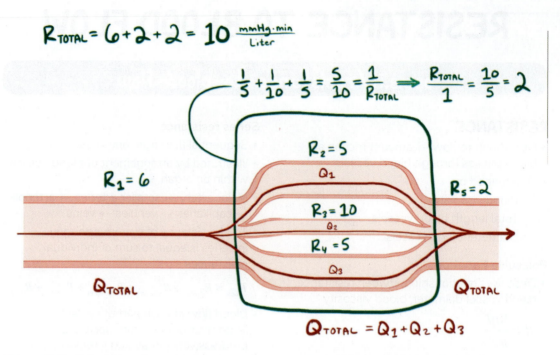

Figure 19.5 Calculating the total resistance for this system involves finding the total parallel resistance first and then adding R_1, $R_{Parallel}$, and R_5. The total blood flow in series, Q, is equal across all parts of the system. Individual vessels in the parallel system have different Qs, since the blood flow is split between each of the vessels, but they add up to Q_{Total}.

LAMINAR FLOW & REYNOLDS NUMBER

osms.it/laminar-flow-and-Reynolds-number

LAMINAR FLOW
- Smooth blood flow through blood vessels → blood velocity highest in center, lowest towards blood vessel walls → zero at walls

TURBULENT FLOW
- Laminar flow disrupted; blood flows axially, radially → kinetic energy wasted → more energy needed to drive blood

Reynolds Number
- Determines whether flow likely to be laminar/turbulent

$$N_R = \frac{\rho d v}{\eta}$$

  - N_R = Reynolds number
  - ρ = blood density
  - d = blood vessel diameter
  - v = blood flow velocity
  - η = blood viscosity
- As viscosity decreases (e.g. anemia), Reynolds number increases
- As velocity increases (e.g. increased cardiac output), Reynolds number increases
- Since velocity depends on diameter
  - $v = 4Q / \pi d^2$
  - Decrease in diameter (e.g. thrombus, atherosclerotic plaque) → velocity increases → Reynolds number increases
- Values of Reynolds number
  - If < 2000 → laminar flow
  - If > 2000 → increased likelihood of turbulent flow
  - If > 3000 → turbulent flow

SHEAR
- Friction between blood, vessel walls
  - Highest at vessel wall, lowest in center → difference in blood flow velocity
- Difference in velocity is parabolic → moving away from walls velocity increases quickly, near middle change in velocity low
- Shear inhibits red blood cell aggregation, lowers viscosity

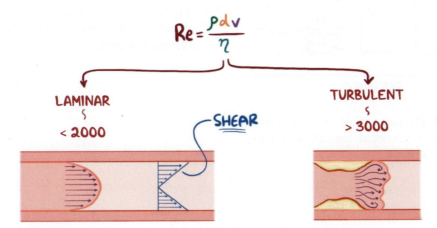

Figure 19.6 Reynolds number is a way to predict whether a fluid is going to be laminar (smooth) or turbulent. Differences in velocity across a blood vessel cause shear.

COMPLIANCE OF BLOOD VESSELS

osms.it/compliance-of-blood-vessels

COMPLIANCE (C)
- AKA capacitance/distensibility: ability of blood vessels to distend, hold an amount of blood with pressure changes
- C = V / P
  - C = compliance of blood vessel (mL/mmHg)
  - V = volume of blood (mL)
  - P = pressure (mmHg)
- High volume, low pressure → high compliance (veins); low volume, high pressure → low compliance (arteries)
- Arteriosclerosis → low compliance → low ability to hold an amount of blood at same pressure → blood backs up in veins
  - Arteries also become less compliant with age
  - If compliance decreases in veins (venoconstriction) → volume decreases (shift from veins to arteries)

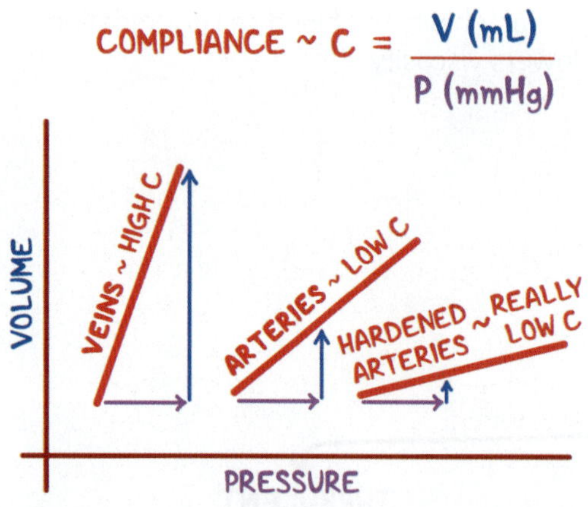

$$\text{COMPLIANCE} \sim C = \frac{V\ (mL)}{P\ (mmHg)}$$

Figure 19.7 The same pressure will expand the volumes of vessels differently depending on their compliance.

ELASTANCE (E)
- Inverse of compliance
  - Blood vessel ability to recoil back after distension
- E = P / V
  - E = elastance of blood vessel (mmHg/mL)
  - P = pressure (mmHg)
  - V = volume of blood (mL)

During systole
- Heart contracts → transfers kinetic energy (140mmHg) to blood → stretches aortic elastic wall, where some kinetic energy stored as elastic energy of walls (form of potential energy) → blood pressure drops to 120mmHg (systolic pressure)

During diastole
- Heart relaxes, aortic valves close → kinetic energy drops to 50mmHg → potential energy of stretched aortic walls adds to kinetic energy again when walls recoil → pressure rises to 60mmHg (diastolic pressure) → allows blood to move forward during diastole
- *Pulse pressure:* 120mmHg - 60mmHg = 60mmHg
- Elastance buffers, dampens pulse pressure → Windkessel effect
- Without elastic properties, blood pressure would be 140/50mmHg with pulse pressure 90mmHg

Chapter 19 Cardiovascular Physiology: Hemodynamics

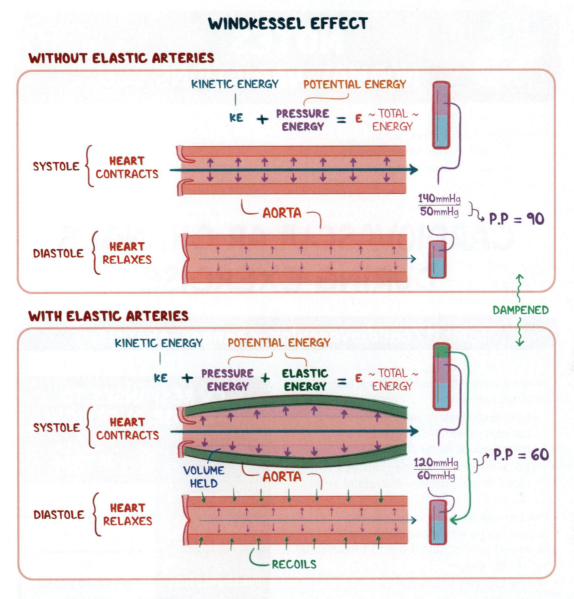

Figure 19.8 *Windkessel effect:* elastance dampens pulse pressure by lowering systolic pressure and increasing diastolic pressure.

Systole: aorta's walls stretch with high pressure contractions and store some energy as elastic energy. Since the total energy is the same as it would be without elastic arteries, there must be less kinetic energy and pressure energy to make room for the elastic energy → lower systolic blood pressure.

Diastole: elastic walls recoil, releasing the stored elastic energy and converting it to pressure energy and kinetic energy → more pressure energy.

NOTES
NORMAL VARIATIONS

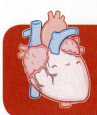

- Physiological adaptations within cardiovascular system in response to changes such as hemorrhage, exercise, postural changes

CARDIOVASCULAR CHANGES DURING EXERCISE

osms.it/cardiovascular-changes-exercise

- Involves central nervous system (CNS), local mechanisms
    - **CNS responses:** changes in autonomic nervous system (ANS) due to inputs from cerebral motor cortex
    - **Local responses:** exercise causes ↑ blood flow, O_2 delivery to skeletal muscles
- Exercise results in ↑ sympathetic (ß1 receptors), ↓ parasympathetic activity to heart → ↑ cardiac output due to ↑ heart rate + ↑ stroke volume
- Muscle changes also occur
    - ↑ metabolites (lactate, potassium, adenosine) are produced → metabolites stimulate local vasodilation → ↑ blood flow → ↓ overall total peripheral resistance (TPR)

OVERALL RESPONSE TO EXERCISE

- **Central command:** ↑ cardiac output (CO), vasoconstriction in some vascular beds (excludes exercising skeletal muscle, cerebral, coronary circulations)
    - ↑ CO → ↑ heart rate, contractility
    - ↑ contractility → ↑ stroke volume → ↑ pulse pressure
    - ↑ CO due to ↑ venous return (sympathetic vein constriction, squeezing action of skeletal muscle on veins)

CV RESPONSES TO EXERCISE OVERVIEW

	RESPONSE
HEART RATE	↑↑
STROKE VOLUME	↑
PULSE PRESSURE	↑ (increased stroke volume)
CARDIAC OUTPUT	↑↑
VENOUS RETURN	↑
MEAN ARTERIAL PRESSURE	↑ (slight)
TPR	↓↓
ARTERIOVENOUS O_2 DIFFERENCE	↑↑ (increased tissue O_2 composition)

Chapter 20 Cardiovascular Physiology: Normal Variations of the Cardiovascular System

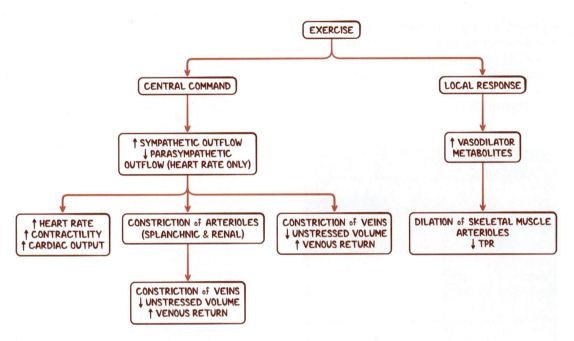

Figure 20.1 Flowchart showing cardiovascular response to exercise.

CARDIOVASCULAR CHANGES DURING HEMORRHAGE

osms.it/cardiovascular-changes-hemorrhage

- Blood loss → ↓ arterial pressure → compensatory responses to restore arterial pressure
  - Response mediated by baroreceptor reflex, renin-angiotensin-aldosterone system (RAAS), vascular actions

Decrease in arterial pressure
- Hemorrhage → ↓ total blood volume → ↓ venous return to heart, ↓ right atrial pressure → ↓ cardiac output → ↓ P_a as a product of cardiac output, TPR

Return of arterial pressure
- Baroreceptors in carotid sinus detect ↓ P_a → relay information to medulla via carotid sinus nerve → ↑ sympathetic outflow to heart, blood vessels; ↓ parasympathetic outflow to heart → ↑ heart rate, ↑ contractility, ↑ TPR, constriction of veins
- ↓ mean arterial pressure → ↓ perfusion to kidney → response via RAAS
  - Kidney secretes renin from renal juxtaglomerular cells → ↑ angiotensin I production → converted to angiotensin II (causes arteriolar vasoconstriction, stimulates aldosterone secretion)
- Capillary changes favor fluid reabsorption
  - ↑ sympathetic outflow to blood vessels, angiotensin II → arteriolar vasoconstriction → ↓ capillary hydrostatic pressure (P_c) → restricts filtration out of capillaries, favors absorption

OTHER RESPONSES IN HEMORRHAGE

- Hypoxemia (↓ arterial P_{O2}): carotid, aortic bodies chemoreceptors sense ↓ P_{O2} → ↑ sympathetic outflow to blood vessels → ↑ vasoconstriction, TPR, P_a
- Cerebral ischemia: local ↑ P_{CO2}

- ↓ blood volume → ↓ return of blood to heart → detection by atria volume receptors → ADH secretion to maintain adequate blood pressure → water reabsorption by renal collecting ducts → arteriolar vasoconstriction

CV RESPONSES TO HEMORRHAGE OVERVIEW	
	RESPONSE
CAROTID SINUS NERVE FINDING RATE	↓
HEART RATE	↑
CONTRACTILITY	↑
CARDIAC OUTPUT	↑
UNSTRESSED VOLUME	↓ (produces increased venous return)
TPR	↑
RENIN	↑
ANGIOTENSIN II	↑
ALDOSTERONE	↑
CIRCULATING EPINEPHRINE	↑ (secreted from adrenal medulla)
ANTIDIURETIC HORMONE (ADH)	↑ (stimulated by decreased blood volume)

Chapter 20 Cardiovascular Physiology: Normal Variations of the Cardiovascular System

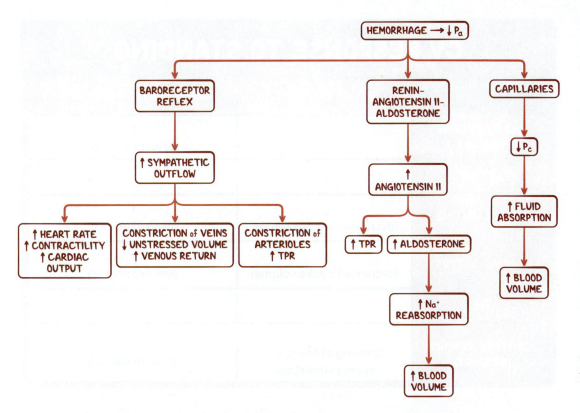

Figure 20.2 Flowchart showing cardiovascular responses to hemorrhage.

CARDIOVASCULAR CHANGES DURING POSTURAL CHANGE

osms.it/cardiovascular-changes-postural

- Standing up quickly → lightheadedness, sometimes fainting (due to delayed constriction of lower extremity blood vessels → orthostatic hypotension)
    - ↓ in systolic blood pressure > 20mmHg/ diastolic blood pressure > 10mmHg within three minutes of standing
- *Initiating event*: pooling of blood in extremities
    - *Moving from supine to standing position*: blood pools in veins of lower extremities → ↓ venous return to heart, ↓ cardiac output → ↓ mean arterial pressure
    - Venous pooling → ↑ hydrostatic pressure in leg veins → ↑ fluid filtration into interstitial fluid, ↓ intravascular volume
    - Severe ↓ blood pressure → syncope

Response of baroreceptor reflex

- Responsible for homeostatic blood pressure maintenance
- Carotid sinus baroreceptors detect ↓ P_a → sends information to medullary vasomotor center → inactivates medulla vagal neurons, activates sympathetic neurons → ↑ sympathetic outflow to heart, blood vessels, ↓ parasympathetic outflow to heart to normalize P_a
- ↑ systemic vascular resistance, cardiac output act in negative feedback mechanism to maintain P_a

CV RESPONSE TO STANDING

	INITIAL RESPONSE	COMPENSATORY RESPONSE
MEAN ARTERIAL PRESSURE	↓	↑ (toward normal)
HEART RATE	–	↑
STROKE VOLUME	↓ (decreased venous return)	↑ (toward normal)
CARDIAC OUTPUT	↓ (decreased stroke volume)	↑ (toward normal)
TPR	–	↑
CENTRAL VENOUS PRESSURE	↓ (pooling of blood in lower extremities)	↑ (toward normal)

Chapter 20 Cardiovascular Physiology: Normal Variations of the Cardiovascular System

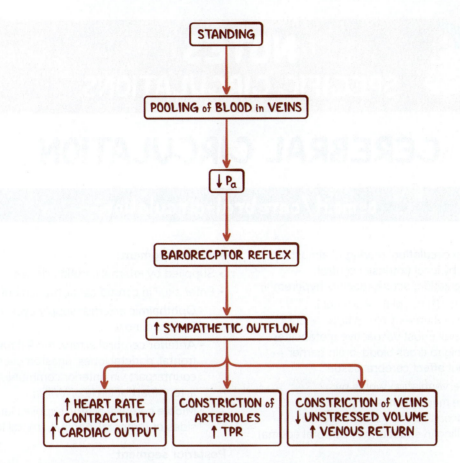

Figure 20.3 Flowchart showing cardiovascular response to postural change.

NOTES
SPECIFIC CIRCULATIONS

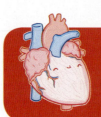

CEREBRAL CIRCULATION

osms.it/cerebral-circulation

- **Cerebral circulation:** managed almost entirely by local (intrinsic) control (autoregulation; active, reactive hyperemia)
  - ↑ pCO_2 (↑H^+, ↓pH) → arteriolar vasodilation → ↑ blood flow → CO_2 removal (most vasoactive metabolites too big to cross blood-brain barrier → do not affect cerebral tissue
  - **Hyperventilation** works by same mechanism → ↓ pCO_2 → vasoconstriction (used to reduce swelling in situations of cerebral edema)

CEREBRAL BLOOD SUPPLY SEGMENTATION

- Cerebral blood supply separated into anterior, posterior segments
- Anterior, posterior circulatory segments join via arterial posterior communicating arteries, form circle of Willis
  - Back-up circulation in case of blood vessel occlusion

Anterior segment
- Supplied by internal carotid arteries
- Enter skull in carotid canal, branch out
  - **Ophthalmic arteries:** supply eyes, orbits, forehead, nose
  - **Anterior cerebral artery:** medial part of frontal, parietal lobes; anastomoses with counterpart via anterior communicating artery (part of circle of Willis)
  - **Middle cerebral artery:** supplies lateral sides of temporal, parietal, frontal lobes

Posterior segment
- Supplied by vertebral arteries
- Enter skull through foramen magnum, branch out
  - Right, left vertebral arteries fuse in skull → basilar artery which supplies brainstem, cerebellum, pons
  - **Posterior cerebral arteries:** supply occipital lobes, inferior parts of temporal lobes

Chapter 21 Cardiovascular Physiology: Specific Circulations

CORONARY CIRCULATION

osms.it/coronary-circulation

- **Coronary arteries:** blood vessels delivering oxygenated blood to heart (myocardium)
- **Cardiac veins:** blood vessels retrieving deoxygenated blood from heart

CORONARY ARTERIES

- Two coronary arteries emerge from base of aorta, surround heart in coronary sulcus

Left coronary artery

- Two branches; supplies left atrium, left ventricle, interventricular septum
  - *Circumflex artery:* supplies left atrium, posterior wall of left ventricle
  - *Anterior interventricular artery:* supplies interventricular septum, anterior walls of ventricles

Right coronary artery

- Two branches; supplies right atrium, right ventricle, part of left ventricle, electrical conduction system
  - *Right marginal artery:* supplies lateral right side of heart, superficial parts of ventricle
  - *Posterior interventricular artery:* supplies interventricular septum, posterior walls of ventricles

CORONARY CIRCULATION CONTROL

- Coronary circulation managed primarily by local (intrinsic) control, secondarily by sympathetic nervous system
- ↑ oxygen demand → ↑ blood flow
- Active hyperemia via local (intrinsic) control triggers
  - Hypoxia → build-up of metabolites ADP, AMP → degraded to adenosine (potent vasodilator) → binds to coronary vascular smooth muscle → ↓ calcium influx into cells → vasodilation → ↑ blood flow, oxygen delivery
- Other intrinsic control of vascular tone provided by endothelial factors
  - *Endothelium-derived nitric oxide:* relaxes arterial smooth muscle
  - *Prostacyclin:* vasodilator
  - *Endothelium-derived hyperpolarizing factor (EDHF):* vasodilator
  - *Endothelin 1:* vasoconstrictor
- Reactive hyperemia
  - Brief arterial occlusion period during systole → ↓ blood flow → ↑ O_2 debt → vasodilation during diastole → ↑ blood flow → O_2 demands are met

CONTROL OF BLOOD FLOW CIRCULATION

osms.it/blood-flow

- Blood flow regulation
    - *Intrinsic (local):* humoral, myogenic control
    - *Extrinsic (systemic):* hormonal, neural

LOCAL (INTRINSIC) BLOOD FLOW CONTROL

Mechanisms

- *Humoral:* mediated by vasoactive substances
    - Histamine, nitric oxide (arteriole dilation)
    - Endothelin, serotonin
- *Autoregulation:* maintains constant blood flow via direct control of arterial resistance
    - Present in organs such as kidneys, brain, heart, skeletal muscle (e.g. ↓ coronary artery pressure → compensatory arteriole vasodilation → ↓ vessel resistance → constant blood flow)
- *Active hyperemia:* ↑ blood flow directed to organ/tissue associated with ↑ metabolic activity (e.g. ↑ blood flow in active skeletal muscle)
- *Reactive hyperemia:* temporary ↑ blood flow following ischemia (↓ blood flow) in organ (e.g. arterial occlusion → ↓ blood flow → ↑ O_2 debt → vasodilation, ↑ blood flow)
- Myogenic hypothesis for autoregulation
    - *Focus on arteriolar resistance:* vascular smooth muscle contracts upon stretching (↑ wall tension) and vice versa
    - ↑ blood flow → arteriole stretching → contraction → ↑ resistance → constant blood flow
    - ↓ blood flow → ↓ arteriole stretching → relaxation → ↓ resistance → constant blood flow
    - *Explained by law of Laplace:* ↑ pressure (P) + ↓ radius (r) → tension (T) remains constant (T=P x r)

- Metabolic hypothesis for autoregulation, active, reactive hyperemia
    - O_2 distribution changes in response to O_2 consumption via altering arteriolar resistance
    - ↑ metabolism → ↑ vasodilating metabolites (CO_2, H^+, K^+, lactate, adenosine) → arteriole vasodilation → ↓ resistance → ↑ blood flow, O_2 distribution
    - Certain tissues more susceptible to certain metabolites (coronary circulation—PO_2, adenosine; cerebral circulation—PCO_2)

NEURAL & HORMONAL (EXTRINSIC) CONTROL

- *Neural:* sympathetic nervous system acts on vascular smooth muscle
    - *α1:* vasoconstriction → skin, intestines
    - *β2:* vasodilation → lungs, skeletal muscles
- *Hormonal:* vasopressin released from anterior pituitary → vasoconstriction

MICROCIRCULATION & STARLING FORCES

osms.it/microcirculation-starling-forces

- **Microcirculation:** vascular network involving capillaries, lymphatic vessels

Capillaries
- **Vessels:** thin walls lined with endothelial cells
- Arterioles → metarterioles → capillaries → venules → veins
    - Metarterioles end in precapillary sphincters → smooth muscle ring controls blood flow/capillary exchange rate by constricting/relaxing
    - Capillary blood flow regulated by intrinsic (local), extrinsic (systemic) control

CAPILLARY EXCHANGE
- **Capillaries:** exchange sites for nutrients, waste, fluids between interstitial, vascular space
    - *Afferent blood:* capillaries → interstitial space → tissue
    - *Efferent blood:* tissue → interstitial space → capillaries

Capillary exchange types
- **Simple diffusion:** substance exchange through lipid bilayer/between capillary wall's epithelial cells
    - Depends on driving force (partial pressure gradient), available diffusion area
    - *Driving force:* substances move across their own partial pressure gradient (towards ↓ concentration area)
    - Lipid soluble substances (O_2, CO_2) pass through lipid bilayer
    - Water soluble substances (ions, glucose, amino acids) pass between endothelial cells through fluid-filled intercellular clefts/fenestrations
- **Vesicular transport:** large molecule exchange (proteins) via pinocytic vesicles (caveolae)
    - In some tissues (kidney, intestine) proteins pass through capillary fenestrations
- **Osmosis:** if capillary wall has aqueous pores, pressure gradient across membrane, driven by Starling forces

STARLING FORCES
- **Capillary filtration/absorption depend on Starling forces:** hydrostatic, colloid osmotic (oncotic) pressure
    - *Filtration:* fluid movement from capillaries → interstitium
    - *Absorption:* fluid movement from interstitium → capillaries

Hydrostatic pressure
- Pressure exerted by fluid against capillary wall
- **Capillary** hydrostatic pressure (P_c)
    - *Favors filtration:* tends to move fluid out of capillaries
    - Blood pressure ↓ throughout capillary beds → arterial (37mmHg) > venous (17mmHg) pressure
- **Interstitial fluid** hydrostatic pressure (P_i)
    - *Opposes filtration:* pressure exerted outside capillary wall
    - Tends to move fluid into capillary
    - Contains very little fluid → P_i considered zero, slightly positive/slightly negative (1mmHg)

Colloid osmotic pressure (oncotic pressure)
- *Pressure gradient:* large non-diffusible molecules (e.g. plasma proteins)
    - Capillary oncotic pressure (π_c) (25mmHg): created by plasma proteins (primarily albumin; reflection coefficient = 1.0); opposes filtration

- Interstitial oncotic pressure (π_i) (0mmHg): contains very little protein; favors filtration

Flow direction
- Arterial end of capillary
  - Blood pressure's outward driving force > inwardly directed oncotic pressure force → fluid moves out of vessel
- Venous end of capillary
  - Oncotic pressure inward driving force > outwardly directed hydrostatic pressure → fluid moves into vessel
- Most fluid leaving capillary at arterial end reenters capillary before leaving venous end
- Fluid remaining in interstitial space recovered by lymphatic vessels
- Fluid movement through capillary wall is dependent on Starling force

Starling equation
- $J_v = K_f [(P_c - P_i) - (\pi_c - \pi_i)]$
  - J_v = fluid movement (mL/min)
  - K_f = hydraulic conductance (wall to water permeability; depends on tissue, wall structure—e.g. fenestrated, non-fenestrated)

LYMPH
- Lymphatic capillaries drain excess fluid + some proteins from interstitial space into venous system
  - Lymphatic capillaries → lymphatic vessels → thoracic duct/right lymphatic duct → subclavian vein
  - One way valves → unidirectional flow

Edema
- Abnormal buildup of fluid in interstitial space
- Causes
  - Imbalance of Starling forces
  - ↑ hydrostatic capillary pressure (↑ volume—e.g. heart failure; obstruction; e.g. thrombosis)
  - ↓ oncotic capillary pressure (↓ plasma protein—e.g. liver failure, malnourishment, nephrotic syndrome
  - ↑ capillary permeability (burns/inflammation)
  - Impaired drainage (immobility; lack of/irradiated lymphatic nodes; parasitic infections of lymphatic nodes—e.g. filariasis)

NOTES
THERMOREGULATION

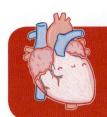

CARDIOVASCULAR TEMPERATURE HOMEOSTASIS

osms.it/cardiovascular-temperature-homeostasis

NORMAL BODY TEMPERATURE
- 37 ± 0.5 °C (98.6 ± 0.9 °F)
- Hypothalamic thermoregulatory center acts as a thermostat
    - Sets temperature set-point
- Thermoreceptors
    - Peripheral (in skin) → sense surface temperature
    - Central (in the body core—e.g. hypothalamus itself) → sense core temperature
- Temperature variations activate thermoreceptors → thermoreceptors inform hypothalamus → hypothalamus activates heat regulation mechanisms → temperature returns to baseline
- Body region variations
    - Core: higher temperature, more stable
    - Skin: lower temperature, more variable
- Core temperature varies with throughout the day
    - Lower during sleep
    - Higher when awake

BODY TEMPERATURE MAINTENANCE
- Body temperature maintained by balancing heat-generation, heat loss

Heat generation
- Activation of sympathetic nervous system
    - Vasoconstriction of skin arterioles → blood bypasses skin → ↓ heat loss
    - Adrenal glands release catecholamines (epinephrine, norepinephrine) → increased metabolic rate → ↑ heat production
    - Piloerection (goosebumps) → heat trapping
- Thyroid hormones released from hypothalamus → ↑ metabolic rate → ↑ heat production
- Non-shivering thermogenesis using brown adipose tissue
    - Activation of primary motor center for shivering in the posterior hypothalamus → skeletal muscle contraction → shivering → ↑ heat production
    - Behavioral changes (adding garments, tightening the arms across the chest, moving around)

Heat dissipation
- Inhibition of sympathetic activity in skin blood vessels → blood goes to skin → ↑ heat loss
- Activation of sympathetic cholinergic fibers innervating sweat glands → ↑ sweating → ↑ heat loss
- Behavioral changes (removing garments, reducing movements, fanning air over body)

Fever
- Body temperature elevation due to change in hypothalamic set-point
- Pyrogens act on hypothalamus → hypothalamus releases prostaglandins → hypothalamic set-point temperature increases → heat-generating mechanisms kicks in → body temperature rises and

reaches new baseline temperature
- Aspirin reduces fever by inhibiting prostaglandins production
- Benefits of fever
  - Inhibit bacterial growth by making growing conditions less favorable
  - Increase efficiency of immune cells

HYPERTHERMIA

- Elevation of body temperature without change in hypothalamic set-point
- Normal mechanisms of thermoregulation are overwhelmed by various factors
  - Excessive environmental temperature
  - Impaired ability to dissipate heat
  - Excessive heat production

Heat exhaustion

- Excessive sweating → significant water and electrolyte loss → ↓ blood volume → ↓ arterial pressure

Heat stroke

- Hyperthermia > 40°C/105.1°F
- Potentially fatal
- Causes
  - High environmental temperature
  - Periods of intense physical activity
- Risk factors
  - *Susceptible individuals*: infants, children (higher metabolic rate; ineffective sweating; physical, psychological limitations); elderly (pre-existing conditions; physical, psychological limitations)
  - *Medications*: ones that inhibit heat-dissipating mechanisms (beta blockers, diuretics)

Malignant hyperthermia

- Genetic alteration of ryanodine receptor 1 (RYR1) in the muscle cells
- *Normally*: cell depolarization → RYR1 activation → calcium release from sarcoplasmic reticulum into cytoplasm → muscle contraction
- *In malignant hyperthermia*: cell depolarization → RYR1 hyperactivation → excessive calcium release → inappropriate muscle contraction, ↑↑ metabolic rate → excessive heat production
- Triggered by drugs
  - *Anesthetic gas*: Alothane, Sevoflurane, Desflurane
  - *Depolarizing muscle relaxants*: Succinylcholine, Decamethonium
- Potentially fatal
- Treatment
  - Dantrolene (skeletal muscle relaxant)

HYPOTHERMIA

- Abnormally low temperature
  - *Diagnosis*: core temperature < 35°C/95°F
- Compensatory mechanisms responding to cold stress are overwhelmed
- ↓ core body temperature → ↓↓ metabolic rate → myocardial irritability, cold diuresis (↓ renal blood flow, water resorption)
  - Progressive oliguria as ↓ core temperature → ↓ intravascular volume, ↑ hematocrit, central nervous system depression

Risk factors

- Prolonged cold exposure
  - E.g. inadequate clothing/shelter, cold water immersion
- Impaired thermoregulation
  - E.g. hypothalamic dysfunction, metabolic derangement
- ↑ heat loss
  - Multisystem trauma, shock, spinal cord transection
- Iatrogenic
  - Cold IV fluid administration, inadequate operating room warming
- ↑ risk populations
  - Older adults (↓ physiologic reserve, ↓ sensory perception, chronic medical conditions)
  - Children (↑ body surface area to body mass ratio, ↓ glycogen stores, young infants unable to use shivering thermogenesis)

Complications

- Cardiac arrhythmias, myocardial infarction, pulmonary edema, pulmonary embolism, lactic acidosis, disseminated intravascular coagulation (DIC), coma, death

Signs & symptoms
- Mild hypothermia
  - Core temperature 32–35°C/90–95°F
  - Shivering, tachypnea, tachycardia, confusion
- Moderate hypothermia
  - Core temperature 28–32°C/82–90°F
  - ↓ shivering and muscle rigidity, hypoventilation, bradycardia, ↓ cardiac output, lethargy, arrhythmias, loss of pupillary reflexes
- Severe hypothermia
  - Core temperature < 28°C/82°F
  - Apnea, ↓ cardiac activity → ventricular arrhythmias → asystole, coma, loss of ocular reflexes, ↓↓ metabolic rate

Rewarming treatment
- Warmed blankets/forced warm-air system; heated, humidified oxygen; warmed crystalloid IV fluid; pleural, peritoneal lavage using warm saline solution; vasopressors
- Extracorporeal blood rewarming
  - Venovenous rewarming, hemodialysis, continuous arteriovenous rewarming (CAVR), cardiopulmonary bypass (CPB), extracorporeal membrane oxygenation (ECMO)

NOTES
CELLULAR STRUCTURES & PROCESSES

CELLULAR STRUCTURE & FUNCTION

osms.it/cellular-structure-and-function

CELL STRUCTURE BASICS
- Basic structural, biological, functional unit that comprise organism
- Smallest self-replicating life-form
- Over 200 types in human body
- Cells → tissue → organ → organ systems → organism

Basic constituents
- Plasma membrane
- Cytoplasm
    - Fluid suspension
    - **Composition:** cytosol, organelles

CYTOSOL
- Intracellular fluid
    - **Composition:** water; dissolved/suspended organic, inorganic chemicals; macromolecules; pigments; organelles
- Site of most cellular activity

ORGANELLES
- Specialized cellular subunits carry out essential functions

Ribosomes
- **Composition:** rRNA, ribosomal proteins
- Can exist freely in cytoplasm/bound to endoplasmic reticulum (forms rough endoplasmic reticulum)
- Turns mRNA into protein via translation
- Organized into two subunits (40s, 60s)
    - *Small subunit:* binding sites for mRNA, tRNA
    - *Larger subunit:* has ribozyme to catalyze peptide bond formation (for bonds between amino acids)

Endoplasmic reticulum
- Membrane-enclosed organelle
- **Appearance:** stack of membranous, flattened disks (cisterns)
- Rough endoplasmic reticulum (RER)
    - Contains bound ribosomes on surface
    - Site of packaging, folding of proteins designated for secretion, lysosomal degradation, plasma membrane insertion; proteins packed into vesicles, sent to Golgi apparatus for further modification
    - RER cisterna continuous with nuclear envelope
- Smooth endoplasmic reticulum (SER)
    - No ribosomes
    - Site of lipid, steroid synthesis, Ca^{2+} ions storage (muscles), glycogen metabolism, detoxification (liver)

Golgi apparatus (complex)
- Membrane-enclosed organelle
    - **Appearance:** collection of fused, flattened sacs (cisterns) with associated vesicles, vacuoles
- Two sides
    - *Cis side:* receives proteins from RER (entry)
    - *Trans side:* opposite side, releases vesicles towards plasma membrane (exit)

- Post-translational modification site (e.g. phosphorylation, glycosylation, sulfonation) of proteins, lipids, hormones → sorted, packaged into secretory vesicles → secreted out of cell/lysosomal fusion/plasma membrane insertion

Mitochondria

- Double membrane-enclosed organelle; synthesizes ATP for cell via aerobic respiration
    - *Outer smooth membrane*: encloses whole organelle
    - *Inner membrane*: forms folds, caverns called cristae (contain proteins needed for aerobic respiration); encloses mitochondrial matrix (contains mitochondrial DNA, ribosomes)
- *Intermembrane space*: space between inner, outer membrane
- In cytoplasm glucose undergoes glycolysis, glucose cleaved into pyruvate
    - Pyruvate enters mitochondria → citric acid cycle (Krebs cycle), electron transport chain (require oxygen)
- In glucose absence, mitochondria can use fatty acids as fuel via beta oxidation (only medium sized fatty acids used; longer ones chopped by peroxisome)
- *Mitochondria number*: correlates with cell activity/energy requirements

Nucleus

- Large, membrane-enclosed organelle present in all cells except mature erythrocytes
- Contains genetic material (DNA, tightly packed into chromatin); coordinates cellular activities
- Most cells contain one nucleus; some cells have more (e.g. skeletal muscle cells, osteoclasts, hepatocytes)
- Usually spherical, may take on other shapes
    - Lobulated (e.g. polymorphonuclear leukocytes)
    - Elongated (e.g. columnar epithelium)

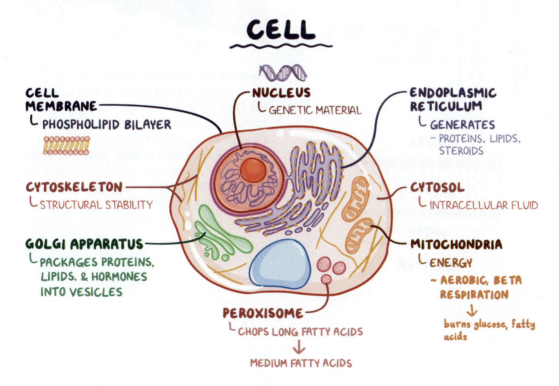

Figure 23.1 Cellular structures and their functions.

CELL MEMBRANE

osms.it/cell-membrane

- Semipermeable membrane made from phospholipid bilayer; surrounds cell cytoplasm

Phospholipid bilayer
- Two-layered polar phospholipid molecules comprising two parts
  - Negatively charged phosphate "head" (hydrophilic; oriented outwards)
  - Fatty acid "tail" (hydrophobic; oriented inwards)

- Semipermeable
  - Allows passage of certain molecules through membrane (O_2, CO_2, etc.)
  - Denies passage of others (large molecules such as proteins, glucose)
- Certain molecule transportation (ions, H_2O) allowed through embedded membrane proteins (ion channels, pumps)

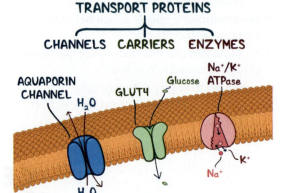

Figure 23.3 Transport proteins move molecules that can't freely diffuse across the cell membrane. Channels form a tunnel through which water and ions flow. Carriers have a binding site for a specific molecule and gates at both ends that open sequentially. Enzymes, or ATPases, actively pump ions in/out of the cell against their concentration gradients.

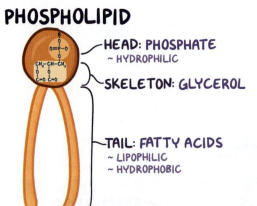

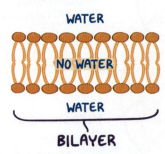

Figure 23.2 Phospholipid parts and their arrangement in a cell membrane.

SELECTIVE PERMEABILITY OF THE CELL MEMBRANE

osms.it/cell-membrane-selective-permeability

- Cell membrane controls which molecules enter, leave
  - *Passive transport*: no energy required
  - *Active transport*: energy required → adenosine triphosphate (ATP)

PASSIVE TRANSPORT

Simple diffusion
- Random molecular motion
- Small, nonpolar molecules move from ↑ concentration → ↓ concentration

Fick's law
- Three factors affect diffusive flux
- Concentration gradient
  - Larger differences in solute concentration on each side of membrane → ↑ driving force → ↑ net diffusion
  - Equal concentrations → no net diffusion (e.g. CO_2, O_2 movement between alveoli, blood)
- Membrane surface area
  - ↑ surface area available for diffusion → ↑ diffusion rate; vice versa (e.g. microvilli in small intestines amplify surface area → ↑ nutrient, water absorption)
- Distance separating each side of membrane (e.g. thickness)
  - ↑ distance molecules must travel → ↓ net diffusion; vice versa (e.g. pulmonary edema → ↑ distance between compartments → ↓ net diffusion)

Facilitated diffusion
- Uses transport proteins (e.g. channels, carrier proteins)
- Allows larger/polar molecules to move across membrane

Channels
- Non-specific; open to allow water, small polar molecules through (e.g. voltage-gated calcium channel)

Carrier proteins
- Very specific, only allow certain molecules to bind (e.g. glucose transporter protein GLUT4)

ACTIVE TRANSPORT

Primary
- Uses ATP
  - Enzymes called ATPases use ATP as fuel; (e.g. Na^+-K^+ ATPase, Ca^{2+} ATPase, H^+-K^+ ATPase)
  - May create concentration/electrochemical gradients

Secondary
- Uses existing electrochemical gradients
  - One solute, normally Na^+, moves with concentration gradient through transporter → supplies energy transporter needs to → another solute against concentration gradient in same/opposite direction as Na^+ (e.g. sodium-glucose SGLT1 transporter)

Bulk transport
- AKA vesicular transport
- Endocytosis
  - Cell membrane invaginates, pulling something in from outside (e.g. pathogen phagocytosis)
- Exocytosis
  - Vesicle inside cell pushes something out (e.g. hormone secretion)

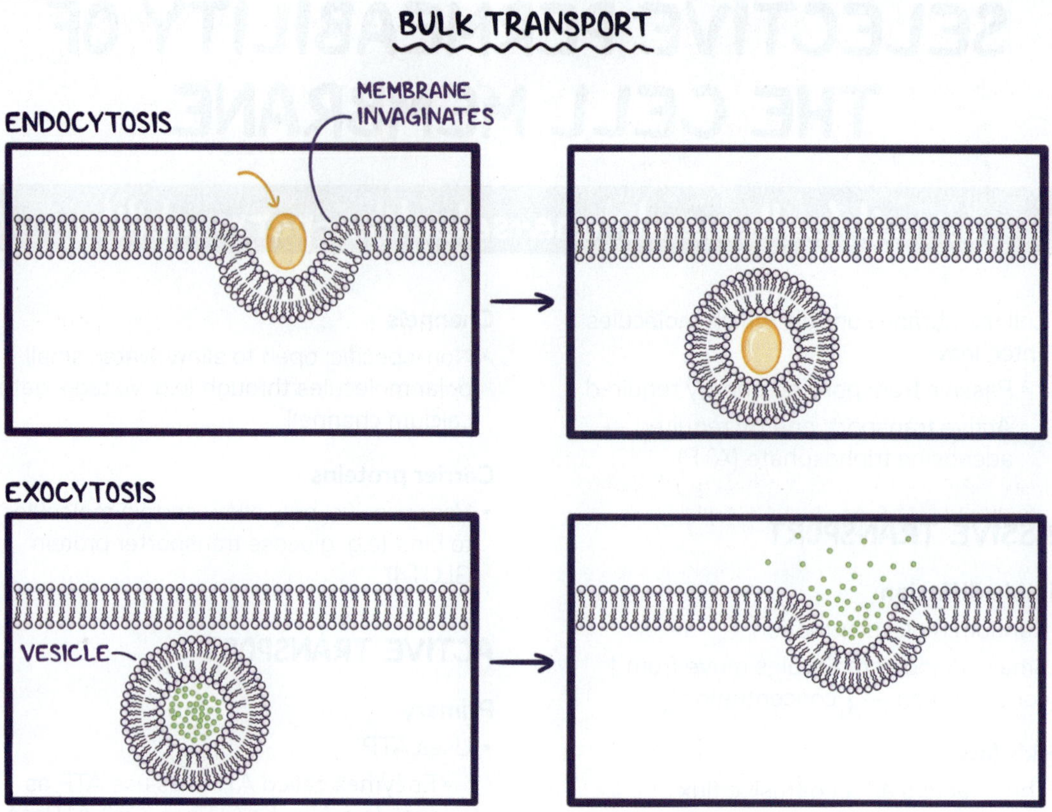

BULK TRANSPORT

ENDOCYTOSIS — MEMBRANE INVAGINATES

EXOCYTOSIS — VESICLE

Figure 23.4 Endocytosis and exocytosis.

EXTRACELLULAR MATRIX

osms.it/extracellular-matrix

- Environment surrounding cells
- Varies between tissues (epithelial, connective, muscular, and nervous)

THREE MAJOR MOLECULES

Adhesive proteins
- Adhere cells together (communication with extracellular fluid)
  - E.g. integrins, cadherins

Structural proteins
- Give tissues tensile, compressive strength
- Collagen
  - Resists tension, can stretch
  - Starts as procollagen → cleaved into tropocollagen → arranged into collagen fibrils
  - **Four types:** type I (bone, skin, tendon), type II (cartilage), type III (reticulin, blood vessels), type IV (basement membrane)
- Elastin
  - Elastic, returns tissue to original shape
- Keratin
  - Tough, found in hair, nails

Proteoglycans
- Fill space between cells, hydrate, cushion cells
  - Consists of protein core with sugar chains

Chapter 23 Cellular Physiology: Cellular Structures & Processes

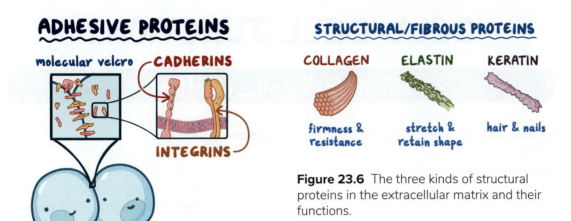

Figure 23.5 Cadherins and integrins are both adhesive proteins which hold cells together.

Figure 23.6 The three kinds of structural proteins in the extracellular matrix and their functions.

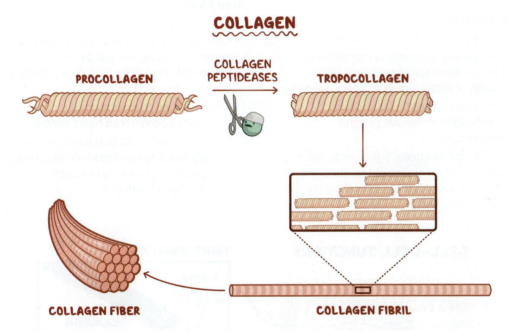

Figure 23.7 Collagen production steps.

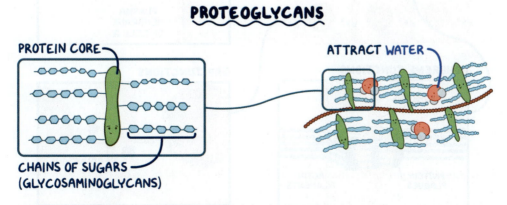

Figure 23.8 Structure of proteoglycans, which hydrate and cushion cells.

OSMOSIS.ORG 165

CELL-CELL JUNCTIONS

osms.it/cell-cell_junctions

- Protein structures that physically connect cells
- Improve cellular communication, tissue structure; allow transport of some substances between cells, create impermeable barrier for others
- Only found between immobile cells; abundant in epithelial tissue (e.g. in skin)

THREE JUNCTION TYPES

Tight junctions
- E.g. in gastrointestinal tract/brain
- Seal adjacent-cell plasma membranes, especially near apical surface; prevent passage of water, small proteins, bacteria
    - Formed by claudins, occludins embedded in cellular plasma membranes
    - In "leaky" epithelia, tight junctions may allow certain molecules to pass (e.g. K^+, Na^+, Cl^- in kidney's proximal tubules—due to ion pores)

Adherens junctions
- E.g. in skin
- Anchor cells together, provide strength; consist of three major components
    - Actin filaments: provide cellular shape
    - Protein plaques: anchor membrane, bind to actin filaments
    - Cadherins: attach to protein plaques, connect to cadherins on other cells

Gap junctions
- E.g. in heart
- Connect adjacent cells, allow rapid communication; formed by connexins → create tubular structure (allows charged particles to pass)
    - In cardiac myocytes: gap junctions create coordinated heart contractions
    - In infected cells: gap junctions send cytokines to neighboring cells, triggering apoptosis, preventing infectious spread ("bystander effect")

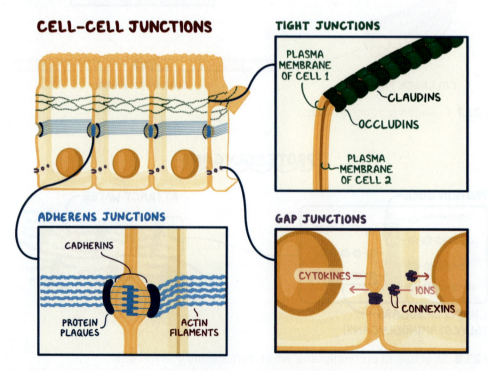

Figure 23.9 The three types of cell junctions.

ENDOCYTOSIS & EXOCYTOSIS

osms.it/endocytosis-and-exocytosis

- Transports material in/out of cell
- Requires adenosine triphosphate (ATP) for energy

ENDOCYTOSIS
- Cells engulf extracellular material

PHAGOCYTOSIS
- AKA cell eating
- Used by white blood cells (e.g. macrophages, neutrophils)

Process
- Cell extends arm-like projects (AKA pseudopods) around target
- Cell membrane slowly engulfs target, invaginates to form vesicle
- Vesicle separates from cell membrane to form phagosome
- Phagosome fuses with lysosome, target is digested
- Debris released by exocytosis

PINOCYTOSIS
- AKA cell drinking
- Used by most cells to take in extracellular fluid; non-specific

Process
- Cell membrane invaginates around extracellular fluid
- Edges of invagination come together to form vesicle
- Motor proteins use ATP to carry vesicle into cytosol

RECEPTOR-MEDIATED ENDOCYTOSIS
- Used by cells to take in specific molecules (e.g. iron, cholesterol)

Process
- Clathrin-covered pits/coated pits with receptors bind certain molecules
- Edges of pit come together, clathrin proteins link up
- Vesicle pinches off; clathrin detaches, returns to cell membrane
- Vesicle merges with endosome to separate receptors into second vesicle

PHAGOCYTOSIS

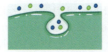
PINOCYTOSIS

RECEPTOR-MEDIATED ENDOCYTOSIS

Figure 23.10 The three types of endocytosis.

EXOCYTOSIS
- Cells expel material into extracellular space (e.g. neurotransmitters, hormones)
- Last phagocytosis step

Process
- Golgi apparatus creates vesicle from various proteins, lipids, hormones
- Motor proteins use ATP to carry vesicle along cytoskeleton
- Vesicle is pressed against cell membrane until rupture → spills contents into extracellular space

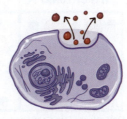

Figure 23.11 Exocytosis: expulsion of material into extracellular space.

OSMOSIS

osms.it/osmosis

- Passive water-flow across selectively permeable (semipermeable) cellular membrane; primarily determined by solute concentration differences (osmotic pressure)

Factors affecting water movement across membrane

- Molecules (e.g. water molecules, ions) tend to move around (kinetic energy) + movement is disordered, random (entropy) → larger solutes tend to block openings in semipermeable membrane
- If solute ions positively charged, they attract slightly negatively charged oxygen atom in water molecule; if solute ions are negatively charged, they attract slightly positively charged hydrogen atoms in water molecule → water molecules partially attached to ion → movement through membrane impeded
- Water molecules tend to move from hypotonic side (more water/less solutes) to hypertonic side (less water/more solutes)

SELECTIVELY-PERMEABLE MEMBRANE

- Allows small molecules (e.g. water) across, but not larger molecules/ions

Isotonic solution

- Side A = side B
- If solute concentration is same on each side of membrane → net water movement across membrane is zero (equilibrium)

Hypertonic/hypotonic solution

- Side A > side B or side B > side A
- If solute concentration is greater on one side (hypertonic) → net water migration across membrane is from hypotonic side toward hypertonic side

CELLULAR EFFECT

- Red blood cell in hypertonic solution → net movement of water molecules out of cell → cell shrinks (crenation)
- Red blood cell in hypotonic solution → net movement of water molecules into cell → cell swells, may burst (lyses)

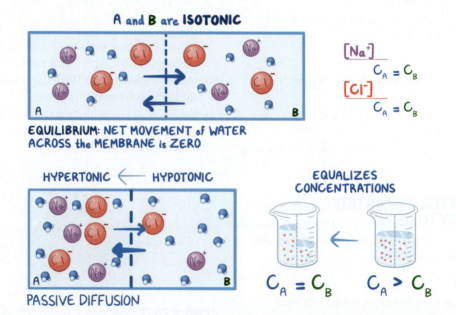

Figure 23.12 Net water molecule movement between isotonic, hyper/hypotonic solutions.

RESTING MEMBRANE POTENTIAL

osms.it/resting-membrane-potential

- Electric potential across cell membrane
  - Given by weighted (based on membrane permeability) sum of equilibrium potentials for all ions
- High concentrations of Na^+, Cl^-, Ca^{2+} outside cell; high concentrations of K^+, A^- (various anions) inside cell → concentration gradients are established
  - Sodium-potassium pump uses ATP to move two K ions into cell, three Na ions out
  - Potassium concentration = 150mMol/L inside cell, 5mMol/L outside
- Concentration gradients establish electrostatic gradients
  - Concentration gradient pushes potassium out through potassium leak channels, inward rectifier channels
  - Anions remain in cell → negative charge builds up → potassium is pulled back into cell
- **Equilibrium (Nernst) potential:** electrostatic gradient equal to concentration gradient (-92mV for potassium)
- **Nernst equation:** equilibrium potential for an ion
  - Single charge: $V_m = 61.5 \times \log\left(\frac{[ION]_{out}}{[ION]_{in}}\right)$
  - Double charge: $V_m = 30.75 \times \log\left(\frac{[ION]_{out}}{[ION]_{in}}\right)$
    - Value is flipped for negative ions
- Resting membrane potential is sum of equilibrium potentials of major ions multiplied by their membrane permeabilities

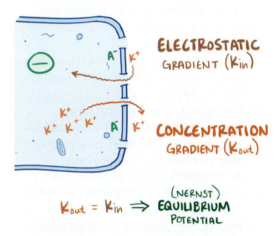

Figure 23.13 Equilibrium potential = electric potential for attracting K^+ back into the cell that's needed to balance the concentration gradient pushing K^+ out of the cell.

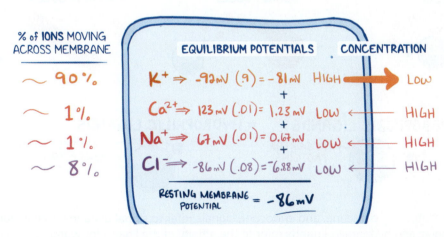

Figure 23.14 The resting membrane potential is closest to the equilibrium potential of the most permeable ion (K^+). Change in permeability → change in resting membrane potential.

CELL SIGNALING PATHWAYS

osms.it/cell-signaling-pathways

INTRACELLULAR SIGNAL CLASSIFICATION

- Classified according to distance between signaling, target cells
    - *Autocrine*: cell signals nearby cells of same type, including itself (e.g. monocytes secrete interleukin-1 β)
    - *Paracrine*: cell signals nearby cells of different type (e.g. ECL cells secrete histamine → signals D cells to secrete somatostatin)
    - *Endocrine*: cell signals distant cells (e.g. pituitary gland secretes TSH → signals thyroid gland)
- Signalling molecules (ligands) bind to receptors; can be hydrophobic/hydrophilic
    - *Hydrophobic*: can't float in extracellular space → brought to target cells by hydrophilic carrier proteins; can diffuse over cell membranes → bind to receptors inside cell
    - *Hydrophilic*: can float in extracellular space → reach target cells themselves; can't diffuse over cell membranes → bind to cell surface (transmembrane) receptors

Cell signalling pathway stages

1. *Reception*: ligand binds to receptor
2. *Transduction*: receptor changes activating intracellular molecules
3. *Response*: signal triggers a response in the target cell

MAJOR TRANSMEMBRANE RECEPTOR CLASSES

G protein-coupled receptors

- Seven-pass transmembrane receptors
- Activate guanine nucleotide-binding (G) proteins inside cell
    - G proteins have three subunits: alpha, beta, gamma
    - Alpha binds guanosine diphosphate (GDP) when inactive
    - When ligand binds, alpha releases GDP, binds guanosine triphosphate (GTP) instead → alpha separates from beta, gamma → alpha interacts with proteins turning GTP back into GDP → reattaches

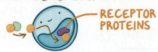
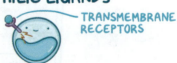

Figure 23.15 Autocrine, paracrine, and endocrine signals refer to signal distance from its target cell. Hydrophobic and hydrophilic ligands refer to the affinity of the ligand for water.

Chapter 23 Cellular Physiology: Cellular Structures & Processes

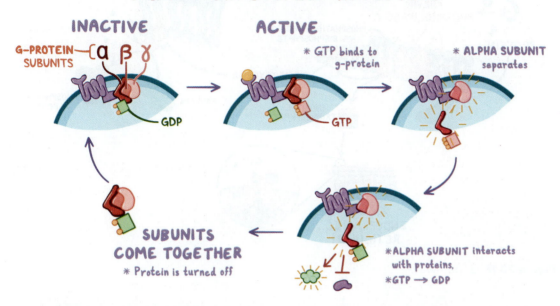

Figure 23.16 Mechanism of action of G-protein coupled receptors.

- Three types of G protein with different pathways
  - G_q: activates phospholipase C in cell membrane → phospholipase C cleaves phosphatidylinositol 4,5-bisphosphate into inositol trisphosphate, diacylglycerol → inositol trisphosphate opens calcium channels in endoplasmic reticulum (calcium flows to cytoplasm, changing electrical charge distribution in cell → cell depolarization); diacylglycerol binds to protein kinase C which phosphorylates target proteins
  - G_s: stimulates adenylate cyclase → adenylate cyclase removes phosphate from adenosine triphosphate (ATP) creating cyclic adenosine monophosphate (cAMP) → cAMP binds to regulatory subunit of protein kinase A → catalytic subunit of protein kinase A phosphorylates target proteins
  - G_i: inhibits adenylate cyclase → negative feedback on G_s

Enzyme-coupled receptors
- Single-pass transmembrane receptors
- Trigger enzymatic activity inside cell when specific ligands bind

- **Composition:** extracellular, ligand-binding domain; intracellular, enzymatic domain
- Three main enzyme-coupled receptor types
  - *Receptor tyrosine kinases:* when ligand binds, these phosphorylate their own tyrosine residues → conformational change creates binding site for other signalling proteins
  - *Tyrosine kinase associated receptors:* when ligand binds, these phosphorylate various proteins to relay signal to tyrosine kinases inside cell
  - *Receptor serine/threonine kinases:* when ligand binds, type II receptors of this kind phosphorylate type I receptors, which in turn phosphorylate various proteins to relay signal to serine/threonine kinase domain inside cell

Ion channel receptors
- Ion channels which open when specific ligands bind
- Allow ions (e.g. chloride, calcium, sodium, potassium) to flow through
- Resulting shift in electric charge distribution triggers response

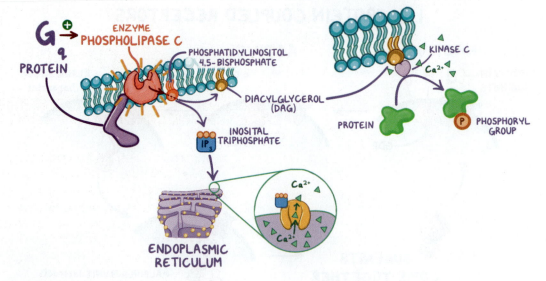

Figure 23.17 G_q pathway.

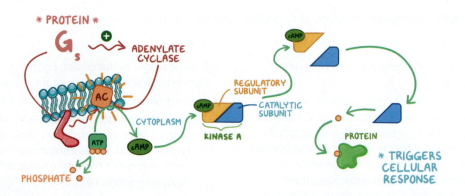

Figure 23.18 G_s pathway.

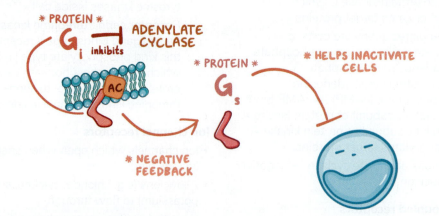

Figure 23.19 G_i pathway.

II. ENZYME-COUPLED RECEPTORS

1. RECEPTOR TYROSINE KINASE

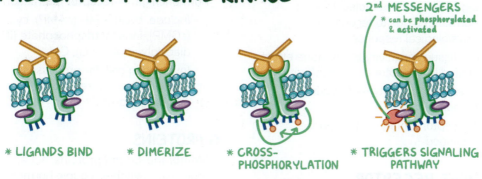

2. TYROSINE KINASE ASSOCIATED RECEPTORS

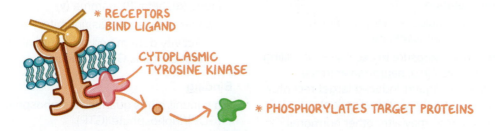

3. RECEPTOR SERINE/THREONINE KINASE

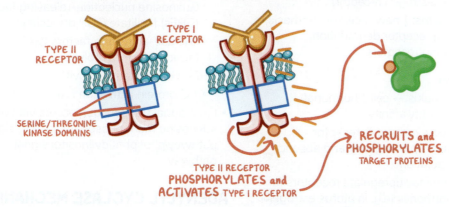

Figure 23.20 Types of enzyme-coupled receptors and their pathways.

III. ION CHANNEL RECEPTORS

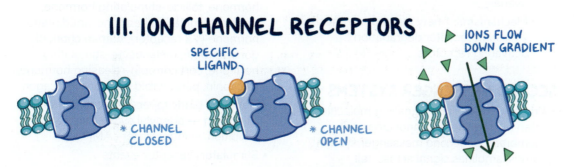

Figure 23.21 Mechanism of action for ion channel receptors.

HORMONAL MECHANISMS

- All cells receive, process outside signals via specific proteins (receptors)
    - Ligand (signalling molecule—e.g. hormone) binds to receptor → physiological response
- Target tissue sensitivity to hormone effect controlled by receptor quantity/affinity
    - ↑ receptor quantity → ↑ maximal response
    - ↑ receptor affinity → ↑ response likelihood

HORMONE RECEPTOR UPREGULATION/DOWNREGULATION

Downregulation

- External stimulus → cell ↓ hormonal receptor quantity/affinity
    - Chronic exposure to excessive signalling molecules (e.g. neurotransmitters/drugs → ligand-induced target receptor desensitization/internalization)
    - Hormones may alter other hormonal receptor sensitivity (e.g. in uterus—progesterone downregulates its own receptor, estrogen receptor)
    - *Mechanisms:* ↓ new receptor synthesis, ↑ existing receptor degradation, inactivating receptors

Upregulation

- External stimulus → cell ↑ hormonal receptor quantity/affinity
    - Repeated exposure to receptor antagonists/prolonged ligand absence → upregulation
    - Hormone may upregulate receptors for other hormones (e.g. in uterus estrogen upregulates its own receptor, also luteinizing hormone (LH) receptors in ovaries)
    - *Mechanisms:* ↑ new receptor synthesis, ↓ existing receptor degradation, activating receptors

SECOND MESSENGER SYSTEMS

- Primary extracellular signalling molecules often hydrophilic → cannot cross cell membrane → second messenger system carries, amplifies signal across cell membrane
- *Second messengers:* intracellular signalling molecules released by cells → triggers physiological changes in response to hormone/ligand–receptor interaction
    - *Include:* cyclic AMP (cAMP), cyclic GMP (cGMP), inositol trisphosphate (IP3), diacylglycerol (DAG), Ca^{2+}
    - *Involved in cellular processes:* proliferation, differentiation, migration, survival, apoptosis

G PROTEINS

- *Membrane-bound proteins:* act as molecular switches, couple hormone receptors to effector enzymes
- Heterotrimeric proteins → three subunits → alpha (α), beta (β), gamma (γ)
- Can be stimulatory (Gs)/inhibitory (Gi)
    - Activity determined by α subunit (αs/αi), that contains GTPase activity

Binding

- α subunit binds guanosine diphosphate (GDP)/triphosphate (GTP)
    - GDP binding → inactive state
    - GTP binding → active state → coupling
    - Guanosine nucleotide-releasing factors (GRFs) facilitate GDP dissociation
    - GTPase-activating factors (GAPs) facilitate GTP hydrolysis
- GRFs, GAPs relative activity
    - ↑ G protein activation rate
- Final signal transduction occurs via cyclic adenosine monophosphate (cAMP) signal pathway/phosphatidylinositol signal pathway

ADENYLYL CYCLASE MECHANISM

- *Hormones acting via cAMP mechanism:* adrenocorticotropic hormone, luteinizing hormone, follicle-stimulating hormone, thyroid-stimulating hormone, antidiuretic hormone (V2 receptor), human chorionic gonadotropin, melanocyte-stimulating hormone, corticotropin-releasing hormone, calcitonin, parathyroid hormone, glucagon
- Hormone binds to receptor coupled to Gs/Gi protein → adenylyl cyclase activation/inhibition → intracellular cAMP ↑/↓
- Stimulatory receptor events
    - Hormone binds to receptor →

conformational change in αs subunit → αs subunit releases GDP → replacement by GTP → αs subunit detaches from Gs protein
- αs subunit-GTP complex migrates within cellular membrane → binds → activates adenylyl cyclase
- Activated adenylyl cyclase catalyzes adenosine triphosphate (ATP) → ↑ cAMP (second messenger)
- Intrinsic GTPase activity in G protein → GTP converts → GDP → αs subunit inactive again
- cAMP acts as second messenger → hormonal signal amplification → final physiological reaction
- Intracellular cAMP → protein kinase A activation → intracellular protein phosphorylation → physiological response
- Phosphodiesterase degrades intracellular cAMP → 5' adenosine monophosphate (inactive metabolite) → hormonal response cessation

PHOSPHOLIPASE C MECHANISM

- *Hormones acting via phospholipase C mechanism:* gonadotropin-releasing hormone, thyrotropin-releasing hormone, growth hormone-releasing hormone, angiotensin II, antidiuretic hormone (V1 receptor), oxytocin
- *Receptor Gq phospholipase C complex:* embedded in cell membrane
- In neutral state (no bound hormone) αq subunit binds GDP → inactive Gq protein
- Hormone binding → GDP release from αq subunit → GTP binding → αq subunit detaches from Gq protein
  - αq-GTP complex migrates within cell membrane → activates phospholipase C → DAG, IP3 released from phosphatidylinositol 4,5-diphosphate (PIP2)
  - IP3 → Ca^{2+} intracellular stores released (from endoplasmic/sarcoplasmic reticulum)
  - DAG, IP3 → activate protein kinase C → protein phosphorylation → physiological response

STEROID HORMONE MECHANISM

- *Hormones acting via steroid hormone mechanism:* glucocorticoids, estrogens, progesterone, testosterone, aldosterone, 1,25-dihydroxycholecalciferol, thyroid hormone
- No cell membrane-mediated transduction step
  - Steroid hormone diffuses across cell membrane → binds to cytosolic (or nuclear) receptor proteins (monomeric phosphoproteins) → DNA transcription, protein synthesis initiated
- Receptor proteins
  - Part of intracellular receptor gene superfamily
  - Each receptor protein has six domains (A–F)
  - Steroid hormone binds E domain near C terminus (central C domain binds to DNA via zinc fingers)
- Steroid-receptor protein complex → conformational change in receptor protein → activation → enters nucleus
- Hormone-receptor complex combines with similar hormone-receptor complex (dimerization)
- New complex binds at C-domain via zinc fingers to specific DNA sequences (steroid-responsive elements), located in target genes' 5' region
- DNA-bound active hormone-receptor complex acts as transcription factor for specific genes → messenger RNA (mRNA) transcription
- mRNA leaves nucleus → translated into new protein with physiological action specific to original hormone

TYROSINE KINASE MECHANISM

- *Hormones acting via tyrosine kinase mechanism:* insulin, insulin-like growth factor 1, growth hormone, prolactin
- *Primary mechanism:* tyrosine kinases phosphorylates protein tyrosine residues
- Two main categories
  - Receptor tyrosine kinases → intrinsic kinase activity within receptor

- Tyrosine kinase–associated receptors → no intrinsic kinase activity, associated noncovalently with proteins without kinase activity

Receptor tyrosine kinases (RTKs)
- Three structural domains
  - *Extracellular binding domain*: binds hormone
  - *Hydrophobic transmembrane domain*: membrane anchor
  - *Intracellular domain*: tyrosine kinase activity
- Hormone binding → activation
  - Activation → phosphorylates itself, other proteins
- Monomer-type RTKs
  - E.g. epidermal growth factor receptors, nerve growth factor
  - Hormone binding to extracellular domain → receptor dimerization → intrinsic tyrosine kinase activation → tyrosine moieties phosphorylation of itself, other proteins → physiological response
- Dimer-type RTKs
  - E.g. insulin, insulin-like growth factor receptors
  - Hormone binding → intrinsic tyrosine kinase activation → tyrosine moieties phosphorylation of itself, other proteins → physiological response

Tyrosine kinase-associated receptors
- E.g. growth hormone
- Three structural domains
  - *Extracellular binding domain*: binds hormone
  - *Hydrophobic transmembrane domain*: membrane anchor
  - *Intracellular domain*: no tyrosine kinase activity; non-covalently associated with tyrosine kinase (e.g. Janus kinase family)
  - Hormone binds to extracellular domain → receptor dimerization → associated protein's tyrosine kinase activated → tyrosine moieties phosphorylation of associated protein, hormone receptor, other proteins

GUANYLYL CYCLASE MECHANISM
- Hormones acting via guanylyl cyclase mechanism include: atrial natriuretic peptide, nitric oxide (NO)
- Extracellular receptor domain binds ligand; intracellular domain has guanylyl cyclase activity
- Ligand binding → guanylyl cyclase activation → GTP to cGMP conversion
- cGMP activates cGMP-dependent kinase → protein phosphorylation (proteins responsible for physiological response)

Intracellular forms (e.g. NO receptor)
- Cytosolic guanylyl cyclase mediates signal conversion
- NO synthase cleaves arginine (in vascular endothelial cells) → citrulline, NO
- NO diffuses from endothelial cells into adjacent vascular smooth muscle → binds, activates soluble (cytosolic) guanylyl cyclase → GTP conversion → cGMP → smooth muscle relaxation

SERINE/THREONINE KINASE MECHANISM
- Involved in cell proliferation regulation, apoptosis, cell differentiation, embryonic development
- G protein-linked receptors → adenylyl cyclase, phospholipase C-linked mechanism
- Hormone binding → protein kinase activation → serine, threonine moieties phosphorylation → physiological response
  - Ca^{2+}-calmodulin-dependent protein kinase (CaMK), mitogen-activated protein kinases (MAPKs) phosphorylate serine, threonine in subsequent reaction cascade

CYTOSKELETON & INTRACELLULAR MOTILITY

osms.it/cytoskeleton-and-intracellular-motility

- Non-membrane-bound organelles comprising complex protein filament network
- Provide structural stability, shape, organization, intracytoplasmic motility, cell motility

TYPES

Microfilaments
- Actin filaments: approx. 7nm
- Dynamic structures made of actin monomers
    - Arranged in long twisting chain
- Form network just below cell membrane
- Functions
    - *Muscle contraction*: slide closer together, further apart
    - *Diapedesis*: create pseudopodia for white blood cells (like neutrophils)
    - *Cell division*: allows cell to pinch-off, divide into two cells during mitosis
    - Microvilli function
    - Mechanical cell membrane support

Microtubules
- Approx. 25nm
- Dynamic structures made of alternating proteins
    - α- and β-tubulins; polymerize to form microtubules
- Stretch across cell
- Functions
    - Intracellular transport (e.g. vesicle movement, melanin transport within pigmented cells)
    - Structural integrity
    - Cell division (form mitotic spindle)
    - Cilia, flagella structural components

Intermediate filaments
- Approx. 8–10nm
- Static structures made of various fibrous proteins (e.g. keratin, desmin, vimentin) depending on cell type
- Rope-like structure; forms branching network
- Functions
    - Organelle, cell-cell anchoring
    - Play key role in providing structural integrity, cell shape

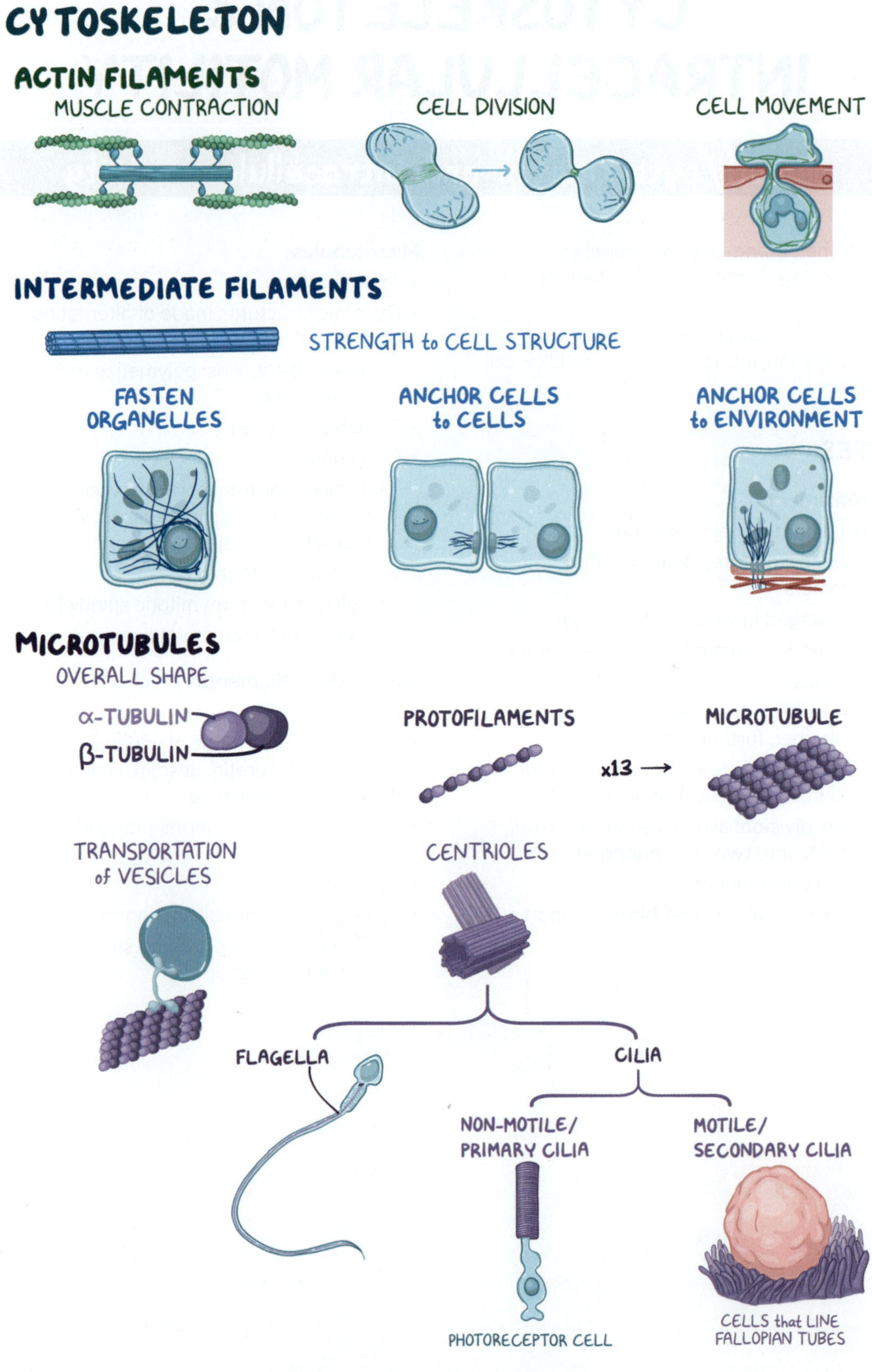

Figure 23.22 Cytoskeleton components and their functions.

NUCLEAR STRUCTURE

osms.it/nuclear-structure

NUCLEAR ENVELOPE
- Encloses, separates nucleus from cytoplasm
- Composed of selectively permeable membrane phospholipid bilayer

Nuclear pores
- Form where membranes fuse together at various intervals
- Each pore lined with nuclear pore complex (nucleoporin) to facilitate communication between nucleus, cytoplasm
- Allow bidirectional macromolecule movement

Outer membrane
- Anchoring proteins that hold nucleus in place within cytoplasm
- Continuous with RER

Inner membrane
- Covered by nuclear lamina
- Thin filamentous protein network, creates web within nucleus; provide support for chromatin

NUCLEOLUS
- Dense non-membrane-bound structure; some cells have more than one nucleolus
- Contains rDNA → transcribed into rRNA
- Assembles ribosomal subunits

NUCLEOPLASM
- Protoplasmic material
    - Composed of complex water, molecule, ion mixture
- Contains nucleolus, chromatin

CHROMATIN
- Helical fiber
    - Composed of 46 DNA molecules wrapped around proteins (histones)
- Histones help regulate DNA, gene expression
- Chromosomes become visible as chromatin fibers become tightly coiled during cellular division

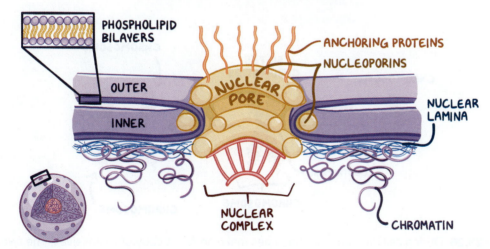

Figure 23.23 Nuclear envelope components.

Nucleosome
- Eight histones packed together in four stacks of two; DNA wraps around them twice
- Strung on strand of DNA-like "beads on string".

Two chromatin types
- *Euchromatin*: loosely packed DNA, actively being transcribed into RNA
- *Heterochromatin*: densely packed DNA, inactive (not being transcribed)

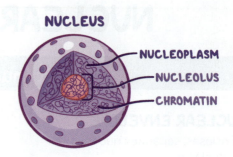

Figure 23.24 The nucleoplasm contains the nucleolus and chromatin.

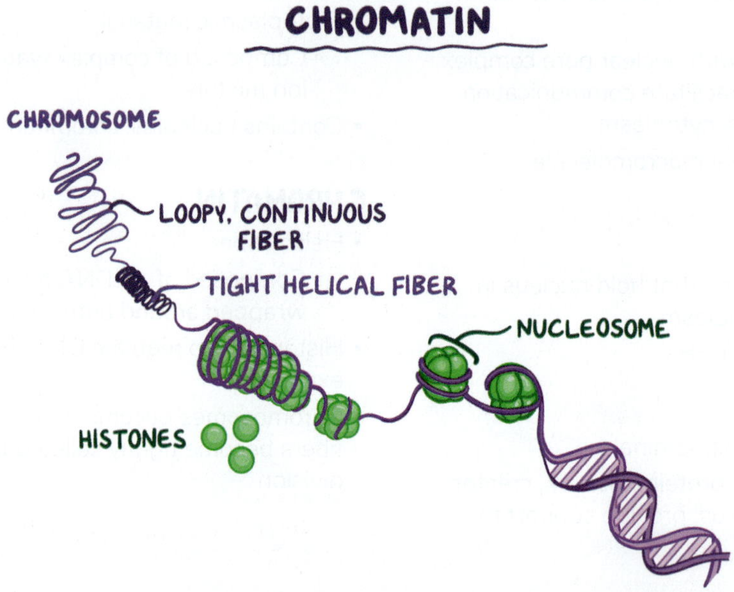

Figure 23.25 In the nucleus, DNA wraps around collections of histone proteins to form nucleosomes.

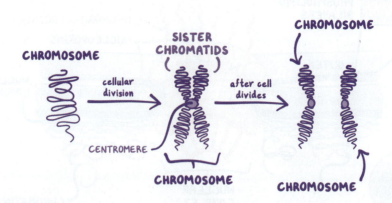

Figure 23.26 During cell division, chromosomes make an exact copy of themselves. The two are connected at the centromere. Each copy is called a sister chromatid. During cell division, the sister chromatids separate so that there is one copy of their genetic material in each daughter cell.

NOTES
CELLULAR PATHOLOGY

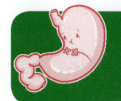

NECROSIS & APOPTOSIS

osms.it/necrosis-and-apoptosis

- Two main ways by which cells die

NECROSIS
- Cell death by injury/disease
    - External triggers (e.g. infection, temperature)
    - Internal triggers (e.g. ischemia)

Coagulative necrosis
- Occurs in hypoxic tissue
- Structural proteins bend out of shape
- Lysosomal proteins become ineffective at removing affected proteins
- Cell dies, some structure remains

Gangrenous necrosis
- Also occurs in hypoxic tissue
- **Dry gangrene:** tissue dries up
- **Wet gangrene:** if infection, liquefactive necrosis also occurs

Liquefactive necrosis
- Hydrolytic enzymes digest dead cells into creamy substance

Caseous necrosis
- Occurs in fungal/mycobacterial infections
- Cell disintegrate (not fully) → cottage cheese consistency

Fat necrosis
- Occurs in response to fatty organ trauma
- Adipose cell membranes ruptured
- Fatty acids combine with calcium, causing dystrophic calcifications
- Can occur in pancreas as result of inflammation (AKA pancreatitis)

Fibrinoid necrosis
- Occurs in malignant hypertension/vasculitis
- Fibrin/inflammation damages blood vessel walls

Also includes oncosis
- Toxins/ischemia damage mitochondria
- ATP can no longer be synthesized (e.g. ionic pumps)
- Sodium, water flow into cell → swelling
- Cell bursts, triggers inflammatory process

APOPTOSIS
- Programmed cell death
- Based on caspase cascade
    - Pro-caspases cleaved into caspases, activating caspase 3
    - Caspase 3 causes activation of cascade of caspase proteins
    - Cleaves various integral proteins, degrading cellular components (e.g. nucleus, organelles, cytoskeleton)
    - Cell loses structure, resulting in blebs, which break off, undergo phagocytosis

Intrinsic/mitochondrial pathway
- Induced by stress (e.g. radiation)
- Process
    - Intracellular proteins BAX, BAK pierce mitochondrial membrane
    - This allows SMACS, cytochrome C to flow out of mitochondria
    - SMACS binds to proteins that otherwise inhibit apoptosis
    - Cytochrome C binds to ATP, APAF-1, forming apoptosome
    - Pro-caspase 9 cleaves into caspase 9, activating caspase 3

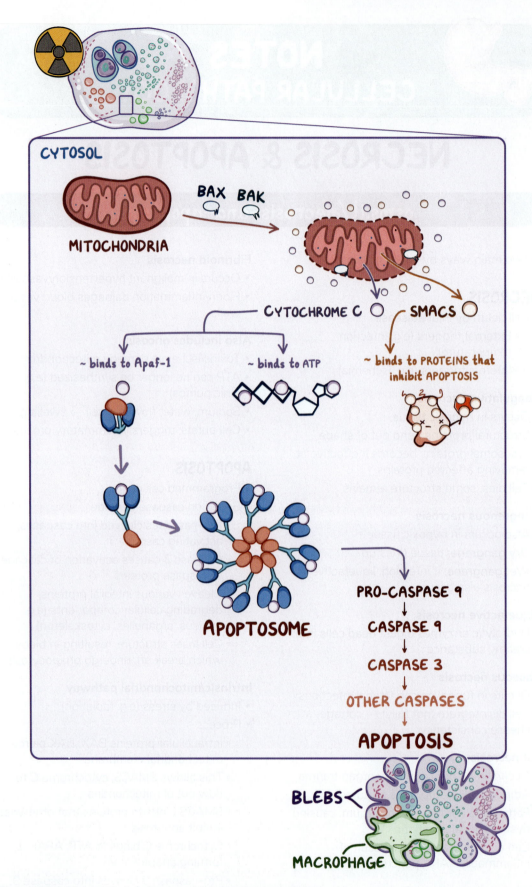

Figure 24.1 The intrinsic/mitochondrial apoptosis pathway.

Extrinsic/death receptor pathway
- Process
  - External cell initiates apoptosis by releasing various signaling proteins
  - Signaling proteins bind to death receptors on cell membrane
  - Cytosolic end of protein dives deep into cell (AKA death domain)
  - Death domain changes shape, binds various proteins to form internal signalling complex
  - Pro-caspase 8 cleaves into caspase 8, activating caspase 3

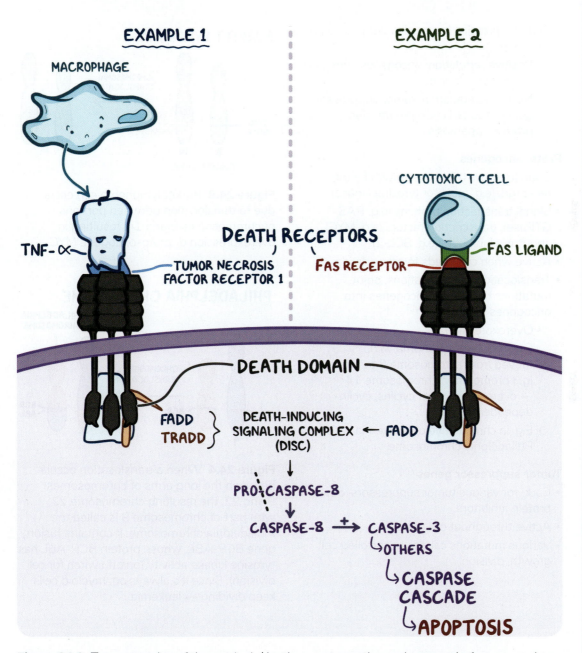

Figure 24.2 Two examples of the extrinsic/death receptor pathway. In example 1, a macrophage recognizes an old cell, a pathogenic cell, or a cell that has completed its task. It releases TNF-α, which binds to the death receptor tumor necrosis factor receptor 1. In example 2, when a cytotoxic T cell detects that a cell is expressing foreign antigens, the T cell expresses FAS ligand on its membrane. FAS ligand binds to the death receptor called FAS receptor. In both cases, the death domain binds other proteins to form DISC and the caspase cascade leads to apoptosis.

ONCOGENES & TUMOR SUPPRESSOR GENES

osms.it/oncogenes-tumor-suppressor-genes

- Code for proteins involved in progression of cell cycle
  - **Positive regulation:** oncogenes stimulate cell growth, division
  - **Negative regulation:** tumor suppressor genes stop cell cycle progression, promote apoptosis

Proto-oncogenes
- Code for growth factors, growth factor receptors (e.g. receptor tyrosine kinase)
- Signal transduction proteins (e.g. RAS GTPase), transcription factors (e.g. MYC), apoptosis inhibitors (e.g. BCL-2)
- Active when cell needs to grow, divide
- Translocations, amplifications, point mutations turn proto-oncogenes into oncogenes
  - Overexpression
  - E.g. in Burkitt lymphoma, MYC moved from chromosome 8 to near IgH promoter on chromosome 14 → overexpression of cyclins, cyclin-dependent kinases
  - E.g. in chronic myeloid leukemia with Philadelphia chromosome

Tumor suppressor genes
- Code for various tumor suppressors, other protein inhibitors
- Active throughout cell cycle
- Various mutations cause uncontrolled cell growth, division

BURKITT LYMPHOMA

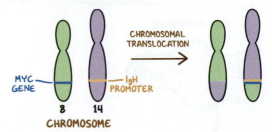

Figure 24.3 Burkitt lymphoma can occur due to translocation between portions of chromosomes 8 and 14, resulting in overexpression of proto-oncogene MYC.

PHILADELPHIA CHROMOSOME

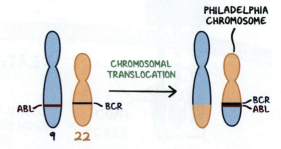

Figure 24.4 When a translocation occurs between the long arms of chromosomes 9 and 22, the resulting chromosome 22 with part of chromosome 9 is called the Philadelphia chromosome. It contains fusion gene *BCR-ABL*, whose protein BCR-ABL has tyrosine kinase activity (on/off switch for cell division). Since it's always on, myeloid cells keep dividing → leukemia.

HYPERPLASIA & HYPERTROPHY

osms.it/hyperplasia-hypertrophy

- Two ways by which cells adapt to stress
- Often happen together in tissues with stem cells

HYPERPLASIA

- Organ/tissue cells ↑ in number
- Only happens in organs with stem cells that can differentiate, mature

Types

- **Compensatory hyperplasia:** in organs that regenerate (e.g. skin)
- **Hormonal hyperplasia:** in organs regulated by hormones (e.g. endocrine)

Causes

- *Physiological processes:* e.g. pregnancy → enlargement of breast
- *Pathological processes:* e.g. excessive hormonal stimulation → excessive endometrial growth
- *Sometimes associated with cancer:* cells mutate → dysplasia

HYPERTROPHY

- Organ/tissue cells ↑ in size

Causes

- *Physiological processes:* e.g. ↑ functional demand → muscle cells produce more myofilaments
- *Pathological processes:* e.g. hypertension → cardiac myocytes produce more myofilaments

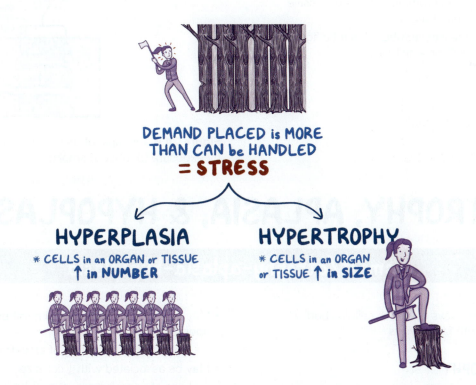

Figure 24.5 An analogy to describe the difference between hyperplasia and hypertrophy. When the workload is bigger than one lumberjack can handle, she gets stressed. Hyperplasia is like hiring more lumberjacks to help; hypertrophy is like the one lumberjack getting bigger and tougher so she can cut down more trees on her own.

METAPLASIA & DYSPLASIA

osms.it/metaplasia-and-dysplasia

METAPLASIA
- Mature differentiated cell transforms into new mature cell type
- Often caused by environmental stressor
  - E.g. tobacco smoke: pseudostratified columnar epithelial cells in airways → stratified squamous epithelium
- Reversible if stimulus reverted

DYSPLASIA
- Tissue develops large number of immature cells
- Precancerous state
- Four pathological changes to cell
  - Anisocytosis (AKA unequal cells)
  - Poikilocytosis (AKA abnormally-shaped cells)
  - Hyperchromatism (AKA excessive pigmentation)
  - Increases number of mitotic figures (AKA more mitosis)

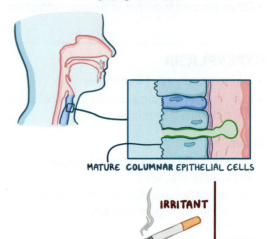

Figure 24.6 Example of metaplasia caused by exposure to tobacco smoke.

ATROPHY, APLASIA, & HYPOPLASIA

osms.it/atrophy-aplasia-hypoplasia

- Three ways by which cellular, bodily growth fails/reverts

ATROPHY
- Cell/organ/tissue size reduction
- Causes include disuse, denervation, ischemia, nutrient starvation, interruption of endocrine signals
- May be associated with ↓ cell number (e.g. apoptosis)
  - E.g. orthopedic casting of an extremity
- May be associated with ↓ cell size
  - Loss of nerve/hormonal supply
  - Ubiquitin proteasome pathway: proteasome destroys polyubiquitinated filaments/vacuoles destroy ubiquitin-

tagged organelles (e.g. muscle atrophy)

APLASIA
- Failure of organ/tissue to form properly
- Growth fails during embryogenesis with no precursor cells

HYPOPLASIA
- Reduced size/abnormal shape of organ/tissue
- Growth fails during embryogenesis in some precursor cells

FREE RADICALS & CELLULAR INJURY

osms.it/free-radicals-and-cellular-injury

FREE RADICAL
- Chemical species with unpaired electron in outer orbit
  - *Physiologic causes:* e.g. oxidative phosphorylation, enzyme activity
  - *Pathologic causes:* e.g. ionizing radiation, inflammation, metal interactions, drugs/chemicals)
- May result in cellular injury

FREE RADICAL CELLULAR INJURY MECHANISMS

Lipid peroxidation
- Free radicals "steal" electron from lipids on cell membrane
- Damages cell membrane, entire cell

Protein oxidation
- Free radicals oxidize proteins, including DNA, inside cell
  - DNA oxidation → mutations → cancer

DEFENSE AGAINST FREE RADICALS

Antioxidants
- E.g. vitamins A, C, E
- Eliminate free radicals by donating electrons

Metal carrier proteins
- E.g. transferrin for iron, ceruloplasmin for copper
- Bind, carry metals to prevent free radical production

Enzymes
- Eliminate various free radical species
  - Superoxide dismutase → superoxide
  - Catalase → hydrogen peroxide
  - Glutathione peroxidase → hydroxyl radical

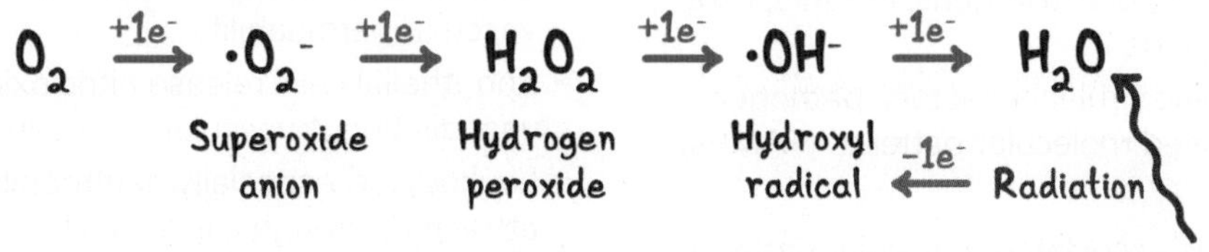

$$O_2 \xrightarrow{+1e^-} \cdot O_2^- \xrightarrow{+1e^-} H_2O_2 \xrightarrow{+1e^-} \cdot OH^- \underset{-1e^-}{\overset{+1e^-}{\rightleftarrows}} H_2O$$

Superoxide anion | Hydrogen peroxide | Hydroxyl radical | Radiation

Figure 24.7 Oxygen is an example of a molecule that can become a free radical.

ISCHEMIA

osms.it/ischemia

- Reduction in blood flow to organ/tissue → oxygen shortage
    - Caused by blockage/compression of blood vessel

Arterial ischemia
- ↓ arterial blood flow → ↓ oxygen received
- *E.g. atherosclerosis*: plaque blocks arteries to heart → ischemic heart disease

Venous ischemia
- ↓ venous blood flow → ↓ drainage → ↓ blood flow → ↓ oxygen received
- *E.g. Budd–Chiari syndrome*: clot blocks hepatic vein → liver ischemia → edema/hepatomegaly

Outcomes
- Sometimes, congestion → ↑↑ pressure → fluid forced out/edema
- ↓↓ oxygen → cell death (e.g. tissue necrosis, infarction)
    - *Ischemic penumbra*: ischemic but still viable tissue
    - *Collateralization*: growth of collateral vessels to serve ischemic tissue
- *Time to reperfusion*: time taken to re-establish perfusion before cells die
    - Short → cells survive → reversible
    - Long → cells die → irreversible

INFLAMMATION

osms.it/inflammation

- Immune response described by four key signs:
    - *Calor*: heat
    - *Dolor*: pain
    - *Rubor*: redness
    - *Tumor*: swelling
- May also involve "functio laesa" (AKA loss of function)
- Triggered by external, internal factors
- External
    - *Non-microbial*: allergens, irritants, toxic compounds
    - *Microbial*: virulence factors, pathogen associated molecular patterns (PAMPs)
- Internal
    - Damage associated molecular patterns (DAMPs)

Example process
- PAMPs, DAMPs recognized by pattern recognition receptors (PRRs) on immune cells
- Activate cells, sparking inflammatory response
- Mast cells contain granules with inflammatory mediators
    - E.g. histamine, serotonin, cytokines, and eicosanoids
- → separate endothelial cells on nearby capillaries
- Macrophages eat any invading pathogens
- Cytokines cause capillaries to enlarge, ↑ vascular permeability
- Endothelial cells release nitric oxide for vasodilation, ↑ vascular permeability
- Leukocytes, especially neutrophils, attracted through capillaries by chemokines, microbial products; squeeze through membrane
    - AKA extravasation
- Leukocyte follows gradient of inflammatory mediators

- Neutrophils phagocytose pathogens immediately before destroying themselves
- Antibodies bound to pathogens activate complement system
  - Aids in opsonization, kills pathogens by lysis
- Dendritic cells phagocytose pathogens, present antigens to T lymphocytes, activating adaptive immune system
- Ends with tissue repair

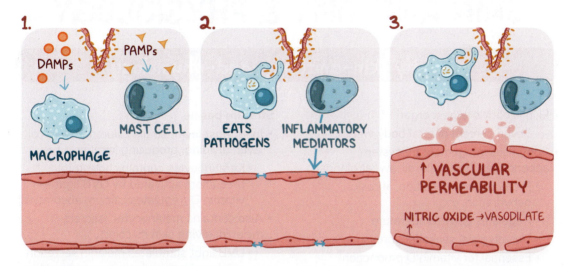

Figure 24.8 1: DAMPs and PAMPs activate immune cells. 2: Macrophages phagocytose pathogens at the site of inflammation. Mast cells release inflammatory mediators that widen the distance between adjacent endothelial cells. 3: Endothelial cells release nitric oxide → ↑ vasodilation, vascular permeability.

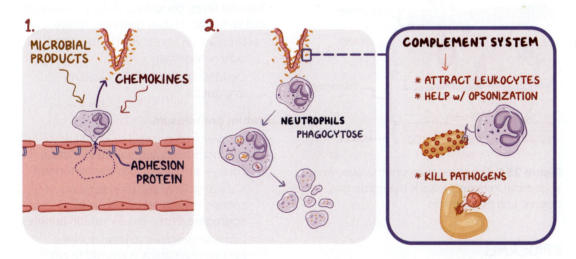

Figure 24.9 1: Neutrophils are the first leukocytes recruited during the acute inflammatory process. They squeeze through the gap between endothelial cells (extravasation) and follow the gradient of inflammatory mediators to the site of inflammation. 2: Neutrophils quickly phagocytose pathogens. While this is happening, complement proteins are activated by the presence of pathogens and help with opsonization (they bind to microbes so leukocytes can more easily eat them). Some can also kill pathogens by forming a channel in their membranes.

NOTES
SKIN STRUCTURES

SKIN ANATOMY & PHYSIOLOGY

osms.it/skin-anatomy-and-physiology

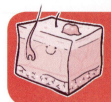

- Skin is body's largest organ
  - Seven percent of total body weight
- Comprises integumentary system, appendages (hair, nails, oil, sweat glands)
  - Protects body (infection, abrasion, dehydration, etc)
  - Regulates body temperature
  - Detects pain, sensation, pressure
  - Essential for vitamin D production
- Three layer division
  - Epidermis, dermis, hypodermis

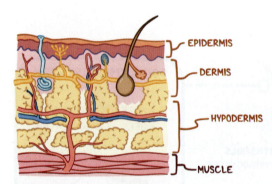

Figure 25.1 The three layers of the skin, from superficial to deep, include: the epidermis, dermis, and hypodermis.

EPIDERMIS

- Epidermis
  - Stratified squamous epithelium
  - Thin outermost layer
- Multiple layers of developing keratinocytes (contain keratin)
  - Make, secrete glycolipids; prevent water seeping into/out of body

Stratum basale
- *Innermost layer:* single columnar stem cell layer; dividing, producing keratinocytes
  - Keratinocytes contain cholesterol precursors activated by UVB light → vitamin D (regulates calcium absorption)
- Also contains melanocytes (secrete melanin, giving skin its color)
  - UVB light stimulates melanin secretion → placed into melanosomes, moved up by keratinocytes → scatters UVB light → natural sunscreen (prevents skin cancer from excessive UVB light)

Stratum spinosum
- *Second layer:* comprises 8–10 keratinocyte cell layers which can no longer divide
  - Proteins on keratinocytes help them adhere together
  - Dendritic cells seek out invading microbes

Stratum granulosum
- *Third layer:* comprises 3–5 keratinocyte cell layers undergoing keratinization (flatten out, die) → epidermal skin barrier formed
  - Keratohyalin granules in keratinocytes contain keratin precursors which aggregate, cross-link → keratin bundles
  - Lamellar granules in keratinocytes contain glycolipids (secreted to cell surface, glues cells together)

Stratum lucidum
- *Fourth layer:* comprises 2–3 dead keratinocyte cell layers that have secreted most of their lamellar granules
  - Only found in thick skin (e.g. palms, soles of feet)

Stratum corneum
- **Uppermost layer:** comprises 20–30 dead keratinocyte cell layers glued together with glycolipids
  - Dead keratinocytes secrete defensins to fight pathogens
  - Cells from stratum lucidum push up → cells from this layer shed → skin flakes/dandruff

- Blood vessels dilate when hot (blood moves closer to surface → allows heat loss)/contract when cold (blood moves away from surface → prevents heat loss)
- Sweat glands ↑ secretion when hot (↑ heat to evaporate sweat)/↓ when cold (↓ heat to evaporate sweat)

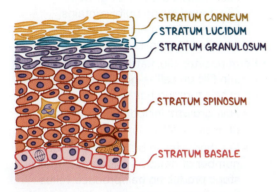

Figure 25.2 The five layers of the epidermis. Stratum basale is the deepest layer and stratum corneum is the most superficial.

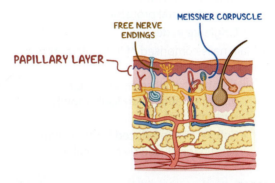

Figure 25.3 The papillary layer of the dermis contains multiple types of nerve endings.

DERMIS
- Dermis
  - Central layer
  - Two layer division (papillary layer; deeper, thicker reticular layer)

Papillary layer
- Fibroblasts (producing collagen) arranged in papillae
- Contains blood vessels, macrophages, nerve endings (e.g. Meissner's corpuscles for fine touch, free nerve endings for pain)
- Responsible for fingerprints (↑ gripping, sensing abilities)

Reticular layer
- Fibroblasts (produces elastin for flexibility)
- Contains oil, sweat glands; lymphatic, blood vessels; hair follicles; macrophages; nerves (e.g. Pacinian corpuscle for pressure, vibration)
- Collagen packed tightly → ↑ support
- Regulates temperature with blood vessels, sweat glands

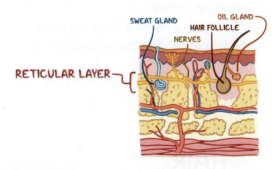

Figure 25.4 Contents of the reticular layer of the dermis.

HYPODERMIS
- Hypodermis (subcutaneous tissue) inner layer
  - Contains adipocytes (store fat), fibroblasts, macrophages, blood vessels, nerves, lymphatics
  - Insulates deeper tissues; provides padding; anchors skin to underlying muscle with connective tissue (e.g. collagen)

HAIR, SKIN, & NAILS

osms.it/hair-skin-and-nails

- Skin appendages include hair, nails, skin glands (oil/sebaceous, sweat/sudoriferous)
  - Regulate body temperature; environmental protection
  - Originate in dermis
- Hair, nails comprised of long, filamentous protein (keratin)
  - *Keratin*: produced by keratinocytes during keratinization (cells rapidly replicate, die)
  - Soft keratin (produced by skin); hard keratin (produced by hair, nails)

HAIR

- Includes vellus hairs (short, thin); terminal hairs (more visible, growth starts at puberty)
- Found everywhere
  - *Exceptions*: palms, soles of feet, lips
- Hair strands sit in follicle; epidermal tissue dips into dermis
  - Associated with sebaceous glands, arrector pili muscles, apocrine glands, nerve receptors
- **Composition**: shaft, root, bulb
  - *Hair matrix*: active hair growth site, found inside bulb; contains keratinocytes, melanocytes; blood supplied by papilla
- Keratinocytes die, flatten out → hard keratin fills up cell → gradually get pushed up follicle forming hair
  - *Hair growth*: includes growth, resting phases
  - Keratinocytes in bulb replicate set number of times → follicle eventually stops producing hair/produce vellus hairs instead (genetically determined) → baldness
- Melanocytes produce melanin (protein pigments that give hair color)
  - Melanocytes move melanin into melanosomes → taken up by keratinocytes

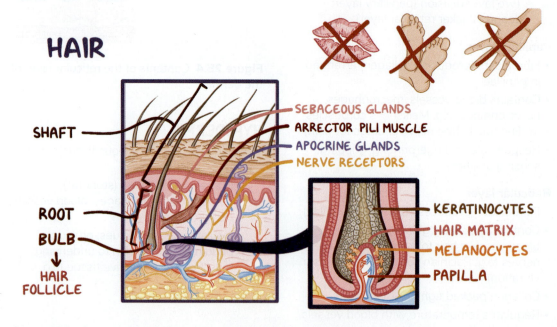

Figure 25.5 Composition of hair and associated structures.

- ↑ age → ↓ melanin → faded, white hair
- Nerve receptors around bulb stimulated when hair shaft moves
- Arrector pili muscle contracts, pulls hair (e.g. cold weather/frightened) → goosebumps

NAILS
- Grow from proximal to distal fingertips/toes
  - Surrounded on either side by nail folds
  - Closed off proximally by eponychium → forms cuticle (dead skin keratinocytes that cover junction between nail, skin)
- *Nail matrix composition:* lunula, nail plate
  - *Lunula:* white, crescent-shaped part of nail near eponychium
  - *Free edge:* nail plate portion hanging over skin
- Modified keratinocytes in matrix form plate by keratinization (similar to hair)
- Nails grow continually through life (unlike hair)

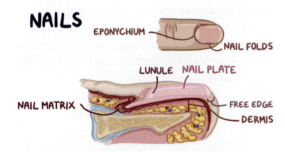

Figure 25.6 Superior view and cross section of a finger illustrating components of the nail.

SEBACEOUS GLANDS
- Secrete sebum (softens hair shaft, prevents moisture-loss, deters pathogens) onto hair follicles/through pores → skin surface
- *During puberty:* ↑ androgen hormones → ↑ sebum production → blocks pores, plugs hair follicles → enclosures allow infection development (e.g. acne, folliculitis)

SUDORIFEROUS GLANDS
- AKA sweat glands

Eccrine (merocrine) glands
- Found everywhere
  - **Exceptions:** lips, ear canal, clitoris, glans of penis
- Coil-shaped structure, in dermis duct opens into pore on skin surface
- **Sweat:** hypotonic (mostly water, electrolytes); dermcidin (destroys bacteria); cools body (evaporation)
- Sympathetic nervous system activation during ↑ cardiovascular activity, fight-or-flight response, fear/anxiety

Apocrine glands
- Found in armpits, genitals
  - Become active during puberty
- Similar to eccrine glands
  - Bigger, fewer; produce secretions with ↑ lipids, proteins
  - Secretions metabolized by bacteria → body odor
- Several modified apocrine gland types
  - *Ceruminous glands:* in ear; produce cerumen; protects eardrum (with ear canal hairs)
  - *Mammary glands:* in breasts; produce milk

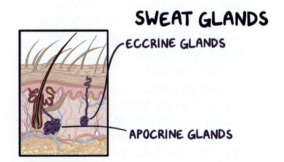

Figure 25.7 The two types of sweat glands (sudoriferous glands).

WOUND HEALING

osms.it/wound-healing

- Damaged tissue repair process
  - Acute wounds heal quickly (days–weeks)
  - Chronic wounds heal slowly (months)

Regenerative tissue capacity
- **Classification:** labile, stable, permanent
- Labile tissues (e.g. skin, connective tissue, intestines)
  - *Heal well:* stem cells constantly divide → rapid, effective healing
- Stable tissues (e.g. liver, endocrine glands, proximal kidney tubules)
  - *Heal slowly:* mature differentiated cells divide/regenerate by hyperplasia
- Permanent tissues (e.g. skeletal muscle, cartilage, neurons)
  - *Heal poorly:* lack of stem cells, no hyperplasia → replaced by scar tissue (fibrosis) → function loss

Open wounds
- Open wounds healed by primary, secondary, tertiary intention
- Primary intention (most surgical wounds)
  - Wound edges fuse (e.g. stitching/gluing) → stem cells (e.g. epidermis) approximate, regenerate damaged tissue (minimal scarring)
- Secondary intention
  - Wound edges too far apart (e.g. pressure ulcers, tooth extraction, severe burns) → stem cells do not approximate → wound replaced by connective tissue growing from base upwards (slower healing; more scar tissue)
- Tertiary intention (delayed closure)
  - Wound cleaned, debrided → purposefully left open (↓ bacterial contamination likelihood) → closed by primary intention/left open for secondary intention

Penetrating trauma wound healing
- Penetrating trauma wound healing steps (e.g. cutting finger → damaged epidermis, dermis, interstitial space)
- Hemostasis (first step)
  - Blood vessels constrict → platelets adhere to site → forms platelet plug → fibrin mesh reinforces platelet plug → forms blood clot
- Inflammation (second step)
  - Damaged cells release chemokines, cytokines → neutrophils, macrophages recruited; blood vessels dilate → immune cells clear debris, digest dead/damaged cells, destroy microbes → blood clot, dead macrophages combine, form scab
- Epithelization/migration (third step)
  - Basal cells (epidermal stem cells) proliferate, replace lost/damaged cells → rejuvenated epidermal layer (approx. 48 hours)
- Fibroplasia (fourth step)
  - Fibroblasts in dermis proliferate, secrete collagen (assemble → form collagen fibrils → collaged bundles) → blood vessel growth stimulated (angiogenesis); fibroblasts also produce glycoproteins, sugars → create granulation tissue in dermal layer
- Maturation (fifth step)
  - *Collagen cross-linking:* covalent bonds form between collagen bundles, improving tensile strength
  - *Collagen remodeling:* fibroblasts degrade subpar collagen
  - *Contraction:* myofibroblasts produce contractile proteins, pulling wound's edges together
  - *Repigmentation:* melanocytes proliferating, restoring color to damaged skin

Chapter 25 Dermatology: Skin Structures

Chronic wounds
- Healing prevention factors → chronic wounds
    - *Narrowed capillaries:* prolonged compression/disease (e.g. diabetes, atherosclerosis) → ↓ blood flow → damaged tissue cannot be reached by immune cells, insufficient oxygen/nutrients → tissue necrosis
    - *Infection:* pathogens compete for oxygen; cause ongoing damage, inflammation
    - *Edema:* disrupts fibroblast activity, collagen deposition, collage cross linking

WOUND HEALING

FIRST STEP

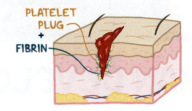

SECOND STEP

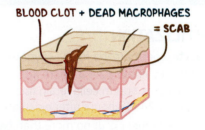

THIRD STEP

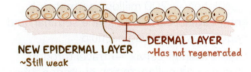

FOURTH STEP

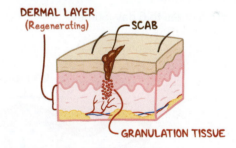

FIFTH STEP

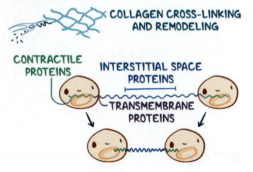

Figure 25.8 The five steps of penetrating trauma wound healing.

NOTES
EARLY WEEKS

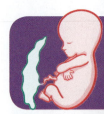

HUMAN DEVELOPMENT DAYS 1-4

osms.it/human_development_days_1-4

FERTILIZATION
- Oocyte, spermatozoa fuse → zygote
  - Oocyte viable 12–24 hours after ovulation; sperm cells retain fertilizing power 24–48 hours after ejaculation
  - Coitus must occur no more than two days before/24 hours after ovulation for fertilization
- Ejaculation → 200 million spermatozoa enter vaginal canal → alkaline seminal fluid neutralizes acidic vaginal fluid
- Only 1% enter cervix → travel through uterus → ampullary region of uterine tube (most likely place for fertilization)
- Cervix → oviduct
  - 30 minutes to 6 day journey
- Ovulation → spermatozoa driven by chemoattractants (produced by cumulus cells of oocytes) to ampulla of uterine tube

Two required processes
- **Capacitation:** epithelial interactions between sperm, uterine wall
  - Glycoprotein coat, seminal plasma proteins covering acrosomal region removed → easier enzyme release → acrosomal reaction
- **Acrosomal reaction:** after binding to zona pellucida
  - Release of enzymes (e.g. acrosin, hyaluronidase) needed to penetrate zona pellucida

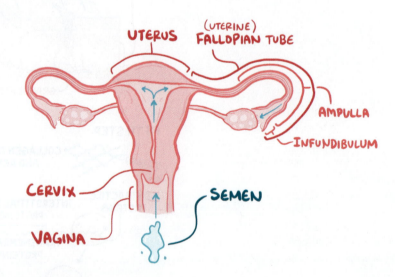

Figure 26.1 Sperm pathway through the uterus.

PHASES OF FERTILIZATION

Phase I: penetration of corona radiata
- Capacitated spermatozoa allowed to pass through corona radiata

Phase II: penetration of zona pellucida, sperm binding
- *Zona pellucida*: glycoprotein layer surrounding oocyte; AKA "jelly coat"
  - Facilitates binding of sperm cell, induces acrosomal reaction mediated by ligand zona pellucida sperm-binding protein 3 (ZP3)
- Approx. 500 spermatozoa arrive at this layer
- Sperm-binding initiates release of acrosin (hydrolytic enzyme) → sperm cell penetrates zona pellucida → sperm makes contact with oocyte → cortical reaction (release of lysosomal enzymes from cortical granules of oocyte) → cortical granules initiate zona reaction, prevent further sperm penetration (polyspermy) by forming protective hyaline layer, inactivate receptor sites on zona pellucida
  - Cortical reaction also activates oocyte to prepare for second meiotic division

Phase III: fusion of oocyte, sperm cell
- Interactions between integrins, ligands → adhesion of sperm, oocyte
  - Fusion of sperm, egg plasma membranes
- Secondary oocyte completes meiosis II → forms female pronucleus, second polar body
- Head, tail of spermatozoa enters oocyte → travels to female pronucleus (containing 23 chromosomes) using tail, energy generated by mitochondria
- Tail, mitochondria detach → sperm nucleus becomes male pronucleus
- Male, female pronuclei move toward each other → merge into single nucleus → cell becomes diploid (zygote contains maternal, paternal genetic information)
- Preparation for mitotic division

ZYGOTE TO BLASTOCYST IMPLANTATION

Cleavage
- Series of fast mitotic divisions of zygote → increase number of cells, decrease size
- 36 hours after fertilization → first cleavage division → two cells (blastomeres)
  - Second division → four blastomeres; third division → eight blastomeres; etc.
- After third cleavage, blastomeres form compact ball of cells connected by tight junctions (compaction)
- Three days after fertilization, cells of compacted embryo divide again → mulberry-shaped 16-cell morula (composed of two zones: inner, outer cell mass)
- Four to five days after fertilization, embryo consists of approx. 100 cells
- Fluid accumulates within internal cavity (blastocoel) → blastocyst
- *Blastocyst*: fluid-filled hollow cell, two zones
  - *Trophoblast*: single layer of large flattened cells, stemming from morula's outer cell mass; gives rise to placenta
  - *Embryoblast*: 20–30 pluripotent cells located on one side, stemming from inner cell mass; gives rise to embryo

PHASES of FERTILIZATION

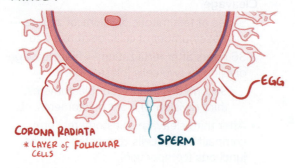

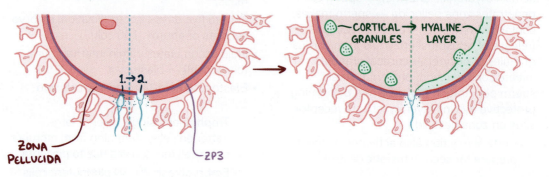

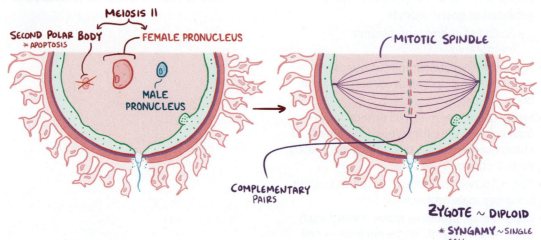

Figure 26.2 Phases of fertilization.
Phase I: sperm penetrates corona radiata.
Phase II: penetration of zona pellucida, sperm binding.
Phase III: fusion of sperm, oocyte; pronuclei fuse to form diploid zygote cell.

Chapter 26 Embryology: Early Weeks

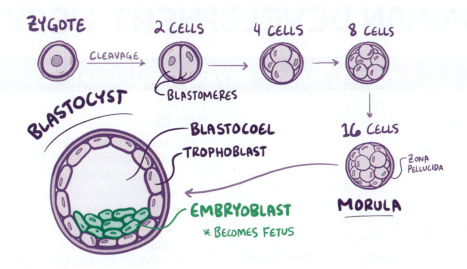

Figure 26.3 Process of going from zygote to blastocyst.

HUMAN DEVELOPMENT DAYS 4-7

osms.it/human_development_days_4-7

DAY 7

Implantation
- Trophoblast binds to uterine wall with L-selectin, integrin receptors
  - Penetrates between epithelial cells
- Uterus at implantation in secretory phase
  - High progesterone released from corpus luteum develops endometrium for implantation
  - Blastocyst implants into decidua basalis, along superior posterior wall of uterus

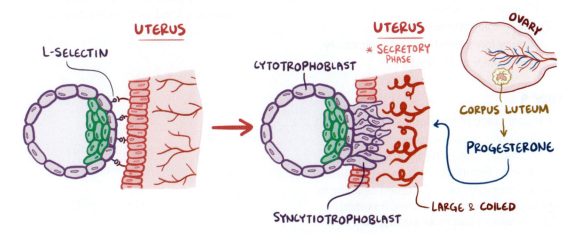

Figure 26.4 Implantation, syncytiotrophoblast proliferation, and development of spiral arteries under the influence of progesterone secreted by the corpus luteum.

HUMAN DEVELOPMENT WEEK 2

osms.it/human-development-week-2

DAY 8

Trophoblast
- Proliferates, forms two layers
- *Cytotrophoblast (cellular trophoblast):* inner layer of mononucleated cells
  - Produces primary chorionic villi, protrudes into syncytiotrophoblast
- *Syncytiotrophoblast:* outer multinucleated mass of cells (without distinct cell boundaries)
  - Invades decidua basalis with finger-like processes; makes enzymes that erode uterine cells; blastocyst burrows into decidua basalis surrounded by pool of blood leaked from degraded blood vessels
  - Human chorionic gonadotropin (hCG) maintains viability of corpus luteum → secretes estrogen, progesterone until week eight (hCG: basis for pregnancy tests)

Embryoblast
- Differentiates into two layers, forms flat disc
- *Hypoblast:* small cuboidal cells adjacent to blastocyst → yolk sac
- *Epiblast:* columnar cells
  - Cavity forms inside → amniotic cavity
  - Lined with amnioblasts

DAY 9

- Lacunar stage of trophoblast development
  - Vacuoles appear in syncytium → vacuoles fuse → form large empty spaces (lacunae)
- At abembryonic pole, flattened cells (from hypoblast) form exocoelomic (Hauser) membrane → line inner surface of cytotrophoblast
  - Hauser membrane, hypoblast line exocoelomic cavity (primitive yolk sac)

DAY 12

- Progesterone levels continue to rise → decidua undergoes decidual reaction
  - Decidual cells enlarge, become coated in sugar-rich fluid (helps sustain embryo)
  - Blastocyst embeds in endometrial stroma
  - Lacunae form within syncytiotrophoblast (erodes endometrial sinusoids)
  - Lacunae fuse with sinusoids → fill with maternal blood → uteroplacental circulation established

DAY 13

- Secondary yolk sac forms within exocoelomic cavity
- *Hypoblast cells:* differentiate into extraembryonic mesoderm cells outside embryo
  - *Mesoderm cells:* line inside of cytotrophoblast, syncytiotrophoblast; line chorionic cavity
- *Epiblast:* gives rise to embryo's germ layers (endoderm, mesoderm, ectoderm)
- Amniotic cavity develops above bilaminar disk, becomes lined with epiblast cells

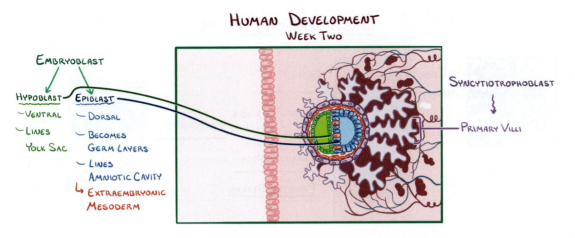

Figure 26.5 Summary of the growth that occurs during the second week of development.

HUMAN DEVELOPMENT WEEK 3

osms.it/human-development-week-3

DAY 14
- Syncytiotrophoblast cells form little protrusions called primary villi
- Villi form around fetus; lacunae form between villi
- Arteries, veins merge within lacunae → form large pool of blood (junctional zone)
- Villi submerged within junctional zone

Gastrulation
- Major event, establishes three germ layers
- Begins with formation of primitive groove (narrow depression into center of epiblast layer)
  - Starts at caudal end, grows towards cranial end → cranial-caudal axis
  - Groove forms on dorsal side of embryo → dorsal-ventral axis
  - **Two sides of groove:** left, right side of body (bilateral symmetry)
- Primitive node forms at cephalic end of primitive groove
  - Contains primitive pit, surrounded by slightly elevated area of ectoderm
- Primitive groove, node, pit → form primitive streak
- Epiblast cells migrate towards primitive groove → move to bottom, slide under (invagination)
- After invagination, cells differentiate into three new layers of embryonic disc (trilaminar disc)
- Cells of trilaminar disc multipotent (ability to differentiate into many tissues, organs)
  - Some epiblast cells displace ventral hypoblast layer, form endoderm
  - Invaginated epiblast cells between newly formed endoderm, epiblast → mesoderm layer
  - Rest of epiblast forms ectoderm layer

DAY 15
- Two areas of ectoderm layer (cranial, caudal region) push ventrally, fuse with endoderm (exclude mesoderm layer) → form two bilaminar regions in otherwise trilaminar disc
  - Cranial bilaminar region develops into oropharyngeal membrane → disintegrates in fourth week to form mouth opening
  - Caudal bilaminar region develops into cloacal membrane → disintegrates in seventh week to form anal opening, genitourinary tracts

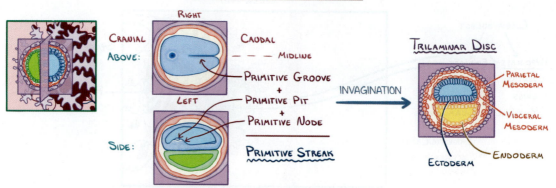

Figure 26.6 Day 14: formation of the primitive streak and trilaminar disc.

DAY 17

- Group of mesoderm cells form solid rod (notochord)
  - *Notochord*: transient embryonic structure (nucleus pulposus of intervertebral disc: remnant in adult life)
  - Solid structure → helps influence how embryo folds
  - Secretes protein called Sonic HedgeHog (SHH) → guides tissue differentiation

DAY 20

- Mesoderm cells around notochord differentiate into three specialized types of cells
  - Paraxial mesoderm, intermediate mesoderm, lateral plate mesoderm; make different tissues, organs
- Notochord starts process called neurulation → stimulates cells of ectoderm to form neural plate
- Neural plate folds, forms neural groove with edges called neural folds
- Neural plate continues to grow, neural folds come together, pinch off from surface of ectoderm to form neural tube between ectoderm, mesoderm
- Trophoblast continues to develop: vasculogenesis
  - *Primary villi*: made up of cytotrophoblastic core covered by syncytial layer
  - *Secondary villi*: form when extraembryonic somatic mesoderm cells penetrate primary villi → grow toward decidua
  - *Tertiary villi*: form when mesodermal cells differentiate into small blood vessels → form villus capillary system → fetal contribution to placenta

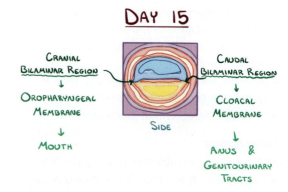

Figure 26.7 Day 15: bilaminar regions of trilaminar disc.

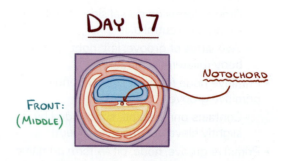

Figure 26.8 Day 17: formation of notochord from mesoderm cells.

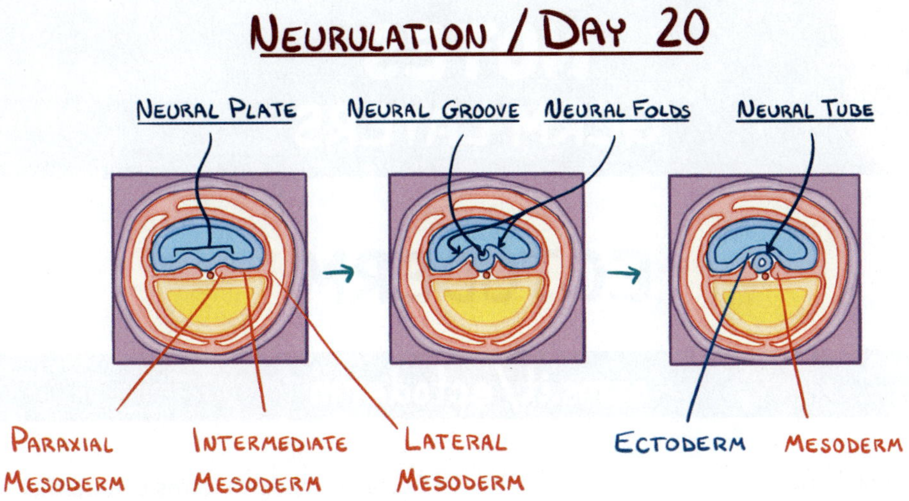

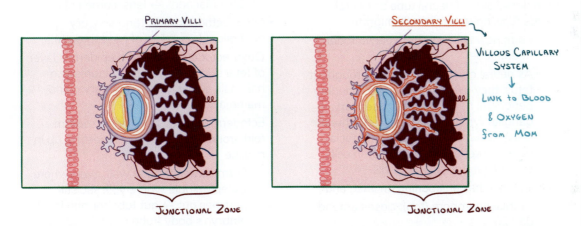

Figure 26.9 Day 20: differentiation of mesoderm near neural plate into paraxial, intermediate, and lateral plate mesoderm; formation of neural tube in process called neurulation.

Figure 26.10 During week 3, extraembryonic mesoderm cells migrate into the primary villi, forming secondary villi. The secondary villi differentiate into fetal vessels known as the villous capillary system, which is the fetal contribution to the placenta.

NOTES
GERM LAYERS

ECTODERM

osms.it/ectoderm

- Beginning of week 3
  - Ectoderm layer broader in cephalic region than in caudal region
- Notochord initiates neurulation, forming neural tube between mesoderm, ectoderm
- On dorsal side of neural tube as neural folds fuse, neural crest cells migrate
  - Form new cell layer between ectoderm, neural tube
  - As neural crest cells migrate throughout fetus, they give rise to tissues including peripheral nervous system (sensory ganglia, sympathetic neurons, Schwann cells), skin melanocytes, part of facial bones, adrenal gland chromaffin cells, thyroid parafollicular (C) cells
- Neural tube has an opening on each end
  - Cranial neuropore (top): closes around day 25
  - Caudal neuropore (bottom): closes around day 28

- Surface ectoderm forms ectodermal thickenings, otic, lens placodes, near cranial end of ectoderm
  - Otic placodes form otic vesicles → cochlea, inner ear
  - Lens placodes → lens, cornea of eyes
- Other ectoderm cells form sensory epithelium (e.g. lining of nose, mouth)
- Other ectoderm cells form epidermis layer of fetal skin, associated structures (e.g. hair, nail, sweat glands, pituitary gland, mammary glands)
- Ectoderm, parietal layer of mesoderm fold around with two sides meeting up in midline
  - Forms anterior body wall, everywhere except middle where yolk sac still pouches out → gut tube formed inside embryo's body (tube inside of tube)

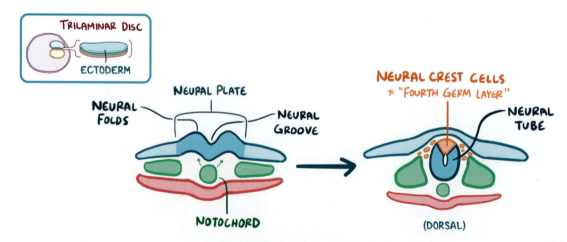

Figure 27.1 Development of neural tube and neural crest cells.

Chapter 27 Embryology: Germ Layers

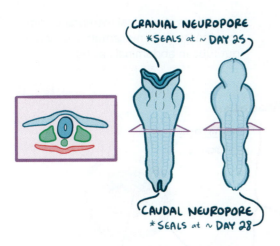

Figure 27.2 The neural tube initially has openings at each end, called cranial and caudal neuropores. Both pores close by around day 28.

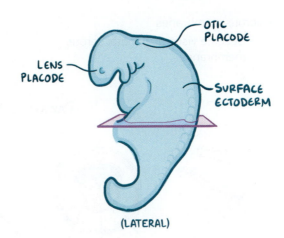

Figure 27.3 The surface ectoderm forms thickenings—the lens and otic placodes—that become eye and ear structures, respectively.

MESODERM

osms.it/mesoderm

- Day 20
  - Mesoderm cells around notochord differentiate into three specialized types of cells that will form different tissues, organs
  - Paraxial mesoderm, intermediate mesoderm, lateral plate mesoderm

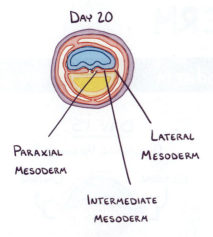

Figure 27.4 The three types of mesoderm that develop around day 20.

Paraxial mesoderm
- Starts to segment into paired tissue blocks called somites, one of each sitting alongside notochord, neural tube above it
  - About three somite pairs form per day in craniocaudal direction
  - By week five, there are 42–44 pairs of somites
  - Number of somites can be used to determine embryo age
- Somites divide into three regions
  - **Sclerotome:** gives rise to bone, cartilage
  - **Myotome:** gives rise to muscles
  - **Dermatome:** gives rise to dermis skin layer

Intermediate mesoderm
- Gives rise to urogenital structures (e.g. adrenal cortex, kidneys, ovaries, testes)

Lateral plate mesoderm
- Gives rise to serous membranes, soft tissues of arms, legs, muscular gut wall, heart, circulatory system

- Serous membranes
  - Become visceral, parietal serous membranes
- Two layers of visceral membrane come together to form mesentery (suspends gut tube in abdominal cavity)

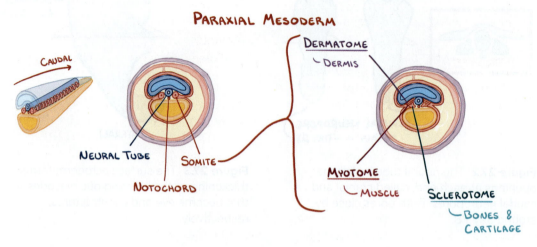

Figure 27.5 The paraxial mesoderm segments into somites. The somites then divide into three regions which develop into distinct body structures.

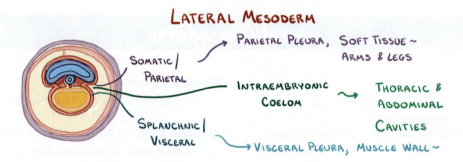

Figure 27.6 Membranes of the lateral mesoderm and their derivatives.

ENDODERM

osms.it/endoderm

- Day 15
  - Cranial, caudal ectoderm regions push ventrally, fuse with endoderm layer
  - Two bilaminar regions formed
  - Cranial bilaminar region → oropharyngeal membrane → mouth
  - Caudal bilaminar region → cloacal membrane → opening of anus, genitourinary tracts

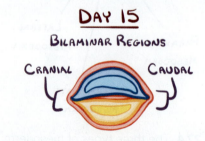

Figure 27.7 Cranial and caudal bilaminar regions of the embryo (lateral view).

- Week 4
  - Embryo folds in two directions
  - *Longitudinal plane*: cranial, caudal folds; embryo begins to curl into fetal position; folding shapes part of yolk sack into gut tube with rest remaining connected in middle via vitelline duct
  - *Transversal plane*: lateral plates of mesoderm split into parietal (somatic) mesoderm layer, visceral (splanchnic) mesoderm layer; parietal mesoderm follows ectoderm, forms chest wall, abdominal body wall; visceral layer of mesoderm follows endoderm, forms gut tube
- Endoderm becomes epithelial cell lining of gastrointestinal tract, while mesoderm becomes muscular wall
- In addition to gastrointestinal, respiratory tract epithelium
  - Endoderm gives rise to tonsils, thyroid, parathyroid glands, thymus, part of liver, gallbladder, pancreas
  - Endoderm cells form parts of ear, epithelial lining of urethra, urinary bladder

GUT TUBE STRUCTURE
- Gut tube divided into foregut, midgut, hindgut

Foregut
- Around week 4
  - Once oropharyngeal membrane breaks down, foregut (including pharynx) connects to primitive mouth (stomodeum)
- Around week 5
  - Foregut gives rise to trachea, lungs

Midgut
- Remains connected to yolk sac which sits outside body via vitelline duct (yolk stalk) which passes through umbilical ring
- Over time vitelline duct gets thinner, collapses; in some people it remains as Meckel's diverticulum

Hindgut
- Around week 7
  - Once cloacal membrane breaks down, upper two thirds of anal canal (derived from endoderm) meet up with lower one third of anal canal, called proctodeum (derived from ectoderm)
  - *Pectinate line*: in adults, the line where the upper two thirds (endoderm) and lower third (ectoderm) of the anal canal meet up

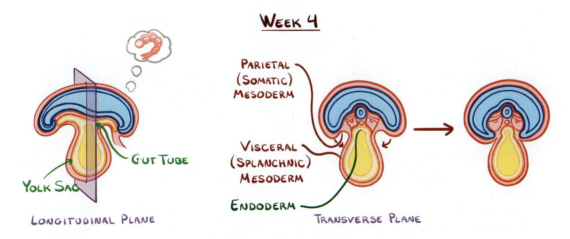

Figure 27.8 Week 4: the embryo folds in the longitudinal and transverse planes.

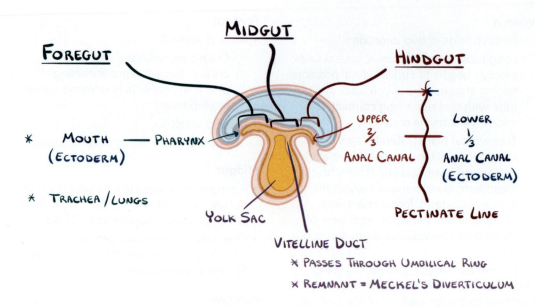

Figure 27.9 Locations and derivatives of the foregut, midgut, and hindgut (lateral view).

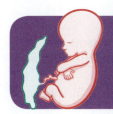

NOTES
EARLY STRUCTURES

DEVELOPMENT OF THE DIGESTIVE SYSTEM & BODY CAVITIES

osms.it/digestive-system-and-body-cavities-development

- Endoderm forms gut tube epithelium
- The rest derives from mesoderm
    - Around week 3 lateral mesoderm splits into parietal (somatic) mesoderm → adheres to ectoderm; visceral (splanchnic mesoderm) → adheres to endoderm
    - Space between the split is called intraembryonic coelom/intraembryonic cavity
    - Eventually becomes thoracic, abdominal cavity
    - Parietal mesoderm → gives rise to serous membrane that lines abdominal, thoracic cavity (parietal pleural, peritoneal, pericardial membrane), soft tissues of arms, legs
    - Visceral mesoderm → gives rise to serous membrane that lines various organs (visceral pleural, peritoneal, pericardial membrane), muscular wall of gut, heart, circulatory system
    - Two visceral peritoneal membranes come together, form mesentery (suspends gut tube in abdominal cavity)

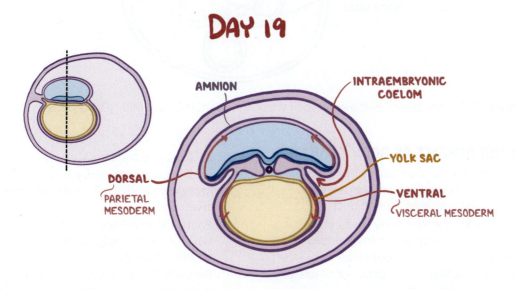

Figure 28.1 During week 3, lateral mesoderm splits into parietal and visceral mesoderm. They give rise to serous membranes that cover various body parts.

OSMOSIS.ORG 209

- During week 4 embryo begins to curl into fetal position
  - Combined visceral mesoderm, endoderm layer folds rostrally, caudally → shapes part of yolk sac forming primitive gut tube
  - The rest of yolk sac is connected in middle via vitelline duct
  - Combined parietal mesoderm, ectoderm folds down with amnion forming lateral body folds
  - Eventually merge, become anterior body wall of embryo

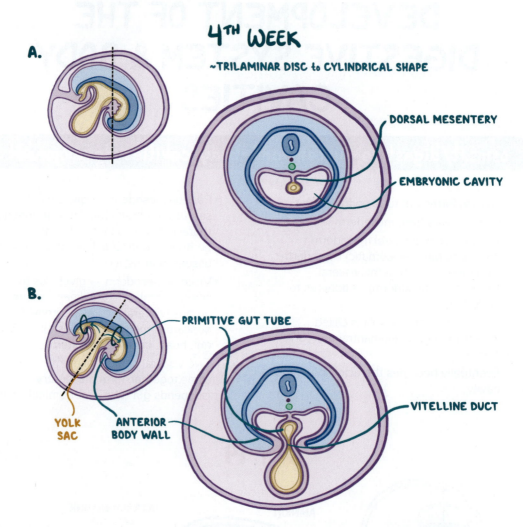

Figure 28.2 Appearance of the embryo in week 4 in caudal (A) and mid- (B) sections.

DEVELOPMENT OF BODY CAVITIES

- Around day 22, thick plate of visceral mesoderm called septum transversum forms just cranial to vitelline duct
  - Divides primitive body cavity into thoracic cavity, abdominal cavities
- Around week 5, two tissue flaps called the pleuropericardial folds, grow out of lateral body wall, fuse together
  - Divides thoracic cavity into two pleural cavities, one pericardial cavity
- In week 7, pleuropericardial folds extend ventrally from body wall, fuse with septum transversum
  - Forms pleuroperitoneal membrane, which seals thoracic cavity from peritoneal cavity
  - Pericardial, pleural cavities in thorax, peritoneal cavity in abdomen

Chapter 28 Embryology: Early Structures

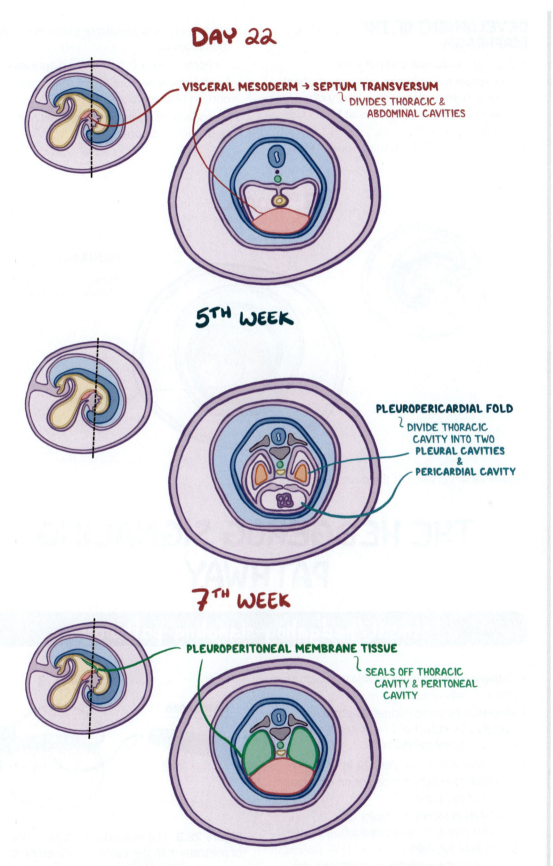

Figure 28.3 Development of body cavities on day 22 and during weeks 5 and 7.

DEVELOPMENT OF THE DIAPHRAGM

- Develops from four components
  - Septum transversum, pleuroperitoneal membranes, dorsal mesentery of esophagus, from somites at levels C3–C5
- Mesodermal cells from third, fourth, fifth pairs of somites penetrate pleuroperitoneal membranes
  - Form muscular portion of diaphragm
- Septum transversum forms tendinous portion of diaphragm
- Mesoderm of lumbar region gives rise to two crura of diaphragm

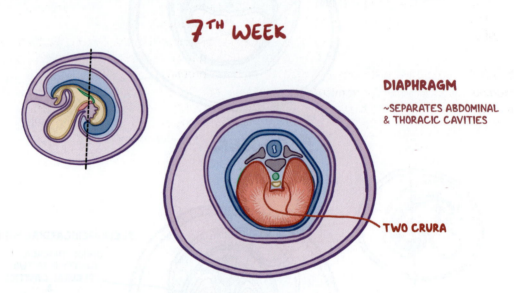

Figure 28.4 Location of the developed diaphragm.

THE HEDGEHOG SIGNALING PATHWAY

osms.it/hedgehog-signaling-pathway

- Pathway which plays key role in structuring general body shape
- Mediated by sonic hedgehog proteins secreted by notochord → proteins diffuse through interstitial fluids
- Functions of sonic hedgehog protein
  - Binds to patched receptor on embryonic cell membrane
  - Patched receptor inhibits cell differentiation; sonic hedgehog protein inhibits patched
  - Inhibits the inhibitor → facilitates cell differentiation

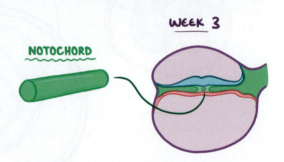

Figure 28.5 The notochord is a solid line of mesoderm at the center of the embryo. It secretes different kinds of hedgehog proteins.

Chapter 28 Embryology: Early Structures

- Sonic hedgehog proteins control gene expression → gene expression depends on amount of sonic hedgehog protein reaching embryonic cells, duration of exposure
- Notochord secretes different kinds of hedgehog proteins
- Embryonic cells are exposed to different combinations of proteins that helps distinguish their position relative to each other (awareness in space), their course of differentiation

REGULATION BY HOMEOBOX GENES

- Homeobox genes code for transcription factors that activate gene cascades which regulate segmentation, craniocaudal patterning
- Homeobox gene products are transcription factors called Hox proteins
- Homeobox genes arranged into four clusters on four different chromosomes
  - HOXA, HOXB, HOXC, HOXD
- Genes toward 3' end of chromosomes control cranial structure development, genes toward 5' end control caudal structure development
- Highly conserved genes across vast evolutionary distances
  - Demonstrated by the fact that a fly can function perfectly well with chicken Hox protein its place
- Mutations in Hox genes can result in body parts, limbs in the wrong place along the body e.g. extra fingers/toes

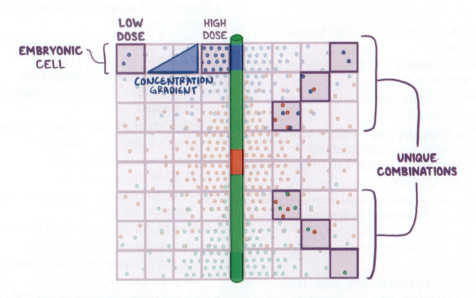

Figure 28.6 SHH and other notochord proteins diffuse through the embryo, creating a concentration gradient that tells embryonic cells where they are located in three dimensional space. The unique combinations of proteins determine into which tissues the cells differentiate.

DEVELOPMENT OF THE PLACENTA

osms.it/placenta-development

- The placenta is co-created by fetus, mother
- Around day 14, syncytiotrophoblast cells form little protrusions called primary villi
  - Villi form all the way around fetus
- Cells clear out from between primary villi
  - Leave behind empty spaces called lacunae
- Maternal arteries. veins grow into decidua basalis, merge with lacunae
  - Maternal arteries fill lacunae with oxygenated blood
  - Maternal veins pick up deoxygenated blood
  - Junctional zone formed as arteries, veins continue to merge
- Formation of feto-placental circulation begins on day 9
  - *Day 9, lacunar stage:* vacuoles form lacunae in syncytiotrophoblast; endometrial sinusoids start to grow into decidua basalis
  - *Day 12:* sinusoids merge with syncytial lacunae, filling them with blood
  - *Day 14:* cells of cytotrophoblast penetrate syncytiotrophoblast, form primary villi
  - *Day 16:* extraembryonic mesoderm cells penetrate into primary villi forming secondary villi, later differentiate into small blood vessels (tertiary villi)
- Around day 17, feto-placental circulation established
  - Fetal mesoderm cells enter primary villi → form fetal arteries, capillaries, veins within each villi
  - Villi capillaries connect to umbilical cord blood vessels → links maternal, fetal circulation

PLACENTAL STRUCTURE
- **Maternal contribution:** derived from uterine endometrium
  - *Basal plate (decidual plate):* thick layer of decidua basalis tissue that maternal spiral arteries, veins pass through to get to junctional zone
- **Fetal contribution:** derived from chorionic plate (trophoblast, extraembryonic mesoderm)
  - *Chorionic frondosum:* numerous villi that emerge from chorionic plate
  - Junctional zone between basal plate, chorionic plate
- Space forms around fetus called chorionic cavity
  - Contains amniotic cavity, yolk sac, embryo
  - *Chorion laeve:* chorionic cavity wall where syncytiotrophoblast villi regressed
  - Outside of chorion laeve, thin layer of decidua (decidua capsularis)
- On ultrasound, chorionic cavity shows up as relatively large, dark space
  - Used to identify pregnancy even before fetus can be seen
- During fourth, fifth months of development, walls called decidual septa form
  - Divide placenta into 15–20 different regions called cotyledons
- Each cotyledon contains about 100 spiral arteries providing steady supply of oxygenated blood
- Oxygen, glucose, molecules like immunoglobulins, hormones, certain toxins are able to move across into fetal capillaries
  - Carbon dioxide moves out of fetal capillaries, enters blood in junctional zone
- Placenta covers about 15–30% of uterine wall at any given time during development
- Placenta grows, thickens
  - At full term, is 20cm/7.9in across (size of frisbee)
- During third stage of labor placenta is expelled from body as afterbirth

Chapter 28 Embryology: Early Structures

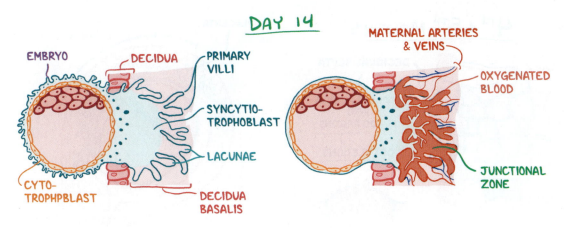

Figure 28.7 Formation of feto-placental circulation: primary villi form. Cells clear out between primary villi, forming lacunae. Tiny maternal arteries and veins merge with lacunae, and the lacunae fill with oxygenated blood. Lacunae merge to form a single pool, the junctional zone.

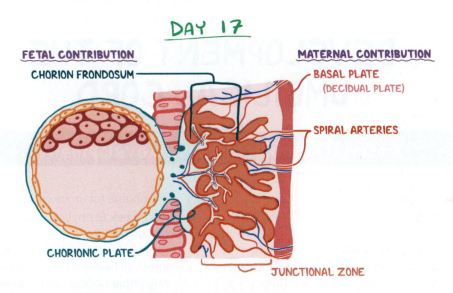

Figure 28.8 Fetal and maternal contributions to the placenta.

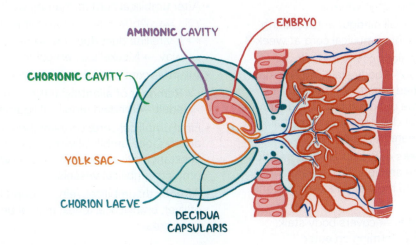

Figure 28.9 Contents of the chorionic cavity.

OSMOSIS.ORG 215

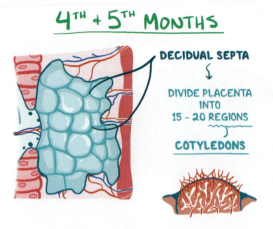

Figure 28.10 Decidual septa form in months four and five that divide the placenta into regions called cotyledons.

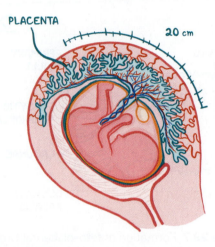

Figure 28.11 The placenta covers approximately 15–30% of uterine wall and is about 20cm/7.9in across at full term.

DEVELOPMENT OF THE UMBILICAL CORD

osms.it/umbilical-cord-development

- Umbilical cord is a long flexible stalk containing two arteries, one vein; connects fetus to placenta
- Forms from three structures
  - *Body (connecting) stalk*: short band of extraembryonic mesoderm that connects embryo to chorion at week 2
  - *Vitelline duct*: open connection between yolk sac, midgut at week 3
  - *Allantois*: small hindgut outpocketing that grows into umbilical cord at week 3
- *In week 4*: amniotic cavity folds down, around embryo → body stalk, vitelline duct, allantois pushed together, form umbilical cord → emerge out of umbilical ring (fibrous tissue ring that develops on abdominal wall at location where they emerge)
- *Between weeks 4–8*: cells lining amniotic cavity produce amniotic fluid → amnion swells, takes up most of space in chorionic cavity
  - Amnion folds → covers body stalk, vitelline duct forming an outer membrane for umbilical cord
- *Around week 6*: physiological umbilical herniation
  - Due to rapid intestinal growth, part of intestine herniates through umbilical ring into umbilical cord; withdraws back into abdominal cavity by end of third month
- After umbilical cord formation, vitelline duct, yolk sac shrink, eventually disappear
  - If vitelline duct does not regress all the way → Meckel's diverticulum
- Allantois continues developing into bladder
  - *Remnant of allantois*: fetus → urachus; adult → median umbilical ligament
- *Final umbilical cord*: contains two umbilical arteries, one umbilical vein, gelatinous substance called Wharton's jelly which protects umbilical vessels
- *After birth*: umbilical vein → round ligament of liver, umbilical arteries; medial umbilical ligaments

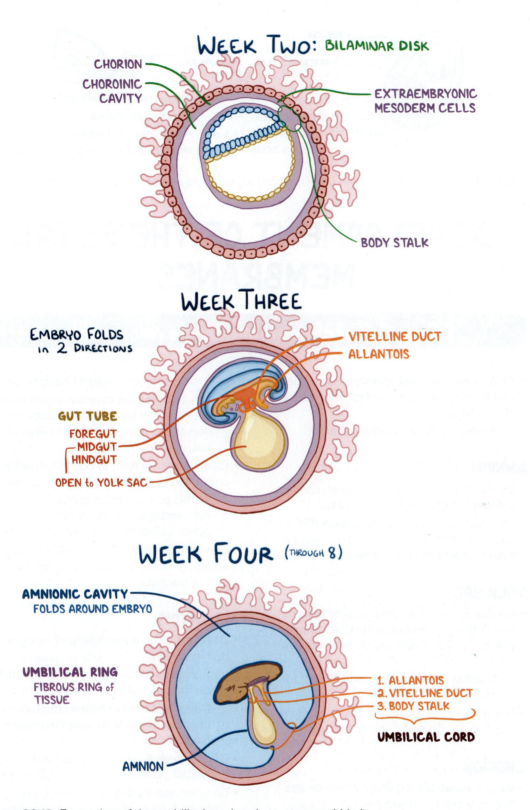

Figure 28.12 Formation of the umbilical cord and structures within it.

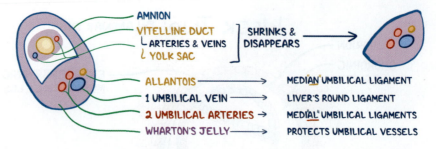

Figure 28.13 Cross section of the umbilical cord revealing its components and their remnants.

DEVELOPMENT OF THE FETAL MEMBRANES

osms.it/fetal-membrane-development

- AKA extraembryonic membranes: tissues that form in uterus during first few weeks of development
    - Amnion, yolk sac, chorion, allantois

AMNION
- On day 8, space appears between epiblast, cytotrophoblast → amniotic cavity
- Cells from epiblast migrate to form thin layer around amniotic cavity, separating it from cytotrophoblast → amnion

YOLK SAC
- On day 9, hypoblast cells migrate to form thin membrane around blastocoel, forming yolk sac walls → yolk sac fills with vitelline fluid
    - Vitelline fluid provides nourishment for embryo
- Nutrients in yolk sac eventually consumed, yolk sac, vitelline duct shrink, disappear

CHORION
- By day 10, epiblast cells differentiate into extraembryonic mesoderm
    - Settle between amniotic cavity/yolk sac, cytotrophoblast → creating thick layer of extraembryonic mesoderm tissue between the two
    - A space forms within this layer → extraembryonic coelom/chorionic cavity
    - Cavity continues to expand until there is only a thin layer of extraembryonic mesoderm lining amniotic cavity/yolk sac, cytotrophoblast
- Cavity does not form at body stalk where embryoblast remains attached to chorion
    - At this point, chorion contains extraembryonic mesoderm, cytotrophoblast, syncytiotrophoblast
- Chorion develops chorionic villi, invades endometrium, eventually helps form fetal part of placenta

ALLANTOIS
- Develops as an outpouching of hindgut during week 3
    - Serves as canal through which urine is eliminated, before urethra develops
    - Degenerates into fibrous structure called urachus, remains attached to urinary bladder
- During week 4, allantois, vitelline duct, body stalk combine to form umbilical cord
- Between weeks 4–8, amnion secretes amniotic fluid → amniotic cavity swells, folds down around embryo → protects, insulates embryo → continues to grow → amnion, chorion fuse together, form amniotic sac

Chapter 28 Embryology: Early Structures

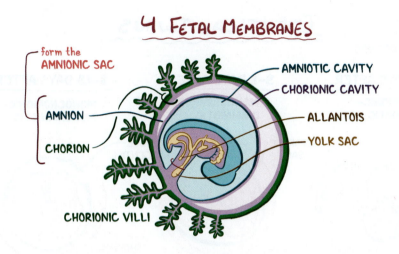

Figure 28.14 Four fetal membranes include: amnion, chorion, allantois, yolk sac.

DEVELOPMENT OF TWINS

osms.it/twin-development

FRATERNAL (DIZYGOTIC) TWINS

- Occur at rate of about 10 per 1,000 births worldwide
- Originate from two separate eggs (hyperovulation) fertilized individually by two different sperms → zygotes have completely different genetic makeups
  - Hyperovulation may be due to an overabundance of follicle-stimulating hormone (FSH)
- Mothers of fraternal twins tend to be older (> 35 years), taller, heavier on average, with shorter, more frequent menstrual cycles → high levels of follicle-stimulating hormone

IDENTICAL (MONOZYGOTIC) TWINS

- Occur at a rate of about 4 per 1000 births worldwide
- Originate from single zygote that splits into two groups of cells → zygotes have identical genetic makeup
- The split can occur at any time during first thirteen days of development
- Identical DNA → identical physical traits that have a strong genetic basis → sex, hair, eye color, blood type, other physical features

IDENTICAL TWIN CATEGORIES

- Categorized by how, when division occurs → affects how identical twins share space, resources in uterus

Dichorionic-diamniotic
- Division occurs within 2–3 days following fertilization
- Embryos develop completely separately from one another
- Have separate placentas, amniotic sacs

Monochorionic-diamniotic
- Division occurs between 3–8 days following fertilization
- Embryos share a single placenta, separate amniotic sacs

Monochorionic-monoamniotic
- Division occurs between 8–13 days after fertilization
- Embryos share both placenta, amniotic sac

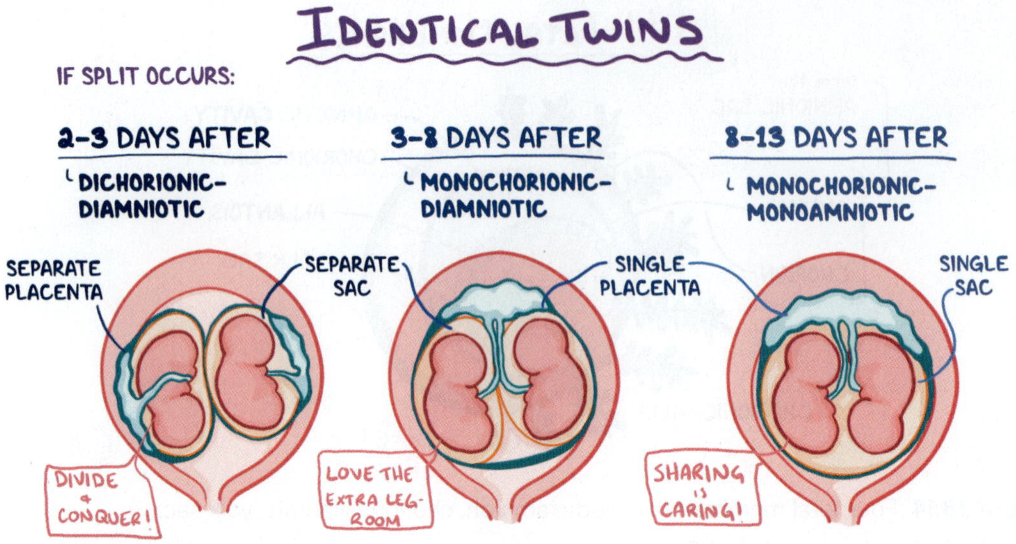

Figure 28.15 The way the womb is shared by identical twins depends on the time frame in which the zygote split in two.

NOTES
BODY SYSTEM STRUCTURES

DEVELOPMENT OF THE SKELETAL SYSTEM

osms.it/axial-skeleton-development

- Follows gastrulation (AKA formation of ectoderm, mesoderm, endoderm)

Axial skeleton
- Skull, vertebrae, rib cage, sternum
- Derived from mesoderm
- *Exception:* some skull bones come from ectoderm

Appendicular skeleton
- Pelvic, shoulder girdles; bones in limbs
- Derived from mesoderm

Pathways of bone development
- AKA ossification
- Two pathways
  - Endochondral, intramembranous

Endochondral ossification
- Almost all bones
  - *Exceptions:* clavicles; parietal, frontal bones of skull; maxilla; mandible; nasal bone; parts of temporal, occipital bones
- Hyaline cartilage serves as bone formation model
  - Mesenchymal cells differentiate into chondrocytes, which form cartilaginous model
  - Bone develops by replacing cartilage

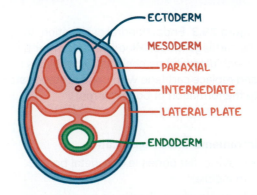

Figure 29.1 Cross section through an embryo demonstrating ectoderm, mesoderm, and endoderm. Paraxial and lateral plate mesoderm give rise to bones and muscles.

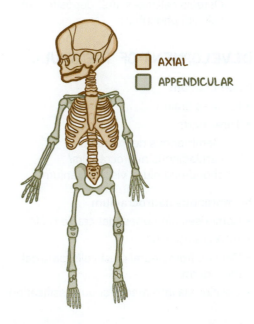

Figure 29.2 Axial and appendicular skeletons.

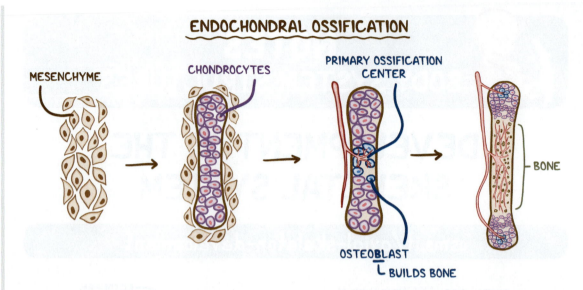

Figure 29.3 Endochondral ossification: the primary ossification center is at the center of the cartilage model. Blood vessels enter the primary ossification center, bringing nutrients, osteoblasts, and osteoclasts. Osteoblasts replace chondrocytes at the primary ossification center and replace cartilage with bone. Osteoclasts start to break down the center of bone, which leads to the formation of bone marrow.

Intramembranous ossification
- Clavicle, flat bones (e.g. parietal bones, mandible)
- Bone develops directly on membranous sheaths
    - Mesenchymal cells differentiate into osteoblasts, secrete osteoid (AKA unmineralized matrix)
    - Osteoid calcifices after deposition of calcium phosphate

DEVELOPMENT OF THE SKULL

Neurocranium
- Encases brain
- Three parts
    - Membranous neurocranium, cartilaginous neurocranium/ chondrocranium, viscerocranium

Membranous neurocranium
- Comprises flat bones that cradle brain
- AKA cranial vault
- Derived from neural crest cells, paraxial mesoderm
- Ossifies via intramembranous ossification

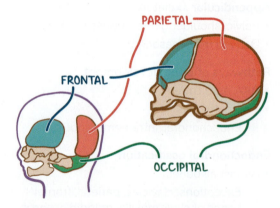

Figure 29.4 Lateral view of membranous neurocranium. It is composed of the flat bones that form a hard, protective shell around the brain.

Cartilaginous neurocranium
- AKA chondrocranium
- Bones around base of skull
- Derived from neural crest cells, paraxial mesoderm; become prechordal, chordal chondrocranium, respectively
- Ossifies via endochondral ossification

Chapter 29 Embryology: Body System Structures

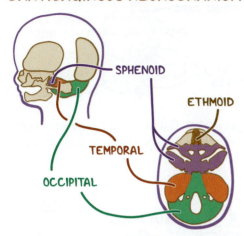

Figure 29.5 Lateral view (left) and superior view (right) of bones comprising cartilaginous neurocranium.

Viscerocranium
- Facial bones
- Six pharyngeal arches; facial bones arise from first arch
  - *Dorsal side*: maxilla, zygomatic bones, parts of temporal bone
  - *Ventral side*: Meckel's cartilage undergoes intramembranous ossification; becomes mandible
  - Dorsal tip of mandibular process, second pharyngeal arch → become incus, malleus, stapes

Temporary skull structures
- Skull bones not fully fused at birth
  - Allows molding of fetal head during passage through birth canal
  - Closes by 18 months old, allows brain growth
- *Sutures*: narrow gaps between bone plates filled with fibrous tissues
- *Fontanelles*: wide sutures where > two bones meet
  - Anterior fontanelle most prominent
  - Where two parietal, two frontal bones meet

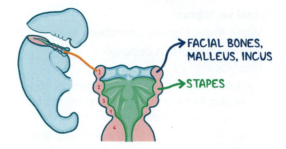

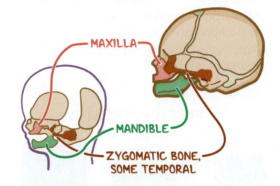

Figure 29.6 The viscerocranium arises primarily from the first pharyngeal arch with stapes arising from the second arch. The viscerocranium is composed of the facial bones (illustrated here in a lateral view).

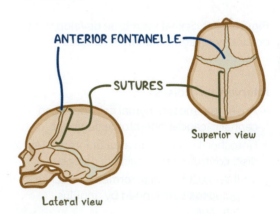

Figure 29.7 Lateral and anterior view of the anterior fontanelle where the frontal and parietal bones meet.

VERTEBRAE, RIBS, & STERNUM

Spinal vertebrae
- **Week 4**: develop from somites
- Sclerotome portion undergoes resegmentation
    - Sclerotome cells from cephalic portion of somite fuse with caudal portion of neighboring somite
- Sclerotome cells surround notochord, spinal cord; transform into mesenchymal cells
- Mesenchymal cells form vertebrae through endochondral ossification
- Ribs then emerge from costal facets of thoracic vertebrae

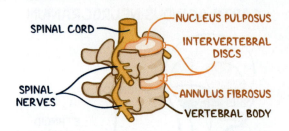

Figure 29.9 Relationship between vertebrae, intervertebral discs, spinal cord, and spinal nerves.

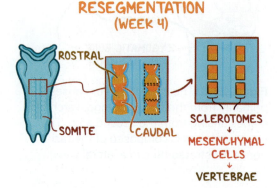

Figure 29.8 Spinal vertebrae development occurs by resegmentation of somites.

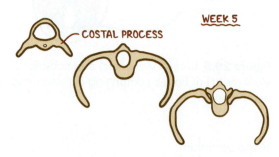

Figure 29.10 Rib development arises from costal processes of thoracic vertebrae.

Intervertebral discs
- Arise from mesenchymal cells between cephalic, caudal sclerotome segment
- Notochord enlarges in area of intervertebral disc, contributing to nucleus pulposus
    - Intervertebral disk formed as nucleus pulposus surrounded by annulus fibrosus
- Myotomes bridge intervertebral discs, form vertebral muscles
- *Primary spinal curves established*: thoracic, sacral

Sternum
- Arises from parietal mesoderm layer in anterior body wall
- Cartilaginous bars form on either side of midline, fuse
    - Differentiate into manubrium, main body of sternum, xiphoid process

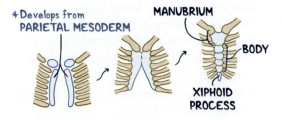

Figure 29.11 Sternum development arises from parietal mesoderm.

DEVELOPMENT OF THE MUSCULAR SYSTEM

osms.it/muscular-system-development

KEY POINTS
- **Mesoderm:** becomes vast majority of muscles
- **Paraxial mesoderm:** becomes skeletal muscle
- **Visceral/splanchnic mesoderm:** becomes cardiac muscle, some smooth muscle
- **Ectoderm:** becomes remaining smooth muscle

DEVELOPMENT OF SKELETAL MUSCLE

Mesodermal cells
- Form myogenic cells, which undergo mitosis
- Form postmitotic myoblasts
    - Synthesize actin, myosin
- Fuse, form multinucleated myotubes
    - Myotubes synthesize actin, myosin, troponin, tropomyosin, other muscle proteins
- Proteins aggregate, form myofibrils (AKA muscle fibers/cells)

Paraxial mesoderm
- Divides into segments, AKA somitomeres, in craniocaudal sequence
- Seven somitomeres form head, neck muscles
    - Contribute to pharyngeal arches' formation
- Remaining somitomeres form 35 pairs of somites for trunk region
- Undergo epithelialization
    - AKA form balls of epithelial cells

Somites
- Ventral region of each somite forms sclerotome
    - AKA bone-forming cells
- Upper region of each somite forms dermatome plus two muscle-forming areas
- Cells of ventrolateral, dorsomedial lip of somites migrate ventral to dermatome, proliferate there to form dermomyotome
    - *Exception:* some cells of ventrolateral lip migrate into parietal mesoderm layer of lateral plate mesoderm; these contribute to abaxial domain, discussed below
- Lateral somitic frontier separates somite clusters from parietal mesoderm into two domains
    - **Primaxial domain:** consists of somites around neural tube; receives signals for differentiation from notochord, neural tube; forms shoulder, back, intercostal muscles
    - **Abaxial domain:** receives signals for differentiation from lateral plate mesoderm; forms infrahyoid, abdominal wall, limb muscles

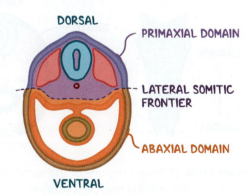

Figure 29.12 Divisions of mesoderm created by lateral somitic frontier.

DEVELOPMENT OF CARDIAC MUSCLE

- Develops from visceral (i.e. splanchnic) mesoderm surrounding endothelial heart tube
- Myoblasts adhere via special attachments, which later become intercalated discs
- Patterning of striations forms branch-like lines
    - Unlike straighter lines of skeletal muscles

DEVELOPMENT OF SMOOTH MUSCLE

- Paraxial mesoderm cells from first seven somite pairs form smooth muscle of head
    - Includes tongue, jaw muscles, throat muscles
    - Develops in response to signals released by neural crest cells
- Visceral/splanchnic mesoderm surrounding gut tube → becomes digestive system muscles
- Ectoderm → becomes sphincter, dilator muscles of pupils, mammary glands, sweat glands
- Proepicardial cells, neural crest cells → becomes smooth muscle of aorta, arteries

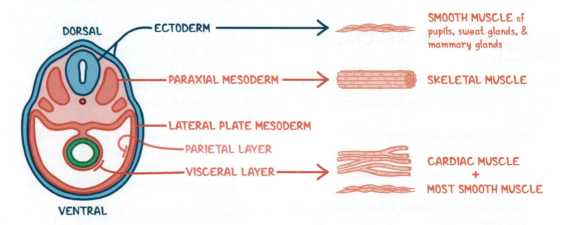

Figure 29.13 Cross section through an embryo demonstrating the origins of skeletal, cardiac, and smooth muscle.

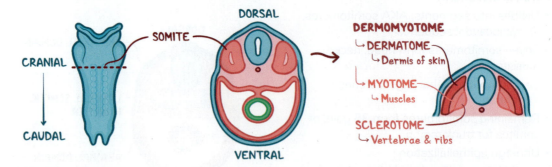

Figure 29.14 Different regions of the somite form different body structures. The myotome is responsible for skeletal muscle formation.

DEVELOPMENT OF THE LIMBS

osms.it/limb-development

Limb buds: overview
- *End of week 4:* limb buds visible on ventrolateral body wall
- Limb bud structure
  - *Mesenchymal core:* forms connective tissue, bones
  - *Myotomes:* form muscles
  - *Ectoderm cover:* forms epidermis of skin

Connective tissue & bones
- Development determined by series of interactions between ectoderm, mesenchyme
- Ectoderm at the limb apex proliferates, forms apical ectodermal ridge (AER) → induces adjacent mesenchyme to remain undifferentiated, rapidly proliferating cells
  - AKA undifferentiated zone
- Ectoderm further influences mesenchyme
- Mesenchyme differentiates into cartilage, muscle; forms three components proximo-distally
  - *Stylopod:* becomes humerus/femur
  - *Zeugopod:* becomes radius/ulna, tibia/fibula
  - *Autopod:* becomes carpals, metacarpals, metatarsals
- Week 6: limb bud apexes flatten, become hand, foot plates
- Fingers, toes formed via localized apoptosis induced by AER
  - Separates hand, foot plates into five parts
- Mesenchyme underneath differentiates into chondrocytes
  - Chondrocytes form primary hyaline cartilage models of future bones
- As chondrogenesis stops, joint formation induced
  - Condensed mesenchyme differentiates into dense fibrous tissue (forms articular cartilage, synovial membrane, menisci, ligaments of joint)

Limb muscle development
- Derived from dorsolateral cells of somites
  - AKA myotomes
  - Myotomes from C4-T2 migrate to upper limb
  - Myotomes from L2-S2 migrate to lower limb
- During migration to limbs, myotomes form two compartments
  - Anterior condensation → flexor, pronator muscles of upper limb; flexor, adductor muscles of lower limb
  - Posterior condensation → extensor, supinator muscles of upper limb; extensor, abductor muscles of lower limb
  - Ventral primary branches of spinal nerves, mesenchyme divide; form dorsal, ventral branches to these compartments
  - Week 7: limbs rotate
- Upper limb rotates 90° laterally
  - Lower limb rotates 90° medially

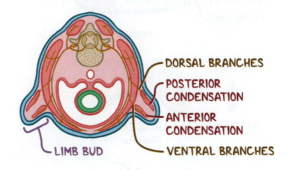

Figure 29.15 Limb muscle development: myotomes migrate to limbs, forming anterior and posterior condensations that are innervated by ventral and dorsal branches of the spinal nerve's primary ventral branches.

DEVELOPMENT OF THE CARDIOVASCULAR SYSTEM

osms.it/cardiovascular-system-development

- Begins during week 3
- Mesoderm cells travel through primitive streak to embryo's head, form horseshoe-shaped area with two limbs
  - AKA primary heart field
- Vascular endothelial growth factor (VEGF) signals limbs' cells to organize into two tubes
- Lateral mesoderm splits into somatic, splanchnic layers
  - Concurrently, primitive pericardial cavity forms lateral to each tube
- At inferior end, each endocardial tube connects to vitelline vein stemming from yolk sac
- Mesoderm cells also form pair of longitudinal vessels (AKA dorsal aortae)

LATERAL FOLDING OF EMBRYO

- Embryo folds into cylindrical shape as lateral borders meet at midline
  - Two endocardial tubes fuse, forming primitive heart tube
- Left, right vitelline veins also fuse, forming sinus venosus
  - AKA inflow tract
- Aortae fuse, forming aortic sac
  - AKA outflow tract
- Primitive pericardial cavities fuse around heart tube, forming pericardial cavity
- Heart tube remains attached to pericardial cavity by sheet of mesoderm called dorsal mesocardium; heart tube now has two layers (endothelial lining, cardiac myoblasts)
- Endothelial lining forms endocardium
- Cardiac myoblasts form myocardium
  - Some myocardial cells in sinus venosus begin to produce rhythmic electrical discharge
- Mesenchymal cells of dorsal mesocardium form proepicardial organ
  - These cells proliferate, migrate over myocardium, form epicardium

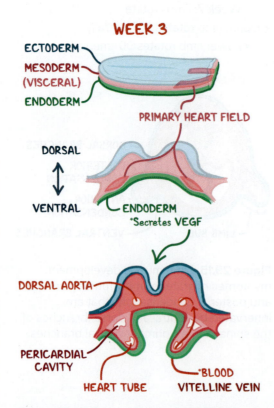

Figure 29.16 Early development of the cardiovascular system starting in week 3.

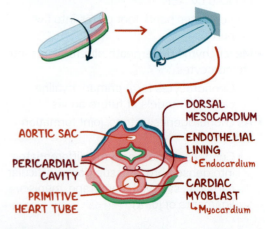

Figure 29.17 Structures formed as a result of lateral folding of the embryo.

Chapter 29 Embryology: Body System Structures

CRANIOCAUDAL FOLDING OF EMBRYO

- Cylindrical embryo folds down its length, forming shrimp-like shape
  - Heart pushed toward chest
- By week 4: heart tube reaches thorax, circulating blood can be seen travelling through heart tube

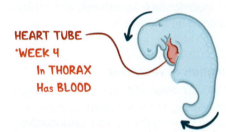

Figure 29.18 Craniocaudal folding of the embryo places heart tube in thorax.

PARTITION OF THE HEART TUBE

Sections of the heart tube

- *Sinus venosus*: left, right sinus horn bring in blood
- Primitive atrium, primitive ventricle separated by atrioventricular sulcus
- *Primitive atrium*: becomes left, right atria
- *Primitive ventricle*: forms left ventricle
  - Separated from bulbus cordis by bulboventricular sulcus
- *Bulbus cordis*: forms right ventricle, outflow tracts for both ventricles
- *Truncus arteriosus*: at top of heart tube
  - Pumps blood through aortic sac into early version of circulatory system

LOOPING OF THE HEART TUBE

- Heart tube folds into "C" shape
- Truncus arteriosus and bulbus cordis move down, to right
  - Form top portion of "C"
- Primitive ventricle bends to right of midline, slightly to front
  - Forms middle portion of "C"
- Primitive atrium, sinus venosus
  - Form bottom of "C"
- Enlarging ventricle moves left
  - Crosses over midline again, covers primitive atrium
- Visceral pericardium attaches to outside of heart, forms epicardium

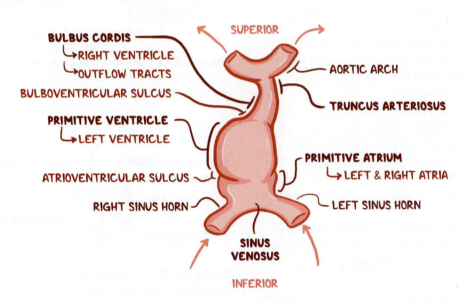

Figure 29.19 Heart tube sections and the structures they become.

LOOPING

BULBUS CORDIS → RIGHT VENTRICLE
PRIMITIVE VENTRICLE → LEFT VENTRICLE
PRIMITIVE ATRIUM → LEFT & RIGHT ATRIA

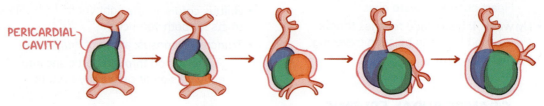

Figure 29.20 During week 4, the heart tube undergoes looping: tube lengthens, walls thicken, and sections move towards appropriate locations to continue development.

FURTHER PARTITIONING OF THE HEART

- Mesoderm proliferates on anterior, posterior walls of atrioventricular canal
  - Forms anterior, posterior endocardial cushion
  - Cushions grow towards each other, fuse
- Heart now separated into left, right atrioventricular canals
- Endocardial cells proliferate on ventricular side of each canal
  - These form leaflets of mitral, tricuspid valves
- Canals now divided into atria, ventricles

Formation of the atria

- Crescent-shaped septum primum grows downward between future left, right atria
  - Opening (AKA ostium primum) remains
- Septum primum continues to grow, fuses with endocardial cushion, closes ostium primum completely
- Ostium secundum appears in center of septum primum
- Septum secundum grows downward just to right of septum primum, covers ostium secundum
  - Leaves small opening (AKA foramen ovale)
- Septum secundum acts as one-way valve, allowing blood flow from left to right atrium
- After birth, closure of foramen ovale is facilitated by
  - ↓ in right atrial pressure due to occlusion of placental circulation
  - ↑ in left atrial pressure due to ↑ pulmonary venous return

Formation of ventricles

- Muscular ridge of tissue grows upward from apex, fuses with thinner membranous region coming down from endocardial cushions
  - Forms left, right ventricles
- **End of week four:** cardiac loop starts to take shape of adult heart

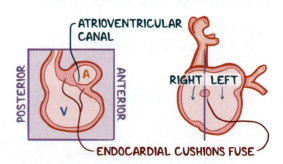

Figure 29.21 Fusion of the endocardial cushions separates the heart into right and left atrioventricular canals.

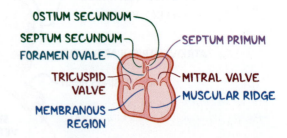

Figure 29.22 Structures contributing to the formation of the atria and ventricles.

Chapter 29 Embryology: Body System Structures

DEVELOPMENT OF THE ARTERIAL SYSTEM

Development of the aorta
- Starts with division of truncus arteriosus
- Two endocardial cushions appear on right-superior, left-inferior walls
- Cushions grow with spiraling trajectory, wrap around each other
- Form aorticopulmonary septum
  - Divides into root of aorta, pulmonary artery
  - Semilunar valves develop shortly after

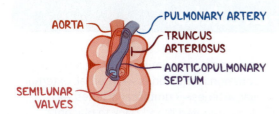

Figure 29.23 Anterior view of heart visualizing development of the aorta and pulmonary artery.

Arteries of head & neck region, pulmonary arteries
- Come from five aortic arches
- 1st arch: maxillary artery
- 2nd arch: stapedial artery
- 3rd arch: two common carotid arteries, part of internal carotid arteries
- 4th aortic arch
  - Left 4th arch: aortic arch
  - Right 4th arch: right subclavian artery
- 6th arch: pulmonary arteries, ductus arteriosus

Remaining arteries
- Develop mainly from right, left dorsal aortae → fuse during lateral folding, form dorsal aorta
- Dorsal aorta sprouts posterolateral arteries; lateral arteries; ventral arteries (AKA vitelline, umbilical)

DEVELOPMENT OF THE VENOUS SYSTEM
- Develops from sinus venosus
- **Week 4**: sinus venosus receives deoxygenated blood from sinus horns, opens in center of primitive atrium
- Each horn receives blood from vitelline/omphalomesenteric veins, umbilical veins, common cardinal veins
- Next, sinus venosus becomes asymmetric, shifts to right
  - Caused by left to right shunts
- Right sinus horn enlarges; becomes smooth-walled part of right atrium; forms openings for superior, inferior vena cavas
- Left sinus horn shrinks; persists as coronary sinus, oblique vein of left atrium

DEVELOPMENT OF THE CONDUCTING SYSTEM
- Special group of myocardial cells in wall of sinus venosus organize, synchronize their electrical discharge, form pacemaker centers
  - *Cells in wall of sinus venosus:* form sinoatrial node
  - *Cells in atrioventricular septum:* form atrioventricular node
  - *Cells in interventricular septum:* form bundle of His
  - *Rest of ventricular myocardium:* form modified cardiac myocytes, which become Purkinje fibers

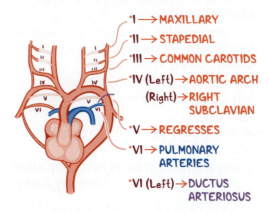

Figure 29.24 Aortic arches and their derivatives. The arches exist from weeks four to six and sprout from aortic sac.

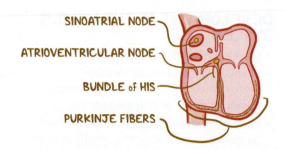

Figure 29.25 The heart's conducting system.

FETAL CIRCULATION

osms.it/fetal-circulation

KEY POINTS
- *Placenta*: low-resistance circuit, organ of gas exchange
- *Fetal systemic circulation*: low-resistance circuit
- *Lungs*: filled with fluid, hypoxic vasoconstriction
    - High-resistance circuit, no role in gas exchange
- Right side of heart pressure > left side of heart pressure
- Ductus venosus, foramen ovale, ductus arteriosus shunt blood away from fetal lungs

Pattern of flow
- Placenta → umbilical vein → divides into left, right umbilical vein
- Left umbilical vein → portal vein → liver → hepatic vein → inferior vena cava → right atrium
- Right umbilical vein → ductus venosus (bypasses liver) → inferior vena cava → right atrium
- Right atrium → left atrium via foramen ovale
    - Small amount of blood from right atrium enters right ventricle, pulmonary artery, lungs
- Blood shunted from pulmonary artery to aorta by small blood vessel
    - AKA ductus arteriosus
- Aorta → oxygenated blood delivered to systemic circulation → right, left common iliac arteries → internal, external iliac arteries → umbilical arteries → deoxygenated blood back to placenta

CHANGES AT BIRTH
- Pulmonary circulatory pressure ↓ while systemic circulation ↑
    - When umbilical cord cut, low-resistance circuit removed → systemic circulation increases
    - Lung fluid replaced by air as neonate takes first breaths/cries
    - Oxygen diffuses into blood vessels surrounding alveoli, pulmonary arterioles relax, pulmonary resistance falls, blood flows into lungs
- Closing of ductus arteriosus
    - Pressure changes cause decreased blood flow through ductus arteriosus
    - *Complete closure*: 12–24 hours after birth
    - *Physical remnant*: ligamentum arteriosum
- Closing of foramen ovale
    - Pressure in right side of heart falls, seals foramen ovale
    - *Physical remnant*: fossa ovalis
- Umbilical vein forms round ligament of liver
- Ductus venosus forms ligamentum venosum of liver

Chapter 29 Embryology: Body System Structures

FETAL CIRCULATION: PATHS TO RIGHT ATRIUM

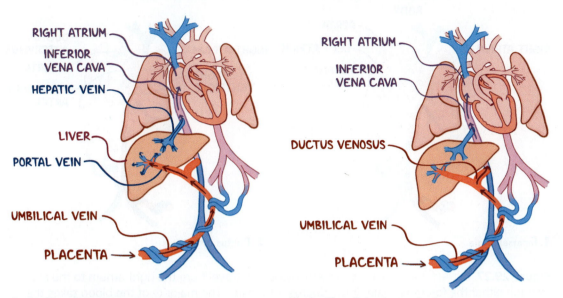

1a. Left umbilical vein to portal vein

1b. Left umbilical vein to ductus venosus

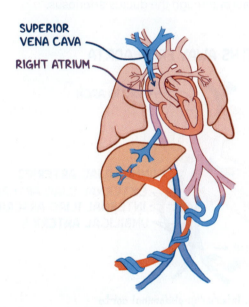

2. Superior vena cava

Figure 29.26 The fetal right atrium receives blood from the inferior vena cava (via liver and ductus venosus) and the superior vena cava.

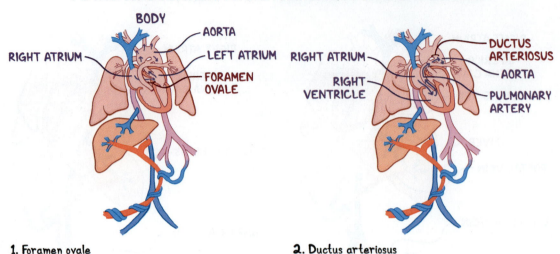

Figure 29.27 In the fetal circulatory system, blood can travel from the right atrium to the aorta through either the foramen ovale or the ductus arteriosus. The majority of the blood takes the first path from the higher pressure right atrium to the lower pressure left atrium, bypassing the right ventricle entirely. The blood that does flow into the right ventricle is shunted from the high pressure pulmonary artery to the lower pressure aorta through the ductus arteriosus.

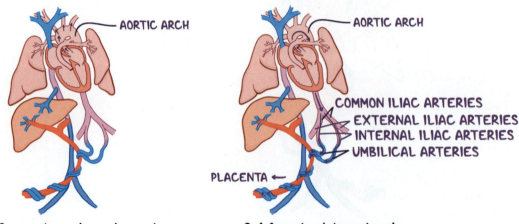

Figure 29.28 The aorta sends blood to the entire body through its various branches. The interior iliac arteries each give rise to an umbilical artery. These arteries travel alongside the umbilical vein and bring deoxygenated blood back to the placenta, where CO_2 is delivered and O_2 is picked up. This cycle repeats until birth.

Chapter 29 Embryology: Body System Structures

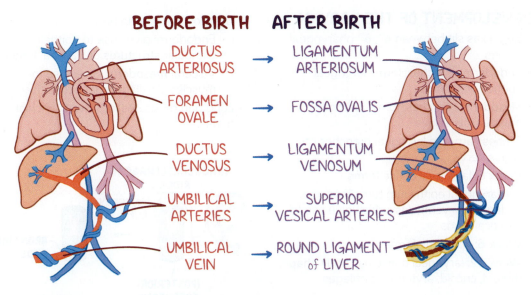

Figure 29.29 The fetal circulatory adaptations and their physical remnants after birth. The umbilical arteries and vein are surrounded by a substance called Wharton's jelly in the umbilical cord. Once exposed to the cold air, Wharton's jelly shrinks and squeezes the umbilical blood vessels, causing them to wither. The arteries constrict and flatten, and are mostly gone within a few months; only a small portion remains and subsequently function as the superior vesical arteries, which supply blood to either side of the bladder.

DEVELOPMENT OF THE RESPIRATORY SYSTEM

osms.it/respiratory-system-development

KEY POINTS
- **Week 4**: starts developing
    - Lung bud sprouts from foregut portion of digestive tract
- **Endoderm, mesoderm**: form lower respiratory tract structures
    - Larynx, trachea, lungs

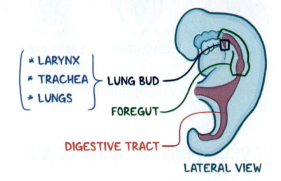

Figure 29.30 Week 4: lung bud sprouts from foregut.

DEVELOPMENT OF THE LARYNX

- Begins as slit between 4th, 6th pharyngeal arches
- *Endoderm of arches:* forms laryngeal epithelium, glands
- *Mesoderm of arches:* forms laryngeal muscles, cartilages
- Arches carry the laryngeal branches of vagus nerve
- Week 5: laryngeal orifice forms
    - Laryngeal epithelium turns into laryngeal ventricles, which give rise to vocal cords
- Week 6: epiglottis forms
- Week 12: laryngeal orifice has adult shape; thyroid, cricoid, arytenoid cartilages

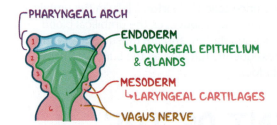

Figure 29.31 The endoderm and mesoderm of the pharyngeal arches contribute to larynx formation.

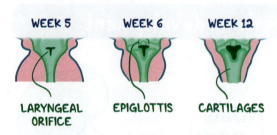

Figure 29.32 Key timing and features in larynx development.

DEVELOPMENT OF THE TRACHEA & LUNGS

- Week 4: two tracheoesophageal ridges grow towards one another, fuse into septum
- Septum divides foregut into two regions
    - Posterior: esophagus
    - Anterior: lung bud
- Composition of lung bud
    - *Endoderm:* gives rise to epithelial, glandular structures of trachea, lungs
    - *Visceral mesoderm:* gives rise to muscles, cartilage, connective tissue
- Lung bud bifurcates into two bronchial buds

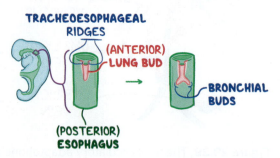

Figure 29.33 At the loose end, the lung bud bifurcates into two bronchial buds which give rise to the lungs.

STAGES OF LUNG DEVELOPMENT

Pseudoglandular stage: weeks 5–16

- Bronchial buds differentiate
    - Left and right main/primary bronchi
    - Three lobar/secondary bronchi for right lung lobes, two for left lung lobes
- *Lobar/secondary bronchi:* divide into 10 segmental/tertiary bronchi on right, eight on left
    - AKA lung segments
- Segmental/tertiary bronchi divide repeatedly until 15–25 terminal bronchioles formed
- Lungs now consist of simple columnar epithelium

Canalicular stage: weeks 16–26

- Terminal bronchioles continue to divide, form respiratory bronchioles
- Respiratory bronchiole divides into three to six alveolar ducts
- Prominent capillary network forms
- Week 24: primitive alveoli appear closer to trachea
- Lungs now consist of simple cuboidal epithelium
    - Unsuitable for gas exchange

Terminal sac stage: week 26–birth
- More primitive alveoli form
- Epithelial lining of terminal sacs differentiate
- Flat cells in direct contact with endothelium of the capillaries
    - AKA type I pneumocytes, form blood-air barrier
    - Also includes basement membrane
- Pulmonary surfactant produced by large, cuboidal cells
    - AKA type II pneumocytes

Alveolar stage: week 36–8 years old
- Terminal sacs partitioned by secondary septae
- Number of adult alveoli increase
    - 0–70 million at birth, 300–400 at eight years old
- Number of respiratory bronchioles increases with lung size

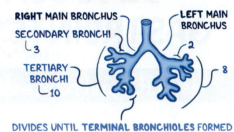

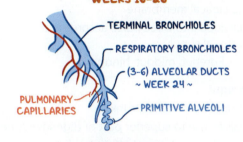

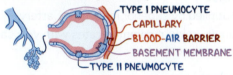

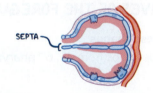

Figure 29.34 The stages of lung development.

DEVELOPMENT OF THE GASTROINTESTINAL SYSTEM

osms.it/gastrointestinal-system-development

Primitive gut tube
- Forms during week 3
- Extends from buccopharyngeal membrane to cloacal membrane
- Divided into three parts according to arterial supply
  - Foregut, midgut, hindgut

Foregut
- Supplied by celiac trunk
- Gives rise to superior part of digestive tube
  - Pharynx to first half of duodenum
  - Also liver, gallbladder, pancreas

Midgut
- Supplied by superior mesenteric artery
- Briefly, midgut communicates with yolk sac via vitelline duct

Hindgut
- Supplied by inferior mesenteric artery

DERIVATIVES OF THE FOREGUT

Pharynx & esophagus
- Pharynx develops from 4th, 6th pharyngeal arches
- **Week 4:** tracheoesophageal septum divides foregut below pharynx into two regions
  - *Esophagus:* posterior
  - *Lung bud:* anterior
- Esophageal epithelium, glands derived from foregut endoderm
  - Epithelium proliferates, initially fills lumen
  - *By week 8:* becomes hollow tube via recanalization
- Esophageal muscles, adventitia derived from surrounding mesoderm

Stomach & duodenum
- Begin as small dilation of foregut
- Ventral mesogastrium attaches ventral border to anterior body wall
- Dorsal mesogastrium attaches dorsal border to posterior body wall
  - *Dorsal border:* grows faster, forms greater curvature
  - *Ventral border:* lesser curvature
- Stomach undergoes 90°, clockwise rotation along its length
  - Pulls dorsal, ventral mesogastria with it

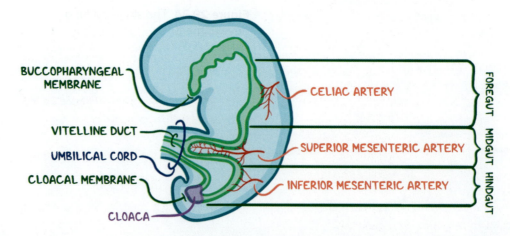

Figure 29.35 The primitive gut tube at week 3, including subdivisions and their blood supplies.

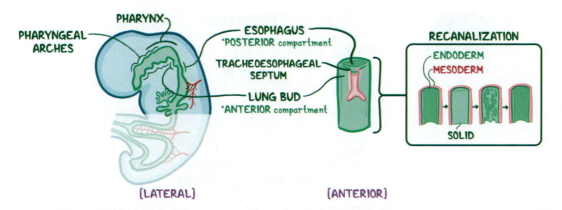

Figure 29.36 The pharynx and esophagus are derivatives of the foregut. The tracheoesophageal septum divides the foregut into the esophagus posteriorly and the lung bud anteriorly. The esophageal endoderm (epithelium) initially proliferates and fills the lumen, but recanalization is complete by week 8.

- Greater curvature moves to right side of body, lesser curvature to left
- Stomach now has anterior, posterior faces
- **Ventral mesogastrium:** becomes lesser omentum
- **Dorsal mesogastrium:** grows, bends as stomach rotates
  - Forms cavity (AKA omental bursa) between stomach, posterior body wall
- **Omental bursa:** communicates with peritoneal cavity through omental foramen
  - Omental bursa grows, fills with peritoneal fluid
  - *Develops two projections:* upper recess, lower recess
- **Upper recess:** extends behind developing liver
- **Lower recess:** extends downward over developing intestines
  - Sheets of dorsal mesogastrium that form lower recess fuse, forming greater omentum
- Stomach rotates once more on frontal plane
  - Repositions superior end of stomach
  - Forms cardiac sphincter, pylorus
  - Turns duodenum into C-shaped loop, with middle of "C" on right side
- **First two sections of duodenum:** derived from last part of foregut
- Tiny tissue buds on last portion of foregut grow, develop into liver, gallbladder, pancreas

Liver & gallbladder
- Liver bud, AKA hepatic diverticulum, gives rise to liver, gallbladder, biliary duct system
  - Forms inside ventral mesogastrium, extends into sheet of mesoderm that separates developing heart from midgut (AKA septum transversum)
  - Contains mesoderm, endoderm
- Foregut endoderm forms hepatocytes
  - *During week 12:* hepatocytes start producing bile during mesoderm
  - Forms Kupffer cells, hematopoietic tissue
  - *During week 6:* produce red blood cells
- Liver bud divides into two parts
  - *Larger, superior portion:* becomes liver
  - *Smaller, inferior part:* becomes gallbladder

Pancreas
- Two pancreatic buds eventually fuse to form entire organ
  - *Dorsal bud:* forms tail, body, part of head
  - *Ventral bud:* forms most of head
- **Week 10:** begins secreting insulin

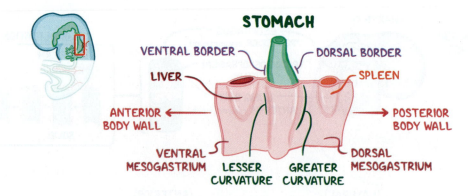

Figure 29.37 Lateral view of the embryo visualizing the stomach and associated structures before any rotation has taken place. The stomach presents as small foregut dilation beneath esophagus. Starting at week 5, the liver grows between the layers of the ventral mesogastrium and the spleen grows between the layers of the dorsal mesogastrium.

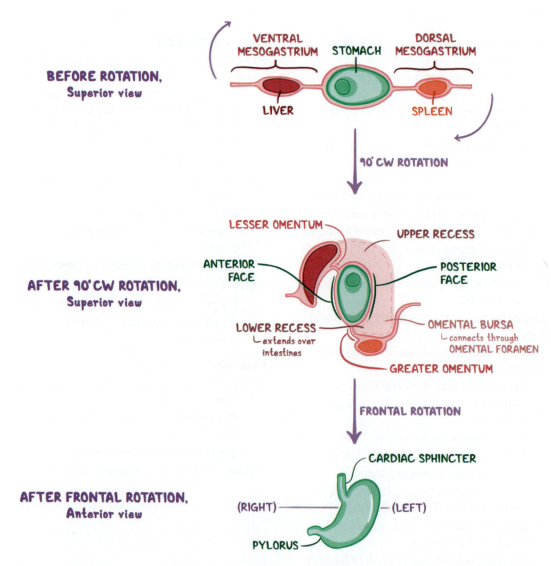

Figure 29.38 The two rotations events in the development of the stomach.

Chapter 29 Embryology: Body System Structures

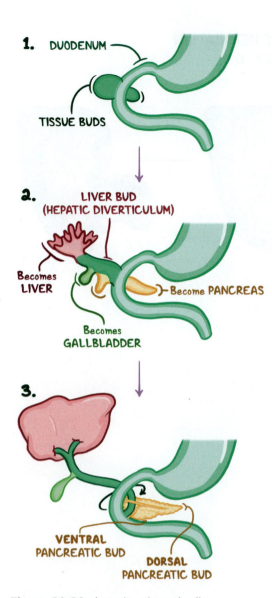

Figure 29.39 Anterior view: the liver, gallbladder, and pancreas develop from tissue buds at the distal end of the foregut.

DERIVATIVES OF THE MIDGUT

- Key elements
- Parts of small, large intestines derive from midgut
  - *Small intestine:* third, fourth sections of duodenum; jejunum; ilium
  - *Large intestine:* cecum, appendix, ascending colon, proximal ⅔ of transverse colon

Physiologic gut herniation
- During rapid gut tube growth, primary intestinal loop herniates through vitelline duct, develops inside umbilical cord
- Primary intestinal loop protrudes inside umbilical cord, superior mesenteric artery grows between loop's two limbs
  - *Cranial limb:* initially develops above superior mesenteric artery
  - *Caudal limb:* develops below superior mesenteric artery
- First, loop rotates 90° counterclockwise around axis of superior mesenteric artery
  - Moves cranial limb to right side of artery, inferior limb to left
- Cranial limb becomes convoluted
  - Marks future jejunal, ileal anses
- Caudal limb develops small dilation
  - Eventually becomes cecum, appendix
- Week 10: loop rotates final 180°, moves into abdominal cavity
  - Formerly caudal limb now frames developing small intestine loops, becomes ascending colon, right ⅔ of transverse colon

DERIVATIVES OF THE HINDGUT

- Left ⅓ of transverse colon, descending colon, sigmoid colon, upper part of anal canal derive from hindgut
- Begins after caudal limb of midgut, extends to cloacal membrane
- Anal canal's lower portion derives from primitive anus (AKA proctodeum)
  - *Proctodeum:* pit of ectoderm that forms below cloacal membrane
- Week 4: Urorectal septum forms
  - Separates cloaca into anterior urogenital sinus, posterior anal canal; covered by urogenital, anal membranes, respectively
- End of week 7: separation completed
  - Anal membrane ruptures, forming continuous anal canal
  - Anal canal opens in embryo's tail-region

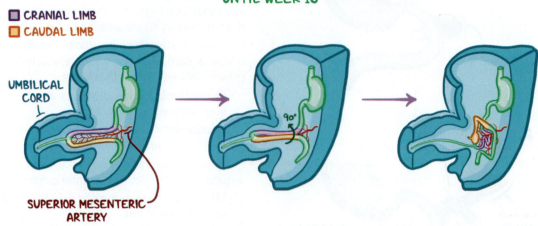

Figure 29.40 The process of physiologic gut herniation.

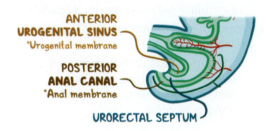

Figure 29.41 Hindgut structures at week 7 when the anal membrane has ruptured to form a continuous anal canal.

DEVELOPMENT OF THE RENAL SYSTEM

osms.it/renal-system-development

- Begins in week 4
- Intermediate mesoderm on each side of embryo condenses, forming cylindrical structure (AKA urogenital ridge)
- Urogenital ridge runs parallel to future spinal column; has two portions
  - *Genital ridge:* becomes gonads
  - *Nephrogenic cord:* becomes urinary structures

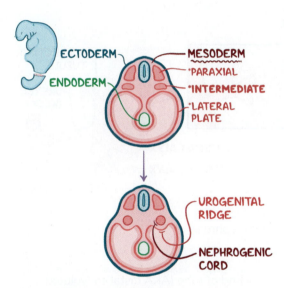

Figure 29.42 Week 4: urogenital ridge formation.

- Three structures emerge from nephrogenic cord in cranio-caudal fashion
  - Pronephros, mesonephros, metanephros

Pronephros
- *Beginning of week 4:* arises in neck region
- *End of week 4:* regresses
- Does not produce urine
- Consists of pronephric duct, nephrotomes
  - *Pronephric duct:* tube that runs length of nephrogenic cord
  - *Nephrotomes:* chunks of tissue that break off nephrogenic cord

Mesonephros
- Arises in thoracic, upper lumbar region of nephrogenic cord
- Consists of mesonephric duct, mesonephric tubules
- *Mesonephric duct:* develops from pronephric duct
  - Extends pronephric duct to cloaca
- *Mesonephric tubules:* hollow, S-shaped tubes
  - Connect to mesonephric duct on one end
  - On other end, form cup (AKA Bowman's capsule) around clump of capillaries (AKA glomerulus)
  - Glomerulus extracts fluid from capillaries, fluid flows down duct, becomes urine, drained through mesonephric duct into cloaca
  - After week 10, permanent kidneys take over, mesonephros regresses

Metanephros
- Week 5: develops in pelvic region
- Forms permanent kidneys
- Intermediate mesoderm near the mesonephric duct differentiates into metanephric mesoderm (AKA metanephric blastema)
- This induces mesonephric duct to sprout ureteric bud
  - Ureteric bud connected mesonephric duct via the ureteric stalk
- Ureteric bud lengthens, secretes growth factors
- This causes metanephric mesoderm to grow (AKA reciprocal induction)
- Ureteric bud grows into metanephric mesoderm
  - Metanephric mesoderm surrounds end

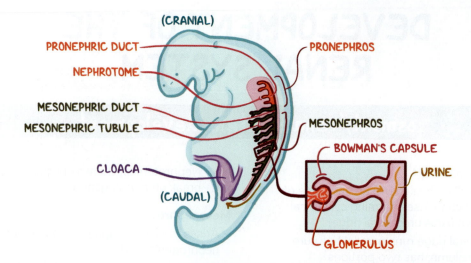

Figure 29.43 Locations and components of the pronephros and mesonephros.

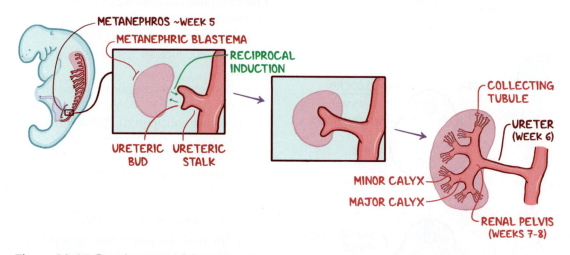

Figure 29.44 Development of the kidney from the metanephros.

of ureteric bud, leaving just ureteric stalk uncovered
- **Week 6:** ureteric stalk lengthens, forms ureter
- **Weeks 7–8:** ureteric bud divides in half, forms renal pelvis
- **Division continues:** two major calyces become minor calyces, then millions of collecting tubules

Nephrons
- **Week 8:** start forming
- Cells in collecting tubules signal adjacent metanephric mesoderm to form round cell clusters (AKA metanephric vesicles)
  - Vesicles elongate, bend into S-shaped tube
  - End of tube (AKA distal convoluted tubule) connects with collecting tubules
  - Other end forms proximal convoluted tubule; becomes Bowman's capsule, glomerulus
  - Portion between distal, proximal convoluted tubules lengthens, forms loop of Henle
- **Week 10:** nephrons start producing urine
- Initially, kidneys nourished by internal iliac arteries
- As permanent kidneys develop, they move up from pelvis to reach upper abdomen
  - Renal arteries form, lower branches degenerate

Chapter 29 Embryology: Body System Structures

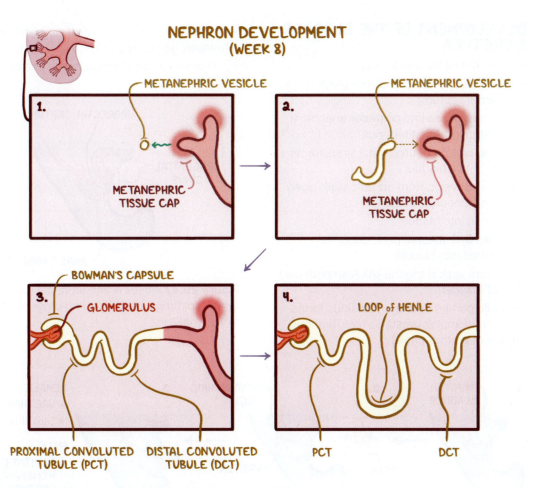

Figure 29.45 Nephron development begins at week 8.

1: Metanephric tissue cap signals adjacent metanephric mesoderm to form round cell clusters called metanephric vesicles.
2: Vesicles elongate, curve; end of tube connects with collecting duct.
3: Proximal and distal convoluted tubules (PCT, DCT).
4: Tube lengthens between PCT, DCT → loop of Henle.

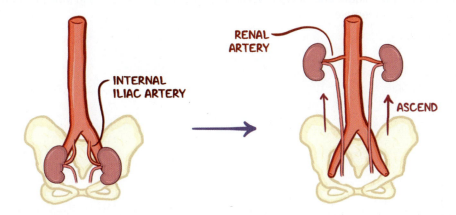

Figure 29.46 The kidneys are originally nourished by the internal iliac arteries. As kidneys ascend, the aorta forms branches at higher and higher levels to supply them. The renal arteries develop once the kidneys have reached their final position and earlier branches degenerate.

DEVELOPMENT OF THE BLADDER & URETHRA

- **Week 4**: begins developing
- Wall of tissue forms in cloaca (AKA urorectal septum)
    - Splits cloaca into posterior anal canal, anterior urogenital sinus
    - Top portion of urogenital sinus forms primitive bladder
- Ureters develop from ureteric stalk, open into mesonephric ducts
    - Drain into bladder
- **Weeks 5–6**: mesonephric ducts get absorbed into bladder
    - Form vesical trigone (AKA smooth part of bladder)
- Middle portion of urogenital sinus forms urethra (female); prostatic, membranous parts of urethra (male)
- Bottom portion of urogenital sinus grows towards genital tubercle
    - Forms clitoris (female), penis (male)

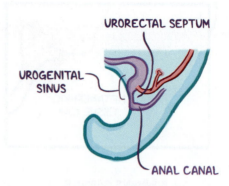

Figure 29.47 Week 4: the urorectal septum forms, splitting cloaca (forming urogenital sinus, anal canal).

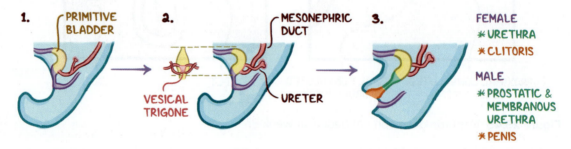

Figure 29.48 Development of the bladder and urethra.

1: Top portion of the urogenital sinus stretches out to form primitive bladder.
2: During weeks 5 and 6, the mesonephric ducts are absorbed into the bladder, forming the smooth part of the bladder wall called the vesical trigone.
3: Outcomes for the middle and bottom portions of the urogenital sinus in individuals who are genetically male and female.

DEVELOPMENT OF THE INTEGUMENTARY SYSTEM

osms.it/integumentary-system-development

DEVELOPMENT OF THE SKIN

Epidermis
- Derived from single layer of surface ectoderm
- *In second month:* cells divide, forms layer of periderm (AKA epitrichium)
- Cells of periderm desquamated during second ½ of prenatal life, form vernix caseosa
- Neural crest cells invade epidermis, form melanocytes
  - Move to keratinocytes in skin, hair bulb
  - Produce skin, hair pigmentation
- Cells in basal layer proliferate, form intermediate zone
- By end of fourth month, four layers complete
  - Basal/germinative layer, spinous layer, granular layer, horny layer
- Hair, nails, glands all develop as epidermal proliferations

Dermis
- Derived from mesenchyme from three sites
- *Lateral plate mesoderm:* produces dermis of limbs, body wall
- *Paraxial mesoderm:* produces dermis of back
- *Neural crest cells:* dermis of neck, face
- During third, fourth months, dermis forms many irregular papillary structures (AKA dermal papillae)
  - Project upward into epidermis
  - Contain Meissner corpuscles (AKA tactile sensory receptors)

Hair
- *Week 12:* hair follicles form from cells of stratum basale
- Begins as epidermal proliferation that penetrates into dermis (AKA hair bud)
- Hair bud invaginates at terminal end, forming hair papillae
- Each hair papilla fills with mesoderm
  - Vessels, nerves develop
- Cells of hair bud's center become keratinized, forming hair shaft
- Peripheral cells form the epithelial hair sheath
- Mesenchyme surrounding hair bud forms dermal root sheath, attached arrector pili muscle
- By end of third month, first hair appears as lanugo
  - Begins to shed at term
- Sebaceous gland forms from small bud in mesoderm
  - Secretes sebum

Nails
- By end of third month, nail fields form from thickenings at tips of digits
- Nail fields form nail root through migration
- Growth proximal, dorsal to each side of digit
- Tissue proliferates around each nail field, forming shallow depression
- Epidermis at nail roots differentiates into fingernails, toenails
  - Reaches tips by ninth month of development

Sweat glands
- Eccrine glands
  - Forms over most of body
  - Buds arise from germinative layer
  - Buds grow into dermis
  - Terminal part coils, forms secretory part of glands
- Apocrine glands
  - Develop during puberty over hairy parts of the body
  - Arise from epidermal buds that produce

hair follicles

Mammary glands
- Modified sweat glands
- Arise as bilateral bands of thickened epidermis (AKA mammary lines/mammary ridges)
- **Week 7**: these lines extend from from base of forelimb to base of hindlimb
  - Most of the line disappears, except in thoracic region
- Mammary lines penetrate mesenchyme, give rise to 16–24 sprouts that form small buds
- By end of intrauterine life, sprouts are canalized, form lactiferous ducts
- Lactiferous ducts initially open into small epithelial pit
  - Shortly after birth, proliferate, transform into nipple
- At puberty, lactiferous ducts stimulated by estrogen, progesterone to form alveoli, secretory cells

NOTES
HEAD & NECK STRUCTURE

PHARYNGEAL ARCHES, POUCHES, & CLEFTS

osms.it/pharyngeal-arches-pouches-clefts

- **Week 4:** pharyngeal apparatus begins to form, develop into various head, neck structures
- Bars of mesoderm form six pharyngeal arches in craniocaudal fashion
  - Numbered from one to six
  - 5th quickly regresses, does not form any structures
- Between pharyngeal arches, four pharyngeal clefts cover each arch's external part with ectoderm
- Four pharyngeal pouches line each arch's internal part with endoderm
- Each pharyngeal arch carries its own cranial nerve

First pharyngeal arch
- Innervated by mandibular branch of trigeminal nerve (CN V_3)
- Bones
  - Forms maxilla, mandible temporal, zygomatic bones
  - Two small portions of mandible form incus, malleus bones of middle ear
- Muscles
  - *Muscles that help with chewing:* temporalis, masseter, pterygoid muscles, tensor tympani muscles
  - *Muscles that help with swallowing:* tensor veli palatini, mylohyoid muscles, anterior belly of digastric muscle

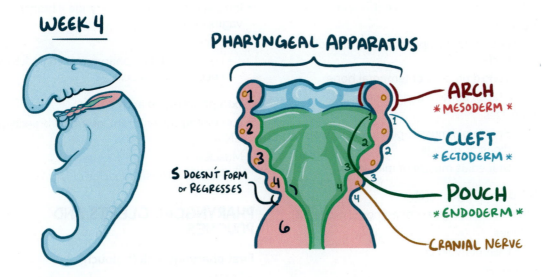

Figure 30.1 Locations of the pharyngeal arches, clefts, and pouches.

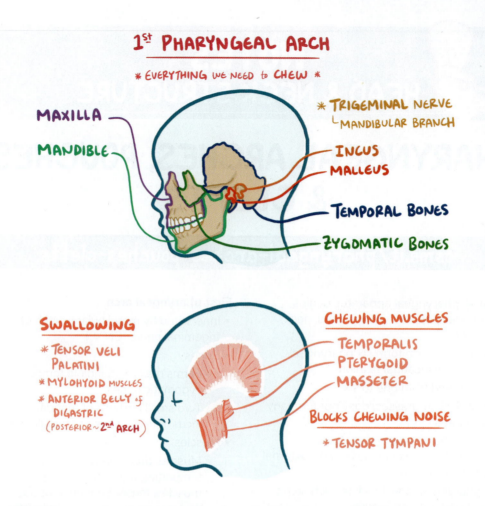

Figure 30.2 Bones and muscles originating from the first pharyngeal arch.

Second pharyngeal arch
- Innervated by facial nerve (CN VII)
- Bones
    - Lesser horns, upper portion of hyoid bone
    - Styloid process of temporal bone
    - Stapes bone of middle ear
- Muscles
    - Stylohyoid muscle, posterior belly of digastric muscle
    - Stapedius muscle of middle ear

Third pharyngeal arch
- Innervated by glossopharyngeal nerve (IX)
- Bones
    - Rest of hyoid bone
- Muscles
    - Stylopharyngeus muscle in throat

Fourth pharyngeal arch
- Innervated by superior laryngeal branch vagus nerve (CN X)
- Muscles
    - Levator palatini, pharyngeal constrictors, cricothyroid muscle

Sixth pharyngeal arch
- Innervated by recurrent laryngeal branch of CN X
- Muscles
    - Rest of intrinsic muscles of larynx

PHARYNGEAL CLEFTS AND POUCHES

First pharyngeal cleft, pouch
- Form ear
- Cleft gives rise to external auditory meatus, ear drums

Chapter 30 Embryology: Head & Neck Structure

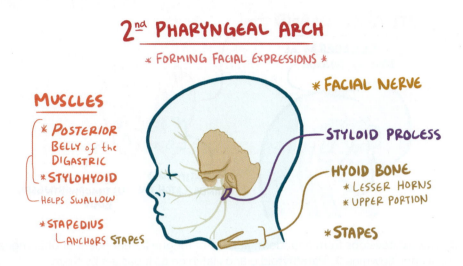

Figure 30.3 Bones and muscles originating from the second pharyngeal arch.

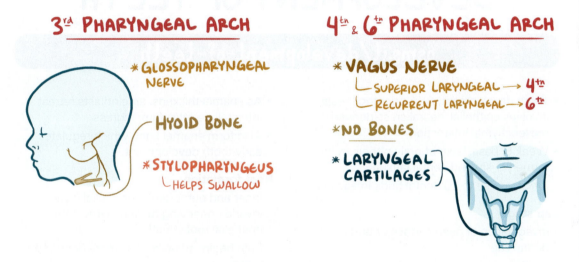

Figure 30.4 Structures originating from the third, fourth, and sixth pharyngeal arches. Muscles from fourth and sixth not shown.

- Pouch gives rise to internal auditory meatus, AKA middle ear, eustachian tube

Second-fourth clefts
- Fade as embryo grows
  - Cells lining second pharyngeal pouch multiply, migrate to form primitive tonsils

Third, fourth pouches
- Both divide into dorsal, ventral portions
- Dorsal portion of third pouch becomes inferior parathyroid gland
- Ventral portion becomes primitive thymus
  - Later descends down to chest

- Dorsal portion of fourth pouch becomes superior parathyroid gland
- Ventral portion becomes ultimo-pharyngeal body
  - Contains cells which differentiate into parafollicular/C-cells, migrate into thyroid

Thyroid and parathyroid glands
- Thyroid develops from endoderm at base of tongue independent of pharyngeal apparatus, descends down neck
- Parathyroid glands latch onto thyroid

OSMOSIS.ORG 251

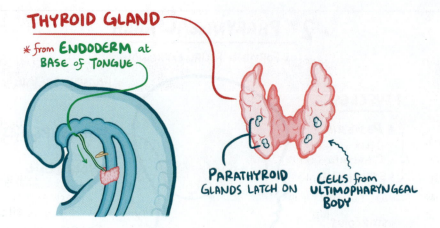

Figure 30.5 Thyroid develops from endoderm at base of tongue independent of pharyngeal apparatus, descends down neck. Parathyroid glands latch on as it passes by them.

DEVELOPMENT OF TEETH

osms.it/development-of-teeth

- Tooth development, AKA odontogenesis, involves epithelial, neural crest-derived mesenchymal interaction
- **Week 6:** basal layer of oral epithelium has formed C-shaped dental lamina
  - Gives rise to 10 dental buds in each jaw

Cap stage

- Invagination of deep surface of buds → dental cap
- Each dental cap consists of:
  - Outer dental epithelium
  - Inner dental epithelium
  - Central core of stellate reticulum
- Mesenchyme forms dental papilla, which form odontoblasts
  - Produce dentin
- Remainder of dental papilla forms pulp

Bell stage

- Dental cap grows, indentation deepens, forming bell-shaped configuration
- Inner dental epithelium cells transform into ameloblasts
  - Produce enamel deposited over dentin
- As enamel thickens, ameloblasts retreat into stellate reticulum, regress
- Also form enamel knot, which regulates early tooth development

Root formation

- Inner and outer dental epithelial layers invade underlying mesenchyme, form epithelial root sheath
- Pulp begins to narrow as more dentin laid down
  - Forms canal containing nerves, blood vessels
- Mesenchymal cell differentiation
  - Cementoblasts produce cementum (AKA type of specialized bone)
  - Periodontal ligament gives structural integrity to tooth
- As root lengthens, it pushes crown into oral cavity
  - Deciduous teeth (AKA milk teeth) arise 6–24 months of age
- Permanent teeth buds form during third month of development, remain dormant until sixth year of life

DEVELOPMENT OF THE BRAIN

osms.it/development-of-the-brain

DEVELOPMENT OF BRAIN VESICLES

- Neural plate folds, forming neural tube
- Rostral region develops into brain
- **Week 4:** primary brain vesicles develop
- **Week 6:** vesicles develop

Primary vesicle: forebrain/prosencephalon
- Secondary vesicles
  - *Telencephalon:* cerebral hemispheres, caudate, putamen, amygdaloid, claustrum, laminal terminalis, olfactory bulbs, hippocampus
  - *Diencephalon:* epithalamus, subthalamus, thalamus, hypothalamus, mammillary bodies, neurohypophysis, pineal gland, globus pallidus, renina, iris, ciliary body, optic nerve (CN II), optic chiasm, optic tract

Primary vesicle: midbrain/mesencephalon
- Secondary vesicle
  - Mesencephalon

Primary vesicle: hindbrain/rhombencephalon
- Secondary vesicles
  - *Metencephalon:* pons, cerebellum
  - *Myelencephalon:* medulla

DEVELOPMENT OF HINDBRAIN/RHOMBENCEPHALON

- Alar, basal plates separated by sulcus limitans

Basal plate
- Contains three groups of motor nuclei
- General somatic efferent
  - Cranial nerves III, IV, VI (metencephalon); XII (myelencephalon)
  - *Innervation:* somatic striated muscle (extrinsic eye muscles, tongue)
- Special visceral efferent
  - Cranial nerves V, VII (metencephalon); IX, X (myelencephalon)
  - *Innervation:* striated muscle of pharyngeal arches, AKA pharynx
- General visceral efferent
  - Cranial nerve III (metencephalon); IX, X (myelencephalon)
  - *Innervation:* parasympathetic pathway to sphincter pupillae; smooth muscles of airways, heart, salivary glands, viscera

Alar plate neuroblasts
- Contain three groups of sensory relay nuclei
- General visceral afferent
  - Cranial nerve X (myelencephalon)
  - *Innervation:* viscera, AKA gastrointestinal tract
- Special afferent
  - Cranial nerves VII, IX (metencephalon, myelencephalon); VIII (metencephalon)
  - *Innervates:* tongue, palate, epiglottis, AKA taste; cochlea, semicircular canals, AKA balance, hearing
- General somatic afferent
  - Cranial nerves V, VII (metencephalon); IX (myelencephalon)
  - *Innervation:* touch, temperature, pain in head, neck

MYELENCEPHALON

- Gives rise to medulla oblongata
  - Transitional zone between brain, spinal cord
- Alar plate sensory neuroblasts give rise to
  - Cochlear nuclei, vestibular nuclei, spinal trigeminal nucleus, solitary nucleus, dorsal column nuclei, inferior olivary nuclei
- Basal plate motor neuroblasts give rise to
  - Nuclei of CN X, IX, XI
- Roof plate lined by ependymal cells covered by vascular mesenchyme, AKA pia mater
  - Collectively known as tela choroidea
  - Projects into ventral cavity, invaginations form choroid plexus

- Choroid plexus produces cerebrospinal fluid

METENCEPHALON

- Develops from rostral rhombencephalon, gives rise to cerebellum, pons

Cerebellum

- Functions as center for coordination, posture
- Neuroectoderm cells proliferate
  - In ventricular zone, form cerebellar nuclei, Purkinje cells, golgi cells
  - In external germinal layer, form basket, granule, stellate cells
  - External, internal germinal layers form astrocytes, oligodendrocytes, Bergmann cells

Pons

- Serves as pathway for nerve fibers between spinal cord, cerebrum, cerebellum
- Base of pons contains
  - Pontine nuclei from alar plate
  - Corticobulbar, corticospinal, corticopontine fibers from cell bodies in cerebral cortex; pontocerebellar fibers
  - Alar plate sensory neuroblasts (CN V, CN II, CN III)
  - Basal plate motor neuroblasts (CN V, CN VI, CN VII)

DEVELOPMENT OF MESENCEPHALON

- Gives rise to midbrain
- Basal plate neuroblasts give rise to motor nuclei
  - Oculomotor (III) nucleus → general somatic efferent column
  - Edinger–Westphal nucleus of oculomotor nerve (III) → general visceral efferent
  - Substantia nigra
  - Red nucleus
  - Trochlear (IV) nucleus, part of CN V migrate to metencephalon
- Alar plate sensory neuroblasts gives rise to superior, inferior colliculi
- Crus cerebri contains corticobulbar, corticospinal, corticopontine fibers

DEVELOPMENT OF THE PROSENCEPHALON

Diencephalon

- Develops from median portion of prosencephalon
- Consists of one roof plate, two alar plates; basal plate regresses
- Alar plates give rise to
  - **Epithalamus**: also develops from roof plate; gives rise to pineal body, habenular nuclei, commissure, posterior commissure, tela choroidea, third ventricle choroid plexus
  - **Thalamus**: gives rise to thalamic nuclei, lateral geniculate body, medial geniculate body
  - **Subthalamus**: gives rise to subthalamic nucleus; zona incerta; lenticular, thalamic fasciculi (AKA fields of Fortel)
  - **Hypothalamus**: also develops from floor plate; gives rise to hypothalamic nuclei, mammillary bodies, neurohypophysis
- Optic vesicles, cups, stalks derivatives of diencephalon
  - Give rise to retina, iris, ciliary body, CN II, optic tract
- Hypophysis (AKA pituitary) develops from two different structures
- Anterior lobe/adenohypophysis
  - Develops from Rathke's pouch
  - Ectodermal diverticulum of primitive oral cavity/stomodeum
- Posterior lobe/neurohypophysis
  - Develops from the infundibulum
  - Neuroectodermal evagination of hypothalamus

Telencephalon

- Gives rise to cerebral hemispheres, caudate, putamen, amygdaloid, claustrum, lamina terminalis, olfactory bulbs, hippocampus
- **Week 5**: cerebral hemispheres begin emerging as two outpocketings of prosencephalon
  - Contain cerebral cortex, white matter, lateral ventricles

Basal ganglia

- Basal part of hemispheres grow, bulge into the lateral ventricles, giving rise to part of hemisphere wall (AKA corpus striatum)

- **Expands:** gives rise to caudate nucleus, putamen, amygdaloid nucleus, claustrum
- Divided by fibers of internal capsule
  - Single layer of ependymal cells form choroid plexus
  - Thickened wall of hemisphere forms hippocampus
  - Only globus pallidum arises from neuroblasts of subthalamus that migrated into the hemispheres

Hemispheres

- Rapid, extensive growth of hemispheres creates many convolutions (AKA gyri)
  - Separated by grooves (AKA sulci) fissures
- Hemispheres develop frontal, parietal, occipital, temporal lobes, which overlie insula

Cerebral cortex

- Develops from paleopallium/archipallium, neopallium
- Initially has neuroepithelial, mantle, marginal layers
- Neuroblasts proliferate, migrate to subpial regions to differentiate into mature neurons
  - Continues until all layers are formed
- Early formed neuroblasts have deep position in cortex, whereas later formed neuroblasts more superficially positioned
- Classified into neocortex, allocortex
  - **Neocortex:** AKA isocortex
  - **Allocortex:** subdivided into 2 parts
    - **Archicortex:** includes hippocampal formation
    - **Paleocortex:** includes olfactory cortex
- Telencephalon also gives rise to olfactory bulbs, tracts

DEVELOPMENT OF COMMISSURES

- Bundles of nerve fibers connecting corresponding areas in right, left hemispheres
- Cross in midline of brain via lamina terminalis (AKA commissural plate)
- Anterior commissure
  - Appears first
  - Connects olfactory bulbs, middle, inferior temporal gyri
- Hippocampal commissure/fornix commissure
  - Appears second
  - Fibers arise in hippocampus → connect to lamina terminalis → mammillary body, hypothalamus
- Corpus callosum
  - Appears third
  - Largest commissure
  - Forms bundle in lamina terminalis, connects two homologous neocortical areas of cerebral hemispheres

DEVELOPMENT OF CRANIAL NERVES & AUTONOMIC NERVOUS SYSTEM

osms.it/development-cranial-nerves-ANS

DEVELOPMENT OF CRANIAL NERVES

- By week 4: nuclei for all cranial nerves present
- Except olfactory (I), optic (II) nerves, all cranial nerves arise from hindbrain
- Motor nuclei derived from rhombomeres produced by neuroepithelium
    - Gives rise to motor nuclei of cranial nerves IV, V, VI, VII, IX, X, XI, XII
    - Motor neurons for these nuclei reside within brain
- Cranial nerve sensory ganglia originate from neural crest cells, ectodermal placodes

DEVELOPMENT OF AUTONOMIC NERVOUS SYSTEM

- Comprised of efferent motor fibers
    - Innervate smooth muscle, cardiac muscle, secretory glands
    - Divided into sympathetic, parasympathetic systems

Sympathetic nervous system

- Ganglia arise from basal plate of neural tube, neural crest cells
    - Basal plate gives rise to preganglionic sympathetic neurons in intermediolateral horns of spinal cord
    - Neural crest cells give rise to postganglionic sympathetic neurons of sympathetic chain ganglia, prevertebral sympathetic ganglia, adrenal chromaffin cells
- Cell bodies of preganglionic neurons reside at T1–L2 of spinal cord
- Preaortic ganglia located at major vessel branches

Parasympathetic nervous system

- Ganglia arise from basal plate of neural tube, neural crest cells
    - Basal plate gives rise to preganglionic parasympathetic neurons of cranial nerve nuclei—CN III (midbrain), CN VIII (pons), CN IX, X (medulla), spinal cord at S2–S4
    - Neural crest cells give rise to postganglionic parasympathetic neurons of ciliary ganglion (CN III), pterygopalatine ganglion (CN VII), submandibular ganglion (CN VII), enteric ganglion (Meissner, Auerbach, CN X), ganglia of abdominal, pelvic cavities
- Neuron cell bodies reside in brainstem, S2–S4 of spinal cord

DEVELOPMENT OF THE SPINAL CORD

osms.it/development-spinal-cord

NEURAL TUBE

- Neural plate folds in cephalocaudal manner, forming neural tube
    - Open at each end, forming cranial, caudal neuropores
- **Three layers:** neuroepithelial cells/ventricular zone, mantle layer/intermediate zone, marginal layer/outermost layer

Neuroepithelial cells

- Form thick layer of pseudostratified epithelium
    - Rapid division forms more neuroepithelial cells, produces neuroepithelium
    - Neuroepithelium gives rise to neuroblasts (AKA primitive nerve cells)

Mantle layer

- Forms around neuroepithelial layer
- Composed of neuroblasts that migrated from neuroepithelial layer
- Gives rise to gray matter of spinal cord

Marginal layer

- Contains neuroblast nerve fibers
- Gives rise to white matter
- Myelination → color

Thickening of mantle layer

- Ventral, dorsal thickening occurs as more neuroblasts form
- Ventral thickening produces basal plates
    - Basal plates form ventral motor horn of spinal cord
- Dorsal thickening produces alar plates
    - Alar plates form dorsal sensory horn of spinal cord
- Sulcus limitans divides basal, alar plates
- Intermediate horn develops between motor, sensory horns
    - Located at T1–T12, L2/L3
    - Contain sympathetic portion of autonomic nervous system
- Dorsal midline portion (AKA roof plate) ventral midline portion (AKA floor plate) of neural tube do not contain neuroblasts
    - Serve as crossover pathways

CELL DIFFERENTIATION

Development of nerve cells

- Start out as round, apolar cells
- Differentiate as primitive axons, dendrites develop
    - Bipolar neuroblast differentiates into multipolar neuroblast
    - Eventually develops into neuron

Development of glial cells

- Glioblasts formed by neuroepithelial cells that migrate to the mantle and marginal layers
- Differentiate into glial cells
    - *Protoplasmic astrocytes, fibrillar astrocytes:* provide support, metabolic functions
    - *Oligodendroglial cells:* myelination in CNS
    - *Microglia cells:* phagocytic activity
- Neuroepithelial cells cease to produce neuroblasts, glioblasts
    - Differentiate into ependymal cells, which line central canal of spinal cord

DEVELOPMENT OF SPINAL NERVES AND GANGLIA

- **Week 4:** development of spinal nerves begins
- Motor nerve fibers arise from cell bodies in basal plates (AKA ventral horns)
    - Form bundles (AKA ventral motor roots)
- Processes from nerve cell bodies in spinal cord ganglia

- Form bundles (AKA dorsal sensory roots)
- Spinal nerves split into rami containing both motor, sensory fibers
- Dorsal primary rami
  - Innervate dorsal axial musculature, vertebral joints, skin of back
- Ventral primary rami
  - Innervate limbs, ventral body wall
  - Form brachial, lumbosacral plexus

MYELINATION OF THE NERVOUS SYSTEM

Myelination in PNS
- Carried out by Schwann cells
  - Originate from neural crest cells
  - Each Schwann cell myelinates just one axon of peripheral nerve, wrapping around axon to form neurilemma (AKA myelin, sheath)

Myelination in CNS
- Carried out by oligodendrocytes
  - One oligodendrocyte can myelinate ≤ 50 axons
  - Myelination of corticospinal tracts incomplete until first one-two years of postnatal life

DEVELOPMENT OF THE EAR

osms.it/development-of-the-ear

- Comprised of internal, middle, outer ear

DEVELOPMENT OF THE INTERNAL EAR
- Around day 22, otic placodes formed
- Ectoderm thickens each side of rhombencephalon
- Sides invaginate, form otic/auditory vesicles (AKA otocysts)
- Otocystic cells of vesicles differentiate into ganglion cells for vestibulocochlear/ statoacoustic ganglia
- Each vesicle divides, forming two components that will become membranous labyrinth
  - **Ventral component:** forms saccule, cochlear duct
  - **Dorsal component:** forms utricle, semicircular canals, endolymphatic duct

DEVELOPMENT OF THE COCHLEA
- **Week 6:** cochlear duct forms as saccule forms tubular outgrowth
  - Cochlear duct spirally penetrates mesenchyme
  - Completes 2.5 turns by week 8
- **Week 7:** cochlear duct cells give rise to spiral organ of Corti
  - Cochlear duct remains connected to saccule via ductus reuniens
  - Mesenchyme surrounding cochlear duct differentiates into cartilaginous shell
- **Week 10:** large vacuoles appear in cartilage
  - Form two perilymphatic spaces: scala vestibuli, scala tympani
  - Cochlear duct now separated from scala vestibuli by vestibular membrane, from scala tympani by basilar membrane
  - Lateral wall of cochlear duct remains attached to cartilage by spiral ligament
  - Median angle of cochlear duct connected to cartilaginous process called modiolus

DEVELOPMENT OF ORGAN OF CORTI
- Epithelial cells of cochlear duct form two ridges
  - Inner ridge gives rise to spiral limbus
  - Outer ridge gives rise to sensory hair cells of auditory system
- Tectorial membrane covers sensory cells

while attached to spiral limbus
- ▫ *Sensory cells, tectorial membrane:* organ of Corti

DEVELOPMENT OF SEMICIRCULAR CANALS

- **Week 6:** flattened outpouchings appear on dorsal component/utricle of otic vesicle
  - ▫ Central portion of their walls eventually disappear, semicircular canals develop
- Each canal has two ends
  - ▫ *Crus ampullare:* dilated end
  - ▫ *Crus nonampullare:* does not dilate
  - ▫ Cells in ampullae form crista ampullaris
- Maculae acusticae develop in walls of utricle, saccule
  - ▫ *Maintenance of equilibrium:* change in position of head, body generates impulses in sensory cells of cristae, maculae; carried by cranial nerve VIII/vestibular fibers

DEVELOPMENT OF THE MIDDLE EAR

- Composed of tympanic cavity, Eustachian tube/auditory tube
- Tympanic cavity develops from first pharyngeal pouch/endoderm
- Pouch expands, reaches floor of first pharyngeal cleft
  - ▫ Distal part of pouch widens, becomes primitive tympanic cavity
  - ▫ Proximal part remains narrow, becomes auditory tube

DEVELOPMENT OF THE OSSICLES

Malleus and incus
- Derived from cartilage of first pharyngeal arch
  - ▫ Tensor tympani muscle innervated by mandibular branch of trigeminal nerve

Stapes
- Derived from cartilage of second arc
  - ▫ Stapedius muscle innervated by facial nerve

Ossicles
- Appear during the first half of fetal life
- Remain embedded in mesenchyme until it dissolves in eighth month
  - ▫ Space around ossicles forms
- Endodermal epithelium of primitive tympanic cavity covers space's wall
  - ▫ Connects ossicles to cavity wall like mesentery
- During late fetal life, tympanic cavity expands dorsally to form tympanic antrum
- After birth, epithelium of tympanic cavity extends to the mastoid process
  - ▫ Forms air sacs (AKA pneumatization)
  - ▫ Mastoid air sacs communicate with tympanic antrum, tympanic cavity

DEVELOPMENT OF THE EXTERNAL EAR

- External auditory meatus derived from dorsal portion of first pharyngeal cleft
- During third month, epithelial cells of meatus' floor proliferate, form solid epithelial plate (AKA meatal plug)
  - ▫ During seventh month meatal plug dissolves, creating definitive eardrum
  - ▫ Meatal plug persists until birth → congenital deafness
- Composition of eardrum
  - ▫ Ectodermal epithelial lining of auditory meatus
  - ▫ Endodermal epithelial lining of tympanic cavity
  - ▫ Intermediate mesoderm layer of connective tissue
- Auricle
  - ▫ Auricle develops from six mesenchymal proliferations/auricular hillocks at dorsal ends of first, second pharyngeal arches surrounding first pharyngeal cleft
  - ▫ These proliferations later fuse, form definitive auricle

DEVELOPMENT OF THE EYE

osms.it/development-of-the-eye

KEY POINTS
- **Day 22:** begins with formation of optic grooves on both sides of forebrain
- As neural tube closes, optic grooves form outpouchings (AKA optic vesicles)
- Optic vesicles reach surface ectoderm, induce lens formation
    - Optic vesicles invaginate, form double layered optic cups
    - Inferior surface of optic cup forms choroid fissure pathway for hyaloid artery
- **Week 7:** choroid fissure closes, gives rise to pupil
- Ectoderm cells elongate, form lens placode
- Lens placode invaginates, forms lens vesicle

DEVELOPMENT OF THE RETINA
- Optic cup has two layers
    - Inner, outer layer initially separated by intraretinal space; obliterated in adult
    - *Outer/pigmented layer:* gives rise to pigmented layer of retina
    - *Inner/neural layer:* gives rise to neural layer of retina
- *Posterior 4/5:* pars optica retinae
- Cells bordering the intraretinal space differentiate into rods and cones
- *Adjacent mantle layer:* gives rise to neurons and supporting cells
    - Outer, inner nuclear layers, ganglion cell layer
- Surface fibrous layer contains nerve cell axons of deeper layers
    - Nerve fibers converge towards optic stalk
    - Optic stalk develops into optic nerve
- *Anterior 1/5:* pars ceca retinae
    - *Pars iridica retinae:* forms inner layer of iris
    - *Pars ciliaris retinae:* forms ciliary body

Iris
- Three layers
- Outer, pigmented layer of optic cup
- Inner, neural layer of optic cup
- Richly vascularized connective tissue layer containing pupillary muscles
    - Sphincter, dilator pupillae develop from ectoderm of optic cup
- Pars ciliaris retinae
    - Externally covered by mesenchyme layer, forms ciliary muscle
    - Internally connected to lens by suspensory ligament/zonula

DEVELOPMENT OF THE LENS
- Cells of optic vesicles elongate, fill lumen of vesicle with primary lens fibers
    - **End of week 7:** fibers reach anterior vesicle wall
    - Secondary fibers area added to central core

DEVELOPMENT OF CHOROID, SCLERA & CORNEA
- **End of week 5:** loose mesenchyme surrounds eye primordium, differentiates into 2 layers
    - *Inner layer:* similar to pia mater, forms highly vascularized pigmented layer, AKA choroid
    - *Outer layer:* continuous with dura mater, forms sclera
- Anterior chamber forms on anterior aspect of the eye
    - Splits loose mesenchyme via vacuolization
    - *Inner layer:* iridopupillary membrane, sits in front of lens, iris
    - *Outer layer:* substantia propria of cornea, continuous with sclera
- Cornea now contains 3 layers
    - Epithelial layer derived from surface ectoderm

- Substantia propria
- Epithelial layer bordering anterior chamber
- **Posterior chamber:** space between iris, lens
- Anterior, posterior chambers filled with aqueous humor produced by ciliary process of ciliary body
  - Aqueous humor circulates from posterior into anterior chamber through pupil
  - In anterior chamber, fluid flows through canal of Schlemm (AKA scleral venous sinus) at iridocorneal angle, resorbs into bloodstream

DEVELOPMENT OF THE VITREOUS BODY

- Mesenchyme invades inside of optic cup through choroid fissure
  - Forms hyaloid vessels, which supply lens during intrauterine life
- Invading mesenchyme also forms fibrous network between lens, retina
  - Interstitial spaces of network fill with vitreous body
- During fetal life, hyaloid vessels eventually disappear, replaced by hyaloid canal

DEVELOPMENT OF THE OPTIC NERVE

- Develops from optic stalk, which connects optic cup to brain
- Initially, optic cup has ventral groove (AKA choroid fissure)
  - Fissure contains hyaloid vessels
  - Nerve fibers of retina line stalk's inner wall
- **Week 7:** choroid fissure closes
  - Narrow tunnel forms inside optic stalk
  - Nerve fibers fill tunnel, forming optic nerve
- Contents of optic nerve
  - Inner layer provides neuroglia supports optic nerve fibers
  - Hyaloid artery later transforms into central artery of retina
- **Choroid:** continuation of pia arachnoid, sclera continuation of dura layer of nerve

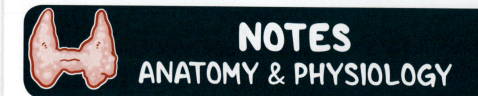

NOTES
ANATOMY & PHYSIOLOGY

ENDOCRINE ANATOMY & PHYSIOLOGY

osms.it/endocrine-anatomy-and-physiology

ENDOCRINE GLANDS
- Secrete hormones directly into bloodstream (exocrine glands use ducts)
- Maintain homeostasis by controlling variables such as body temperature, fluid balance
  - Especially with negative feedback mechanisms

HORMONES
- Can be classified as steroids/non-steroids

Steroid hormones
- Derived from cholesterol; produced in adrenal glands, gonads (testes/ovaries)
- Hydrophobic/non-polar → travel through bloodstream with transport proteins, diffuse across target cell phospholipid membrane

Non-steroid hormones
- Derived from peptides/proteins or single amino acids
- Peptidic hormones are hydrophilic → bind surface receptor proteins instead of passing through target cell membrane
- Amino acid hormones derived from tyrosine; generally hydrophilic (e.g. adrenaline/epinephrine and noradrenaline/norepinephrine), apart from thyroid hormones

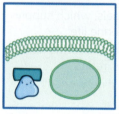
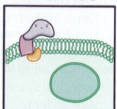

Figure 31.1 Steroid hormones diffuse across the target cell membrane and bind to an intracellular receptor. Peptide hormones bind to a cell surface receptor. Both methods result in changes in gene expression.

HORMONE SECRETION & REGULATION

Paracrine signaling
- Effects of hormones released by nearby cells; e.g. glucagon → activates alpha cells, inhibits beta cells

Sympathetic nervous system
- Epinephrine/norepinephrine alter secretion depending on adrenergic receptor type;
- e.g. β2: activates beta cells

Parasympathetic nervous system
- Acetylcholine activates alpha cells and beta cells via M3 receptors

Chapter 31 Endocrine Physiology: Endocrine Anatomy & Physiology

GLAND LOCATIONS & FUNCTIONS

- Endocrine glands scattered throughout body

Hypothalamus

- Located at base of brain
- Hypothalamus, brain work closely to make hormones that control other endocrine glands
- Made up of several nuclei (neuron clusters) which secrete hormones

Pituitary gland

- Located just below brain; physically connected to hypothalamus by pituitary stalk (infundibulum)
- Made up of anterior, posterior lobe
- Anterior pituitary: AKA adenohypophysis
    - Made of glandular tissue
    - Receives stimulatory, inhibitory hormones from hypothalamus via hypothalamo-hypophyseal-portal system
- Posterior pituitary: AKA neurohypophysis
    - Made of axons from hypothalamic supraoptic, paraventricular nuclei
    - Receives hormones directly from hypothalamus
    - Instead of producing own hormones, posterior pituitary stores hormones for later release
    - Herring bodies: axon dilations which store hormones
    - Hormones include antidiuretic hormone (ADH/vasopressin), oxytocin
    - ADH signals: ↑ blood osmolarity, ↓ blood volume (ADH retains water from urine, constricts blood vessels → negative feedback)
    - Oxytocin signals: childbirth (dilates cervix, stimulates uterine contractions), breastfeeding (contracts breast cells), social interaction, orgasm
- Stimulatory pituitary hormones
    - Thyrotropin releasing hormone (TRH): pituitary secretes thyroid-stimulating hormone (TSH) → thyroid produces thyroid hormones
    - Corticotropin releasing hormone (CRH): pituitary secretes adrenocorticotropic hormone (ACTH) → adrenal glands produce cortisol
    - Gonadotropin releasing hormone (GnRH): pituitary secretes gonadotropins, e.g. follicle-stimulating hormone (FSH), luteinizing hormone (LH) → gonads produce gametes (sperm for testes, oocytes for ovaries), sex hormones (testosterone, estrogen, progesterone)
    - Growth hormone releasing hormone (GHRH): pituitary secretes growth hormone → growth of long bones, tissues in body
- Inhibitory pituitary hormones
    - Growth hormone inhibiting hormone (GHIH/somatostatin): pituitary secretes less/no growth hormone

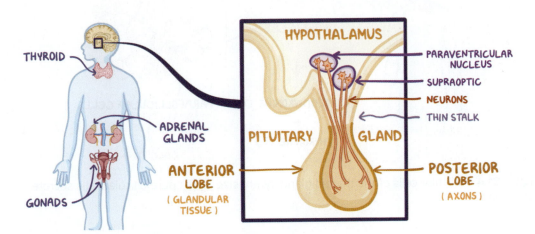

Figure 31.2 Endocrine glands' location and the relationship between the hypothalamus and the the pituitary gland's two lobes.

- **Prolactin inhibiting hormone (dopamine):** pituitary secretes less/no prolactin (no milk is produced whenever not breastfeeding)

Pineal gland
- Located behind hypothalamus, pituitary gland
- Contains pinealocytes which synthesize melatonin
  - Melatonin mostly secreted during night, regulates body's circadian rhythm (body clock)

Thyroid gland
- Located at front of neck
- Left, right lobe
- Made of thousands of follicles which synthesize triiodothyronine (T_3), thyroxine (T_4)
  - In the cell $T_4 \rightarrow T_3$
  - $T_3 \rightarrow \uparrow$ basal metabolic rate
- Parafollicular cells (C-cells) between follicles secrete calcitonin
- Two parathyroid glands on back of each thyroid lobe (four in total) secrete parathyroid hormone
- Calcitonin, parathyroid hormone work similarly
  - Control calcium, phosphate, bone metabolism
- Regulated by blood calcium levels

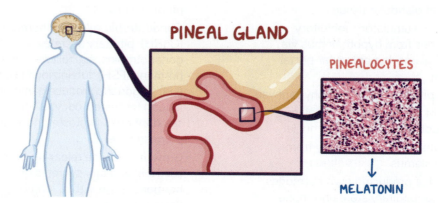

Figure 31.3 Pineal gland location and histological appearance of pinealocytes.

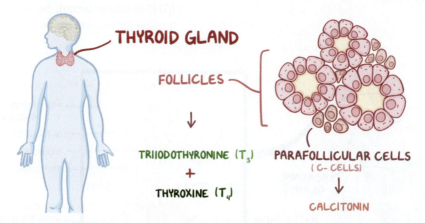

Figure 31.4 Follicular cells of the thyroid gland synthesize T_3, T_4; parafollicular cells secrete calcitonin.

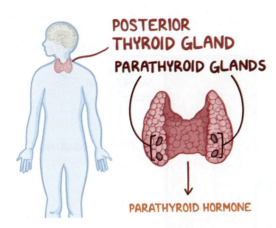

Figure 31.5 The parathyroid glands are found on the back of the thyroid. They secrete parathyroid hormone.

Adrenal glands
- Two glands situated retroperitoneally inside renal fascia, each surrounded by fibrous capsule; sit on top of kidneys
    - Connective tissue separates them from kidney, renal fascia from diaphragm
    - One of the most vascularized tissues
    - Differ in shape (right shaped as pyramid, left shaped as crescent moon)
- Outer layer (cortex) surrounding a core (medulla)
- **Medulla:** neuroectodermal origin; secretes catecholamines (e.g. adrenaline, noradrenaline) during "fight or flight" situations
    - ↑ blood pressure, ↑ cardiac output, ↑ bronchial dilation, ↑ glycogenolysis
- **Cortex:** makes up 80% of gland, mesodermal origin, secretes adrenocortical steroid hormones
    - **Three zones:** zona glomerulosa (makes mineralocorticoids—e.g. aldosterone), zona fasciculata (makes glucocorticoids), zona reticularis (makes sex hormone precursors)
    - **Aldosterone:** regulates extracellular fluid volume, potassium homeostasis; involved in renin-angiotensin-aldosterone system (RAAS); ↑ renal water and sodium reabsorption, ↑ renal potassium excretion → ↑ blood pressure
    - **Cortisol:** integral to stress response; also has metabolic, anti-inflammatory, immunosuppressive, vascular effects; regulated via hypothalamic-pituitary-adrenal (HPA) axis
    - **Androgens:** adrenals only source of androgens in biologically-female individuals; effects include ↑ libido, pubic hair development, sebaceous gland hypertrophy; minor role in biologically-male adults

ENDOCRINE PANCREAS
- Located behind stomach
- Three sections
    - Head, body, tail
- Has both endocrine, exocrine functions
- Contains hormone-producing cell clusters
    - Islets of Langerhans (1–2% of pancreas)
- Produce hormones secreted directly into bloodstream that regulate blood glucose

Cell types
- Alpha (α) cells
    - 15–20% of total islet cells
    - Produce glucagon
    - ↓ blood glucose → glucagon secreted → hepatic glycogenolysis and gluconeogenesis → glucose released into bloodstream
- Beta (β) cells
    - 65–80% of total islet cells
    - Produce insulin, amylin
    - ↑ blood sugar → insulin secreted → anabolic functions: promotes glucose entry into cells, ↑ glycogen synthesis, ↓ lipolysis
- Gamma (γ) cells/PP cells
    - 3–5% of total islet cells
    - Produce pancreatic polypeptide
    - Secretion stimulated by meals high in protein, hypoglycemia, physical activity, fasting; inhibits pancreatic exocrine (enzymes) and endocrine (insulin) activity
- Delta (δ) cells
    - 3–10% of total islet cells
    - Produce somatostatin
    - Paracrine function of suppressing both insulin and glucagon
- Epsilon (ε) cells
    - < 1% of total islet cells
    - Produce ghrelin
    - Functions in appetite stimulation

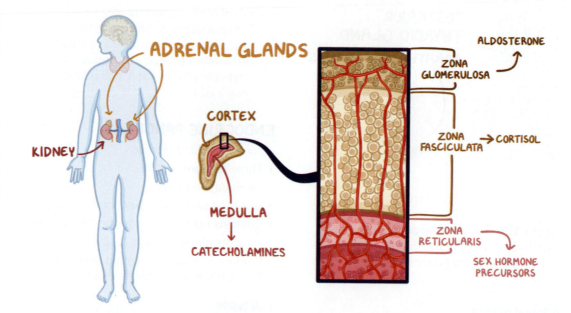

Figure 31.6 Location of the adrenal glands and the hormones secreted by the cortex, medulla.

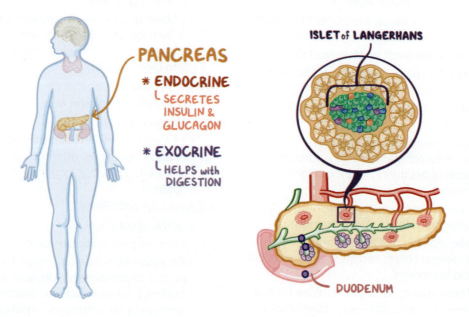

Figure 31.7 The pancreas has both endocrine and exocrine functions. It has hormone-producing clusters of cells called Islets of Langerhans.

MAJOR HORMONES AND THEIR FUNCTIONS

GLAND	HORMONE	TYPE	REGULATED BY	TARGET	FUNCTION
HYPOTHALAMUS	Oxytocin	Peptide	Bonding, motherhood	Uterus, mammaries	Uterine contractions, milk ejection
	ADH	Peptide	Blood osm., volume	Kidneys	↑ water reabsorption
ANTERIOR PITUITARY	Growth hormone	Peptide	GHRH, GHIH	Muscles, liver	Muscle growth, bone growth (by IGF-1)
THYROID	T₃, T₄	Amine	TSH	Cells	↑ metabolism
	Calcitonin	Peptide	Calcium in blood	Bones, kidneys, etc.	↓ blood calcium levels
PARATHYROID	Parathyroid	Peptide	Calcium in blood	Bones, kidneys, etc.	↑ blood calcium levels
ADRENAL CORTEX	Cortisol	Steroid	ACTH	All tissues	↑ blood glucose, inflammatory response
	Aldosterone	Steroid	↓ blood pressure, ↑ blood potassium	Kidneys	↓ urine sodium, ↑ urine potassium
	Sex hormones	Steroid	Puberty, ongoing	Gonads	Sex characteristics
ADRENAL MEDULLA	Epinephrine, norepinephrine	Modified amino acid	"Fight or flight" situations	All tissues	"Fight or flight" response
PANCREAS	Insulin	Protein	↑ blood sugar	Liver, muscle, fat	↓ blood sugar
	Glucagon	Protein	↓ blood sugar	Liver, muscle, fat	↑ blood sugar
TESTES	Testosterone	Steroid	FSH, LH	Gonads	Male sex characteristics and function
OVARIES	High	High	FSH, LH	Gonads	Female sex characteristics and function

NOTES: PITUITARY HORMONES

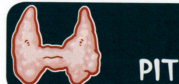

GENERALLY, WHAT ARE THEY?

- *Pituitary gland*: AKA hypophyseal gland/hypophysis
- Connected to hypothalamus via pituitary stalk (infundibulum) which controls pituitary secretory actions
- Consists of two embryologically, functionally different parts that secrete different hormones

ANTERIOR PITUITARY (ADENOHYPOPHYSIS)

- Connects to hypothalamus via blood vessels (hypophyseal portal system)
- Hypothalamus produces releasing hormones → pituitary secretes tropic hormones that regulate target tissues

Corticotropin-releasing hormone (CRH)
- Adrenocorticotropic hormone (ACTH) → adrenal medulla

Gonadotropin-releasing hormone (GnRH)
- Luteinizing hormone (LH), follicle-stimulating hormone (FSH) → ovaries, testes

Growth hormone releasing hormone (GHRH)
- Stimulates release of somatotropin/growth hormone (GH) → various tissues throughout body

Thyrotropin-releasing hormone (TRH)
- Thyroid-stimulating hormone → thyroid gland

Prolactin (PL)
- Acts on breasts (lactogenesis)
    - Hypothalamus inhibits prolactin production via dopamine
    - TRH, estrogen, progesterone, oxytocin stimulate prolactin

POSTERIOR PITUITARY (NEUROHYPOPHYSIS)

- Represents an extension of hypothalamus
- Does not secrete its own hormones
- Stores, releases neurohormones synthesized in hypothalamus

Vasopressin/antidiuretic hormone (ADH)
- Acts on kidney tubules, arterioles

Oxytocin
- Acts on uterus, breasts

ADRENOCORTICOTROPIC HORMONE (ACTH)

osms.it/adrenocorticotropic-hormone

- Hormone secreted by anterior pituitary corticotropic cells
- Main action of ACTH involves stimulating adrenocortical cells of zona fasciculata of the adrenal cortex to secrete glucocorticoids (primarily cortisol)
  - Anti-inflammatory effects
  - Increases blood glucose levels
  - Increases fat and protein breakdown

SYNTHESIS

- Pre-pro-opiomelanocortin (pre-POMC) → proopiomelanocortin (POMC) → ACTH, gamma lipotropin, beta endorphin, melanocyte-stimulating hormone

STIMULATION OF ACTH RELEASE

- Corticotropin releasing hormone (CRH) secreted by hypothalamus
  - Stress, low blood glucose, low glucocorticoid levels, increased sympathetic activity, normal diurnal rhythm
  - Release of ACTH demonstrates circadian rhythm affected by suprachiasmatic nucleus → low evening concentrations, high in morning

ACTH RELEASE REGULATION

- ACTH release is regulated by hypothalamic-pituitary-adrenal axis negative feedback
  - Hypothalamus releases CRH → CRH stimulates pituitary to release ACTH → ACTH stimulates adrenal cortex to secrete cortisol → ↑ cortisol inhibits hypothalamic release of CRH → ↓CRH decreases ACTH secretion → closed loop

ACTH SIGNALING PATHWAY

- ACTH binds to ACTH receptor on adrenal cortex adrenocorticotropic cells, primarily zona fasciculata; also expressed in skin, both white, brown adipocytes
- ACTH receptor is a seven-membrane-spanning G-coupled receptor
- ACTH binds to receptor → activates G_s protein → α subunit released → activates adenylate cyclase → ↑ cAMP → activates protein kinase A → phosphorylation cascade → transcription factor activation → effects

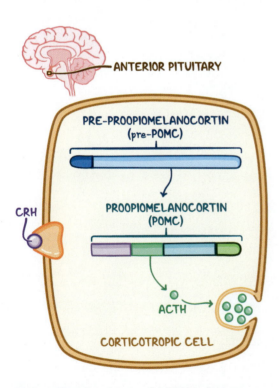

Figure 32.1 Synthesis of ACTH in the anterior pituitary. Corticotropin releasing hormone (CRH) stimulates the cell to release ACTH.

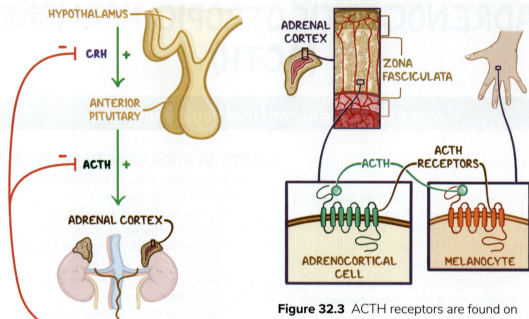

Figure 32.2 The negative feedback loop which regulates ACTH release.

Figure 32.3 ACTH receptors are found on adrenocortical cells in the zona fasciculata of the adrenal cortex, as well as on melanocytes in the skin.

Chapter 32 Endocrine Physiology: Pituitary Hormones

GROWTH HORMONE (GH)

osms.it/growth-hormone

- AKA somatotropin
- Peptide hormone secreted by somatotropic cells of anterior pituitary
  - Regulates tissue growth
- Released in pulsatile manner every two hours; peaks one hour after falling asleep

REGULATION OF SECRETION

Induction of GH release
- Hypoglycemia, ↑ estrogen, testosterone (puberty), stress (e.g. trauma, fever), exercise, sleep stages III, IV

Three negative feedback loops
- ↓ GH stimulates hypothalamus to release GHRH → ↑ GHRH stimulates pituitary to release GH → ↑ GH inhibits release of GHRH → absence of GHRH inhibits GH release → closed loop
- ↑ GH stimulates somatomedins production in the liver, bones, muscles → somatomedins inhibit GH release
- ↑ GH and somatomedins stimulate somatostatin production in hypothalamus → somatostatin inhibits GH release

GH SIGNALING PATHWAY
- Growth hormone receptor (GHR) belongs to cytokine receptor family
- To activate intracellular signaling, GH must bind to two GH receptors → dimerization of GHR
- GH binds to receptor → conformational change → key tyrosine residue phosphorylation → activation of tyrosine kinase JAK2 → STAT5, Src family kinases, insulin receptor substrate (IRSs) signalling molecule activation → gene transcription, effects

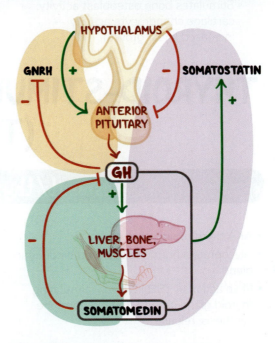

Figure 32.4 The three negative feedback loops that regulate GH secretion, each highlighted in a different colour. GH and somatomedin together stimulate somatostatin production in the hypothalamus, which inhibits GH release.

EFFECTS OF GH
- Primary effect of GH is cell metabolism stimulation, growth, division

Direct effects
- Anti-insulin-like effects
- *Carbohydrates*: ↑ blood glucose levels
  - Stimulates gluconeogenesis, glycogenolysis in liver
  - Increases tissue insulin resistance
- *Fats*: ↑ fatty acids in blood
  - Stimulates adipose tissue lipolysis

Indirect effect
- Insulin-like effects through insulin-like growth factors (e.g. somatomedins like IGF-1)
- Stimulates cell growth, division, and differentiation; reduces apoptosis

- **Proteins**: anabolic effect
  - Stimulates amino acid, protein uptake
  - Stimulates protein synthesis
  - Decreases protein breakdown
- Epiphyseal plates, cartilage
  - Stimulates bone osteoblast activity, cartilage chondrocyte activity → increased linear growth

THYROID-STIMULATING HORMONE (TSH)

osms.it/thyroid-hormone

- AKA thyrotropin
- Glycoprotein hormone secreted by pituitary gland
- Main action of TSH involves stimulating thyroid gland growth, thyroid hormone synthesis, release

STIMULATION OF TSH RELEASE

- Thyrotropin-releasing hormone (TRH) secreted by hypothalamus
  - Low T_3, T_4 blood levels
  - Decreased metabolism
  - Cold stress
  - Conditions that increase ATP demand

REGULATION OF SECRETION

- TRH secreted by hypothalamus, stimulates pituitary thyrotropic cells to release TSH
- Thyroid hormones, specifically T_3, down-regulate TRH receptors on thyrotropic cells, inhibiting TSH secretion
- TSH release, thyroid hormone is regulated by negative feedback loop
  - Hypothalamus releases TRH → TRH stimulates pituitary to release TSH → TSH travels to thyroid follicle → stimulates thyroid hormones synthesis, secretion → thyroid hormones inhibit both TRH, TSH release → absence of TRH, TSH inhibits further thyroid hormone secretion → closed loop

TSH SIGNALING PATHWAY

- TSH binds TSH receptor primarily found on thyroid gland follicular cells
  - Also found on adipose tissue, fibroblasts
- TSH receptor is integral membrane receptor coupled with G_s protein
- TSH binds to receptor → activates G_s protein → α subunit released → activates adenylate cyclase → ↑ cAMP → activates protein kinase A → phosphorylation cascade → transcription factor activation → effects

EFFECTS OF TSH

- TSH has two effects on the thyroid gland
  - Stimulates all the steps in thyroid hormone synthesis, secretion
  - **Trophic effect**: increases growth of thyroid gland

THYROID HORMONE

osms.it/thyroid-hormone

- Glycoprotein hormones T_3 (triiodothyronine), T_4 (tetraiodothyronine) secreted by thyroid follicular epithelial cells
- Less active form thyroid hormone (T_4) is secreted, converted in target tissue into more active form (T_3)

SYNTHESIS OF THYROID HORMONES

Six steps

- Thyroglobulin (TG) synthesized in follicular cell rough endoplasmic reticulum (RER), secreted into lumen (colloid)
- Iodine from blood enters follicular cells on basolateral side via Na^+/I^- symport
- Iodine exits cell on apical side via transporter pendrin
- Inside follicle lumen at apical side, iodine oxidized by enzyme thyroid peroxidase ($I^- \rightarrow I_2$)
- I_2 iodinates TG tyrosyl residues (organification of I_2), catalyzed by thyroid peroxidase, forms monoiodotyrosine (MIT), diiodotyrosine (DIT)
- On TG, two DIT molecules coupled to form T_4 (faster reaction); MIT coupled with DIT to form T_3 → TG now contains T_3, T_4, MIT, DIT residues

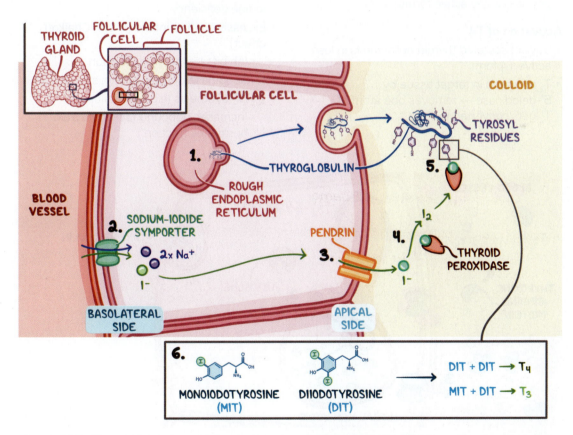

Figure 32.5 Thyroid hormone synthesis overview. 1. Thyroglobulin (TG) is synthesized in rough endoplasmic reticulum, secreted into colloid. 2. Iodine enters cell from blood via Na^+/I^- symporter. 3. Iodine exits cell into colloid via pendrin. 4. Iodine is oxidized by thyroid peroxidase, become I_2 5. I_2 iodinates tyrosyl residues on TG, forming monoiodotyrosine (MIT), diiodotyrosine (DIT). 6. Two DITs combine to form T_4; MIT combines with DIT to form T_3.

THYROID HORMONE SECRETION AND TRANSPORT

Thyroid hormone secretion
- Thyroid hormones stored in colloid until stimulated for secretion
  - TSH stimulation → endocytosis of iodinated TG by follicular epithelial cells → TG transportation to basal membrane → TG fuses with lysosome → TG hydrolysis, T_3, T_4, MIT, DIT residue release → T_3 (10%), T_4 (90%) secreted into circulation
  - Iodide from MIT, DIT residues recycled for next synthesis

Transport of thyroid hormones
- Once in circulation, most thyroid hormones travel bound to thyroxine-binding protein (TBP)
  - Some bound to prealbumin, albumin
- Small fraction travels unbound → physiologically active forms

Activation of T4
- 90% of secreted thyroid hormone is in less active T4 form
- T_4 activated in target tissue by 5'-deiodinase → removes one atom of I_2 → T_4 gets converted to T_3
- Starvation inhibits 5'-deiodinase in target tissue, except in brain → lowers O_2 consumption, basal metabolic rate (BMR)

REGULATION OF SECRETION

Negative feedback loop
- Regulated by negative feedback loop in hypothalamic-pituitary-thyroid axis
  - Thyrotropin-releasing hormone (TRH) secreted by hypothalamus, stimulates thyrotropic cells of pituitary to release thyroid-stimulating hormone (TSH)

Effects of TSH on thyroid gland
- Two effects
  - Stimulates all steps in thyroid gland synthesis, secretion
  - **Trophic effect:** increases thyroid gland growth

Other regulatory factors
- Iodine deficiency
- Excessive iodine intake (Wolff–Chaikoff effect)
  - Inhibits iodine organification
- 5'-deiodinase deficiency (e.g. starvation)
- ↓ TBP synthesis (e.g. liver failure)
  - Increases unbound (active) thyroid hormones fraction

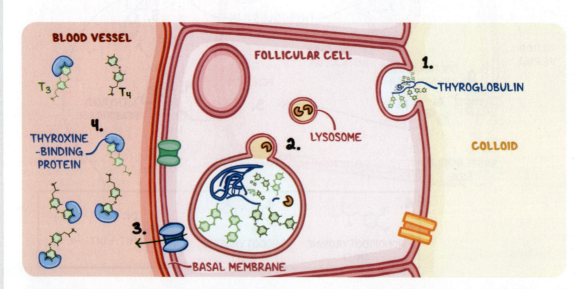

Figure 32.6 Thyroid hormone secretion overview. 1. TG in colloid is endocytosed into follicular cell. 2. Lysosome fuses with vesicle; thyroid hormones are cleaved from TG. 3. Hormones are released into blood. 4. In blood, most thyroid hormones travel bound to a protein, thyroxine-binding protein being most common.

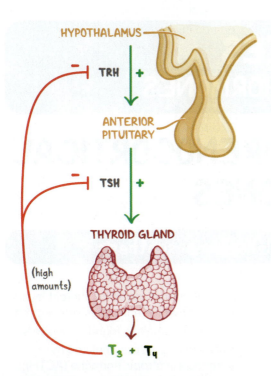

Figure 32.7 The negative feedback loop which regulates thyroid hormone secretion.

- ↑ catecholamine, glucagon, growth hormone activity → ↑ proteolysis, lipolysis, gluconeogenesis
- Cardiovascular system
  - ↑ β1 adrenergic receptors, Ca^{2+} ATPase → ↑ inotropic (contractility), chronotropic (heart rate) effect → ↑ cardiac output
- Central nervous system (CNS)
  - Gestational period → CNS development
  - Adult period → ↑ brain activity, attention span, memory
- Growth
  - ↑ osteoblast, osteoclast activity → ↑ bone formation, maturation

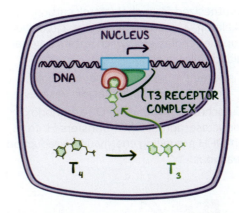

Figure 32.8 In the target cell, T_4 is converted to T_3, which enters the nucleus and binds to a receptor. The receptor complex binds to DNA to stimulate transcription.

SIGNALING PATHWAY

- Thyroid hormones act on all organ systems
- Inside target cells, T_4 converts to T_3 → T_3 enters nucleus, binds nuclear receptor → T_3 receptor complex binds DNA, stimulates transcription → translation → protein synthesis
- T_3 stimulates synthesis of Na^+-K^+ ATPase, Ca^{2+} ATPase, transport proteins, proteolytic, lysosomal enzymes, β1 adrenergic receptors, structural proteins

EFFECTS OF THYROID HORMONE

- Key hormone in regulating body metabolism; also important for embryological growth
- *General effect*: all tissues except brain, spleen and gonads
  - ↑ Na^+-K^+ ATPase → ↑ oxygen consumption → ↑ basal metabolic rate (BMR), body temperature
- *Catabolic effect*: metabolism of macromolecules
  - ↑ transport proteins → ↑ glucose absorption from GI tract

NOTES

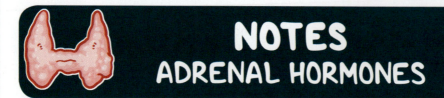

NOTES
ADRENAL HORMONES

SYNTHESIS OF ADRENOCORTICAL HORMONES

osms.it/adrenocortical-hormone-synthesis

- **Synthesized from cholesterol:** carbon skeleton, 21-carbon molecules; circulation supplies cholesterol which enters adrenal gland cells via endocytosis
  - Some synthesized de novo → both forms stored in cytoplasmic vesicles
- Cytochrome p450 using O_2, adrenodoxin reductase, adrenodoxin transfers H^+ from NADPH producing energy using reduction reactions
- Different enzymes found in different layers according to which hormones synthesized
- Cholesterol desmolase found in all layers
  - Rate-limiting step; stimulated by adrenocorticotropic hormone (ACTH); converts cholesterol to pregnolone
- Corticosteroid is common name for steroid hormones made in cortex: include mineralocorticoids, glucocorticoids

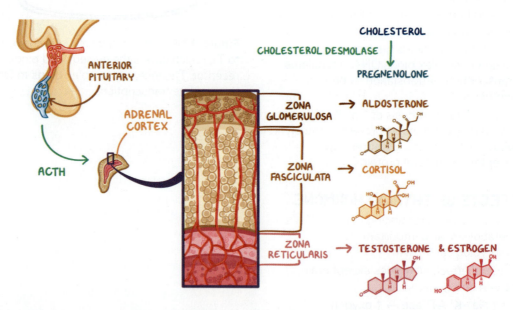

Figure 33.1 Three zones of adrenal cortex secrete steroid hormones under control of ACTH, which is released by anterior pituitary. Adrenal cortex cells first convert cholesterol to prognenolone using enzyme cholesterol desmolase. Prognenolone is then converted into aldosterone in zona glomerulosa, cortisol in zona fasciculata, and testosterone and estrogen in zona reticularis.

Chapter 33 Endocrine Physiology: Adrenal Hormones

Mineralocorticoids
- Synthesized in zona glomerulosa
- *Example:* aldosterone
- Aldosterone synthase required and found only in zona glomerulosa, converts cortisone → aldosterone

Glucocorticoids
- Synthesized in zona fasciculata
- Examples: cortisol, corticosterone
- 17α-hydroxylase (if deficient corticosterone can be formed) → 3β-hydroxysteroid dehydrogenase → 21β- and 11β-hydroxylase

Androgens
- Synthesized in zona reticularis
- *Examples:* dehydroepiandrosterone (DHEA), androstenedione
- 17,20-lyase responsible for conversion of glucocorticoids into androgens
- DHEA, androstenedione have a weak androgenic effect
  - *Male:* converted to testosterone in testes
  - *Female:* main source of androgens
- Low quantity of testosterone, 17β-estradiol

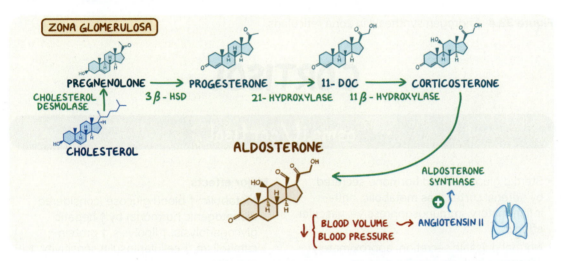

Figure 33.2 Aldosterone synthesis in zona glomerulosa. Aldosterone synthase is stimulated by hormone angiotensin II, which is produced in lungs in response to low blood pressure, volume.

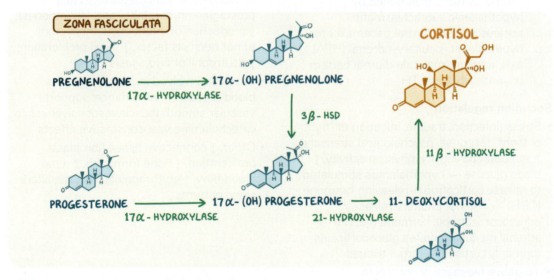

Figure 33.3 Cortisol synthesis in zona fasciculata.

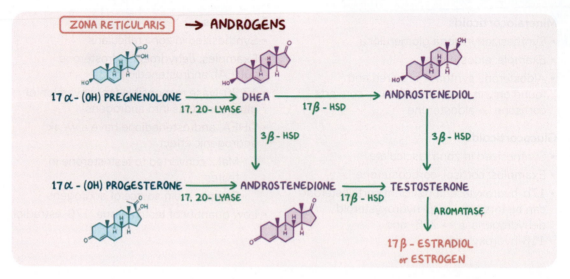

Figure 33.4 Androgen synthesis in zona reticularis.

CORTISOL

osms.it/cortisol

- Steroid glucocorticoid hormone secreted by adrenal cortex; has metabolic, anti-inflammatory, immunosuppressive, vascular effects
- Normal pulsatile secretion, approximately 10 surges in diurnal (daily) pattern
    - Concentration highest in morning, lowest in evening
    - *Diurnal pattern:* maintained by hypothalamic suprachiasmatic nucleus; acts as central pacemaker for hypothalamic-pituitary-adrenal (HPA) axis; adrenals maintain diurnal pattern of sensitivity to ACTH

Secretion regulation
- Stress (infection, trauma, initiation of "fight or flight" response, psychological stressors), ↑ sympathetic activity, physical activity, ↓ blood glucose → hypothalamus stimulated to release corticotropin-releasing hormone (CRH) → anterior pituitary releases adrenocorticotropic hormone (ACTH) → adrenal medulla secretes glucocorticoids (primarily cortisol) → target tissues
- Negative feedback of cortisol to hypothalamic-pituitary axis → ↓ cortisol

Major effects
- *Metabolic:* ↑ blood glucose (considered diabetogenic hormone) by ↑ hepatic glycogenolysis, ↑ lipolysis, ↑ protein catabolism, ↓ cellular insulin sensitivity, ↑ appetite
- *Immune:* ↓ intensity of immune, inflammatory responses by ↓ production of arachidonic acid metabolites (e.g. prostaglandin, thromboxane, leukotrienes), ↓ production of interleukins, interferon, tumor necrosis factor; ↓ T cell proliferation; ↓ neutrophil phagocytosis
- *Vascular:* involved in normal vascular blood pressure maintenance; supports vascular smooth muscle responsiveness to catecholamine vasoconstrictive effects
- *Other:* ↓ connective tissue fibroblast proliferation, ↓ bone formation, ↑ renal blood flow, ↑ erythropoietin release, alters sleep patterns

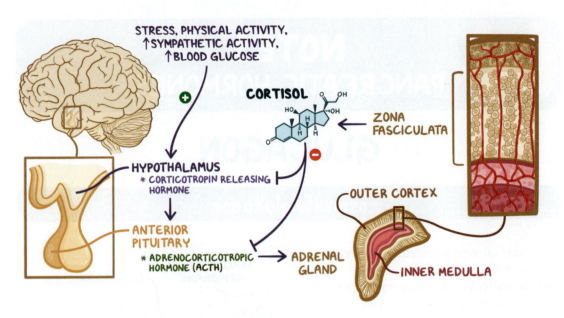

Figure 33.5 Cortisol secretion regulation.

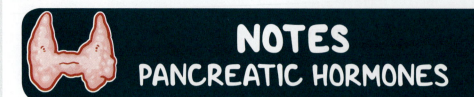

NOTES
PANCREATIC HORMONES

GLUCAGON

osms.it/glucagon

- Peptide hormone secreted by pancreatic alpha cells
- Important for blood glucose regulation, along with insulin
- Synthesis
  - Preproglucagon → proglucagon → glucagon

Secretion regulated mainly by glucose
- ↓ glucose levels between meals or while sleeping → ↓ insulin → glucagon secretion stimulation → hepatic glycogenolysis, gluconeogenesis → ↑ blood glucose levels

Other factors that regulate glucagon secretion
- Sympathetic nervous system
  - Adrenaline (α_2 receptors)
- Parasympathetic nervous system
  - Acetylcholine (M_3 receptors)
- Alanine, arginine
  - E.g. from high protein meal
- Cholecystokinin, somatostatin
- Exercise

GLUCAGON SIGNALING PATHWAY
- Glucagon receptor is a heterotrimer
  - G-protein coupled receptor that contains α, β, γ subunits
- Glucagon binds to receptor → activates G_s protein → α subunit released → activates adenylate cyclase → ↑ cAMP → activates protein kinase A → phosphorylation cascade → transcription factor activation → effects

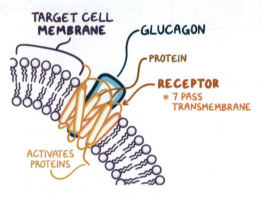

Figure 34.1 Glucagon exerts its effects by binding to G-protein coupled receptors on the membranes of liver and adipose cells.

EFFECTS OF GLUCAGON
- Primary action is to increase blood glucose when it falls below normal range
- **Carbohydrates:** ↑ blood glucose levels
  - Stimulates glycogenolysis in liver, muscle
  - Stimulates gluconeogenesis in liver, kidney
  - Inhibits hepatic glycolysis
- **Fats:** ↑ fatty acids, keto acid levels in blood
  - Inhibits fatty acid synthesis, oxidation in liver
  - Inhibits fat deposition in adipose tissue
  - Stimulates lipolysis
  - Stimulates keto acid production

Chapter 34 Endocrine Physiology: Pancreatic Hormones

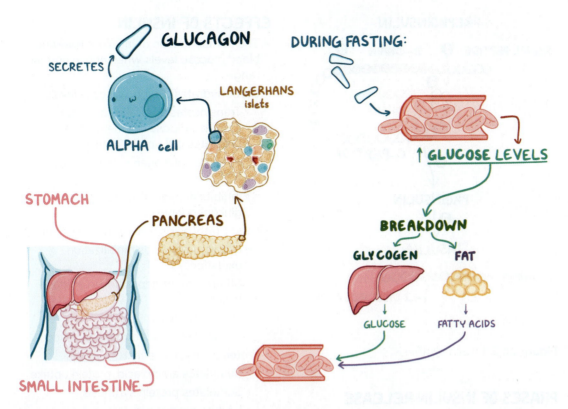

Figure 34.2 Glucagon is secreted by pancreatic alpha cells when glucose levels are low. It increases glucose levels in the bloodstream by inducing the breakdown of storage molecules in the liver and adipose cells.

INSULIN

osms.it/insulin

- Peptide hormone secreted by pancreatic beta cells
- Important for blood glucose regulation
- Consists of A and B amino acid chains connected with two disulfide (-S-S-) bonds

SYNTHESIS

- Preproinsulin → proinsulin → insulin
- During insulin synthesis, protein called C-peptide cleaved off, secreted together with insulin in equimolar amounts within secretory vesicles → C-peptide used to measure insulin levels

SECRETION

Secretion regulated mainly by glucose

- Carbohydrates consumption → ↑ glucose → passive diffusion into beta cells through GLUT2 transporters → stimulation of insulin secretion

Other factors that stimulate insulin secretion

- ↑ fatty acid, amino acid levels in blood
- Parasympathetic nervous system
    - Acetylcholine (M_3 receptors)
- Sympathetic nervous system
    - Adrenaline (β_2 receptors)
- Growth hormone (GH), adrenal corticotropic hormone (ACTH)

OSMOSIS.ORG 281

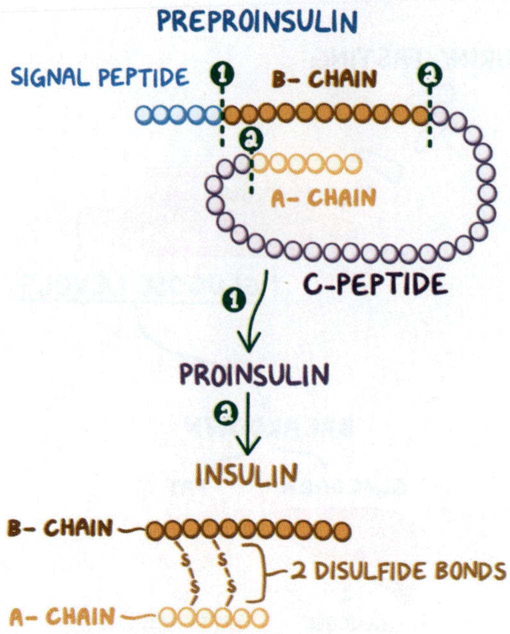

PREPROINSULIN

Figure 34.3 Insulin synthesis.

PHASES OF INSULIN RELEASE

- Two phases

First phase

- Involves L-type Ca^{2+} channels
- Rapidly triggered release of preformed secretory vesicles
- Lasts 10 minutes

Second phase

- Involves R-type Ca^{2+} channels
- Slow release of newly formed secretory vesicles
- Lasts 2–3 hours

INSULIN SIGNALING PATHWAY

- Insulin receptor is a tetramer
  - Contains two extracellular α subunits connected by disulfide bonds, two intracellular β subunits connected to each α subunit
- Insulin binds to α subunits → activates tyrosine kinase activity in β subunits → β subunit autophosphorylation → insulin receptor substrates (IRS) phosphorylation cascade → transcription factor activation → effects

EFFECTS OF INSULIN

- The primary action of insulin is lowering blood glucose levels when above normal range
- *Carbohydrates:* ↓ blood glucose levels
  - Translocates GLUT4 transporters to muscle, adipose cell membranes → facilitates cell uptake of glucose
  - Activates glycogen synthesis in liver, muscles
  - Inhibits hepatic glycogenolysis, gluconeogenesis
- *Fats:* ↓ fatty acids, keto acid levels in blood
  - Inhibits fatty acids mobilization, oxidation
  - Stimulates fat deposition in adipose tissue
  - Inhibits lipolysis
  - Inhibits keto acid formation in liver
- *Proteins:* anabolic effect
  - Stimulates amino acid, protein uptake
  - Stimulates protein synthesis
  - Inhibits proteolysis
- *Other:* ↓ K^+ levels in blood
  - Increases potassium uptake
  - Stimulation of cell growth, gene expression

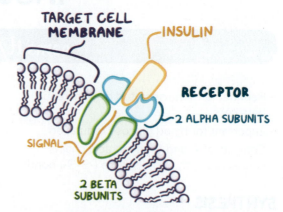

Figure 34.4 Insulin exerts its effects by binding to alpha subunits of insulin receptor, which leads to signal transduction within cell.

Chapter 34 Endocrine Physiology: Pancreatic Hormones

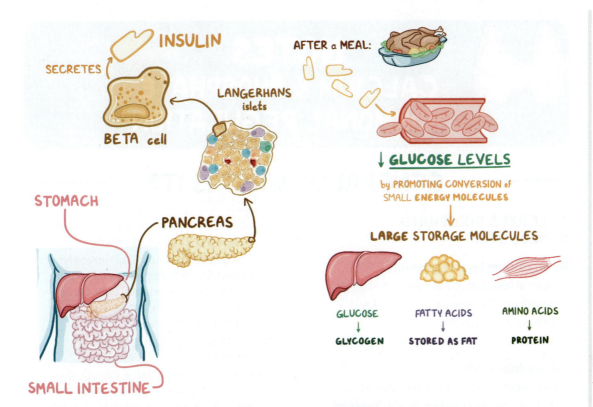

Figure 34.5 Insulin is secreted by pancreatic beta cells when glucose levels are high. It promotes conversion of glucose → glycogen in liver, fatty acids → fat, and amino acids → protein.

SOMATOSTATIN

osms.it/growth-hormone-and-somatostatin

- Peptide hormone secreted by pancreatic delta cells

Factors that regulate somatostatin secretion
- Ingestion of glucose, fatty acids, amino acids
- Glucagon
- Sympathetic nervous system
    - β-adrenergic agonists

SOMATOSTATIN SIGNALING PATHWAY
- Somatostatin receptor is a G-protein coupled receptor
- Somatostatin binds to receptor → activates G_i protein → inhibits adenylate cyclase → ↓ cAMP → ↓ Ca^{2+} → inhibitory effect

EFFECTS OF SOMATOSTATIN
- Inhibits secretion of insulin, glucagon
- Inhibits pancreatic exocrine secretion
- Inhibits secretion of all gastrointestinal hormones (gastrin, cholecystokinin, secretin, motilin etc.)
- Decreases gastrointestinal motility, blood flow, gastric emptying

NOTES

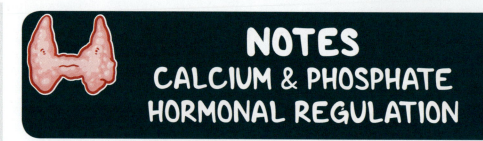

NOTES
CALCIUM & PHOSPHATE HORMONAL REGULATION

GENERALLY, WHAT IS IT?

CALCIUM & PHOSPHATE HOMEOSTASIS

Blood calcium level regulation
- Normal total blood calcium: 8.5–10mg/dl
- Parathyroid hormone: ↑ calcium level
- Vitamin D: ↑ calcium level
- Calcitonin: ↓ calcium level

Extracellular calcium
- Diffusible: can cross cell membranes
    - Free-ionized calcium (Ca^{2+}): involved in cellular processes → neuronal action potential, muscle contraction, hormone secretion, blood coagulation
    - Complexed calcium: Ca^{2+} ionically bound to other negatively-charged molecules (e.g. oxalate, phosphate → electrically-neutral molecules, do not partake in cellular processes)
- Non-diffusible: cannot cross cell membranes
    - Calcium bound to large negatively charged proteins (e.g. albumin → protein-albumin complex too large to cross cell membranes → not involved in cellular processes)

CALCITONIN

osms.it/calcitonin

CALCITONIN STRUCTURE
- Polypeptide hormone involved in blood calcium regulation
    - Not primary calcium regulator, even if thyroid gland removed, remaining regulatory mechanisms able to maintain calcium homeostasis
- Produced by thyroid gland's parafollicular cells (C cells)
- C cells synthesize preprocalcitonin (141 amino acid polypeptide) → successive enzymatic cleavage steps produces procalcitonin → immature calcitonin (33 amino acids) → mature calcitonin (32 amino acids) → stored/readied for release in secretory granules within C cells

CALCITONIN RELEASE
- Calcium-sensing receptors on C cells' surface monitor blood calcium levels → if calcium drifts above normal range → calcitonin released

CALCITONIN ACTION
- Lowers blood calcium level

Bone
- ↓ bone resorption → ↓ blood calcium concentration
    - When attaching to bone matrix osteoclast membranes form multiple arms (ruffled border) → aids attachment, increases surface area → arms secrete acid → assists bone breakdown

- Calcitonin binds to calcitonin receptor on basal osteoclast surface → G-protein coupled receptor activation → adenylate cyclase activation → adenosine triphosphate (ATP) converted to 3',5'-cyclic AMP (cAMP) → ↑ cAMP levels → ↓ number of osteocyte arms formed → ↓ bone resorption

Kidneys
- ↓ calcium, phosphate reabsorption by principal cells of distal convoluted tubules

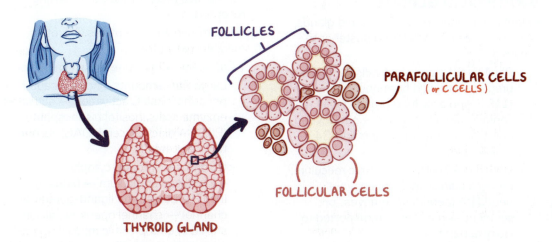

Figure 35.1 Calcitonin is made and stored in thyroid gland's C cells.

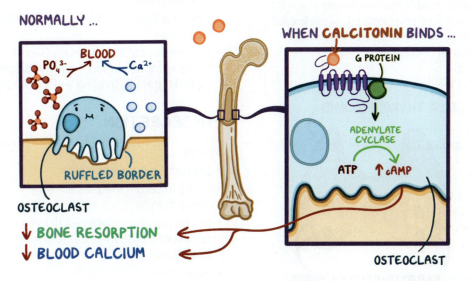

Figure 35.2 When calcitonin binds to its receptor on an osteoclast, it reduces number of osteoclast arms formed, decreasing bone resorption and blood calcium.

PARATHYROID HORMONE

osms.it/parathyroid-hormone

- Primary blood-calcium level regulator

PARATHYROID GLANDS

- Hormone produced by parathyroid glands, four pea-sized glands found posterior to thyroid
  - Parathyroid gland chief cells synthesize preproparathyroid hormone (preproPTH) (115 amino acid-long protein chain → contains biologically-active parathyroid hormone segment in N-terminal 34 amino acids)
  - Within chief cell endoplasmic reticulum, protein chain cleaved by enzyme peptidase (peptidase removes "pre" segment → proPTH → transported to Golgi apparatus)
  - Final processing in Golgi apparatus (trypsin-like enzyme cleaves off six amino acid "pro" segment → functional parathyroid hormone (single chain 84 amino acid polypeptide) → packaged into secretory vesicles → eventual release)

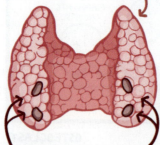

Figure 35.3 Location of the parathyroid glands which produce parathyroid hormone.

CA^{2+} CHANGES

- Ca^{2+} level changes detected by parathyroid cell surface receptor (calcium-sensing receptor)
- Calcium-sensing receptor is G-protein mediated receptor
- ↑ Ca^{2+} level → hormone release inhibition
  - Large Ca^{2+} amounts bind to receptor → phospholipase C activation → activated enzyme splits inositol bisphosphate (PIP_2) → diacylglycerol (DAG), inositol triphosphate (IP_3)
  - IP_3 diffuses through cytoplasm to endoplasmic reticulum → binds to Ins3PR receptor on ligand-gated Ca^{2+} channel → channel opens → calcium stored in endoplasmic reticulum released into cytoplasm → ↑ intracellular calcium → stops binding of PTH-holding granules to chief cell membrane → no PTH release
- ↓ extracellular Ca^{2+} levels → PTH release facilitation
  - Little/no calcium-sensing G-protein receptor activation → no inhibition of PTH granule binding → PTH release

PTH SECRETION

Stimuli

- ↓ serum Ca^{2+} concentration
- Mild ↓ in serum magnesium (Mg^{2+}) concentration
- ↑ in serum phosphate → calcium phosphate complex formation → calcium receptor stimulation ↓
- Adrenaline
- Histamine

Inhibitors

- ↑ serum Ca^{2+} concentration
- Severe ↓ serum Mg^{2+} concentration
- Calcitriol

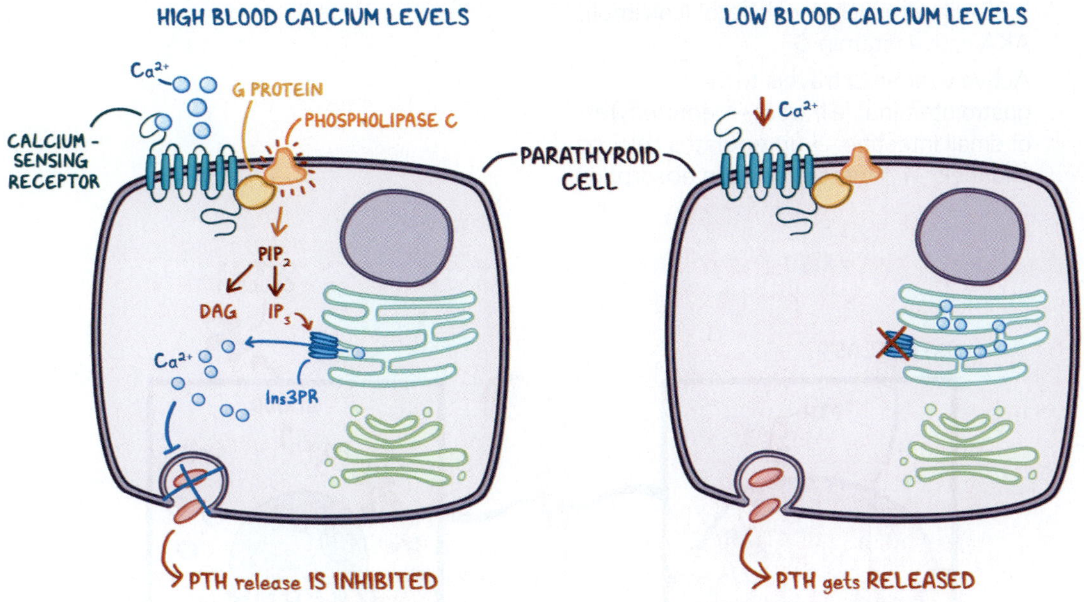

Chapter 35 Endocrine Physiology: Calcium & Phosphate Hormonal Regulation

Figure 35.4 High calcium levels in blood inhibit PTH release from parathyroid cells, while low calcium levels in blood facilitate PTH release from parathyroid cells.

Magnesium

- Involved in stimulus-secretion coupling
- Moderate ↓ serum Mg^{2+} concentration promotes action of PTH on renal mineral resorption
- Severe hypomagnesemia (e.g. alcoholism) inhibits PTH secretion, causes PTH resistance

EXTRACELLULAR CALCIUM INCREASE

- PTH → ↑ extracellular calcium levels (three target organ systems)

Bones

- PTH receptors on osteoblasts
- PTH binding → ↑ cytokine release
  - Receptor activator of nuclear factor κB ligand (RANKL)
  - Macrophage colony-stimulating factor (M-CSF)
  - Inhibits osteoprotegerin (OPG) secretion (inhibition absence → free OPG binds to RANKL (decoy receptor) → prevents RANK-RANKL interaction
  - PTH-induced cytokine release permits RANK-RANKL interaction → multiple macrophage precursors fuse → osteoclast formation (bone breakdown)
- Bone breakdown → release of calcium, phosphate into blood (initially forms physiologically-inactive compound)

Kidneys

- PTH binds to receptors on cells of proximal convoluted tubules → inhibits sodium-phosphate co-transporters on apical surface → ↓ sodium, phosphate reabsorption → ↑ urinary phosphate excretion
- PTH binds to receptors on principal cells of distal convoluted tubules → sodium/calcium channel upregulation → ↑ calcium reabsorption from urine

Intestines

- PTH promotes vitamin D_3 (cholecalciferol) conversion → active form
  - Cholecalciferol synthesized by keratinocytes in skin epidermis when exposed to UV light (also found in foods) → cholecalciferol travels to liver, enzyme 25-hydroxylase catalyzes conversion to 25-hydroxycholecalciferol (calcidiol)
  - 25-hydroxycholecalciferol travels to kidney's proximal tubular cells → enzyme 1-alpha-hydroxylase (upregulated by PTH) converts it to

1,25-dihydroxycholecalciferol (calcitriol), AKA active vitamin D
- Active vitamin D travels to gastrointestinal (GI) tract → enterocytes of small intestine → upregulates calcium channels → ↑ dietary calcium absorption

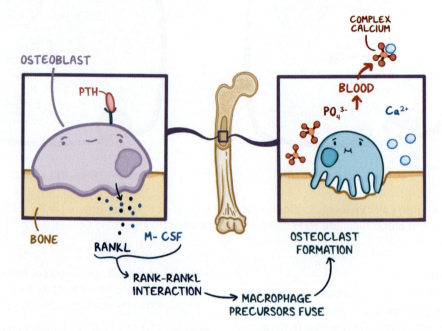

Figure 35.5 One way PTH increases extracellular calcium levels is by stimulating osteoclast formation in bone.

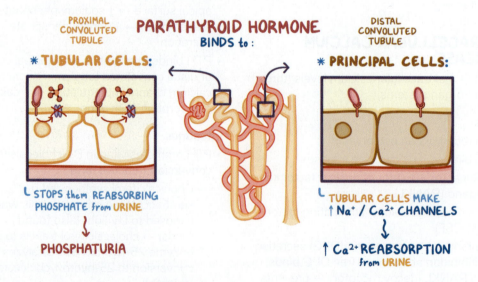

Figure 35.6 The second way PTH increases extracellular calcium levels is by ↑ urinary phosphate excretion and ↑ calcium reabsorption from urine.

Chapter 35 Endocrine Physiology: Calcium & Phosphate Hormonal Regulation

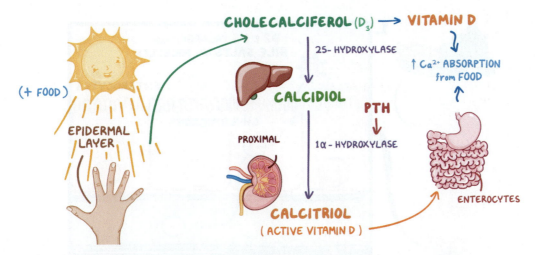

Figure 35.7 The third way PTH increases extracellular calcium levels is by helping convert cholecalciferol into vitamin D. It does so by upregulating enzyme 1α-hydroxylase.

VITAMIN D

osms.it/vitamin-D

- Steroid hormone (derived from cholesterol, fat soluble) → gene transcription stimulation
  - Promotes new bone mineralization
  - ↑ serum Ca^{2+}, phosphate concentration → ↑ available substrate concentration for bone mineralization

VITAMIN D SOURCES

Intestine
- Absorbs precursors (biologically inactive)
  - Vitamin D_2 (ergocalciferol) is derived from dietary plant sources
  - Vitamin D_3 (cholecalciferol) is derived from dietary animal sources

Skin
- Skin keratinocyte exposure (stratum basale, stratum spinosum) to UV light → vitamin D_3 production
  - 7-dehydrocholesterol reacts with UVB light (wavelengths between 270–300nm) → vitamin D_3

PRECURSOR ACTIVATION
- Ergocalciferol, cholecalciferol reach small intestine lumen → packaged in small fat-soluble sacs (micelles) with aid of bile salts → diffuse through apical membrane of absorptive intestinal cells (enterocytes)
- Within enterocytes inactive vitamin D precursors integrate into lipoproteins (chylomicrons) → exit into lymphatic system → drain into blood circulation (hepatic portal vein) → bind to carrier proteins (vitamin D-binding protein/albumin) → transported to liver
- Hepatocytes contain 25-hydroxylase → hydroxyl group added to carbon 25 (C25) of ergocalciferol, cholecalciferol → 25-hydroxycholecalciferol (calcifediol) → calcifediol (primary vitamin D circulating form) reenters blood bound to carrier proteins
  - Hepatic hydroxylation requires NADPH, O_2, Mg^{2+} (not cytochrome P-450)
- Blood transports calcifediol to renal proximal tubules → proximal tubule cell mitochondria contain 1α-hydroxylase → hydroxyl added to C1 → 1,25 dihydroxycholecalciferol (calcitriol—active vitamin D form)

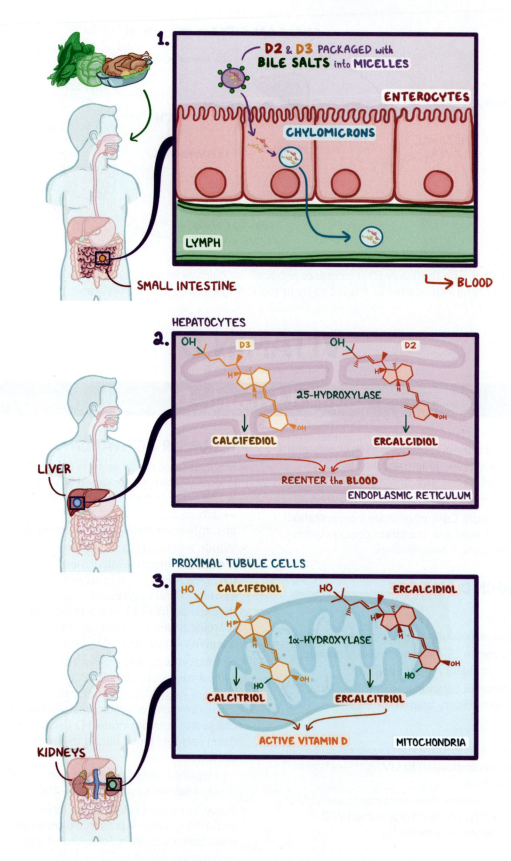

Figure 35.8 Conversion of vitamins D_2 and D_3 into active vitamin D.

Alternative pathway

- Hydroxylation at C24 → biologically inactive 24,25-dihydroxycholecalciferol
- Pathway choice regulated by blood calcium level, parathyroid hormone
  - C1 hydroxylation occurs as response to ↓ calcium/phosphate levels
  - 1α-hydroxylase activity ↑ through ↓ plasma Ca^{2+} concentration, ↑ circulating PTH levels, ↓ plasma phosphate concentration
  - C1 phosphorylation requires NADPH, O_2, Mg^{2+}, cytochrome P-450 pathway
  - If calcium levels sufficient, inactive metabolite preferentially produced

Kidney

- Stimulates Ca^{2+}, phosphate reabsorption

Intestine

- Increases Ca^{2+}, phosphate absorption
- Induces vitamin D-dependent Ca^{2+} binding-protein synthesis (calbindin D-28K)
  - Systolic protein → binds four Ca^{2+} ions
- Intestinal Ca^{2+} absorption mechanism
  - Ca^{2+} *diffusion*: intestinal lumen → cell (through electrochemical gradient)
  - *Inside cell*: calbindin D-28K binds Ca^{2+} → Ca^{2+} pumped across basolateral membrane by Ca^{2+}-ATPase

VITAMIN D ACTIONS

Bone

- Acts synergistically with PTH → osteoclast activity stimulation → bone resorption → old bone demineralization → ↑ Ca^{2+}, phosphate concentration for new bone mineralization

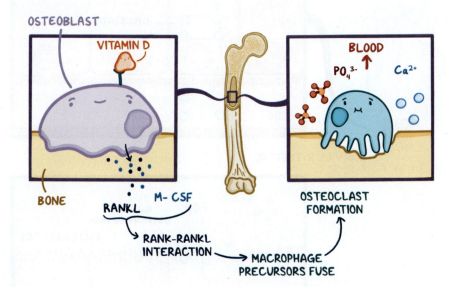

Figure 35.9 Vitamin D stimulates osteoclast formation, increasing blood calcium and phosphate concentrations.

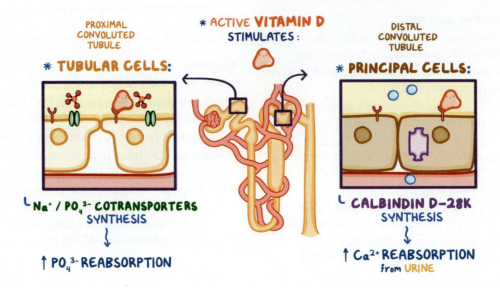

Figure 35.10 Vitamin D stimulates calcium and phosphate reabsorption in kidneys.

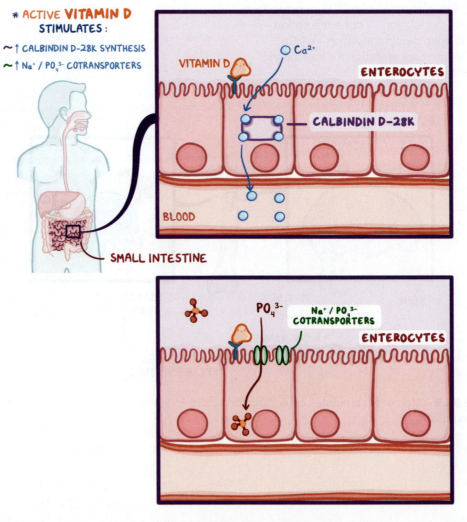

Figure 35.11 Vitamin D stimulates calcium and phosphate absorption in the small intestine by increasing synthesis of calbindin D-28K and sodium/phosphate cotransporters.

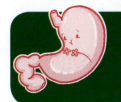

NOTES
ANATOMY & PHYSIOLOGY

ANATOMY

osms.it/gastrointestinal-anatomy-physiology

- **Alimentary/GI tract:** continuous muscular tube from mouth to anus
- Many digestive organs reside in abdominal, pelvic cavity; covered by mesentery

PERITONEUM
- Thin connective tissue composed of mesothelium, connective tissue supporting layer, simple squamous epithelium
- Lines abdominal, pelvic cavities; binds organs together, holds them in place
- Contains blood vessels, lymphatics, nerves innervating abdominal organs
    - *Parietal peritoneum:* lines abdominal, pelvic cavities
    - *Visceral peritoneum:* covers organ surfaces
    - *Peritoneal cavity:* potential space between parietal, visceral layers
- *Intraperitoneal organs:* digestive organs; keep mesentery during embryological development, remain in peritoneal cavity (e.g. stomach)
- *Retroperitoneal organs:* lose mesentery during embryological development, lay posterior to peritoneum (e.g. kidneys, pancreas, duodenum)
- *Mesentery:* double layer of parietal peritoneum on dorsal peritoneal cavity, provides routes for vessels, lymphatics, nerves to digestive organs

Omentum
- Visceral peritoneum layer covering stomach, intestines; contains adipose tissue, many lymph nodes
    - Expands during weight gain; "fat skin"
- *Lesser omentum:* double layer arises from lesser curvature of stomach, extends to liver
- *Greater omentum:* four layers (double sheet folds back upon itself); arises from greater curvature of stomach, covers intestines

GI tract layers
- Four basic tissue layers from esophagus to anus
- Serosa/adventitia
    - Outermost layer of intraperitoneal organs; also visceral peritoneum
    - Primarily composed of simple squamous epithelial cells, connective tissue
    - Secretes slippery fluid, prevents friction between viscera, digestive organs
    - Esophagus has adventitia instead of serosa
    - Retroperitoneal organs have serosa, adventitia
- Muscularis propria
    - Outer longitudinal, inner circular smooth muscle for involuntary contractions; regions of thickened circular layer forms sphincters
    - Skeletal muscle in esophagus for voluntary swallowing
    - Contains myenteric plexus (between longitudinal, circular layers of smooth muscle)
    - Myenteric plexus responsible for peristalsis, mixing
- Submucosa
    - Connective tissue that binds muscularis, provides elasticity, distensibility
    - Contains Meissner's plexus
    - Richly vascularized, innervated

- Mucosa
  - Innermost layer composed of epithelial membrane lining entire GI tract
  - *Functions:* exocrine glands secrete water, mucus, digestive enzymes, hormones; absorb digested nutrients; provides protective surface
  - *Muscularis mucosae:* smooth muscle layer responsible for mucosa movement; contains folds to increase surface area
  - *Lamina propria:* loose areolar connective tissue; contains blood, lymphatic vessels; contains MALT (lymphoid tissue that protects against pathogens)
  - *Epithelium:* mouth, esophagus, anus composed of stratified squamous cells; rest of GI tract simple columnar with mucus secreting cells

BLOOD CIRCULATION
- Splanchnic circulation
- *Celiac trunk:* supplies stomach, liver, spleen
- *Superior mesenteric artery:* supplies small intestine
- *Inferior mesenteric artery:* supplies large intestine

INNERVATION
- Supplied by autonomic nervous system (ANS)
- *Sympathetic component:* thoracic splanchnic nerves → celiac plexus
- *Parasympathetic component:* vagus nerve
- Enteric division provides local control of GI activity; "the brain in the gut"; can function independently of ANS

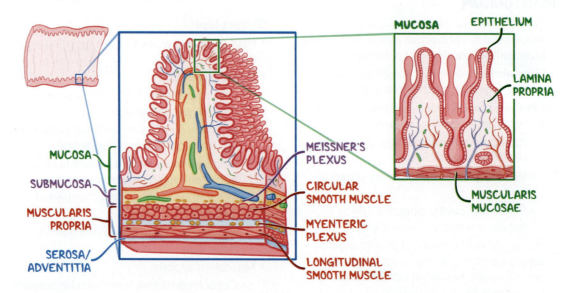

Figure 36.1 Cross section from small intestine showing the four basic tissue layers that line gastrointestinal tract: (from the outermost) serosa/adventitia, muscularis propria, submucosa, and mucosa.

Chapter 36 Gastrointestinal System: Anatomy & Physiology

STRUCTURES

osms.it/gastrointestinal-anatomy-physiology

ORAL (BUCCAL) CAVITY

Function
- Ingestion, mechanical, chemical digestion, propulsion
- Saliva contains antibacterial properties that cleanses, protects oral cavity, teeth from infection
- *Propulsion*: swallowing (performed by tongue) propels food into pharynx, starts propulsion through GI tract
- *Mechanical digestion*: via mastication by teeth, tongue
- *Chemical digestion*: salivary amylase starts carbohydrate chemical breakdown

Secretions
- *Chemical digestion*: salivary amylase starts carbohydrate chemical breakdown; mucin, water provide lubrication
- *Lysozyme*: kills some microbes
- *Lingual lipase*: digests some lipids

ESOPHAGUS
- Muscular tube extending from laryngopharynx to stomach
- *Esophageal hiatus*: diaphragm opening where esophagus, vagus nerve pass through to abdominal cavity
- *Cardiac orifice*: junction of esophagus, stomach

Function
- Propulsion/peristalsis
- Epiglottis closes larynx, routes food into esophagus
- Lower end of esophagus contains mucous cells to protect esophagus from stomach acid reflux

Sphincters
- *Upper esophageal sphincter*: skeletal muscle; regulates movement from pharynx to esophagus
- *Cardiac sphincter*: AKA lower esophageal sphincter; smooth muscle at cardiac orifice that prevents acidic contents of stomach from moving upward into esophagus

Histology
- Mucosa
    - Nonkeratinized stratified squamous epithelium (simple columnar epithelium near cardiac orifice)
- Mucosa, submucosa form longitudinal folds when empty
- Submucosa
    - Mucus secreting glands
- Muscularis externa
    - *Superior ⅓*: skeletal muscle
    - *Middle ⅓*: skeletal, smooth muscle
    - *Inferior ⅓*: smooth muscle
- Adventitia instead of serosa

Secretions
- *Mucus*: lubrication, protection from gastric acid

STOMACH
- Located in upper left abdominal cavity quadrant
- Contains rugae (mucosa, submucosa) when stomach empty → expands to accommodate food

Function
- Churning, digestion, storage
- Beginning of chemical digestion turning food into chyme to be delivered into small intestine

Regions
- *Cardia*: most superior area surrounding cardiac orifice where food from esophagus enters stomach
    - Defined by Z-line of gastroesophageal junction
    - *Z-line*: epithelium changes from stratified squamous → simple columnar

OSMOSIS.ORG

- **Fundus:** area lying inferior to diaphragm, upper curvature
  - Food storage
- **Body:** central, largest area of the stomach
- **Pylorus:** connects to duodenum via pyloric sphincter
  - Controls gastric emptying, prevents backflow from duodenum into stomach

Histology
- Muscularis contains regular GI tract layers with three-layered muscularis propria unique to stomach allowing for vigorous contractions, churning
  - Inner oblique layer
  - Middle circular layer (contains myenteric plexus)
  - Outer longitudinal layer

Glands
- Lined with simple columnar epithelium; forms gastric pits (tube-like opening for gastric glands)
- Cardia, pylorus glands mainly secrete mucus
- Fundus, body glands secrete majority of digestive stomach secretions
- Pyloric antrum glands mainly secrete mucus, hormones (mainly gastrin)

Secretions
- **Mucous cells:** neck, basal regions of glands; produce mucus that protects stomach lining, lubricates food
- **Parietal cells:** gland apical region amongst chief cells; produce HCl, intrinsic factor
- **Chief cells:** gastric gland base; produce pepsinogen (protein digestion)
- **Enteroendocrine cells (ECL cells):** located deep in glands; secretes histamine, somatostatin, serotonin, ghrelin
- **G-cells:** gastrin
- **D-cells:** somatostatin

SMALL INTESTINE

Function
- Primary organ of digestion, nutrient absorption; segmentation (localized mixing area), peristalsis
- **Absorption:** food breakdown products absorbed
- Contains circular folds, villi, microvilli to maximize absorption surface area
  - Circular folds are permanent, composed of mucosa, submucosa

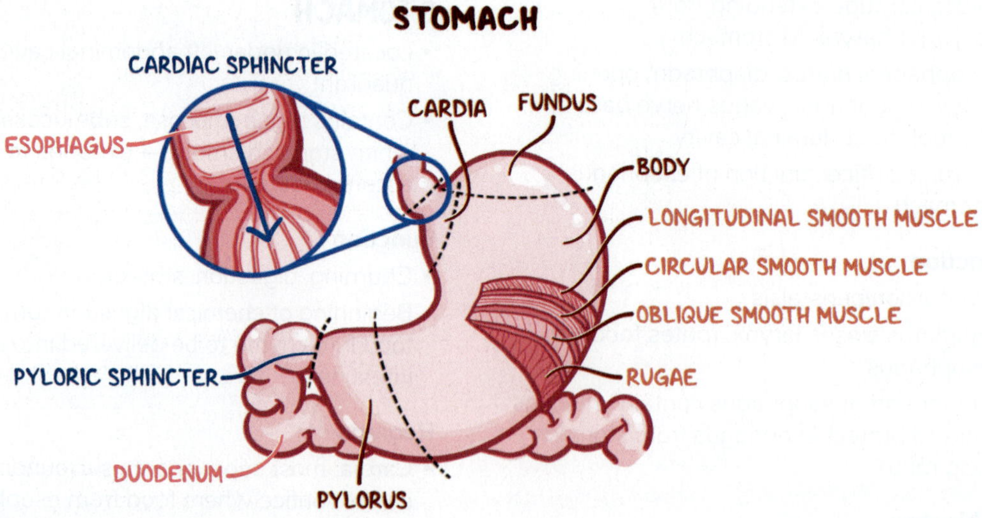

Figure 36.2 Stomach anatomy.

Chapter 36 Gastrointestinal System: Anatomy & Physiology

Innervation
- Relayed through celiac, superior mesenteric plexus
- *Sympathetic:* thoracic splanchnic
- *Parasympathetic:* vagus

Blood supply
- *Arterial:* superior mesenteric artery
- Veins from small intestine → hepatic portal vein → liver

Histology
- *Epithelium of villus:* simple columnar absorptive cells
  - Main function is absorbing nutrients
- Mucus secreting goblet cells in epithelium
- Mucosa contains pits called intestinal crypts
  - *Crypt cells:* secrete intestinal juice containing mucus
  - *Enteroendocrine cells:* within crypts, intraepithelial lymphocytes (T cells)
  - *Paneth cells:* located deep in crypts, release defensins, lysozyme to protect against pathogens

Sections
- Duodenum
  - Mostly retroperitoneal
  - Curves around head of pancreas, receives bile from liver via bile duct, pancreatic secretions from pancreas via main pancreatic duct
  - *Ampulla of vater:* bulb-like point where bile duct, main pancreatic duct unite, deliver secretions into duodenum
  - *Major duodenal papilla:* ampulla opening into duodenum releasing bile/pancreatic secretions
  - *Hepatopancreatic sphincter:* controls bile entry, pancreatic secretions
  - Duodenal glands (Brunner's) in duodenal submucosa secrete alkaline mucus to neutralize acidic chyme
- Jejunum
  - Intraperitoneal
  - Suspended from posterior abdominal wall by mesentery
- Ileum
  - Intraperitoneal
  - Joins large intestine at ileocecal valve
  - Suspended from posterior abdominal wall by mesentery
  - *Peyer's patches:* lymphatic tissue sections composed predominantly of proliferating B lymphocytes, mostly located in ileal lamina propria as protection against pathogenic bacteria; B lymphocytes release IgA

Secretions
- Brush border enzymes on microvilli complete food digestion (e.g. mucus, water, peptidases, disaccharidases)
- Pancreas, liver contribute to most small intestine digestion

LARGE INTESTINE
- Retroperitoneal except for transverse, sigmoid parts
  - Intraperitoneal transverse, sigmoid sections anchored to posterior abdominal wall by mesocolon (mesentery)
  - Connects ileum via ileocecal valve, sphincter

Function
- Digestion, absorption, propulsion, defecation
- *Digestion:* enteric bacteria digests remaining food
  - Bacteria also produce vitamin K, other B vitamins
- *Absorption:* absorbs mainly water, electrolytes, vitamins to concentrate, form feces
- *Propulsion:* propels feces towards rectum
- *Defecation:* stores, eliminates feces from body

Unique features
- *Tenia coli:* three longitudinal ribbons of smooth muscle on ascending, transverse, descending, sigmoid colons that contract to produce haustra
- *Haustra:* small pouches/segments of large intestine created by tenia coli
- *Epiploic appendages:* small pouches of peritoneum filled with fat

Regions
- Cecum → ascending colon → right colic/hepatic flexure → transverse colon → left colic/splenic flexure → descending colon → sigmoid colon → rectum → anal canal → anus
    - *Cecum*: pouch that lies below ileocecal valve at large, small intestine junction; beginning of large intestine
    - *Appendix*: pouch of lymphoid tissue (part of MALT) located in cecum, harbors bacteria to recolonize gut when needed
- Anal canal has two sphincters
    - *Internal anal sphincter*: involuntary, composed of smooth muscle
    - *External anal sphincter*: voluntary, composed of skeletal muscle

Histology
- Muscularis mucosae consists of inner circular, outer longitudinal layers
- Large intestine mucosa: simple columnar epithelium
- Anal canal: stratified squamous epithelium
- Does not contain folds, villi, microvilli as in small intestine
- Many crypts with goblet cells

Pectinate line
- Divides upper ⅔ from lower ⅓ of anal canal where many distinctions made
- Embryological origin
    - Above: endoderm
    - Below: ectoderm
- Epithelium
    - Above: columnar epithelium
    - Below: stratified squamous epithelium
- Innervation
    - Above: inferior hypogastric plexus
    - Below: inferior rectal nerves
- Lymph drainage
    - Above: internal iliac
    - Below: superficial inguinal lymph nodes
- Vascularization
    - Above: superior rectal artery, superior rectal vein (drains into inferior mesenteric vein → hepatic portal system)
    - Below: middle, inferior rectal arteries; middle, inferior rectal veins

Flora
- Large intestine contains largest bacterial ecosystem in body
- Function of bacteria
    - Synthesize vitamins (vitamin K, some B vitamins)
    - Ferment indigestible carbohydrates (e.g. cellulose)
    - Metabolism/digestion of certain molecules (e.g. hyaluronic acid, mucin)
    - Live symbiotically with host
    - Present pathogens to nearby lymphoid tissue (MALT)

Secretions
- Mucus

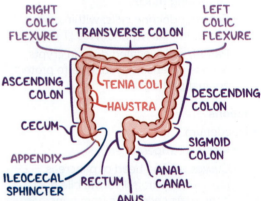

Figure 36.3 Large intestine anatomy.

ACCESSORY ORGANS

- Gallbladder, liver, pancreas
- Liver
  - Hepatocytes produce bile which emulsifies lipid globules, aids in absorption
  - Stores glucose in form of glycogen
- Gallbladder
  - Bile storage; releases bile into small intestine in response to hormonal stimulus
- Pancreas
  - *Exocrine function:* acini secrete various digestive enzymes; "pancreatic juice;" e.g. secretin, cholecystokinin (CCK)
  - *Endocrine function:* islets produce glucagon, insulin to maintain normal glucose levels; somatostatin, pancreatic polypeptide production

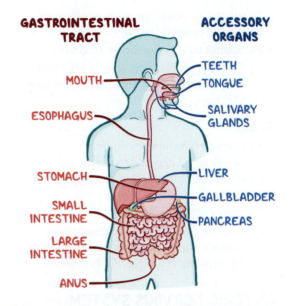

Figure 36.4 Overview of gastrointestinal tract, accessory organs structures.

PHYSIOLOGY

osms.it/gastrointestinal-anatomy-physiology

PROCESSING OF FOOD

1. Ingestion
2. Mechanical digestion
   - Carried out by teeth; increases surface area to facilitate enzymatic digestion
3. Propulsion
   - Movement, mixing of food through GI tract, starts with swallowing
4. Secretion
   - Exocrine glands secrete various digestive juices into digestive tract lumen
5. Digestion
   - Complex food broken down via enzymes
6. Absorption
   - Digested nutrients absorbed by GI mucosal cells into blood/lymph
7. Elimination
   - Indigestible substances eliminated via anus in form of feces

GI MUSCLE PROPERTIES

- Smooth muscle of GI tract acts as syncytium
  - Muscle fibers connected by gap junctions allowing electrical signals to initiate muscle contractions from one muscle fiber to next rapidly along length of bundle
- Normal resting membrane potential of GI smooth muscles: -50mV to -60mV
- Two types of electrical waves contributing to membrane potential

Slow waves

- Generated, propagated by interstitial cells of Cajal (pacemaker cells)
- *Slow-wave threshold:* potential that must be reached by slow wave to propagate smooth muscle
- Does not cause smooth muscle contraction
- Slow-wave threshold reached → L-type calcium channels activated → calcium influx → motility initiation

- Occur at 12 cycles/minute in duodenum, decreases towards colon
- Regulated by innervation, hormones
  - Excitatory stimulants (e.g. acetylcholine, substance P), inhibitory stimulants (e.g. VIP, nitric oxide)

Spikes
- True action potentials occurring automatically when GI smooth muscle potential becomes more positive than -40mV
- Digestive activity controls
  - Involves regulation by autonomous smooth muscle, intrinsic nerve plexuses, external nerves (ANS), GI hormones

ENTERIC NERVOUS SYSTEM
- Intrinsic nervous system of the GI system
- Division of ANS
- Provides major nerve supply to GI tract controlling GI function, motility
  - Parasympathetic system activates digestion
  - Sympathetic system inhibits digestion
  - Also capable of self-regulation, autonomous function

Receptors and plexus
- Chemoreceptors respond to chemicals from food in gut lumen
- Stretch receptors respond to food distending GI tract wall
- Two plexus consist of motor neurons, interneurons, sensory neurons
  - *Submucosal (Meissner's) nerve plexus:* innervates secretory cells → controls digestive secretions
  - *Myenteric nerve plexus:* innervates smooth muscle layers of muscularis → controls GI motility
- Segmentation, peristalsis mostly automatic mediated by pacemaker cells, reflex arcs

Reflex mediation
- *Short reflexes:* intrinsic control (enteric nervous system)
- *Long reflexes:* extrinsic control outside of GI tract (e.g. CNS, autonomic nerves)

GASTROINTESTINAL MOTILITY

Gastric motility
- Peristaltic contractions originate in upper fundus, move to pyloric sphincter
- Moves gastric chyme forward → gastric emptying into duodenum

Small intestinal motility
- Mix chyme, digestive enzymes, pancreatic secretions, bile → digestion
- Expose nutrients to mucosa → maximize absorption
- Advance chyme along small intestine via segmentation actions → ileocecal valve → ileocecal sphincter → large intestine

Large intestinal motility
- Unabsorbed small intestine material → large intestine
  - Contents now feces (destined for excretion)
- Segmental contractions (cecum, proximal colon) associated with haustra (sac-like segments characteristic of large intestine) mixes contents
- Mass movements
  - *Function:* move contents long distances (e.g. transverse → sigmoid)
  - Occur 1–3 times daily
  - *Water absorption:* fecal contents → increasingly solid (hard to mobilize)
  - Final mass movements propel contents to rectum → stored until defecation
- Gastrocolic reflex
  - Stomach distension → ↑ colonic motility → ↑ mass movements
  - Afferent limb (from stomach) → parasympathetic nervous system mediates → efferent limb → CCK, gastrin production → ↑ colonic motility

- Defecation
  - Rectum 25% full → defecation urge
  - Rectum fills with feces → rectal wall distends → stretch receptors send afferent signals to spinal cord → to brain (awareness of need to defecate) + afferent signals to myenteric plexus → peristaltic waves → move feces forward → internal anal sphincter relaxes → external anal sphincter remains tonically contracted (striated skeletal muscle under voluntary control) → when appropriate, external anal sphincter relaxed voluntarily → rectal smooth muscle contracts → ↑ pressure → Valsalva maneuver (expire against closed glottis) → ↑ intra-abdominal pressure → ↑ defecation pressure → feces forced out through anal canal

SECRETORY PRODUCTS OF THE GASTRIC MUCOSA GLANDS

	STIMULUS FOR SECRETION	SECRETORY PRODUCTS	FUNCTION
CHIEF	Gastrin Acetylcholine	Pepsinogen (converts to pepsin in presence of HCl) Gastric lipase	Breaks down protein into peptide chains Initiates lipolysis
D	HCl	Somatostatin (paracrine)	Modulates HCl secretion by inhibiting gastrin, histamine release
ECL	Gastrin Acetylcholine Surges before meals (cephalic stimulation)	Histamine Ghrelin	Primary stimulator of HCl secretion by parietal cells Stimulates appetite Increases gastric secretion, motility
G	Partially digested protein	Gastrin	Increases secretion of HCl Relaxes ileocecal valve
MUCOUS	Mechanical stimulation by stomach contents	Mucus Bicarbonate	Protective alkaline barrier for gastric epithelium Lubrication
PARIETAL	Gastrin (endocrine) Histamine (paracrine) Acetylcholine (neural)	HCl Intrinsic factor	Activates pepsinogen Inactivates amylase Denatures proteins - Kills microorganisms Binds with vitamin B12 for intestinal absorption

NOTES
GASTROINTESTINAL FUNCTION

ENTERIC NERVOUS SYSTEM

osms.it/enteric-nervous-system-and-slow-waves

- Intrinsic component of gastrointestinal (GI) innervation that can function without extrinsic innervation
- Communicates with sympathetic nervous system, parasympathetics
- Ganglia located in myenteric, submucosal plexuses
    - *Myenteric/Auerbach's plexus*: located between longitudinal, circular smooth muscle layers; GI movement function
    - *Submucosal/Meissner's plexus*: located in submucosa; function in GI secretions, blood flow
- Neurons of extrinsic system release neurocrines
    - Neurochemicals consisting of neurotransmitters, neuromodulators
- Extrinsic branch of GI innervation
    - Sympathetic, parasympathetic divisions

PARASYMPATHETIC INNERVATION
- Parasympathetic ganglia located within myenteric, submucosal plexuses
- Parasympathetic preganglionic, postganglionic neurons either cholinergic (release acetylcholine) or peptidergic (release substance P/vasoactive intestinal peptide)
- Vagus nerve innervates upper GI
    - Upper ⅓ of esophagus, stomach, small intestine, ascending, proximal transverse colon
    - Consists of 75% afferent, 25% efferent fibers
    - *Vagovagal reflexes*: reflexes in which both afferent, efferent limbs originate from vagus nerve

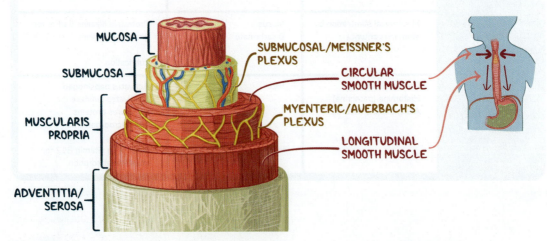

Figure 37.1 Locations of the myenteric (Auerbach's) and submucosal (Meissner's) plexuses within the four layers of the gastrointestinal tract. The myenteric plexus is located between the circular and longitudinal smooth muscle layers, which produce different movements in the GI tract.

- Pelvic nerves innervate lower GI
  - Distal transverse colon, descending, sigmoid colon

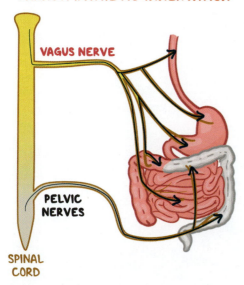

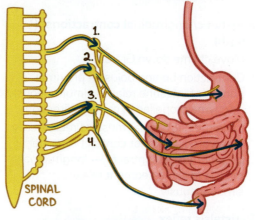

1. CELIAC GANGLION
2. SUPERIOR MESENTERIC GANGLION
3. INFERIOR MESENTERIC GANGLION
4. HYPOGASTRIC GANGLION

Figure 37.3 Sympathetic preganglionic neurons synapse outside the GI tract, in the four ganglia shown above.

Figure 37.2 The vagus nerve provides parasympathetic innervation from the upper esophagus to the proximal transverse colon. The pelvic nerve provides innervation from the distal transverse colon to the rectum.

SYMPATHETIC INNERVATION
- Sympathetic preganglionic neurons synapse in ganglia outside GI tract
  - Celiac, superior mesenteric, inferior mesenteric, hypogastric ganglia
- Sympathetic postganglionic neurons either synapse on ganglia in myenteric/submucosal plexuses or directly innervate target organs
- Sympathetic preganglionic neurons are cholinergic; sympathetic postganglionic neurons are adrenergic (release norepinephrine)

MECHANISMS
- Slow waves
  - Duodenum: 12 waves/minute
  - Ileum: 9 waves/minute
- Migrating myoelectric complexes every 90 minutes clears any remaining chyme

- Sympathetic via fibers from celiac/superior mesenteric ganglia → ↓ contractions
- Two forms of contractions; coordinated by enteric nervous system

Innervation
- Parasympathetic via vagus nerve (CN X)
  - ↑ contractions; most nerves cholinergic, some release neurocrines (e.g. peptidergic)
- Motilin
  - Secreted by endocrinocytes in proximal small intestine, regulate contractions
- Vasoactive intestinal peptide (VIP)
  - Induces smooth muscle relaxation (e.g. sphincters); induces water secretion into pancreatic juice, bile; inhibits gastric acid secretion
- Enkephalins
  - Inhibitory modulators in myenteric, submucosal plexuses

Segmental contractions (↓ diameter)
- Mix, expose chyme to secretions, enzymes
- Contraction → splits chyme → both orad, caudad directions → relaxation → merging of chyme → repeated

- No forward/propulsive movement along small intestine

Peristaltic/longitudinal contractions (↓ length)
- Move chyme down GI tract
- Contraction behind bolus → proximal portion of intestine relaxes simultaneously → chyme propelled in caudad direction
- Longitudinal, circular muscles reciprocally innervated → do not contract together; if circular muscle contracts → longitudinal muscle in same segment relaxes simultaneously

Peristalsis reflex
- Enterochromaffin-like (ECL) cells in intestinal mucosa sense food bolus → secrete serotonin (5-HT) → binds to intrinsic primary afferent neuron receptors → activates peristalsis reflex → excitatory neurotransmitters (acetylcholine, substance P, neuropeptide Y) released behind bolus → ↑ circular muscle contraction → ↓ longitudinal muscle activation → segment narrows, lengthens → in front of bolus, circular muscle inhibitory mechanisms (VIP, nitric oxide) activate, excitatory pathways in longitudinal segment activate → segment shortens, widens → chyme propelled forward in caudad direction

GASTROINTESTINAL HORMONES

osms.it/gastrointestinal-hormones

SOMATOSTATIN

- Members of G protein coupled-receptor superfamily

Function
- ↓ secretion of many other hormones (e.g. gastrin, bicarbonate, digestive enzymes)
- ↓ nutrient absorption from gut by prolonging gastric emptying time
- ↓ pancreatic secretions
- ↓ visceral blood flow

Secretion and activation
- Central nervous system, pancreatic delta cells, enteroendocrine delta cells
- Somatostatin binds receptors → activates inhibitory G protein → inactivate adenylate cyclase → ↓ cAMP production → protein kinase not activated → ↓ Ca^{2+} → inhibitory effect
- Site of action
    - Stomach, pancreas, small intestine, gallbladder, liver
- Secretory stimulants
    - Glucose, arginine, leucine, glucagon, vasoactive intestinal peptide (VIP), cholecystokinin (CCK)

GASTRIN

Function
- Induces gastric acid secretion

Secretion and stimulation/inhibition
- Secreted by enteroendocrine G cells of stomach, duodenum
- Secretory stimulants
    - Presence of acidic content, partially digested food in duodenum, vagus nerve stimulation
- Inhibited by somatostatin

MOTILIN

Function
- Stimulates gastric, pancreatic enzyme secretion

Secretion and stimulation/inhibition
- Secreted by enteroendocrine M cells of proximal small intestine
- Secretory stimulants
    - Duodenal alkalinization, gastric distension
- Inhibited by duodenal nutrients

PANCREATIC PEPTIDE (PP)

Function
- ↓ gastric emptying, slows small intestine motility

Secretion and stimulation/inhibition
- Secreted by endocrine cells in pancreatic islets
- Secretory stimulants: intraluminal nutrients, vagal nerve activation, hypoglycemia

PEPTIDE Y (PPY)

Function
- Inhibits gastric acid secretion, gastric motility, slows intestinal motility
- Inhibits pancreatic exocrine secretion

Secretion and stimulation/inhibition
- Secreted by pancreatic islet alpha cells, enteroendocrine cells
- Secretory stimulants
    - Ingestion of nutrition, bile acids, fatty acids

SECRETIN

Function
- ↓ acidity to improve pancreatic enzyme function
- ↑ pancreatic secretion, biliary bicarbonate, water
- Regulates pancreatic enzyme secretion
- ↓ gastric emptying, gastrin release, gastric acid secretion

Secretion and stimulation/inhibition
- Secreted by enteroendocrine S cells in proximal small intestine
- Secretory stimulants
  - Gastric acid, bile salts, peptides, fatty acids, ethanol
- Inhibited by somatostatin

CHOLECYSTOKININ (CCK)

Function
- Promotes food delivery from stomach into small intestine
- Regulates nutrient-stimulated enzyme secretion
- ↑ gallbladder contraction
- ↑ enzymatic pancreatic secretion output

Secretion and stimulation/inhibition
- Secreted by enteroendocrine I cells
- Secretory stimulants
  - Nutrition ingestion, fatty acids, amino acids

INSULIN

Function
- Major anabolic hormone
- ↓ blood glucose
- Promotes liver, muscle glycogen storage
- Fatty acids, triacylglycerol storage in adipose tissue
- Protein synthesis, glucagon suppression

Secretion and stimulation/inhibition
- Secreted by beta cells of pancreatic islet cells
- Secretory stimulants
  - High blood glucose, glucose, arginine, leucine, glucagon, VIP, CCK
- Inhibited by somatostatin

GLUCAGON

Function
- Counteracts insulin
- ↑ blood glucose, promotes glycogenolysis, gluconeogenesis, ketogenesis
- Works mainly on liver

Secretion and stimulation/inhibition
- Secreted by alpha cells of islet cells, L-cells of intestine
- Inhibited by somatostatin

INCRETINS
- Includes glucagon-like peptide-1 (GLP-1), glucose-dependent insulinotropic peptide (GIP)

Function
- ↑ insulin release from pancreatic beta-cells
- ↑ levels of cAMP in islets leading to expansion of beta-cells

GASTRIC INHIBITORY PEPTIDE (GIP)
- AKA glucose-dependent insulinotropic peptide

Function
- Weakly inhibits HCl production, stimulates insulin release

Secretion and stimulation/inhibition
- Secreted by duodenal mucosa
- Secretory stimulant
  - Fatty chyme

HISTAMINE

Function
- Activates parietal cells to release HCl

Secretion and stimulation/inhibition
- Secreted by stomach mucosa
- Secretory stimulant
  - Food in stomach

SEROTONIN

Function
- Stomach muscle contraction

Secretion and stimulation/inhibition
- Secreted by stomach, duodenal mucosa
- Secretory stimulant
    - Food in stomach

VASOACTIVE INTESTINAL PEPTIDE (VIP)

Function
- Dilates intestinal capillaries
- ↑ secretions, ↓ acid secretion
- Relaxes intestinal smooth muscle
- Site of action
    - Small intestine, pancreas, stomach

Secretion and stimulation/inhibition
- Secreted by enteric neurons/parasympathetic ganglia
- Secretory stimulant
    - Chyme, parasympathetic stimulus

ENKEPHALINS

Function
- Smooth muscle constriction causing ↓ fluid flow into intestines (opiates acting on enkephalin receptors ↓ fluid flow to intestines, cause constipation)
- Site of action
    - Intestine
- Secreted by
    - GI tract neurons

GHRELIN

Function
- Stimulate hunger
- Site of action
    - Hypothalamus lateral nucleus

Secretion and stimulation/inhibition
- Secreted by gastric cells
- Secretory stimulant
    - Empty stomach
- Inhibited by stomach stretching when food present

LEPTIN

Function
- Stimulate satiety
- Site of action
    - Ventromedial nucleus of hypothalamus

Secretion and stimulation/inhibition
- Secreted by adipocytes

SATIETY

osms.it/satiety

- Hypothalamus controls appetite, satiety
  - *Ventral posteromedial nucleus (VPN) of hypothalamus*: activates satiety
  - *Lateral hypothalamic area*: activates hunger, feeding

HORMONES

Leptin
- Stimulates satiety, decreases appetite
- Secreted by fat cells in proportion to fat amount in adipocytes

Ghrelin
- Increases appetite, hunger
- Secreted by gastric cells before meal
- Starvation, weight loss stimulates ghrelin release

Insulin
- Stimulates satiety, decreases appetite
- Fluctuates throughout day

Peptide YY (PYY)
- Stimulates satiety, decreases appetite directly (via hypothalamus), indirectly (via inhibiting release of ghrelin)

GLP-1
- Stimulates satiety, decreases appetite
- Secreted by intestinal L cells

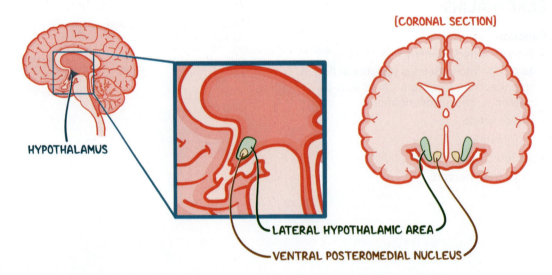

Figure 37.4 Locations of two areas in the hypothalamus that control appetite and satiety.

NOTES
UPPER GASTROINTESTINAL TRACT

CHEWING & SWALLOWING

osms.it/chewing-and-swallowing

CHEWING
- First step to process ingested food to prepare for digestion, absorption
- Three functions
  - ↓ food particle size → facilitate swallowing
  - Mix food with saliva → lubrication
  - Mix food particles with amylase → begin carbohydrate digestion
- Teeth move, masticate food into small fragments, tongue functions to taste, roll food around in oral cavity → compact into small ball (bolus)

Oral cavity walls
- *Roof:* soft, hard palate
- *Floor:* tongue, mylohyoid muscles
- *Sides:* cheeks
- *Front:* lips, teeth

- Involuntary component of chewing
  - Mouth mechanoreceptors → sensory information to brainstem → reflex oscillatory pattern to muscles of mastication
- Voluntary component
  - Can override reflex chewing at any time

Muscles involved with mastication
- *Temporalis muscle:* fan-shaped muscle on both sides of head
- *Masseter muscle:* connects mandible to zygomatic arch of temporal bone
- *Medial pterygoid muscle:* connects mandible to medial pterygoid plate
- *Lateral pterygoid muscle:* located at condylar process
- All muscles of mastication innervated by branches of trigeminal (CN V)

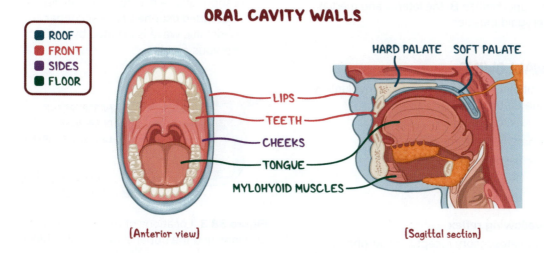

Figure 38.1 The structures that make up the walls of the oral cavity.

- All muscles coordinate, work together to grind, mechanically break down food
- Tongue moves from side to side to reposition food → push it between teeth to be chewed, mixed with saliva → soft, mushy bolus ready for swallowing

MUSCLES of MASTICATION

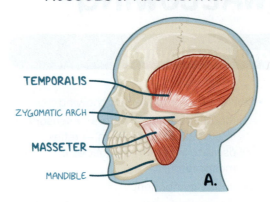

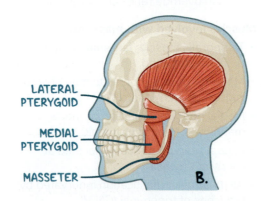

Figure 38.2 The muscles of mastication. A: The temporalis and masseter muscles are superficial to B: the laterial and medial pterygoid muscles.

SWALLOWING

- Initiated voluntarily in mouth, involuntary thereafter
  - AKA deglutition
- Pharynx has three parts
  - Nasopharynx
  - Oropharynx
  - Throat

Swallowing reflex

- Somatosensory receptors near pharynx → detect sensory information (e.g. food in mouth) → travel via vagus and glossopharyngeal nerves → swallowing center in medulla → sends efferent, motor information via glossopharyngeal, vagus nerves → directs coordinated movement of pharyngeal striated muscle, upper esophagus

Three phases
- Oral (voluntary)
  - Tongue presses against hard palate → forces bolus towards oropharynx → pharynx contains high density of somatosensory receptors → activation → swallowing reflex initiation in medulla
- Pharyngeal (swallowing reflex)
  - Soft palate, uvula moves upwards → creates narrow passage → prevents food reflux into nasopharynx → epiglottis closes down over laryngeal opening → larynx moves upwards against epiglottis → act as seal to prevent food entering trachea → upper esophageal sphincter relaxes → food passes from pharynx to upper esophagus → peristaltic wave initiation → food propelled through open upper esophageal sphincter
  - Breathing inhibited during this phase
- Esophageal (swallowing reflex/enteric nervous system)
  - Swallowing reflex closes upper esophageal sphincter → food cannot reflux back into pharynx → primary peristaltic wave (coordinated by swallowing reflex) → propels food along esophagus → if all food not cleared → distended esophagus → secondary peristaltic wave is initiated by enteric nervous system

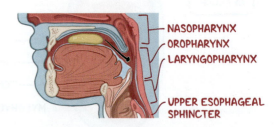

Figure 38.3 Locations of the three pharynx divisions and the upper esophageal sphincter.

Chapter 38 Gastrointestinal Physiology: Upper Gastrointestinal Tract

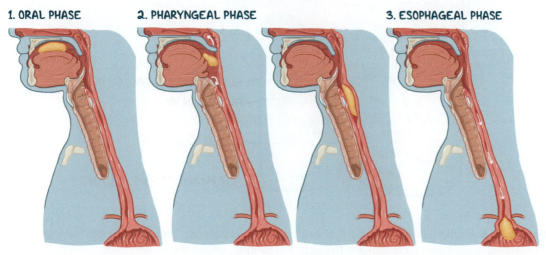

Figure 38.4 Mastication muscles. A: The temporalis and masseter muscles are superficial to B: the lateral and medial pterygoid muscles.

SALIVARY SECRETION

osms.it/salivary-secretion

SALIVARY GLANDS
- Three major salivary glands exist outside oral cavity
  - *Parotid*: composed of serous cells → secrete fluid composed of ions, enzymes, water
  - *Submandibular, sublingual*: composed of serous, mucous cells → stringy, viscous solution of aqueous fluid, mucin glycoprotein for lubrication
- Minor salivary glands (e.g. buccal) scattered throughout oral cavity mucosa
- Each gland is paired; all produce saliva which are delivered to oral cavity via ducts
- *Appearance*: cluster of grapes
  - Each grape = single acinus
  - Blind end of branching duct system
- Saliva formation is two-step process
  - Acinus lined with acinar cells → produces initial saliva → passes through intercalated duct → striated duct lined with ductal cells → modify initial saliva → myoepithelial cells stimulated neurally → contract → saliva ejected into mouth
- Cell types
  - *Acinar cells*: produce initial isotonic saliva (mixture of water, ions, enzymes, mucus)
  - *Ductal cells*: modify electrolyte concentrations in initial saliva to produce final saliva
  - *Myoepithelial cells*: present in acini, intercalated ducts; contract to eject saliva into oral cavity
- Innervation of salivary glands
  - Saliva production stimulated by both parasympathetic (dominant), sympathetic activation (unique feature)
- Blood supply
  - Saliva production stimulated → unusually high blood flow
  - When corrected for organ size, blood flow is ↑ 10x more than exercising skeletal muscle

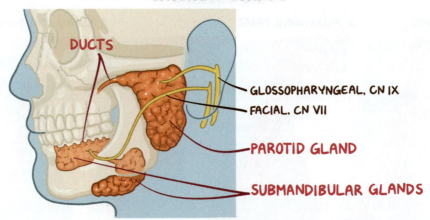

Figure 38.5 Protid glands sit in front of each ear. Submandibular glands sit under the mandible. Sublingual glands (not pictured) are beneath the tongue, under the mouth floor.

SALIVA
- Produced by salivary glands; rate of 1L/ daily

Functions
- Initial digestion of starches/lipids by salivary enzymes
- Lubricating ingested food to allow movement through esophagus
- Diluting, buffering ingested foods (which may be harmful)
- Cleanses mouth
- Dissolves food chemicals so it can be tasted

Saliva composition
- Water (97–99.5%)
- Electrolytes
- *Alpha-amylase*: initial carbohydrates digestion, like potatoes/rice
- *Lingual lipase*: initial lipid digestion
- Mucus
- Immunoglobulin A
- *Kallikrein*: protease enzyme; cleaves high molecular weight kininogen → bradykinin → vasodilation → increased blood flow during salivary activity
- *Lysozyme*: enzyme inhibiting bacterial growth, prevents tooth decay
- *Defensin*: acts as local antibiotic
- pH 6.5–7.5
  - Usually maintained by $NaHCO_3$

Saliva formation
- Initial saliva is isotonic
  - Concentrations of K^+, HCO_3^-, Na^+, Cl^- similar to plasma
- Final secreted saliva is hypotonic (↓ osmolarity), when compared to plasma
  - ↑ K^+, HCO_3^-, ↓ Na^+, Cl^-
- Modification of saliva by ductal cells
  - Complex transport system
- Luminal membrane has three transporters
  - Na^+-H^+ exchange
  - H^+-K^+ exchange
  - Cl^--HCO_3^- exchange
- Basolateral membrane has two transporters
  - Na^+-K^+ ATPase
  - Cl^- channel
- Overall action of all transporters together
  - Absorption of Na^+, Cl^- → ↓ Na^+, Cl^- concentration in saliva
  - Secretion of K^+, HCO_3^- → ↑ K^+, HCO_3^- concentration in saliva
  - Net absorption of solute (NaCl > $KHCO_3$)
- Process of isotonic saliva → hypotonic saliva
  - Ductal cells are water impermeable
  - Due to net absorption (solutes leave saliva, water does not travel with)
- Saliva tonicity depends on flow rates
  - Depends on amount of time saliva in contact with ductal cells (↑ Na^+, Cl^-

- absorption, ↑ K⁺ secretion)
  - **↑ flow rate (4mL/min):** composition parallels plasma, initial saliva produced by acinar cells
  - **↓ flow rate (1mL/min):** most dissimilar composition to plasma
  - **Exception:** HCO₃⁻ remains constant, despite flow changes; selective parasympathetic stimulation; ↑ flow rate → ↑ HCO₃⁻ parasympathetic stimulation → ↑ HCO₃⁻ secretion

Saliva secretion regulation
- Minor salivary glands continuously secreting small amounts to keep oral cavity moist
- When food enters → major glands activated → large amounts of saliva produced
- Two unique features
  - Exclusive neural control by autonomic nervous system (other gastrointestinal secretions controlled both neurally, hormonally)
  - Saliva secretion ↑ by both sympathetic + parasympathetic
- Parasympathetic innervation
  - Activity ↑ with visual stimulus of food, smell, nausea, conditional reflexes (e.g. Pavlov's salivating dog)
  - Activity ↓ with fear, sleep, dehydration
  - Chemoreceptors, mechanoreceptors in oral cavity stimulated → signal carried via facial (CN VII), glossopharyngeal (CN IX) nerves → salivatory nucleus in brain stem (medulla and pons)
  - Vinegar and citric juice → strongest chemoreceptor stimulus
  - Postganglionic neurons → release acetylcholine (ACh) → bind muscarinic receptors → ↑ IP₃ + intracellular Ca²⁺ → saliva secretion
- Sympathetic innervation
  - Thoracic segments T₁–T₃ → preganglionic nerves → synapse on superior cervical ganglion → postganglionic sympathetic neurons release norepinephrine (NE) → bind to beta-adrenergic > alpha-adrenergic receptors on acinar/ductal cells → stimulation of adenylyl cyclase → ↑ cAMP → ↑ saliva secretion

SLOW WAVES

osms.it/enteric-nervous-system-and-slow-waves

ENTERIC NERVOUS SYSTEM
- AKA 'gut brain'
- Contains over 100 million neurons (more than spinal cord)
- Intrinsic/"in-house" nerve plexuses spread throughout GI tract like chicken wire
- Semiautonomous enteric neurons made up of two nerve plexuses (ganglia connected by unmyelinated tracts)
  - Submucosal nerve plexus → located in submucosa; innervates secretory cells; controls local digestive secretions
  - Myenteric nerve plexus → located between circular, longitudinal muscle layers in muscularis externa; major controller of gastrointestinal (GI) tract motility
- Enteric nervous system connected to central nervous system (CNS) via
  - Afferent visceral fibers
  - Sympathetic, parasympathetic branches
  - Synapse with intrinsic plexus neurons

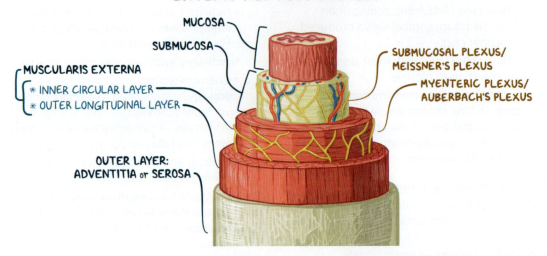

Figure 38.6 The enteric nervous system is found within the walls of the entire gastrointestinal tract. The submucosal plexus is found in the submucosa and the myenteric plexus is found within the muscularis externa between the longitudinal and circular muscle layers.

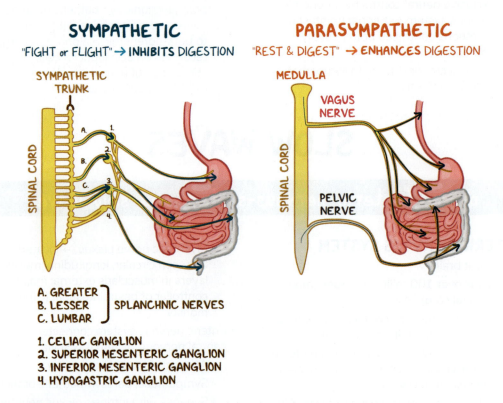

Figure 38.7 The gastrointestinal portions of the visceral motor system.

Sympathetic division: preganglionic fibers are in the lower thoracic and upper lumbar segments of the spinal cord, and they synapse in ganglia located near the spinal cord.

Parasympathetic division: preganglionic fibers arise from the brainstem (vagus nerve) and sacral component of the spinal cord (pelvic nerve), and synapse in a neural plexus on or very near the target organ.

SLOW WAVES

- Unique feature of GI tract electrical activity
  - Oscillating depolarizations, repolarization of membrane potential of GI smooth muscle cells
- Depolarization → membrane potential becomes less negative → moves towards threshold → burst of action potentials (APs) occur on top of slow wave (plateau) → contraction/smooth muscle tension → membrane potential becomes more negative → moves away from threshold → repolarization → smooth muscle relaxation

Frequency

- Intrinsic rate is 3–12 slow waves/minute
- Not determined by hormonal/neural input, however can modulate amount of APs at plateau → ↑/↓ contraction strength
- Each part of GI tract has characteristic frequency
  - Stomach → slowest (3/min), duodenum → fastest (12/min)

Mechanism

- Cyclic opening of Ca^{2+} channels → Ca^{2+} influx → depolarization
- Plateau phase maintained by continuous Ca^{2+} influx
- Opening of K^+ channels → K^+ outflux → repolarization

Slow wave origin

- Myenteric plexus is network of nerves, located between longitudinal, circular layers in muscularis externa
- Interstitial cells of Cajal located in myenteric (Auerbach) plexus
  - Referred to as 'pacemaker' cells of GI tract smooth muscle
  - Cyclic, spontaneous depolarizations, repolarization occur in these cells → rapid spread to adjacent smooth muscle cells via gap junctions
- Pacemaker → frequency → AP rate → coordinated smooth muscle contraction
- Slow waves to contractions
- Subthreshold slow waves → can produce weak contraction
- Even without AP occurrence → smooth muscle not completely relaxed/tonically contracted
- Above threshold slow waves → APs occur on top of slow wave → stronger contraction → phasic contraction
- ↑↑ APs on top of slow wave → ↑↑ phasic contraction strength
- Unlike skeletal muscle, where each AP results in twitch/separate contraction, smooth muscle APs summate into one long contraction

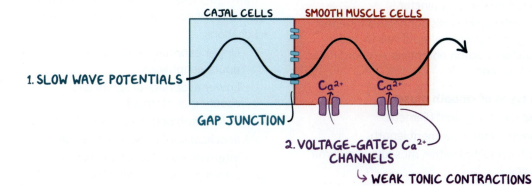

Figure 38.8 Slow wave origin and mechanism. Slow waves are generated by spontaneous depolarization and polarization of Cajal cells, which are attached to smooth muscle cells via gap junctions. The slow wave potentials travel through the smooth muscle cells → voltage-gated calcium channels open → weak depolarization of smooth muscle cells → weak tonic contractions that maintain the tone of the gastrointestinal tract.

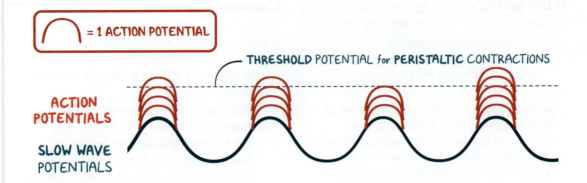

Figure 38.9 Slow wave potentials from enteric nervous system + action potentials from extrinsic nervous system → threshold potential for peristaltic contractions. Strength of contraction is determined by number of action potentials above each slow wave; rate of contraction is determined by the rate of the slow waves.

ESOPHAGEAL MOTILITY

osms.it/esophageal-motility

GI MOTILITY

- Generally, GI motility refers to contraction, relaxation of GI walls, sphincters
- GI contractile tissue is all smooth muscle except
    - Pharynx
    - Upper ⅓ esophagus
    - External anal sphincter
- Smooth muscle cells connected together via gap junctions → rapid cell-to-cell transfer of action potentials → coordinated contractions

Two types of smooth muscle
- *Circular:* ↓ segment diameter
- *Longitudinal:* ↓ segment length
- Both contained within muscularis externa layer

Two types of contractions
- *Phasic:* periodic → relaxation
    - Located in esophagus, small intestine
- *Tonic:* constant level of contraction, without regular intervals of relaxation
    - Located in lower esophagus, upper stomach, ileocecal valve, internal anal sphincter

Sphincters
- Specialized circular muscle separating adjacent GI tract regions
- Maintain positive pressure → anterograde, retrograde flow prevented
- Smooth muscle contraction → peristalsis of GI contents to sphincter → sphincter transiently lowers pressure → relaxation → passage of contents to adjacent organ
- Locations
    - *Upper esophageal sphincter:* pharynx-upper esophagus
    - *Lower esophageal sphincter:* esophagus-stomach
    - *Pyloric sphincter:* stomach-duodenum
    - *Ileocecal sphincter:* ileum-cecum
    - *Internal and external sphincters:* preserves fecal continence

ESOPHAGUS

Key features
- Muscular 25cm/9.8in tube divided into three regions
- *Cervical:* connects with pharynx behind trachea; separated by upper esophageal sphincter

Chapter 38 Gastrointestinal Physiology: Upper Gastrointestinal Tract

- **Thoracic:** suprasternal notch to esophageal hiatus in diaphragm
- **Abdominal:** esophageal hiatus to esophageal opening into stomach; separated by lower esophageal sphincter

Layers
- Adventitia
  - Thick fibrous connective tissue; outermost
- Muscularis externa
  - Outer longitudinal, inner circular muscle layers; myenteric plexus lies between
- Submucosa
  - Dense layer of connective tissue containing blood vessels, lymphatics, mucus glands secreting mucus to lumen via ducts; contains submucosal (Meissner) plexus
- Mucosa → three layers
  - Muscularis mucosa (outermost layer of longitudinal muscle)
  - Lamina propria
  - Epithelial layer

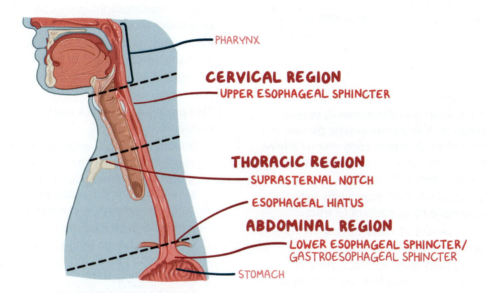

Figure 38.10 Regions of esophagus, associated structures.

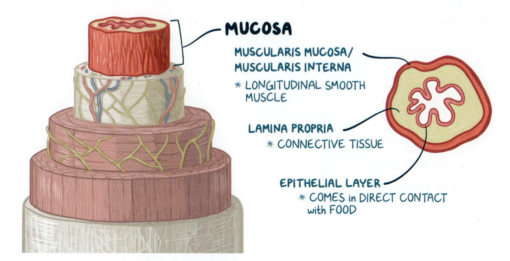

Figure 38.11 Layers of esophageal mucosa.

Innervation
- *Intrinsic:* Vagus nerve (CN X)
- *Extrinsic:* Myenteric plexus in muscularis externa

Function
- Esophageal motility propels food bolus from pharynx → stomach
    - Food bolus formed in oral cavity → upper esophageal sphincter opens → bolus passes pharynx to upper esophagus → upper esophageal sphincter closes → primary peristaltic contraction → series of coordinated sequential contractions → each segment contracts → creates area of high pressure behind bolus → pushed down esophagus
- If not all food pushed through → distension of esophageal wall → activation of mechanoreceptors in mucosal layer → afferent, sensory information to enteric nervous system and myenteric plexus → coordination of muscle contractions above site of distension + relaxation below it → secondary peristaltic wave
- Esophagus has thick muscularis externa compared to other parts of GI tract
- Primary peristaltic wave travels approximately 3cm/sec
    - Solid food takes approximately 10 seconds to travel from cervical region → stomach
    - Liquids approximately 1–2 seconds
    - Accelerated by gravity (sitting/standing > lying supine)
- Food bolus approaches lower esophageal sphincter → opening mediated by peptidergic fibers of vagus nerve, release vasoactive intestinal peptide (VIP) → lower esophageal sphincter smooth muscle relaxation → at same time, orad region of stomach relaxes (phenomenon referred to as receptive relaxation) → pressure decreases in orad stomach → food bolus propelled into stomach → lower esophageal sphincter closes immediately, returns to high pressure resting tone → prevents reflux

Intrathoracic esophagus
- Upper, middle esophagus located in thorax, only lower esophagus located in abdomen
- Intraesophageal pressure = intrathoracic pressure which is < atmospheric pressure
- Intraesophageal pressure < intra abdominal pressure
- This pressure difference causes two problems
    - Inhibiting air from entering upper esophagus (air will travel down pressure gradient, esophagus essentially sucking air in); prevented by upper esophageal sphincter (always in closed resting state)
    - Inhibiting gastric contents from entering lower esophagus (reflux); prevented by lower esophageal sphincter (always in closed resting state)
    - Conditions where intraabdominal pressure ↑↑ (e.g. pregnancy, morbid obesity) → gastroesophageal reflux

Chapter 38 Gastrointestinal Physiology: Upper Gastrointestinal Tract

GASTRIC MOTILITY

osms.it/gastric-motility-and-secretions

STOMACH
- Anatomy differentiated based on motility, stomach can be divided into orad (proximal), caudad (distal)
    - *Orad region*: fundus, proximal body; thin-walled
    - *Caudad region*: distal body, antrum; thick-walled (stronger contractions to mix chyme, propel to small intestine)

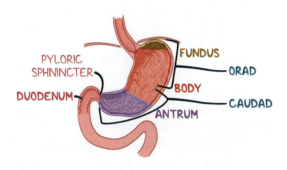

Figure 38.12 Divisions of the stomach.

Layers
- *Mucosa*: innermost layer; modified → contains various glands filled with different cells → secrete components of gastric juice
- *Submucosa*: contains submucosal plexus → controls secretions and gastric blood flow, contains blood vessels
- *Muscularis externa*: modified
- *Serosa*: outermost layer
- Three layers of stomach muscles that involuntarily contract to produce peristalsis
    - Outer longitudinal layer
    - Middle circular layer
    - Inner oblique layer (unique to stomach)

Innervation
- *Extrinsic*: autonomic nervous system
- *Intrinsic*: myenteric receives parasympathetic innervation (via vagus nerve), sympathetic innervation (via fibers from celiac ganglion); submucosal plexuses

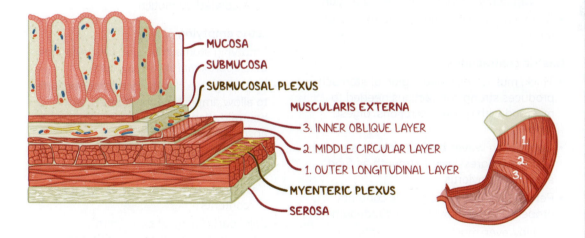

Figure 38.13 Layers of the stomach.

COMPONENTS OF GASTRIC MOTILITY

- Three components
- Receptive relaxation
    - Relaxation of lower esophageal sphincter, orad stomach region to receive food bolus from esophagus
- Gastric contractions to break up bolus, mix with gastric secretions → initiate digestion
- Gastric emptying → propelling chyme to small intestine
    - Gastric emptying rate hormonally determined → allows adequate time for small intestine digestion/absorption
    - Liquids (faster); solids (slower)

Receptive relaxation

- **Vasovagal reflex:** both afferent, efferent limbs of reflex carried within vagus nerve
    - Lower esophageal distension → relaxation, opening of lower esophageal sphincter → mechanoreceptors detect distension → send afferent sensory information to CNS through sensory neurons → CNS transmits efferent information to orad stomach smooth muscle wall → postganglionic peptidergic vagal nerve fibers release VIP → orad stomach ↓ pressure, ↑ volume → allows food bolus passage
    - Vagotomy inhibits receptive relaxation
- Stomach can accommodate up to 1.5L of food

Gastric contractions

- Thick, muscular caudad region of stomach produces strong contractions needed to mix food with gastric secretions, digest food
- Contraction waves begin in middle stomach body → progressively ↑ strength as food approaches pylorus
- Periodically, portion of gastric contents propelled through pylorus to duodenum
    - However, most gastric contents undergo retropulsion (propelled back into stomach for further mixing)
- Majority of the chyme not initially injected through pylorus to duodenum since contraction wave closes pyloric sphincter
- Frequency of slow waves in caudad stomach; bringing membrane potential to threshold so APs can occur
    - 3–5/min → frequency of caudad stomach contraction approximately same
    - Slow wave frequency not influenced by neural/hormonal input
    - Frequency of APs, contraction force are influenced by neural/hormonal input
- Frequency of APs, force of contraction ↑↑ by
    - Parasympathetic stimulation
    - Gastrin
    - Motilin
- Frequency of APs, force of contraction ↓↓ by
    - Sympathetic stimulation
    - **Secretin:** hormone produced by duodenal S cells; regulates water homeostasis, GI tract secretions
    - **Gastric inhibitory peptide (GIP):** hormone secreted by intestinal K cells; inhibits gastric acid secretion, stimulates insulin secretion
- Migrating myoelectric complexes
    - Periodic gastric contractions during fasting
    - **Function:** clear stomach of remaining content from last meal
    - 90-minute intervals
    - Mediated by motilin

Gastric emptying

- Emptying stomach of 1.5L postmeal can take approximately three hours
- Emptying rate closely monitored/regulated to allow ample time for stomach acid neutralization in duodenum, digestion/absorption of nutrients
- Emptying speeds
    - Liquids > solids
    - Isotonic contents > hyper/hypotonic contents
- Solid particles must be < $1mm^3$; retropulsion continues until this size reached
- Factors that ↑ gastric emptying time (slows gastric emptying process)
    - ↓ pH in duodenum (presence of H^+ ions); mediated by enteric nervous system
    - H^+ receptors in duodenal mucosa detect ↓ pH of intestinal contents → activate

Chapter 38 Gastrointestinal Physiology: Upper Gastrointestinal Tract

interneurons in myenteric plexus → relay info to gastric smooth muscle → ↑ gastric emptying time/slows gastric emptying process → allows time to neutralize acid by pancreatic HCO_3^-.
- ↑ fatty acids (highly fatty meal)

- The hormone cholecystokinin (CCK) secreted from duodenal I cells when fatty acids present in duodenum → slows gastric emptying (↑ gastric emptying time) → allow adequate time for fat to be digested/absorbed

GASTRIC SECRETION

osms.it/gastric-motility-and-secretions

- Altogether gastric mucosa secretes fluid referred to as 'gastric juice'
- Four major components
    - HCl
    - Pepsinogen
    - Intrinsic factor (needed for vitamin B_{12} absorption in ileum)
    - Mucus (protects gastric mucosa from corrosive acids, lubricates)
- Oxyntic glands
    - Found in body of stomach
    - Empty secretions via ducts into lumen of stomach
    - Opening of duct in gastric mucosa referred to as pits, lined by epithelial cells superficially

GASTRIC CELLS OVERVIEW

	LOCATION	SECRETION
CHIEF CELLS	Body	Pepsinogen
PARIETAL CELLS	Body	HCl + Intrinsic factor
MUCOUS CELLS	Antrum	Mucus + Pepsinogen
G CELLS	Antrum	Gastrin (to circulation)

Secretory cells
- Found in gastric glands
- Mucous neck cells
    - Scattered around neck, basally
    - Produce thin watery mucus (different from mucous cells of surface epithelium)
- Parietal (oxyntic) cells
    - Found more apically; scattered around chief cells
    - Produce HCl, intrinsic factor
- Chief cells
    - Found basally
    - Produce pepsinogen (inactive form of pepsin); activated by HCl
    - Also produce lipases (15% of GI lipolysis)
- Enteroendocrine cells
    - Found deep in gland
    - Release various chemical messengers directly into lamina propria (e.g. histamine, serotonin act via paracrine mechanism, somatostatin acts via paracrine/hormone mechanism)
- G cells
    - Secrete gastrin → bloodstream → ↑ HCl secretion by parietal cells, ↑ pepsinogen secretion by chief cells + ↑ contraction of stomach muscles
- Pyloric glands found in antrum of stomach
    - Similar configuration to oxyntic glands but with deeper pits
    - Mucous neck cells secrete mucus, HCO_3^-, pepsinogen → pyloric ducts
    - G cells secrete gastrin → circulation

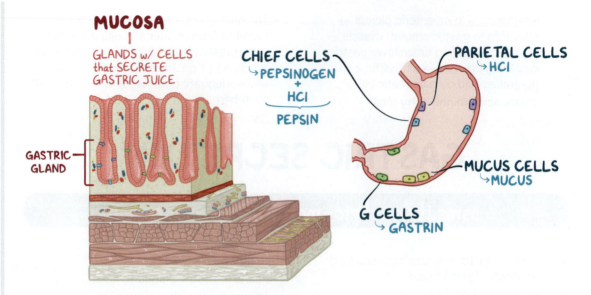

Figure 38.14 Location of secretory cells within gastric glands and in the stomach, as well as secretory products.

Mucosal barrier
- Stomach is harshest, most corrosive environment in entire GI tract
  - Due to HCl, protein-digesting enzymes
- To combat these conditions
  - Thick bicarbonate-rich mucus
  - Tight junctions joining epithelial cells together (prevents gastric juice leakage)
  - Undifferentiated stem cells → shed and replace damaged epithelial mucosal cells

HCl secretion and mechanism
- Parietal cells → HCl secretion → gastric content pH 1–2
- Functions to convert inactive pepsinogen (secreted by chief cells) → active pepsin → protein digestion; also functions to kill ingested bacteria
- Apical membrane of gastric gland has two transporters
  - H^+-K^+ ATPase: H^+ secreted into stomach lumen; primary active process (H^+ and K^+ flow against electrochemical gradient); site of action by proton pump inhibitors (e.g. omeprazole)
  - Cl^- channel: Cl^- follows H^+ into lumen; passive process

- Basolateral membrane has two transporters
  - Na^+-K^+ ATPase
  - Cl^--HCO_3^- exchanger
- Basolateral membrane cells contain carbonic anhydrase
  - $CO_2 + H_2O \rightarrow H_2CO_3 \rightarrow H^+ + HCO_3^-$
  - H^+ then secreted with Cl^- into lumen of stomach
  - HCO_3^- is absorbed into blood → 'alkaline tide' (↑ blood pH in gastric venous blood after meal)
- Overall net HCl secretion, net HCO_3^- absorption

HCl secretion modulation
- Gastrin (secreted into systemic circulation by gastric antral G cells)
  - Reaches parietal cells via endocrine mechanism
  - Binds to CCK_B receptors of parietal cells (affinity for gastrin = CCK)
  - Stimulates H^+ secretion via IP_3/Ca^{2+} second messenger mechanism
  - *Triggers for gastrin secretion*: stomach distension, small peptides, amino acids in stomach, vagus nerve stimulation
  - Can indirectly stimulate H^+ secretion by ↑ histamine release from endochromaffin-like (ECL) cells

- Histamine
  - Released from ECL cells in gastric mucosa
  - Paracrine diffusion mechanism to nearby parietal cells
  - Binds to H_2 receptors coupled to G_s protein → stimulation of adenylyl cyclase → ↑ cAMP → activation of protein kinase A → ↑ secretion of H^+ by parietal cells
  - Site of action of the H_2 blockers (e.g. cimetidine)
- ACh
  - Released by vagus nerve (directly innervate parietal cells)
  - ACh directly binds to parietal cell M_3 receptors → activation of phospholipase C → releases diacylglycerol (DAG) and IP_3 from membrane phospholipids → ↑ intracellular Ca^{2+} → Ca^{2+} and DAG → activate protein kinases → ↑ H^+ secretion by parietal cells
  - Site of action of antimuscarinics (e.g. atropine); atropine does not block HCl secretion completely
  - Will block direct vagal effects on parietal cells
  - Will not block indirect vagal effects on gastrin secretion since neurotransmitter is gastrin-releasing peptide (GRP), not ACh
  - Can indirectly stimulate H^+ secretion by ↑ histamine release from ECL cells
- Rate of H^+ secretion is regulated by individual actions of gastrin, histamine, ACh or by the combination of them via potentiation (ability of two or more stimuli to interact together to produce a greater combined response than sum of individual effects)

Cephalic phase of gastric secretion
- 30% of total HCl secretion
- *Stimuli*: smell and taste of food, chewing, swallowing, conditional reflexes in anticipation of eating (ex. Pavlov's dog)
- Two physiological mechanisms
  - Direct vagal stimulation of parietal cells
  - Indirect vagal stimulation of parietal cells via gastrin

Gastric phase of gastric secretion
- 60% of total HCl secretion
- *Stimuli*: gastric distension, amino acid/small peptide presence

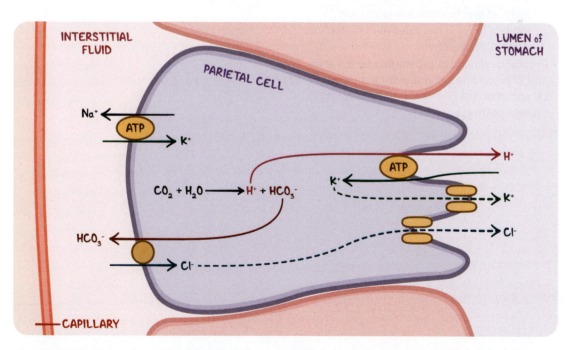

Figure 38.15 Mechanism of HCl secretion by parietal cells in the stomach's gastric glands. Dotted lines indicate passive diffusion, whereas solid lines indicate active transport.

- Four physiological mechanisms
  - Distension → direct vagal stimulation
  - Distension → indirect vagal stimulation (via gastrin)
  - Antral distension → local gastrin release reflex
  - Amino acids/small peptides → G cells → gastrin release
- Caffeine, alcohol are also HCl secretion stimulants

Intestinal phase of gastric secretion
- 10% of total HCl secretion
- Mediated by protein digestion products

Inhibition of HCl secretion
- First major factor is ↓ pH of gastric contents
  - Gastrin secretion inhibited by low pH
  - Chyme moved to small intestine → no longer requirement of pepsinogen → pepsin
- Second major factor is somatostatin
  - Secreted by D cells in stomach
  - Inhibits H^+ secretion from parietal cells
  - **Direct mechanism:** somatostatin → binds to receptor on parietal cell coupled with Gi protein → ↓ adenylyl cyclase → ↓ cAMP → ↓ H^+ secretion
  - **Indirect mechanism:** somatostatin inhibits ECL, G cell release of histamine, gastrin, respectively
- Prostaglandins (e.g. prostaglandin E_2) also inhibit histamine's stimulatory action on H^+ secretion via G_i protein → ↓ adenylyl cyclase pathway

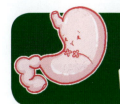

NOTES: DIGESTION & ABSORPTION

DIGESTION & ABSORPTION
- *Digestion*: breakdown of large food molecules into monomers for absorption in gastrointestinal (GI) tract
- Chemical digestion accomplished by enzymes secreted into alimentary canal by glands

Mechanical digestion
- Mastication
    - Mouth ingests food, begins mechanical, chemical digestion (mastication, salivation), initiates propulsion by swallowing
    - Partly voluntary, partly reflexive (e.g. stretch reflexes, pressure inputs)

Deglutition (swallowing)
- Movement of food from mouth to stomach
- *Buccal phase*: voluntary
    - Occurs in mouth
    - Tongue pushes against hard palate forcing food bolus into oropharynx
- *Pharyngeal-esophageal phase*: involuntary
    - Controlled by brainstem swallowing center
    - Cranial nerves (mainly Vagus) activate muscles of pharynx, esophagus
    - Soft palate rises, closes nasopharynx, epiglottis covers larynx, upper esophageal sphincter relaxes → peristalsis moves food through pharynx, esophagus → gastroesophageal sphincter relaxes allowing food to enter

Two absorption pathways
- *Cellular pathway*: substance crosses apical/luminal membrane to enter intestinal epithelial cell, then crosses basolateral membrane to enter into blood
- *Paracellular pathway*: move across tight junctions between intestinal epithelial cells to enter blood
- Absorptive surface maximized by villi, microvilli, folds (folds of Kerckring) in small intestine
    - Most digestion occurs in duodenum, least amount of digestion occurs in ileum (as reflected by length of villi - longest villi in duodenum, shortest in ileum)
    - *Brush border*: surface of microvilli containing digestive enzymes

HYDRATION

osms.it/hydration

- Total body water
    - Intracellular fluid (inside cells) + extracellular fluid (outside cells—e.g. blood, interstitium)
- Water functions
    - Bodily secretions, digestion, detoxification (urination), thermoregulation (sweating)
- Total body water balanced by intake, elimination

Water intake
- Water ingested in fluid/food form
    - 80% → fluid; 20% → food
- Bloodstream absorption in small, large intestines

Water loss
- Breathing; sweating; urinating, defecating

DEHYDRATION
- Occurs when water loss > water intake
- Causes
    - Vigorous exercise, decreased oral intake, dry air, vomiting, diarrhea, excessive sweating, inability to swallow, diuretics
- Symptoms
    - Thirst, dry mouth/lips, nausea, fatigue, lightheadedness, darkened/decreased urine
- High risk groups
    - *Children:* lower stores of water, ↑ surface area to body mass, thirst sensors not fully developed, depend on caregivers
    - *Elderly:* decreased thirst sensation, medication, chronic diseases affecting kidneys

CARBOHYDRATES & SUGARS

osms.it/carbohydrates-and-sugars

DIGESTION

Mouth
- Begins carbohydrate digestion
- *Enzyme:* salivary alpha amylase
    - Starts starch digestion → dextrins, maltose, maltotriose

Stomach
- Salivary amylase inactivated
- Relatively no breakdown of starch

Small intestine
- Majority of carbohydrate digestion
- Enzymes include
    - *Pancreatic amylase:* digests starch → disaccharides; hydrolyzes interior 1,4-glycosidic bonds in starch yielding disaccharides
    - *Intestinal brush border enzymes:* digest oligosaccharides, disaccharides → lactose, maltose, sucrose → galactose, glucose, fructose; e.g. dextrinase, maltase, glucoamylase, lactase, sucrase

ABSORPTION
- *Primary site of absorption:* small intestine

Pathway of absorption
- *Glucose, galactose:* absorbed into enterocytes via sodium ion cotransport (secondary active transport) → GLUT2 transporter extrudes glucose, galactose across basolateral membrane into blood

- **Sodium-glucose cotransporter (SGLT1):** moves glucose inside enterocytes against electrochemical gradient using ATP created from sodium gradient created by sodium-potassium ATPase on the basolateral membrane
- **Fructose:** absorbed into enterocytes via facilitated diffusion by GLUT5 transporter in apical membrane → GLUT2 transporter extrudes fructose across basolateral membrane into blood; fructose absorption cannot occur against electrochemical gradient
- Monosaccharides leave epithelial cells via facilitated diffusion → enter villi capillaries → hepatic portal vein → liver

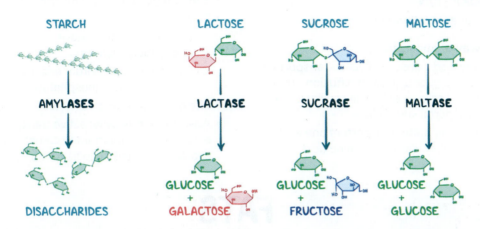

Figure 39.1 Overview of the actions of some of the enzymes involved in carbohydrate digestion.

PROTEINS

osms.it/proteins

- Proteins can be absorbed in the form of amino acids, dipeptides, or tripeptides (as opposed to carbohydrates)

DIGESTION

- Proteins → large polypeptides → smaller polypeptides/peptides → individual amino acids/dipeptides/tripeptides

Stomach

- **Gastric pepsin (with HCl):** digests proteins → large polypeptides
  - Protein digestion starts with gastric pepsin
  - Secreted by chief cells, activated by low pH
- **Proteases** (endopeptidases, exopeptidases)
  - **Endopeptidases:** trypsin, chymotrypsin, pepsin; hydrolyze interior peptide bonds (pepsin, trypsin, chymotrypsin)
  - **Exopeptidases:** hydrolyze individual individual amino acids from carboxyl end (carboxypeptidases A, B)

Small intestine

- Pancreatic, intestinal brush border enzymes continue digestion
- Pancreatic enzymes
  - **Zymogens:** trypsinogen, chymotrypsinogen, procarboxypeptidase A, B
  - **Active forms:** trypsin, chymotrypsin, carboxypeptidase
  - Enterokinase activates trypsinogen → trypsin → trypsin autocatalyzes itself, activates additional pancreatic zymogens

- Digest large polypeptides → small polypeptides/peptides
- Intestinal brush border enzymes
  - Dipeptidase, aminopeptidase, carboxypeptidase
  - Digest small polypeptides/peptides → amino acids/dipeptides/tripeptides

ABSORPTION
- *Site of absorption:* small intestine

Pathway of absorption
- *Amino acids:* absorbed via cotransport with sodium ions or facilitated diffusion out of epithelial cells → enter villi capillaries → hepatic portal vein → liver
  - Four separate transporters one each for neutral, acidic, basic amino acid
- *Dipeptides, tripeptides:* absorbed into enterocytes via cotransport with protons → broken down into amino acids/transcytosis

NUCLEIC ACID DIGESTION & ABSORPTION
- Nucleic acids → pentose sugars, nitrogen-containing bases, phosphate ions
- *Site of digestion:* small intestine only
- Enzymes
  - Pancreatic ribonuclease, deoxyribonucleases
  - Intestinal brush border enzymes (nucleosidases, phosphatases)
- *Site of absorption:* small intestine
- *Absorption pathway:* active transport into enterocytes by membrane carriers → villi capillaries → hepatic portal vein → liver

FATS

osms.it/fats

- Unemulsified triglycerides → monoglycerides/diglycerides, fatty acids
- *Site of digestion:* mouth, stomach, small intestine
- Lipid digestion begins with lingual, gastric lipases hydrolyzing triglycerides → glycerol, fatty acids
  - CCK slows gastric emptying, allowing adequate time for pancreatic enzymes to work
- Pancreatic enzymes (pancreatic lipase, cholesterol ester hydrolase, phospholipase A2), colipase finish digestion in small intestine
  - Bile salts, lysolecithin surround, emulsify dietary lipids to create large surface area for pancreatic enzymes
  - Pancreatic lipase secreted as active enzyme, hydrolyzes triglyceride → monoglyceride + 2 fatty acids
  - Colipase (secreted as inactive procolipase, activated by trypsin) binds to pancreatic lipase protecting it from being inactivated by bile salts

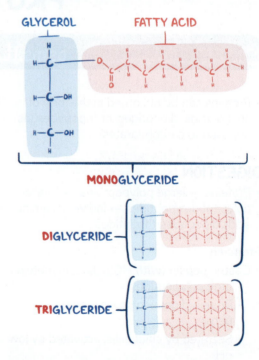

Figure 39.2 Fats are comprised of glycerol backbone and one or more fatty acid chains. A few examples of fats shown above.

- Cholesterol ester hydrolase (secreted as active enzyme) hydrolyzes cholesterol ester → free cholesterol, fatty acids; hydrolyzes triglycerides → glycerol
- Phospholipase A2 (secreted as proenzyme, activated by trypsin) hydrolyzes phospholipids → lysolecithin, fatty acids
- *Final products of lipid digestion:* monoglycerides, cholesterol, glycerol, fatty acids, lysolecithin
  - Since products are hydrophobic (except glycerol), must be solubilized in micelles before transport to enterocyte apical membrane for absorption
  - *Micelles:* products of lipid digestion surrounded by bile salts
- *Site of absorption:* small intestine

Pathway of absorption
- Fatty acids, monoglycerides absorbed via
  - Diffusion
  - Fatty acids, monoglycerides leave micelles → enter epithelial cells → triglyceride formation → chylomicrons formation (fat globules plus surface apoproteins) → chylomicrons enter lacteals → lymph in lacteal transports chylomicrons into systemic circulation
- Apoproteins are essential for absorption of chylomicrons (specifically Apo B)
- Short chain fatty acids diffuse into villi capillaries → hepatic portal vein → liver

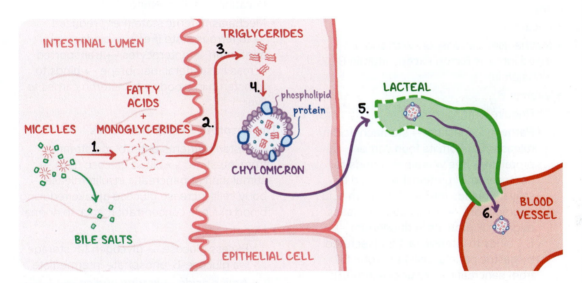

Figure 39.3 Overview of the fat absorption pathway.
1. Fatty acids and monoglycerides leave micelles and
2. enter epithelial cells.
3. They form triglycerides.
4. Chylomicrons containing the fats are then formed.
5. The chylomicrons enter lacteals, and
6. are transported into systemic circulation.

VITAMINS

osms.it/vitamins

- With the exception of vitamin K, which is produced by intestinal bacteria, vitamins are not synthesized in body therefore must be attained by diet

Fat soluble (Vitamins A, D, E, K)
- **Location:** small intestine
- **Mechanism:** incorporated into micelles along with products of lipid digestion, absorbed into enterocytes

Water-soluble (B vitamins, vitamin C, biotin, folic acid, nicotinic acid, pantothenic acid)
- **Location:** ileum
- **Mechanism:** cotransport with sodium (need intrinsic factor) except vitamin B_{12} (cobalamin)
- Vitamin B_{12}
    - Requires intrinsic factor
    - **Pathway:** ingestion → stomach acidity releases B_{12} from its food carrier proteins → free vitamin B_{12} binds to haptocorrin (R proteins) secreted by salivary glands (protects B_{12} from acid degradation) → pancreatic proteases degrade R proteins in duodenum → B_{12} binds to intrinsic factors (secreted by gastric parietal cells) to protect it from pancreatic enzymes → intrinsic factor-B_{12} complex resistant to degradation from pancreatic enzymes → absorbed in ileum

Absorption of calcium
- Active form of vitamin D, 1,25-dihydroxycholecalciferol, required for calcium absorption
- Dietary vitamin D_3 (cholecalciferol) is inactive
- Cholecalciferol → 25-hydroxycholecalciferol (inactive) in liver → 1,25-dihydroxycholecalciferol in kidney by 1alpha-hydroxylase → synthesizes calbindin D-28K (vitamin D-dependent calcium binding protein → promotes calcium absorption from small intestine
- *Decreased by:* oxalic acid, tannins, magnesium, phosphorus, phytates
- *Increased by:* acidic conditions in intestine, vitamin D, estrogen, lactose
- **Location:** small intestine (primarily duodenum)
- **Mechanism:** vitamin D-dependent calcium binding protein

Absorption of iron
- **Location:** small intestine
- **Mechanism:** ferric state (Fe^{3+}) reduced → to ferrous state (Fe^{2+}) → binds apoferritin in enterocytes → transported across basolateral membrane → binds to transferrin in blood → transferrin carries to liver

The absorptive state: hormones
- Digested nutrients enter blood stream from intestines → blood glucose rises → stimulation of pancreatic insulin release → body cells increase glucose uptake reducing blood glucose concentration back to normal
- Hepatocytes
    - Excess glucose → glycogen for storage via glucose-6-phosphate intermediate
    - Amino acids → ketone bodies (converted to acetyl CoA if needed later)
- Myocytes
    - Excess glucose → glycogen for storage via glucose-6-phosphate intermediate
    - Amino acids → actin, myosin → muscle fibers
- Adipocytes store excess lipids increasing fat reserves

Chapter 39 Gastrointestinal Physiology: Digestion & Absorption

INTESTINAL FLUID BALANCE

osms.it/intestinal-fluid-balance

- Along with nutrient digestion, GI tract re-absorbs large amounts of fluid, electrolytes (Na^+, Cl^-, HCO_3^-, K^+)
- Small, large intestine together absorb approximately 9L/2.38 gallons daily
    - Diet → 2L/0.44 gallons; pancreatic, biliary, intestinal secretions → 7L/1.85 gallons
    - Approximately 100–200mL /0.03–0.06 gallons) excreted in feces
    - Absorptive mechanisms disrupted → diarrhea (enormous potential body-water, electrolyte loss)

Villi
- Line intestinal epithelial cells
    - *First step:* solute absorbed; *second step:* water follows
    - Fluid absorbed = isosmotic (water, solute absorption: parallel proportions)
    - Similar to renal proximal tubule
    - Absorptive mechanisms vary by intestinal part

Jejunum
- Major site of Na^+ absorption
    - Enters epithelial cell → Na^+-dependent coupled transporters on apical membrane (Na^+-monosaccharide cotransporters (Na^+-glucose/Na^+-galactose), Na^+-amino acid cotransporters, Na^+-H^+ exchanger)
    - Translocates across basolateral membrane via Na^+-K^+ ATPase
    - H^+ source (for Na^+-H^+ exchanger) = intracellular CO_2 + H_2O → carbonic anhydrase converts to H^+, HCO_3^- → H^+ secreted into lumen → blood absorbs HCO_3^- ("alkaline tide")

Ileum
- Same transporters as jejunum + Cl^--HCO_3^- exchanger on apical membrane
- Cl^- transporter in basolateral membrane
- H^+ secreted into lumen + HCO_3^- secreted into lumen (via Cl^--HCO_3^- exchanger; not absorbed into blood) → Cl^--HCO_3^- exchanger, Na^+-H^+ exchanger → net NaCl movement into cell → net NaCl absorption

Colon
- Apical membrane contains Na^+, K^+ channels
- Net Na^+ absorption + K^+ secretion
- Aldosterone induces Na^+ channel synthesis → ↑ Na^+ absorption, secondary to K^+ secretion

Fluid, electrolyte secretion
- Epithelial cells lining crypts of small intestine → secrete fluid, electrolytes (mucus, lubricating fluids assisting in mixing, digestion) → must also be absorbed more distally
- Electrolyte, fluid secretion route
    - *Small intestine:* paracellular route → "leaky" tight junctions (↓ resistance)
    - *Colon:* cellular route → "tight" tight junctions (↑ resistance)
- Electrolyte, fluid secretion mechanism
    - *Apical membrane:* Cl^- channel
    - *Basolateral membrane:* Na^+-K^+-$2Cl^-$ cotransporter (similar to thick ascending loop of Henle)
    - Na^+, K^+, Cl^- ions move into cells from blood → Cl^- diffuses into lumen via Cl^- channel on apical membrane → Na^+ follows Cl^- passively, paracellularly → H_2O secretion follows NaCl secretion
    - Apical Cl^- channels closed in resting state → opens after various hormones/neurotransmitters (ACh, VIP) bind
    - Bind to basolateral receptor → activate adenylyl cyclase → ↑ cAMP in crypt cells → cAMP opens Cl^- channels
    - Adenylyl cyclase can be maximally activated in cholera → severe, life-threatening diarrhea

NOTES

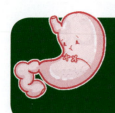

NOTES
LIVER, GALL BLADDER, & PANCREAS

BILE SECRETION & ENTEROHEPATIC CIRCULATION

osms.it/bile-secretion-enterohepatic-circulation

SYNTHESIS OF BILE, BILIRUBIN

- Hemoglobin from old red blood cells taken up by macrophages → biliverdin → unconjugated bilirubin → released into plasma, combines with albumin → unconjugated bilirubin absorbed into hepatic cells, released from albumin → liver conjugates unconjugated bilirubin → conjugated bilirubin excreted from hepatocytes into intestines → some conjugated bilirubin converted by bacteria into urobilinogen (soluble) → some urobilinogen reabsorbed through intestinal mucosa back into blood → re-excreted by liver back into gut/excreted by kidneys into urine → urobilinogen becomes urobilin → stercobilin in feces

RECYCLING OF BILE

- Bile transported from ileum into portal blood after digestion → portal blood delivers bile salts to liver → liver extracts bile salts from portal blood, adds to hepatic bile salt/acid pool → bile returned to gallbladder
- Some bile excreted into feces as stercobilin
- Only excreted bile needs to be replaced

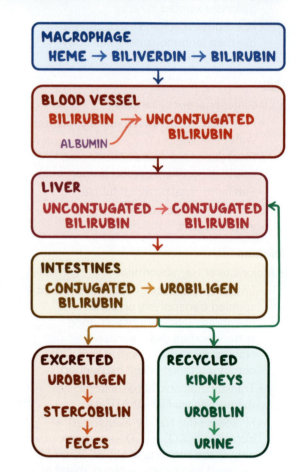

Figure 40.1 Bile synthesis to excretion/recycling pathway.

Chapter 40 Gastrointestinal Physiology: Liver, Gall Bladder, & Pancreas

LIVER ANATOMY & PHYSIOLOGY

osms.it/liver-anatomy-physiology

LIVER ANATOMY

Functions
- Bile production, storage (e.g. glycogen), detoxification, nutrient interconversion, synthesis (e.g. albumin, clotting factors), phagocytosis (Kupffer cells)

Location
- Located in right upper quadrant (RUQ) under diaphragm, almost entirely within rib cage
  - Largest internal organ
- Covered by visceral peritoneum
  - Except superior-most region (bare area), contacts inferior surface of diaphragm
- Falciform ligament: mesentery separates right, left lobes; suspends liver from diaphragm, anterior abdominal wall
- Round ligament/ligamentum teres: inferior to falciform ligament, remnant of fetal umbilical vein

Four lobes
- Right lobe (largest)
- Left lobe
- Caudate lobe
- Quadrate lobe

Blood supply
- 75% from nutrient rich, oxygen poor portal vein
- 25% from nutrient poor, oxygen rich hepatic artery
- Enterohepatic circulation gives liver first access to nutrients, toxins, medications from gut

Liver lobule
- Functional unit of liver
  - Hexagonal liver lobule made of hepatocytes
- Each liver lobule surrounded by six portal triads on each point withlobes central vein in center

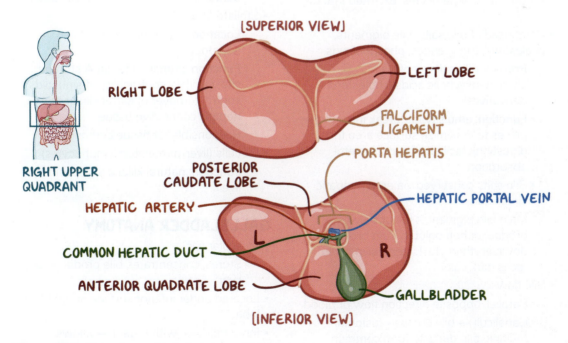

Figure 40.2 Superior and inferior view of liver.

OSMOSIS.ORG 333

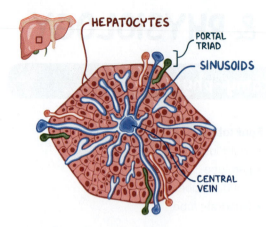

Figure 40.3 Liver lobule.

- Portal triad
  - Portal venule + portal arteriole + bile duct

Sinusoids
- Mixing of portal vein, hepatic arterial blood
- Lined with leaky endothelial cells
- Pathway of blood flow
  - Blood from hepatic portal vein, artery → sinusoids → central vein → hepatic vein → inferior vena cava

Bile
- Produced by hepatocytes, excreted into bile ducts
- Composed of bile salts, bile pigments, cholesterol, triglycerides, phospholipids
  - *Primary bile salts*: cholic, chenodeoxycholic acids (cholesterol derivatives)
  - *Function*: emulsify fat (break into smaller pieces to maximize surface area for digestion); facilitate fat, cholesterol absorption
  - Bile salts conserved via enterohepatic circulation
  - Main bile pigment is bilirubin (waste product of hemoglobin from broken down erythrocytes), stercobilin gives feces dark color
- Bile flow
  - Parallel, opposite direction flow of blood
  - Canaliculi → bile ducts → fusion of multiple bile ducts to form common hepatic duct → fusion with cystic duct draining gallbladder → bile duct → ampulla of vater

Major fuels
- Glucose, fructose, galactose (after meal); fatty acids (after fasting)
  - Amino acids can also be used
  - *Long-chain fatty acids*: major source of fuel during prolonged fasting

Cell types
- Hepatocytes
  - *Function*: carry out most metabolic pathways
  - Majority cell type in liver
  - Contain large amounts of rough, smooth endoplasmic reticulum (ER), Golgi bodies, peroxisomes, mitochondria
- Endothelial cells
  - *Location*: sinusoidal lining
  - *Function*: release growth factors; secrete cytokines, endocytose ligands
  - Contain fenestrations → free diffusion of blood, nutrients between sinusoids, hepatocytes
- Kupffer cells
  - *Location*: sinusoidal lining
  - *Function*: macrophages specific to liver protect against gut-derived pathogens, release cytokines, secrete mediators of inflammatory response, remove damaged erythrocytes from circulation
- Stellate (Ito) cells
  - *Location*: scattered amongst hepatocytes
  - *Function*: primary vitamin A storage site; regulate contractility of sinusoids; control turnover of extracellular matrix, hepatic connective tissue
  - Responsible for tissue cirrhosis
- Pit cells (liver-associated lymphocytes)
  - *Function*: natural killer cells specific to liver

GALLBLADDER ANATOMY
- Muscular sac
  - Stores, concentrates bile produced by liver
- Located under inferior surface of right liver lobe
- Inner mucosa (with rugae) → allows expansion
- Smooth muscle layer → allows contraction

Chapter 40 Gastrointestinal Physiology: Liver, Gall Bladder, & Pancreas

to occur in response to cholecystokinin (produced by duodenum) → bile released into small intestine
- Also contracts in response to vagal stimulation
- Flow of bile
  - Cystic duct → common bile duct → ampulla of vater → duodenum

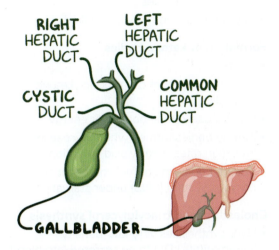

Figure 40.4 Gallbladder.

PANCREAS ANATOMY
- Located retroperitoneal posterior to stomach, duodenum

Four regions
- Head: right side nestled into curve of duodenum
- Neck: thin portion between head, body
- Body: tapered left side
- Tail: ends near spleen

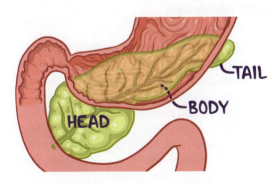

Figure 40.5 Pancreatic location relative to stomach and duodenum.

Acinar gland
- Exocrine gland
- Acinar cells
  - Contain zymogen granules full of proenzymes for digestion
- Stimulated by secretin, cholecystokinin (from duodenum), vagus nerve
- Secretes digestive enzymes into duodenum
  - Amylase, lipase, nuclease secreted as active enzymes
  - Proteases (trypsinogen, chymotrypsinogen, procarboxypeptidase) secreted in zymogen form, must be cleaved to be activated

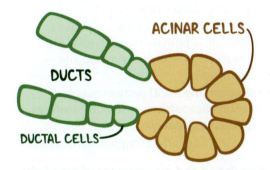

Figure 40.6 Acinar gland.

Islets of Langerhans
- Endocrine gland
- Responsible for glucose homeostasis
  - Beta cells → insulin
  - Alpha cells → glucagon
  - Delta cells → somatostatin → inhibits insulin, glucagon secretion

Ducts
- Main pancreatic duct: located centrally, fuses with bile duct to drain into duodenum
- Accessory pancreatic duct: smaller duct; empties directly into duodenum
- Ductal cells: responsible for aqueous secretions (water, HCO_3^-, sodium)
  - Secretion of bicarbonate ions neutralizes acidic chyme entering duodenum, provides optimal pH for activation of digestive enzymes

LIVER PHYSIOLOGY

Efficient exchange of compounds between sinusoidal blood, hepatocytes
- Fenestrated endothelial cells
- Lack of basement membrane between endothelial cells, hepatocytes
- Slow blood flow

Biotransformation of xenobiotics
- Principal site for processing xenobiotics, toxins
- *Phase I reactions*: oxidation, reduction, hydroxylation, hydrolysis
    - Introduces reactive functional groups to increase compound polarity
- *Phase II reactions*: conjugation, sulfation, glucuronidation, methylation
- *Detoxification*: xenobiotic → phase I reaction → primary metabolite → phase II reaction → secondary metabolite → excretion
- *Cytochrome P450 system*: major xenobiotic metabolizer in body; oxidizes substrates, adds oxygen to structures
    - First pass effect for pharmaceuticals

Regulation and maintenance of blood glucose levels
- ↑ *blood glucose:* → secretion of insulin by pancreas → ↑ uptake of glucose, amino acids by cells; inhibition of glycolysis, activation of glycogen synthesis, inhibition of gluconeogenesis, inhibition of glycogenolysis, inhibition of fatty acid oxidation → ↓ blood glucose
- ↓ *blood glucose:* ↑ breakdown of glycogen → secretion of glucagon, activation of glycolysis, inhibition of glycogen synthesis, activation of gluconeogenesis, activation of glycogenolysis, activation of fatty acid oxidation → ↑ blood glucose

Elimination of ammonia via urea cycle
- Liver
    - Main organ responsible for eliminating ammonia via urea cycle
- Ammonia transported to liver on glutamine, alanine → converted by liver into urea for excretion in urine

Amino acid metabolism/protein synthesis and regulation
- Liver produces plasma proteins (mainly albumin), coagulation factors, metal-binding proteins (transferrin, ceruloplasmin), lipid transporters (apoproteins), protease inhibitors (antitrypsin), glycoproteins, proteoglycans
- Can convert amino acids into glucose, fatty acids, ketone bodies
- Sugars produced by liver O-linked

Formation of ketone bodies
- Liver
    - Only organ that can produce ketone bodies
- Cannot use ketone bodies for energy
- Ketone bodies formed when glucose levels low, high rates of fatty acid oxidation
- Ketone bodies major fuel source for central nervous system (CNS) under starvation

Cholesterol and triacylglycerol synthesis
- Liver synthesizes very low-density lipoprotein (VLDL) to be secreted into blood
- Food plentiful → liver activates synthesis of fatty acid, triacylglycerol, cholesterol → reduces hepatic cholesterol synthesis
- Also sends excess dietary cholesterol to peripheral tissue

Nucleotide biosynthesis
- Liver can synthesize, salvage nucleotides for use by other cells
- Salvage pathway
    - Liver converts free bases to nucleotides for secretion into circulation as needed by peripheral tissues

Lipid metabolism
- Long-chain fatty acids
    - Liver's major fuel source during fasting
    - Triacylglycerols from adipose tissue → fatty acids bound to albumin → liver → activated via fatty Acyl-coenzyme A (acyl-CoA) synthetases → fatty-acyl-CoA → fatty-acyl-carnitine → carnitine crosses inner mitochondrial membrane → fatty-acyl-carnitine → carnitine, fatty-acyl-CoA → beta oxidation
    - Enzymes in beta oxidation, fatty-acid activation specific for length of fatty acid carbon chains

- Medium-chain-length fatty-acid oxidation
  - 4–12 carbons
  - Liver, kidney is site of oxidation
  - Activating enzyme is medium-chain-length fatty acid-activating enzyme (MMFAE)
  - Oxidation begins with medium-chain-length acyl-CoA dehydrogenase
- Very-long-chain fatty-acid oxidation
  - \> 20 carbons
  - Oxidized by peroxisomes to octanoyl-Coa
  - Generates hydrogen peroxide instead of flavin adenine dinucleotide (FADH2), in contrast to mitochondrial beta-oxidation
- Long-chain fatty acids
  - 12–20 carbons
  - Most common type of lipid used for oxidation by liver

PANCREATIC SECRETION

osms.it/pancreatic-secretion

FLOW RATE, COMPOSITION OF PANCREATIC JUICE

High flow rate
- High HCO_3^- concentration, low Cl^- concentration

Low flow rate
- High Cl^- concentration, low HCO_3^- concentration

REGULATION OF BILE, PANCREATIC SECRETION

- Hormones, neural stimuli regulate secretion of bile, pancreatic juice into duodenum

Hormones
- Secretin
  - Released by intestinal cells in response to acidic chyme; stimulates secretion of bile, pancreatic juice
- Cholecystokinin (CCK)
  - Major stimulus for gallbladder to release bile into duodenum; stimulates secretion of enzyme-rich pancreatic juice

Neural stimuli
- Parasympathetic stimulation by vagus nerve stimulates secretion
  - Bile from gallbladder, pancreatic juice

Bile salt
- Major stimulus for more bile secretion via stimulation of secretin release

ACTIVATION OF PANCREATIC PROTEASES

- Enteropeptidase cleaves, activates trypsinogen to trypsin → trypsin activates chymotrypsinogen into chymotrypsin, procarboxypeptidase into carboxypeptidase

NOTES

NOTES
POPULATION GENETICS

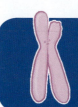

MENDELIAN GENETICS & PUNNETT SQUARES

osms.it/mendelian-genetics-punnett-squares

- **Genetics:** science of inheritance
- **Parental generation ("P")** → 1st filial generation ("F1") → 2nd filial generation ("F2")
- **Homozygous:** male, female alleles are same
- **Heterozygous:** male, female alleles differ
- **Phenotype:** observable trait from genotype

Mendel's laws

- **Law of segregation:** alleles segregate, offspring acquire one allele from each parent
- **Law of dominance:** alleles can be dominant/recessive
  - Dominant traits appear when ≥ one dominant allele is present
- **Law of independent assortment:** separate genes assort independently
  - **Genetic linkage:** proximity of genes on chromosome can cause joint assortment

Punnett square

- Table showing possible combinations of genotypes

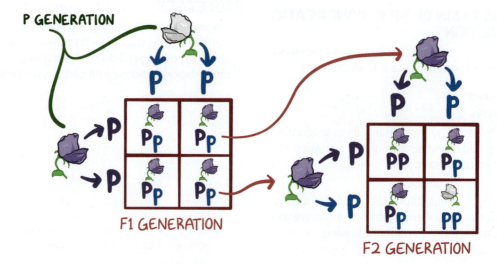

Figure 41.1 2x2 Punnett squares showing the allele combinations for one gene: flower color in pea plants. The parent plants are homozygous for the flower color trait. When they are crossbred (first Punnett square), each offspring in the F1 generation gets one dominant allele (P) and one recessive allele (p). The dominant P allele masks the recessive p allele, so all the flowers appear violet. When any two of the heterozygous F1 generation plants are bred (second Punnett square), the three plants in the F2 generation with at least one P allele have a violet flower phenotype and the one plant with the homozygous pp genotype has a white flower phenotype.

Chapter 41 Genetics: Population Genetics

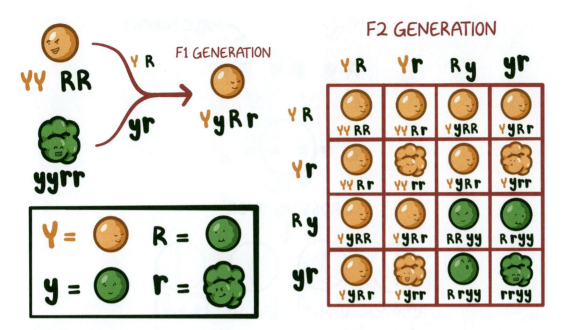

Figure 41.2 4x4 Punnett square showing the allele combinations for two genes: seed color (Y = yellow, y = green) and texture (R = round, r = wrinkly). One parent (P) plant is homozygous dominant (YYRR; yellow, round seeds), the second is homozygous recessive (yyrr; green, wrinkled seeds). When these plants are crossbred, all the F1 generation plants have the genotype YyRr and the phenotype of yellow, round seeds. When the F1 generation plants are bred (Punnett square), there are four possible combinations of the alleles for each parent: YR, Yr, yR, and yr. We can expect the F2 generation to have four phenotypes: yellow and round (≥ one Y and ≥ one R), yellow and wrinkled (≥ one Y and two r), green and round (two y and ≥ one R), green and wrinkled (yyrr). They appear in the ratio 9:3:3:1.

INDEPENDENT ASSORTMENT OF GENES & LINKAGE

osms.it/independent-assortment-and-linkage

- **Independent assortment:** separate genes assort independently
    - Apart from in genetic linkage
    - **Genetic linkage:** proximity of genes on chromosome can cause joint assortment
- **Crossing-over:** in prophase 1 of meiosis, genes can be exchanged between adjacent chromosomes
    - Homozygous genes can occur on different gametes
    - Even repetitions of crossing-over can reverse this effect

- Linked genes have < 50% chance of occurring on different gametes
    - **Parental gametes:** linked genes inherited together
    - **Recombinant gametes:** linked genes between which crossing-over has occurred

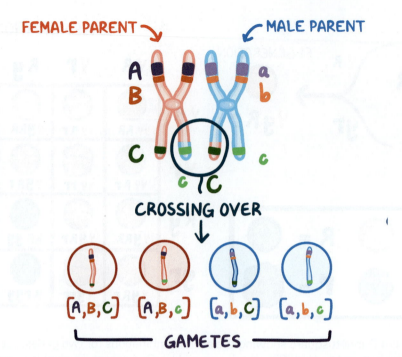

Figure 41.3 Red chromosome from female parent originally carried all dominant alleles for genes A, B, C; blue chromosome from male parent originally carried all recessive alleles for genes A, B, C. If crossing over occurs between the ends of the two chromosomes, dominant allele C from female parent ends up in the chromosome from male parent, vice versa.

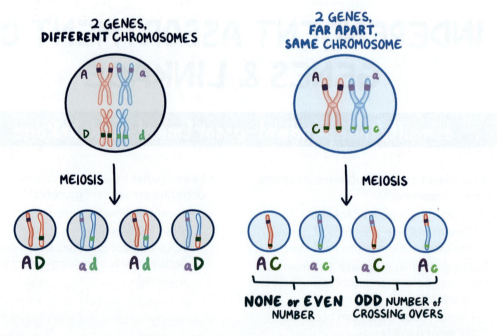

Figure 41.4 Any two genes on different chromosomes always have a 50% chance of going through crossing over in meiosis and showing up in the same gamete. The same is true for two genes very far apart on the same chromosome, because ending up in the same or a different gamete depends on whether there are an odd or even number of crossing over events.

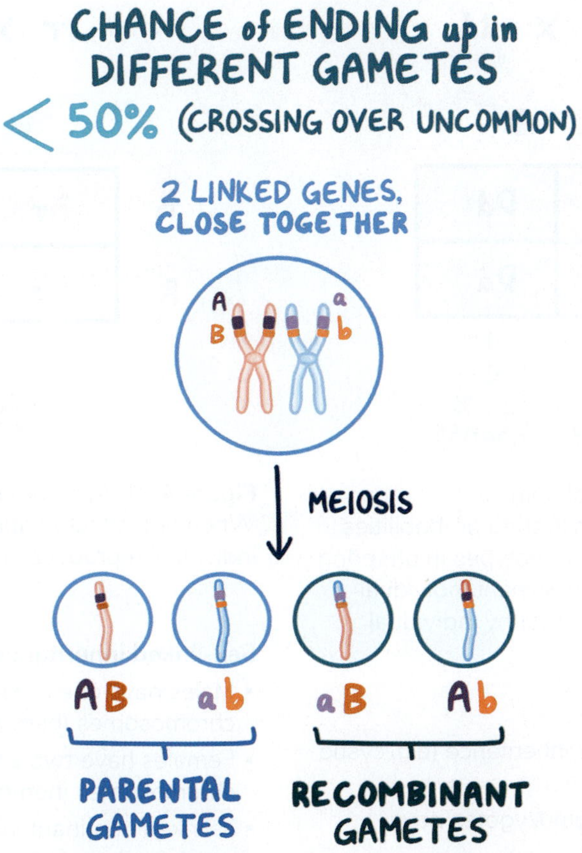

Figure 41.5 It is unlikely for a cut to occur in the small space between linked genes, which is why the chance of them crossing over and ending up in different gametes is < 50%. When linked genes are inherited together, the gametes are called "parental" because they carry same the alleles as the original chromosomes. When crossing over occurs, they are called "recombinant."

INHERITANCE PATTERNS

osms.it/inheritance-patterns

Dominant vs. recessive inheritance patterns

- *Dominant inheritance*: mutation affects dominant allele → one copy causes disease
- *Recessive inheritance*: mutation affects recessive allele → two copies cause disease

Autosomal vs. sexual vs. mitochondrial patterns

- *Autosomal inheritance*: mutation affects somatic chromosome
- *Sexual inheritance*: mutation affects sex chromosome; X-linked/Y-linked
- *Mitochondrial inheritance*: mutation on egg's mitochondrial DNA

Autosomal inheritance

- Autosomal dominant inheritance (e.g. Huntington's disease)
    - Dominant homozygotes (RR), heterozygotes (Rr) have disease
    - Recessive homozygotes (rr) unaffected
    - Disease too severe in homozygotes → don't reproduce

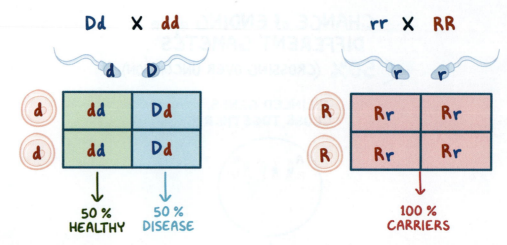

Figure 41.6 Autosomal dominant inheritance. Punnett square demonstrating probabilities of healthy and disease genotypes in offspring when a heterozygous dominant individual (Dd) reproduces with a healthy individual (dd).

- Autosomal recessive inheritance (e.g. cystic fibrosis)
  - Only recessive homozygotes have disease
  - Heterozygotes carriers
  - Tendency to skip generation
  - *Children of consanguineous unions:* ↑ likelihood of disease

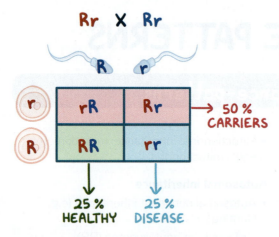

Figure 41.7 Autosomal recessive inheritance. Punnett square demonstrating probabilities of healthy, disease, and carrier genotypes in the offspring when two healthy carriers reproduce.

Figure 41.8 Autosomal recessive inheritance. When one affected and one unaffected individual reproduce, all offspring are carriers.

Sex-linked inheritance

- Males have one allele for genes on X, Y chromosomes (hemizygous)
- Females have two alleles for genes on X chromosomes (homozygous/heterozygous)
- X-linked dominant inheritance (e.g. fragile X syndrome)
  - Dominant hemizygotes, dominant homozygotes, heterozygotes have disease
  - Males reproducing with healthy females have 100% chance to pass onto female children, 0% chance to pass onto male children
  - Females reproducing with healthy males have 50% chance to pass onto children of both sexes
- X-linked recessive inheritance (e.g. hemophilia)
  - Recessive homozygotes, recessive hemizygotes have disease; heterozygotes are carriers
  - Males reproducing with healthy females have 100% chance of female children being carriers, 0% chance of passing disease onto male children
  - Heterozygous females reproducing with healthy males have 50% chance of female children being carriers, 50% chance of passing disease onto male children
- Y-linked inheritance (e.g. baldness)
- Only male heterozygotes have disease

- Always passed from biologically-male parent to biologically-male child

Mitochondrial inheritance
- Mitochondrial inheritance (e.g. DAD, AKA diabetes mellitus and deafness)
  - Males, females can develop disease
  - Only females can pass disease to offspring

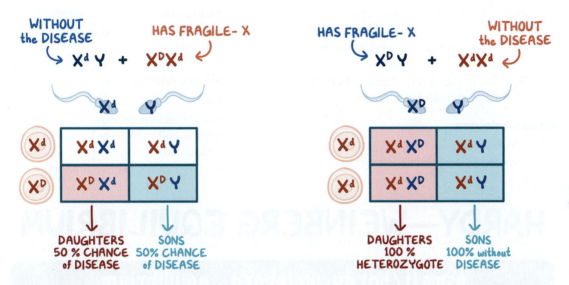

Figure 41.9 Punnett squares demonstrating the inheritance patterns for fragile X syndrome, an X-linked dominant disease, with different combinations of parental genotypes.

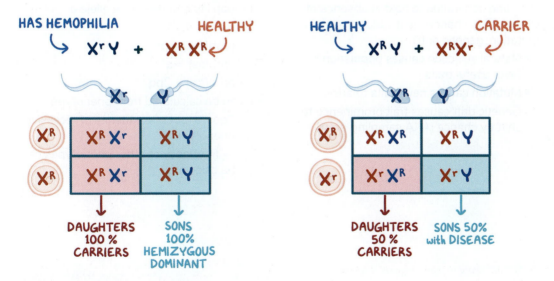

Figure 41.10 Punnett squares demonstrating the inheritance patterns for hemophilia, an X-linked recessive disease, with different combinations of parental genotypes.

EVOLUTION & NATURAL SELECTION

osms.it/evolution-natural-selection

Evolution
- Process by which populations change over time
  - **Population:** group of organisms within species that live in same place
  - **Species:** group of organisms with similar characteristics, ability to breed

Natural selection
- Premises
  - Individuals in species have different traits
  - Some individuals survive, reproduce
  - Some traits → ↑ survival, reproduction (AKA fitness)
  - → more offspring with these traits (AKA differential reproduction)
- Conclusion
  - Population slowly changes over time to favor useful traits (e.g. ↑ survival, reproduction)
- Artificial selection = selective breeding

HARDY—WEINBERG EQUILIBRIUM

osms.it/hardy-weinberg_equilibrium

- Population's genetic traits remain same from one generation to next in absence of evolutionary changes (e.g. natural selection, mutation, genetic drift)
  - Natural selection causes population to favor useful traits
  - Mutation causes new traits to arise
  - Genetic drift causes trait prominence to shift by chance (AKA sampling error)
- Given probability p of dominant allele A, probability q of recessive allele a
  - $p + q = 1$
  - $prob(AA) = p^2$
  - $prob(aa) = q^2$
  - $prob(Aa) = 2pq$
- q can be calculated from phenotype
  - Square root of frequency of recessive phenotype
  - → frequency of other phenotypes can be calculated

EPIGENETICS

osms.it/epigenetics

- Mechanisms to selectively activate/silence genes without modifying nucleotide sequence

Histone modification
- Acetylation
  - Removes positive charge → less attraction to negative DNA phosphates → ↑ gene transcription
- Methylation
  - One methyl group → loosens histone tails → ↑ access for transcription factors → ↑ gene transcription
  - 2-3 methyl groups → tightens histone tails → ↓ access for transcription factors → ↓ gene transcription
- Direct DNA modification
  - Usually occurs in long sequences of cytosine, guanine nucleotides (AKA CpG)
  - Cytosine residues undergo methylation, silencing gene expression
- Modifications occur throughout lifetime
- Affected by environmental factors (e.g. drug usage, diet, exercise)
- Changes are reversible

LAC OPERON

osms.it/lac-operon

- Collection of genes in E. coli, other bacteria that code for proteins required to transport, metabolize lactose
- Includes structural genes like *lacZ*, *lacY*, *lacA* as well as regulatory genes like promoter, operator
  - *lacZ*: β-galactosidase (AKA lactase)
  - *lacY*: β-galactosidase permease
  - *lacA*: β-galactosidase transacetylase
  - *Promoter*: start transcription
  - *Operator*: prevent transcription with repressor (coded by *lacI*)
- Glucose, lactose concentrations can be used to regulate lac operon expression
  - ↑ glucose → repressor stays bound to operator, blocking RNA polymerase
  - ↑ glucose → catabolite activator protein inhibits transcription
  - ↓ glucose → repressor falls off
  - ↓ glucose → catabolite activator protein stimulates transcription

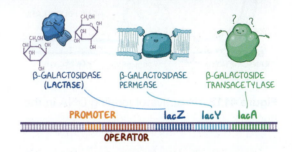

Figure 41.11 The lac operon. β-galactosidase breaks down lactose into glucose and galactose; β-galactosidase permease allows lactose to enter the cell; β-galactosidase transacetylase's function is not clearly understood.

GENE REGULATION

osms.it/gene-regulation

- Natural regulation of gene expression
- Occurs at transcription/post-transcription/translation level
- Transcriptional regulation
    - *Epigenetics:* chemical modifications activate/silence genes without modifying nucleotide sequence (e.g. by methylation/acetylation of histones)
    - *Activators:* bind to DNA enhancer → facilitate binding of general transcription factors, recruit histone acetyltransferases
    - *Repressors:* bind to DNA silencer → prevent RNA polymerase from binding to promoter, recruit histone deacetylases
- Post-transcriptional regulation
    - *Splicing:* spliceosomes remove introns (AKA non-coding sequences) from RNA → resulting mRNA codes for proteins more effectively
    - *Capping:* 5' end of RNA capped with protective 7-methyl-guanine → exonucleases unable to cleave off nucleotides
    - *Editing:* proteins convert certain nucleotides (e.g. ADAR: adenosine → inosine; CDAR: cytosine → uracil) to create sequence variation
- Translation regulation
    - Mainly occurs during initiation
    - Regulatory proteins (AKA initiation) factors must bind before ribosome can begin translation
    - Conditions like starvation, stress inhibit initiation factors to save energy

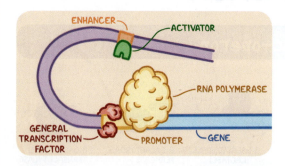

Figure 41.12 An activator looping DNA in the nucleus.

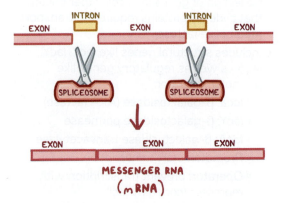

Figure 41.14 Illustration depicting the action of spliceosomes.

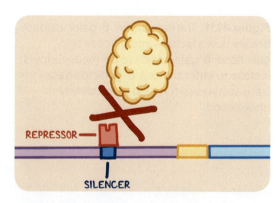

Figure 41.13 A repressor protein in the nucleus binding the DNA sequence called the silencer, which is on the same DNA strand as the gene.

Chapter 41 Genetics: Population Genetics

GEL ELECTROPHORESIS & GENETIC TESTING

osms.it/gel-electrophoresis-genetic-testing

- Method of separating, analyzing macromolecules (e.g. DNA, RNA, proteins), their fragments based on size, charge

Apparatus
- Clear box filled with gel, often agarose
  - Small depressions (AKA "wells") at one end
  - Sample macromolecules placed separately in wells
- Power source connected to gel

Premise
- Current applied → macromolecule fragments move through gel
- Charge of fragments determines
  - **Direction:** opposites attract
  - **Speed:** greater magnitude → faster
- Fragment size also determines speed
  - Gel contains small pores; smaller size → faster
- Fast-moving fragments travel further over given period → production of multiple bands (one per fragment)

Applications
- DNA analysis (e.g. genetic fingerprinting)
  - DNA chopped up with restriction enzymes (e.g. EcoRI cuts at GAATTC)
  - Fragments poured into wells, current applied
  - Fragments move towards positive terminal, form bands at isoelectric point
- Identifying DNA mutations
  - Mutation → restriction enzymes create different fragments → bands change
  - Smaller fragments → bands are further apart
  - More abundant fragments → bands (thicker, brighter)
- **Other applications:** estimation of molecule size, macromolecule separation

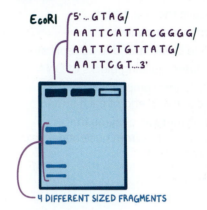

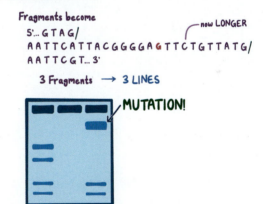

Figure 41.15 Identifying DNA mutations using EcoRI. A mutation in a single nucleotide from A to G in the EcoRI binding site prevents the enzyme from binding and cutting at that location. Now, in gel electrophoresis, there will be only three lines (instead of four) and one fragment will be longer, indicating that the DNA contains a mutation.

POLYMERASE CHAIN REACTION

osms.it/polymerase-chain-reaction

- Technique used to amplify desired DNA segment
- Based on DNA melting, enzyme-driven DNA replication
- Takes place in thermal cycler
- Four essential components
  - **Template DNA:** strand to be replicated
  - **Nucleotides:** building blocks of DNA
  - **Primers:** short complementary DNA strands to the 3' end of each strand
  - **DNA polymerase:** enzyme that synthesizes DNA from nucleotides (e.g. Taq polymerase)

Process
- **Denaturation:** sample heated to 96°C/205°F → bonds between DNA strands separate, forming two template strands
- **Annealing:** sample cooled to 55°C/131°F → primers bind to template strands
- **Extension:** sample heated to 72°C/162°F → Taq polymerase synthesizes complete complementary DNA strands, starting from end of each primer

Applications
- Cloning DNA into plasmids, replicating DNA for analysis (e.g. research and practice)

NOTES
TRANSCRIPTION, TRANSLATION, & REPLICATION

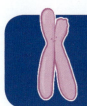

DNA STRUCTURE

osms.it/DNA-structure

DNA (DEOXYRIBONUCLEIC ACID)
- Two polynucleotide chains (double helix shape)

Nucleotides
- 5-carbon sugar, phosphate group, nitrogenous base

Sugar
- Deoxyribose in DNA, ribose in RNA

Nucleobases
- **Purines:** adenine (A), guanine (G)
   - *Pure silver:* purines (pure), adenine, guanine (AG)
- **Pyrimidines:** cytosine (C), thymine (T) for DNA, uracil (U) for RNA
   - *Mnemonic:* CUT the PYE

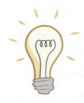

MNEMONIC: CUT the PYE
Pyrimidines
Cytosine
Uracil
Thymine
The
PYrimidin**E**s

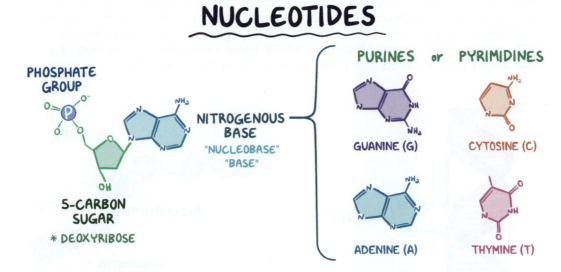

Figure 42.1 Nucleotides consist of a phosphate group, 5-carbon sugar (deoxyribose for DNA) and a nitrogenous base. The base can be a purine, which has two rings (adenine, guanine), or a pyrimidine, which has one ring (cytosine, guanine).

Nucleotide binding and bonding

- Nucleotides bind using sugar, phosphate groups (phosphate group on 5th carbon of sugar binds covalently to 3rd carbon of sugar) → sugar-phosphate backbone
- Nucleotides form hydrogen bonds with bases on opposing strand
    - *Complementary base pairing:* A pairs with T/U (two hydrogen bonds), C pairs with G (three hydrogen bonds)

DNA structure and packing

- Strands coil around each other once every 10 base pairs → major, minor grooves
- In order to be packed tightly, DNA wrapped around histones (positive charge attracts to negative charge of phosphate backbone) → nucleosomes
- Nucleosomes further packed as chromatin fibers
    - *Euchromatin:* loosely packed (genes frequently used)
    - *Heterochromatin:* densely packed (genes rarely used)

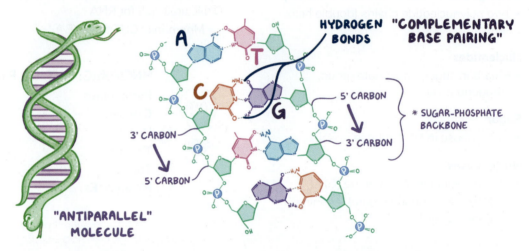

Figure 42.2 *Nucleotide binding:* phosphate group on 5th carbon of sugar on one nucleotide (called 5 prime carbon) binds covalently to 3rd carbon of sugar on another nucleotide (called 3 prime carbon. This gives each DNA strand a sugar-phosphate backbone and a direction (5' to 3' and 3' to 5'). *Nucleotide bonding:* nucleotide bases form hydrogen bonds with the complementary base on the opposing strand, A with T (U in RNA) and C with G.

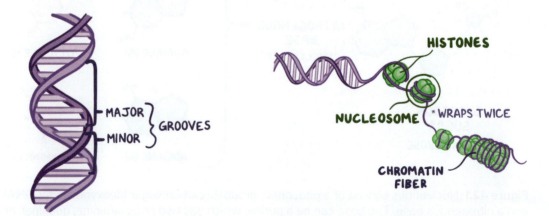

Figure 42.3 Major and minor grooves: larger/smaller spaces between DNA strands where proteins can bind to regulate functions.

Figure 42.4 DNA wraps around histone proteins to form nucleosomes, which pack tighter again to form chromatin fibers.

Chapter 42 Genetics: Transcription, Translation, & Replication

DNA REPLICATION

osms.it/DNA-replication

- Occurs in S phase of cell cycle (before cell division)
- 46 chromosomes duplicated → each daughter cell gets genetic material
- DNA replication semiconservative → each strand of double helix template

PROCESS

Initiation
- Pre-replication complex seeks origin of replication, DNA helicase splits strands → replication fork
  - Single-stranded DNA binding proteins improve stability of lone strands
  - DNA topoisomerase prevents overwinding of later DNA

Elongation
- RNA primase creates multiple RNA primers → randomly bind → DNA polymerase adds complementary nucleotides in 3', 5' direction
  - Forms single leading strand
  - Forms single lagging strand by attaching (with DNA ligase) multiple Okazaki fragments

Termination
- DNA polymerase leaves strand at telomere (TTAGGG nucleotide sequences)
- *Hayflick limit*: maximum number of times cell's DNA can be replicated
  - Due to repeated shortening of telomeres during termination step

DNA CLONING
- Technique used to duplicate segment of DNA within host organism
- Uses "plasmids": genetic structures outside of chromosomes, replicate independently

Process
- Extract desired DNA segment using specific restriction enzymes
- Paste segment into plasmid with DNA ligase → "recombinant DNA"
- Insert plasmid into host organism (e.g. E. coli), encouraging uptake with shock (e.g. heat)
- Identify bacteria carrying plasmid with antibiotics (plasmids given antibiotic resistance gene)
- Leave bacteria to replicate DNA segment, mass-manufacture protein(s)

Applications
- Producing biopharmaceuticals (e.g. insulin), gene therapy (e.g. cystic fibrosis)

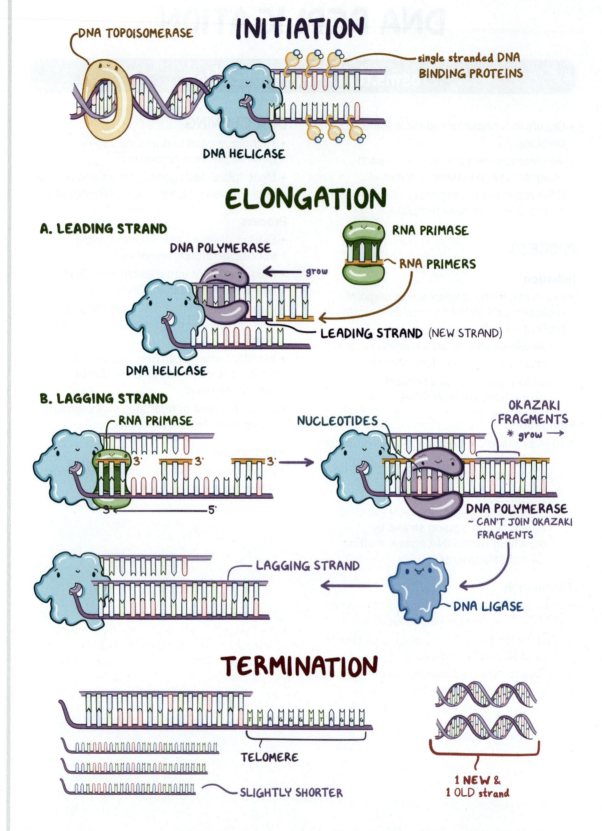

Figure 42.5 Three steps of DNA replication: initiation, elongation, and termination. DNA replication results in two sets of identical DNA, each containing one old strand and one new one.

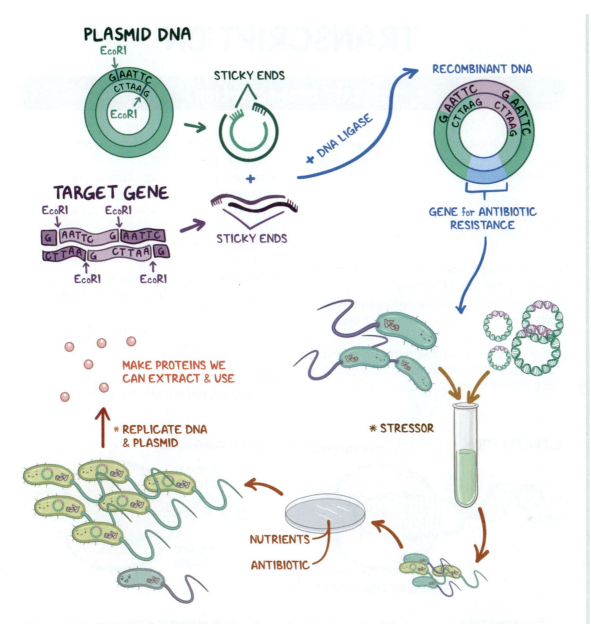

Figure 42.6 DNA cloning. Restriction enzyme (in this case, EcoRI) cleaves a known sequence surrounding a target gene and a plasmid, creating pieces with sticky ends. When DNA ligase is added, these pieces form recombinant DNA (plasmid containing target gene), as well as a gene for antibiotic resistance. A host, in this case E. coli, is combined with recombinant plasmids and subjected to a stressor so that some bacteria take up plasmid. Bacteria are allowed to replicate on plate containing antibiotic, so that only ones that have taken up plasmid can survive. These bacteria produce desired protein from target gene in plasmid.

TRANSCRIPTION

osms.it/transcription

- First step in creating protein from gene
- Gene read, copied on individual messenger RNA (mRNA)

PROCESS

- DNA unpacked from chromatin, undergoes dehelicization
- Promoter region identifies starting point for transcription (e.g. TATA box)
- RNA polymerase shears hydrogen bonds between two strands → transcription bubble
- RNA polymerase follows template strand to assemble mRNA molecule (complementary to template strand)
- Hydrogen bonds reform on nucleotides (already transcribed)
- Termination sequences contains two complementary sequences → resulting mRNA binds with itself forming hairpin loop
- RNA polymerase detaches, DNA closes back up
- Polyadenylate polymerase adds 7-methyl guanosine cap to 5', polyadenine tail to 3' end of mRNA
- Spliceosomes remove introns (don't code proteins) to leave behind exons (do code proteins)
- Resulting mRNA processed by ribosome to create desired protein (translation)

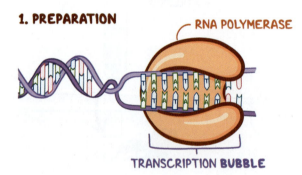
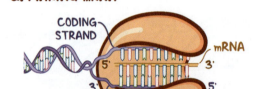
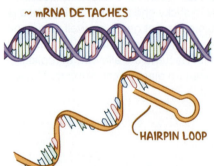

Figure 42.7 Transcription. 1: DNA unpackaging, dehelicization; promoter region identified (TATA box); RNA polymerase shears hydrogen bonds between strands → transcription bubble. 2: RNA polymerase assembles mRNA strand complementary to template strand. Hydrogen bonds reform between DNA nucleotides already transcribed. 3: Termination sequence causes mRNA to form hairpin loop, detach. 4: Cap and tail added, introns spliced out.

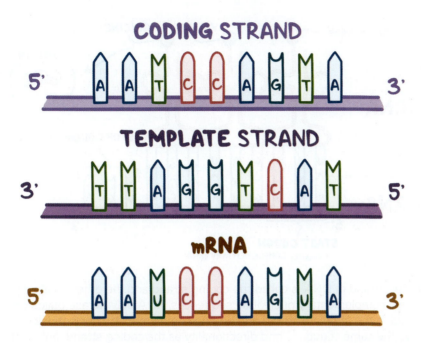

Figure 42.8 One strand of DNA is called the coding strand and the other is called the template strand. They have complementary nucleotide sequences. RNA polymerase builds an mRNA molecule by reading the template strand and adding complementary nucleotides. Therefore, the mRNA will have the same sequence and directionality as the coding strand, only with U instead of T.

TRANSLATION

osms.it/translation

- Second step in creating protein from gene
- Ribosomes assemble protein from mRNA template produced in transcription

PROCESS
- mRNA floats out of nucleus through pore
- *Initiation*: ribosome grabs mRNA, finds start codon (e.g. AUG)
- *Elongation*: ribosome moves along mRNA, producing specific amino acid for each codon
- *Termination*: ribosome reaches stop codon, releases polypeptide (e.g. UGA)

TRANSFER RNA (tRNA)
- Finds, carries amino acids to ribosome
- Three-letter coding sequence (complementary to mRNA)

- Binds to ribosome on aminoacyl/peptidyl/exit site
    - *Aminoacyl*: binds transfer RNA (tRNA) with complementary mRNA codon
    - *Peptidyl*: holds tRNA with polypeptide
    - *Exit*: holds tRNA after amino acid released

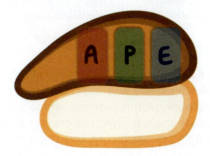

Figure 42.9 Ribosome binding sites.

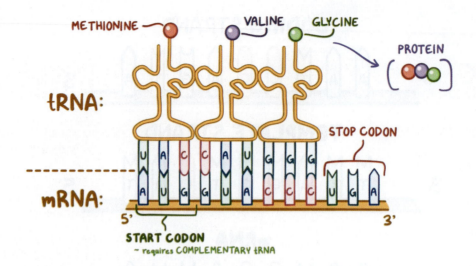

Figure 42.10 One strand of DNA is called the coding strand and the other is called the template strand. They have complementary nucleotide sequences. RNA polymerase builds an mRNA molecule by reading the template strand and adding complementary nucleotides. Therefore, the mRNA will have the same sequence and directionality as the coding strand, only with U instead of T.

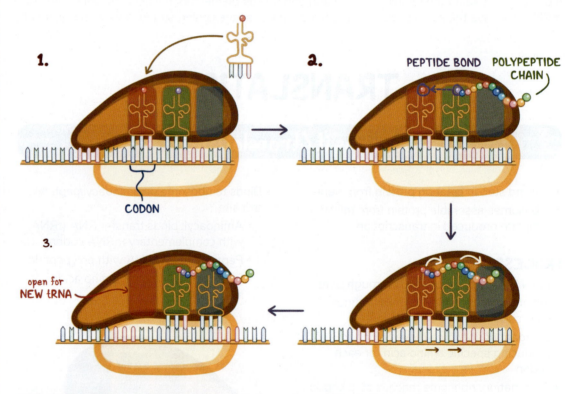

Figure 42.11 Translation extending an existing polypeptide chain.
1: tRNA with amino acid and codon complementary to that of mRNA binds at ribosome A site.
2: Peptide bond forms between amino acid on new tRNA and tRNA in P site holding polypeptide chain, polypeptide chain is transferred to tRNA in A site.
3: Everything moves by one site. A site is now open for a new tRNA.

Chapter 42 Genetics: Transcription, Translation, & Replication

CELL CYCLE

osms.it/cell-cycle

- Sequence of events between formation, division of somatic cell
- Two phases
  - *Interphase:* preparatory phase; cell performs basic functions, replicates DNA
  - *Mitosis:* cellular division

G0 (G-ZERO) PHASE

- Cells function but not dividing/preparing to divide
- Considered outside cell cycle

INTERPHASE

- *Three subphases:* G1, S, G2 phases

Gap/Growth 1 (G1) phase

- Longest phase
- Cell grows while organelles function as usual
- Terminates with G1 checkpoint
  - Cells with damaged DNA → G0 phase/apoptosis

Synthesis (S) phase

- DNA replicated (identical chromatids created)

Gap/Growth 2 (G2) phase

- Organelles duplicated
- Terminates with G2 checkpoint

MITOSIS (M) PHASE

- Cell divides into two daughter cells

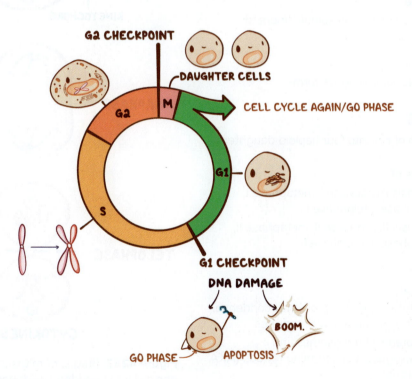

Figure 42.12 Cell cycle summary.

MITOSIS & MEIOSIS

osms.it/mitosis-and-meiosis

- Two processes of cell division

MITOSIS
- Division of cell into two identical daughter cells
- Part of cell cycle
- Consists of prophase, metaphase, anaphase, telophase

Prophase
- Chromatin fibers condense
- Centrioles align chromosomes between centrosomes

Metaphase
- *Prometaphase:* nuclear membrane, nucleolus disintegrate
- *Metaphase:* chromosomes align along metaphase plate, spindle fibers attach to kinetochores

Anaphase
- Centrosomes pull on spindle fibers to separate chromatids

Telophase
- New nuclear envelopes form

MEIOSIS
- Division of cell into four haploid daughter cells
- Consists of
  - *Meiosis I:* prophase I, metaphase I, anaphase I, telophase I
  - *Meiosis II:* prophase II, metaphase II, anaphase II, telophase II

Meiosis I
- Prophase I
  - *Leptotene:* 46 chromosomes condense, nuclear membrane disintegrates
  - *Zygotene:* chromosomes find homologues, bind, forming tetrads (AKA synapsis)

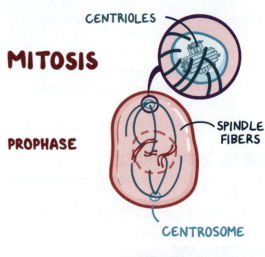
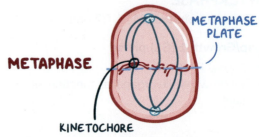
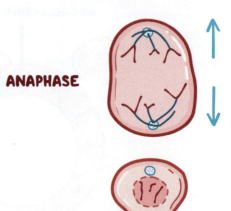
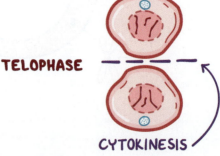

Figure 42.13 Stages of mitosis: division of one cell into two identical daughter cells.

Chapter 42 Genetics: Transcription, Translation, & Replication

- *Pachytene:* homologous chromosomes exchange genetic material (AKA crossing-over)
- *Diplotene:* homologous chromosomes uncoil, slide toward ends (AKA chiasmata)
- *Diakinesis:* terminalization completed
- Metaphase I
  - Tetrads migrate to metaphase plate
- Anaphase I
  - Tetrads split up
  - Chromosomes pulled to each pole by spindle fibers
  - Diploid cell → haploid cell
- Telophase I
  - Cleavage furrow appears, cytokinesis occurs
- Followed by interphase without chromosome duplication in S phase

Meiosis II
- Meiosis II progresses exactly as mitosis
  - Two haploid cells → four haploid cells
  - Same phase names

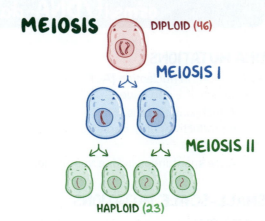

Figure 42.15 Meiosis produces haploid daughter cells with 23 chromosomes each.

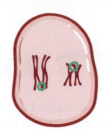

Figure 42.14 Steps of meiosis I, prophase I.

GENETIC MUTATIONS & REPAIR

osms.it/DNA-mutations
osms.it/DNA-damage-and-repair

DNA MUTATIONS
- Alterations in nucleotide (A, T, G, C) sequence of ≥ one gene
  - Affect somatic cells (AKA non-reproductive cells), gametes → germline mutations
  - Arise spontaneously/due to mutagens

SMALL-SCALE MUTATIONS
- Single gene
- *Substitutions*: nucleotide replaced by another
- May result in
  - *Silent mutation*: same amino acid
  - *Missense mutation*: different amino acid (e.g. sickle cell disease)
  - *Nonsense mutation*: stop codon

INSERTIONS & DELETIONS
- Nucleotide added/removed from sequence
- Multiples of three → nonframeshift mutation
  - Reading frame displaced by entire codon → remaining amino acids unchanged → similar resulting protein
- *Frameshift mutation*: resulting protein abnormally long/short, most likely nonfunctional

LARGE-SCALE MUTATIONS
- Often occur due to errors in gamete formation

Abnormal number of chromosomes
- Aneuploidy
  - Additional chromosomes (e.g. Down syndrome)
  - Missing chromosomes (e.g. Turner's syndrome)
- *Polyploidy*
  - Increased number of chromosomes per set (e.g. triploidy)

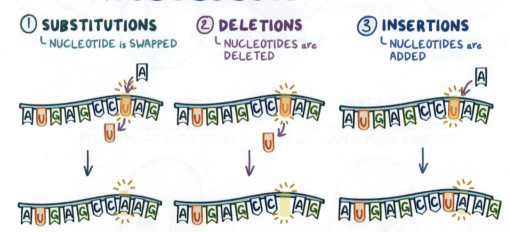

Figure 42.16 Small-scale mutations include: substitutions, deletions, and insertions. They may have a small or large effect on protein function depending on how the new nucleotide affects the translation of the codon sequence into amino acids.

Chapter 42 Genetics: Transcription, Translation, & Replication

Structurally abnormal
- Movement of sections of chromosomes
- *Deletion*: part of chromosome goes missing (e.g. cri du chat syndrome)
- *Duplication*: part of chromosome duplicated
- *Inversion*: part of chromosome breaks off, reattaches
- *Translocation*: parts of two chromosomes switched

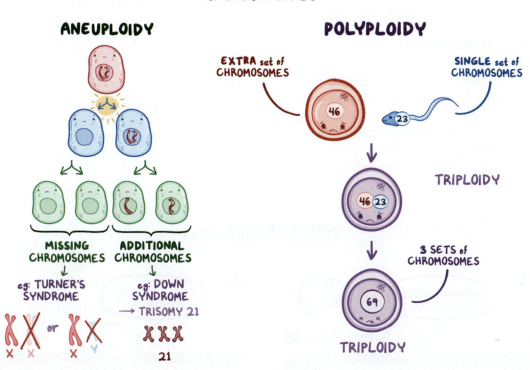

Figure 42.17 Aneuploidy and polyploidy are types of large-scale mutations which result in an abnormal number of chromosomes.

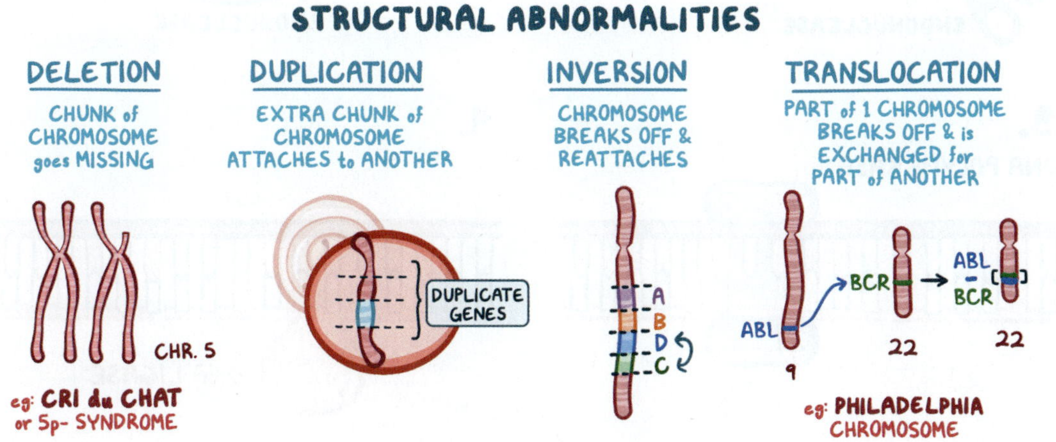

Figure 42.18 Illustration of types of structural abnormalities.

DNA DAMAGE

- DNA damaged by endogenous, exogenous (environmental) factors
- If damaged DNA cannot be fixed → multiple paths
  - *Senescence*: stops dividing
  - *Apoptosis*: programmed cell death
  - *Uncontrolled cell division*: develops into tumor
- If damaged DNA can be fixed → G0 phase

Single strand damage
- Causes
  - Endogenous (errors in DNA replication)
  - Exogenous (harmful chemical/physical agents)
- Repaired with mismatch/base excision/nucleotide excision repair
  - Endonucleases cleave damaged segment
  - Exonucleases remove damaged segment
  - DNA polymerase rebuilds segment
  - DNA ligase glues new segment

Double stranded breaks
- May be due to ionizing radiation

Repair mechanisms
- Non-homologous end joining
  - DNA protein kinase binds to each end of the broken DNA → artemis cuts off rough ends → ends are rejoined with DNA ligase
- Homologous end joining
  - MRN protein complex binds to each end and removes affected nucleotides → DNA polymerase copies genetic information from sister chromatid

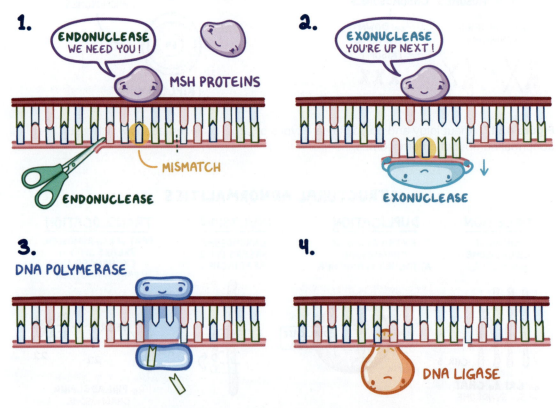

Figure 42.19 Repair of a mismatched nucleotide on a newly synthesized DNA strand. **1:** Endonucleases cleave either side of damaged segment; **2:** Exonucleases remove damaged segment; **3:** DNA polymerase rebuilds segment; **4:** DNA ligase connects new segment to strand.

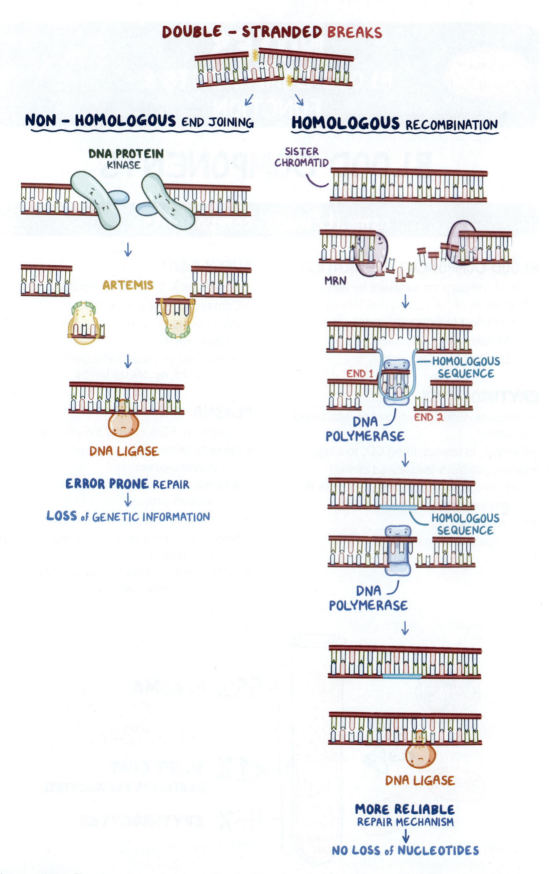

Figure 42.20 Two repair mechanisms for double-stranded breaks: non-homologous end joining and homologous recombination.

NOTES

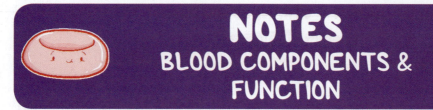

NOTES
BLOOD COMPONENTS & FUNCTION

BLOOD COMPONENTS

osms.it/blood-components

BLOOD COMPONENT SEPARATION
- Blood components separate by density in centrifuge
  - *Heaviest layer*: erythrocytes
  - *Middle layer*: buffy coat
  - *Lightest layer*: plasma

ERYTHROCYTES
- Comprise 45% (hematocrit) of total blood volume
- Carry O_2 to tissues; bring CO_2 to lungs
- Biconcave discs (depressed center)
  - Fit through vessels, ↑ surface area (for gas exchange)
- No organelles
  - ↑ space for hemoglobins

BUFFY COAT
- Comprises < 1% of total blood volume
- Contains platelets, leukocytes
- Platelets clump together → seal damaged blood vessels
- Leukocytes ward off pathogens, destroy cancer cells, neutralize toxins

PLASMA
- Comprises 55% of total blood volume
- *No cells*: 90% water + proteins, electrolytes, gases
- *Albumin*: maintains oncotic pressure, acts as transport protein
- *Globulins*: antibodies, transport proteins
- *Fibrinogen*: involved in clot formation (helps platelets attach)
- *Electrolytes*: include sodium, potassium, calcium, chloride, carbonate

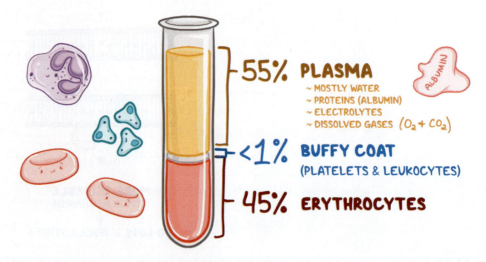

Figure 43.1 Blood components and their relative proportions.

PLATELET PLUG FORMATION (PRIMARY HEMOSTASIS)

osms.it/platelet-plug-formation-primary-hemostasis

- **Hemostasis:** blood-loss prevention
- **First two hemostasis steps:** platelets clump, form plug around injury site in five steps

PLATELET PLUG FORMATION STEPS

1. Endothelial injury
- Nerves, smooth muscle cells detect injury
- Trigger reflexive contraction of vessel (vascular spasm) → ↓ blood flow, loss
- Secretion of nitric oxide, prostaglandins stop; secretion of endothelin begins → further contraction

2. Exposure
- Damage to endothelial cells exposes collagen
- Damaged cells release Von Willebrand factor (binds to collagen)

3. Adhesion
- GP1B surface proteins on platelets bind to Von Willebrand factor

4. Activation
- Platelet changes shape (forms arms to grab other platelets), releases more von Willebrand factor, serotonin, calcium, ADP, thromboxane A2 (positive feedback loop)
- ADP, thromboxane A2 result in GPIIB/IIIA expression

5. Aggregation
- GPIIB/IIIA binds to fibrinogen, links platelets → platelet plug

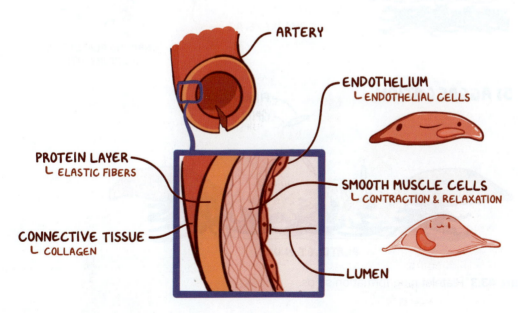

Figure 43.2 Layers of an arterial wall.

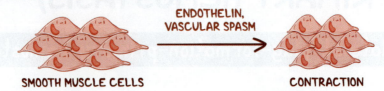
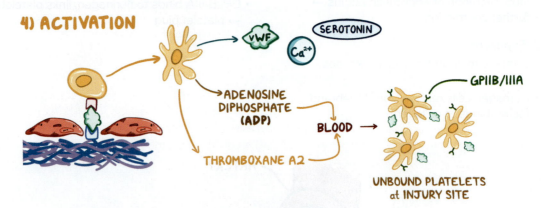
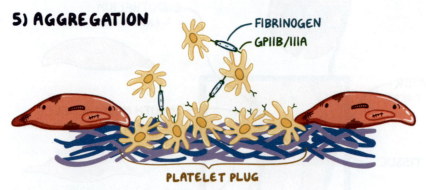

Figure 43.3 Platelet plug formation steps.

COAGULATION (SECONDARY HEMOSTASIS)

osms.it/coagulation-secondary-hemostasis

- **Last two hemostasis steps**: clotting factors activate fibrin, build fibrin mesh around platelet plug
- Begins with either extrinsic/intrinsic pathway; factor X activation → coagulation cascade (common pathway)

EXTRINSIC PATHWAY

1. Trauma damages blood vessel, exposes cells under endothelial layer
   - Tissue factor (factor III) embedded in membrane
2. Factor VII in blood binds to tissue factor, calcium → VIIa-TF complex

INTRINSIC PATHWAY

1. Circulating factor XII contacts negatively charged phosphates on platelets/subendothelial collagen → factor XIIa
2. Factor XIIa cleaves factor XI → factor XIa
3. Factor XIa + calcium cleaves factor IX → factor IXa
4. Factor IXa + factor VIIIa (binds to Von Willebrand factor) + calcium → enter the common pathway

COMMON PATHWAY

1. Factor X is cleaved → factor Xa
2. Factor Xa cleaves factor V → factor Va
3. Factor Xa + factor Va + calcium → prothrombinase complex
   - Prothrombin (factor II) → thrombin (factor IIa)
4. Thrombin activates platelets, cofactors (V, VIII, IX); cleaves fibrinogen, stabilizing factor (→ factor XIIIa + calcium → cross-links in mesh)

COAGULATION TESTS

- **Prothrombin time (PT)**: tests extrinsic pathway
- **Activated partial thromboplastin time (aPTT)**: tests intrinsic pathway

ROLE OF VITAMIN K IN COAGULATION

osms.it/vitamin-k-in-coagulation

- Vitamin K regulates blood coagulation
  - Converts coagulation factors into mature forms
- 12 coagulation factors: (I–XIII, no factor VI); factors II, VII, IX, X require vitamin K
- Quinone reductase reduces vitamin K quinone (dietary form) into vitamin K hydroquinone
- Vitamin K hydroquinone donates electrons to γ-glutamyl carboxylase, converting non-functional forms of II, VII, IX, X into functional forms
  - Adds chemical group made of one carbon, two hydrogens, one oxygen to glutamic acid residues on proteins
- After carboxylation step, vitamin K (as vitamin K epoxide) is converted back into vitamin K quinone via epoxide reductase
- Coagulation factors appear in all coagulation pathways

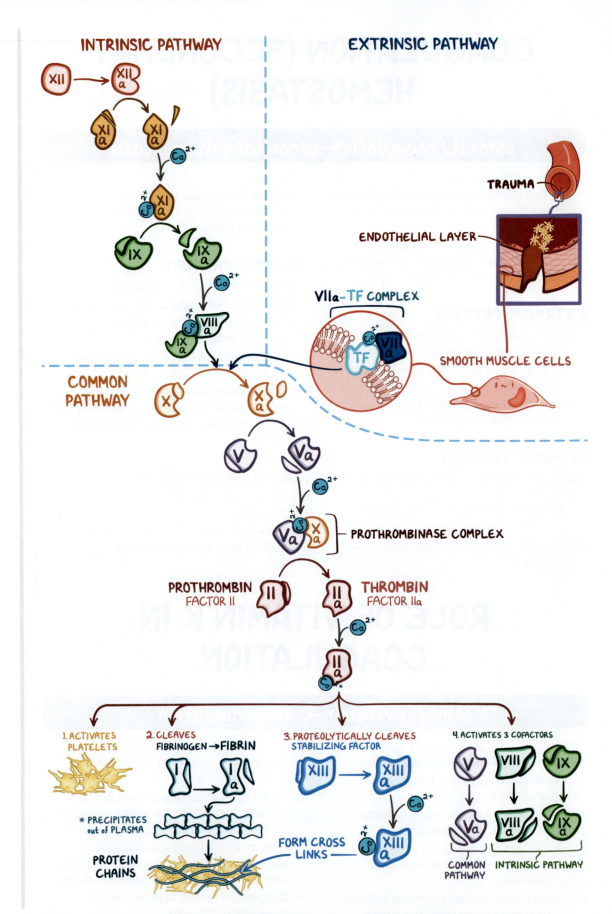

Figure 43.4 Coagulation steps, including the intrinsic, extrinsic, and common pathways.

Chapter 43 Hematology: Blood Components & Function

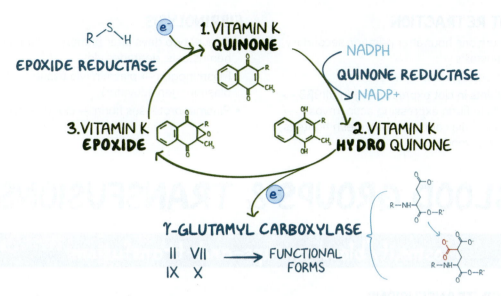

Figure 43.5 Vitamin K cycle. A single molecule of Vitamin K can be reused many times.

ANTICOAGULATION, CLOT RETRACTION & FIBRINOLYSIS

osms.it/clot-retraction-and-fibrinolysis

ANTICOAGULATION

- Occurs during primary, secondary hemostasis; regulates clot formation
- Prevents clots from growing too large → block blood flow, form emboli
- Regulation starts with thrombin (factor II)
  - Multiple pro-coagulative functions
  - Proteins C, S bind thrombomodulin-thrombin → cleaves, inactivates factors V, VIII
  - Antithrombin III binds thrombin/factor X → inactivates both (plus factors VII, IX, XI, XII with lower affinity)
- Other factors prevent platelets adhering during primary hemostasis
  - Nitric oxide, prostacyclin → ↓ thromboxane A2

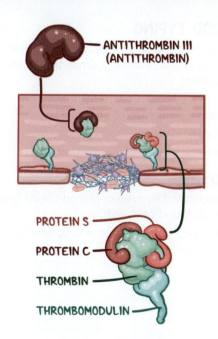

Figure 43.6 Proteins involved in anticoagulation. Thrombomodulin is found on the surface of intact epithelial cells lining blood vessels.

CLOT RETRACTION
- Occurs one hour after primary, secondary hemostasis
    - Contracts clot
- Platelets in clot express integrin αIIBβ3 → binds to fibrin expressing actin, myosin → lamellipodia contract, fibrin mesh tightens closing wood

FIBRINOLYSIS
- Occurs two days after primary, secondary hemostasis; degrades clot
- Plasminogen → plasmin (via tissue plasminogen activator)
- Plasmin proteases fibrin → clot dissolves

BLOOD GROUPS & TRANSFUSIONS

osms.it/blood-groups-and-transfusions

BLOOD TRANSFUSIONS
- *Blood transfusion*: person receives blood/elements of blood (usually through intravenous infusion)
    - *Homologous transfusion*: anonymous donor
    - *Autologous transfusion*: self-donor (e.g. in planned surgery)
- Blood is mixed with calcium oxalate to prevent coagulation, refrigerated/frozen for storage

BLOOD TYPING
- Transfusion blood types not compatible → autoimmune reaction (hemolytic transfusion reaction)
- Two classification systems (based on presence/absence of proteins)
    - ABO system
    - Rh system

ABO system
- Determined by type of glycoproteins found on red blood cells (RBCs)
    - Type A; type B; type A & B; type O (neither)
- Immune system produces antibodies against absent glycoproteins
- *Type AB*: no antibodies → universal recipients
- *Type O*: no antigens → universal donors

Rh system
- Determined by presence of Rh protein
    - Rh positive; Rh negative
- Rh+ can receive blood from either group
- Rh- can only receive Rh- blood

CROSS MATCHING
- Test to confirm donor's blood is safe for recipient
- Recipient serum is mixed with donor blood
    - *Agglutination reaction*: cannot receive

Chapter 43 Hematology: Blood Components & Function

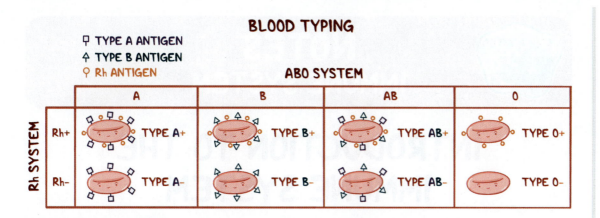

Figure 43.7 Blood types are reported as ABO group and Rh + or -. When both classification systems are combined, there are eight possible blood types: A+, A-, B+, B-, AB+, AB-, O+, O-.

NOTES
IMMUNE SYSTEM

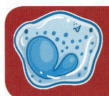

INTRODUCTION TO THE IMMUNE SYSTEM

osms.it/immune-system-introduction

- Includes organs, tissues, cells, molecules
- Protects from microorganisms, removes toxins, promotes inflammation, destroys tumor cells
- Two branches
  - Innate, adaptive

INNATE IMMUNE RESPONSE

- *Nonspecific* cells: phagocytes, natural killer (NK) cells; no immunologic memory
- "Feverishly" fast (minutes to hours)

Noncellular components
- Physical, chemical barriers (e.g. lysozymes in tears, cilia in airways)
- *Inflammation*: stops spread of infection, promotes healing
  - *Four cardinal signs*: redness, heat, swelling, pain
- *Complement system*: cascade of proteins; triggers inflammation, kills pathogens by cytolysis, tags cells for destruction

ADAPTIVE IMMUNE RESPONSE

- Highly specific cells; immunologic memory, need priming
- Significantly slower, esp. initially (weeks)
- *Clonal expansions*: cells replicate
- *Clonal deletion*: cells die off after immune response; some survive as memory cells

CELLS OF THE IMMUNE SYSTEM

Leukocytes (white blood cells)
- Formed by hematopoiesis in bone marrow
  - Starts with multipotent hematopoietic stem cells
  - Cells develop into myeloid/lymphoid progenitor cells
- *Myeloid cells*: contribute to innate response
  - *Neutrophils*: phagocytes, granulocytes, polymorphonuclear cells (nucleus segmented into 3–5 lobes); stain light pink/reddish-purple; most numerous leukocyte
  - *Eosinophils*: phagocytes, granulocytes, polymorphonuclear cells (nucleus usually bilobed); stain pink with eosin; larger cells fight parasites
  - *Basophils*: nonphagocytes, granulocytes, polymorphonuclear cells (nucleus bilobed/segmented); stain blue-purple with hematoxylin; aid in fighting parasites; granules contain histamine, heparin; involved in inflammatory response; least numerous leukocyte
  - *Mast cells*: nonphagocytes, granulocytes; involved in inflammatory response
  - *Monocytes*: phagocytes, antigen-presenting cells; release cytokines to recruit other cells; only circulate in blood; differentiate into macrophages/dendritic cells
  - *Dendritic cells*: phagocytes, antigen-presenting cells; release cytokines to recruit other cells; circulate in lymph,

blood, tissue; consume large proteins in interstitial fluid; break bloodborne pathogens into small amino acid chains → move to lymph node → present antigens to T cells
- Macrophages: phagocytes, antigen-presenting cells; release cytokines to recruit other cells; stay in connective tissue, lymphoid organs; not in blood
- Lymphoid cells: contribute to the adaptive response (except NK cells)
  - NK cells: contribute to innate response; complete development in bone marrow; large, contain granules; primarily target infected, cancer cells; kill target cells with cytotoxic granules (punch holes in target cell membranes by binding to phospholipids → enter cell, trigger apoptosis, programmed cell death)
  - B cells: contribute to adaptive response; complete development in bone marrow; bind to specific antigens (antigen presentation not needed); capable of phagocytosis, antigen presentation; load antigens on major histocompatibility complex (MHC) II, display to T cells; T-cell activation → B cells mature into plasma cells; secrete lots of antibodies/immunoglobulins (B cell receptors in secreted-form, mark pathogens for destruction → "humoral immunity")
  - T cells: contribute to adaptive response; complete development in thymus; responsible for cell-mediated immunity; bind to specific antigens (antigen presentation needed); naive T cells primed by antigen presenting cells (usually dendritic cells); generally categorized into $CD4^+$, $CD8^+$ T cells; $CD4^+$ (helper) T cells secrete cytokines to coordinate immune response, only see antigens on MHC II; $CD8^+$ (cytotoxic) T cells kill target cells, cells with antigens on MHC I

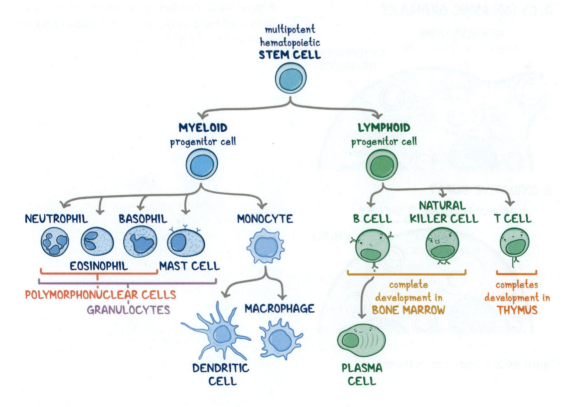

Figure 44.1 Family tree of immune system cells.

CLASSIFICATION OF IMMUNE CELLS

Phagocytes
- Reach around pathogens with cytoplasm, swallowing whole (phagosome)
- Destroy some pathogens with cytoplasmic granules (phagosomes fuse with granules → phagolysosomes; pH in vesicle drops killing pathogens)
- Continue to swallow pathogens before oxidative burst → produces highly reactive oxygen (e.g. H_2O_2; destroys proteins, nucleic acids, killing pathogens, phagocyte)

Granulocytes
- Contain granules in cytoplasm
- All cells (except mast cells) polymorphonuclear

Antigen-presenting cells
- Present antigens to T cells

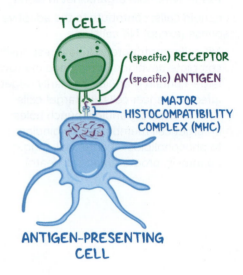

Figure 44.3 Antigen-presenting cell (depicted here as dendritic cell) presenting an antigen to a T cell.

1. PHAGOCYTOSIS

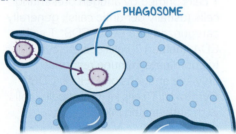

2. CYTOPLASMIC GRANULES

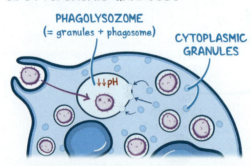

3. OXIDATIVE BURST

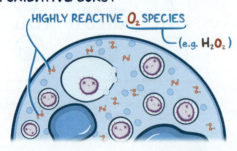

Figure 44.2 Phagocyte activities.

IMMUNE CELL CLASSIFICATIONS

	CLASSIFICATIONS		
BASOPHILS		Granulocytes	
MAST CELLS			
NEUTROPHILS	Phagocytes		
EOSINOPHILS			
MONOCYTES			
DENDRITIC CELLS		Agranulocytes	Antigen-presenting cells
MACROPHAGES			
LYMPHOCYTES			

VACCINES

osms.it/vaccines

- Generate protective adaptive immune response against microbes by exposure to nonpathogenic forms/components of microbes
    - Differs from passive immunity (body creates own antibodies)
- Administration: intramuscularly, intradermally, intranasally, subcutaneously, orally
- Immunoglobulin response depends on route, type of vaccine
    - Intramuscular vaccinations → IgG
    - Rotavirus vaccine (oral) → IgA
- Four main types of vaccines
    - Live attenuated, inactivated (whole cell vaccines)
    - Subunit, toxoid (fractionated vaccines)

LIVE ATTENUATED VACCINES

- Attenuated → pathogen weakened (but still replicates)
- Measles, mumps, rubella, varicella (MMRV); rotavirus; smallpox; yellow fever

INACTIVATED VACCINES

- Pathogen killed using heat/formalin
- Response humoral/antibody-mediated; no cellular immunity → ↓ response
- Hepatitis A; polio; rabies; influenza

SUBUNIT VACCINES

- Contain immunogenic portions of pathogens (polysaccharides/proteins)
- Combination of proteins from different pathogens → conjugate subunit vaccines
- Polysaccharide vaccines
    - T cell independent (only respond to protein antigens)
    - Not effective in children < two years old
    - Memory B cells never formed → repeated doses needed
    - *Haemophilus influenzae* type B; hepatitis B; HPV; *Bordetella pertussis* (pertussis); *Streptococcus pneumoniae*; *Neisseria meningitidis*; Varicella zoster

TOXOID VACCINES
- Against specific toxins (main cause of illness)
- Toxoid fixed/inactivated using formalin
- Often combined with subunit vaccines
- Tetanus, diphtheria, and pertussis (TDaP), diphtheria, tetanus, and pertussis (DTap) vaccine

CONTRAINDICATIONS
- Moderate/severe infection
- Allergy to eggs/previous vaccines
- Guillain–Barré syndrome (vaccines against influenza, DTaP)
- Weakened immune system
  - Pregnant (live attenuated vaccines)

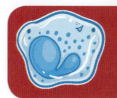

NOTES
B & T CELLS

ANTIBODY CLASSES

osms.it/antibody-classes

- B cell receptor, major component of humoral immunity
- Heavy, light chain; fragment antigen-binding region; constant region (Fc)
- B cell develops into plasma cell → B cell receptor secreted as antibody
- **Antibodies:** monomers, polymers
  - **Valence:** number of antigen-binding fragments

FIVE TYPES
- Coded by heavy chain genes

Immunoglobulin M (IgM)
- 1st antibody response
- Monomer as B cell receptor (valence: 2)
- Pentamer as antibody held together by joining (J) chain (valence: 10)
- Works against carbohydrate, lipid antigens
- Most effective at activating complement pathway

Immunoglobulin G (IgG)
- Monomer (valence: 2)
- Four subclasses
  - IgG1, IgG2, IgG3, IgG4 (differ in constant regions)
- Serves as opsonin
- Activates classical complement pathway

Immunoglobulin A (IgA)
- Monomer (valence: 2)
- Serves as opsonin (eosinophils, neutrophils, some macrophages)
- Main immunoglobulin in mucosal sites; sometimes occurs as dimer (valence: 4)
- Two forms
  - IgA1, IgA2 (differ in constant regions)

Immunoglobulin E (IgE)
- Monomer (valence: 2)
- Production primarily induced by interleukin 4 (IL-4)
- Triggers granule release from mast cells, eosinophils, basophils
- Responds to nonpathogenic targets (e.g. peanuts) → allergies

Immunoglobulin D (IgD)
- Monomer (valence: 2)
- Found alongside IgM antibodies, signals maturation of B cells

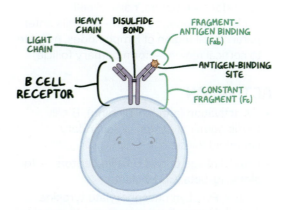

Figure 45.1 B cell receptor components.

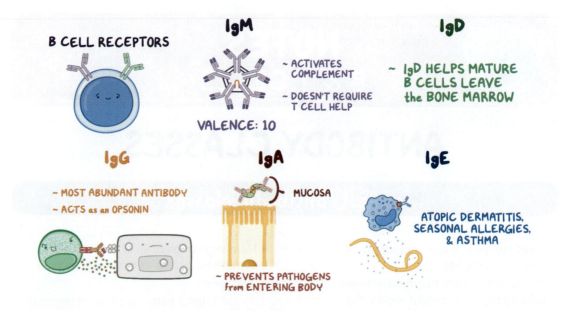

Figure 45.2 Summary of the five classes of antibodies. IgM and IgD can act as B cell receptors.

B CELL ACTIVATION & DIFFERENTIATION

osms.it/b-cell-activation-and-differentiation

- Developing B cell receptor expresses μ heavy chain → B cell receptors IgM
- Alternative splicing → IgM, IgD expressed on surface → mature, naive B cell explores lymphatic system → B cells enter paracortical region of lymph nodes, migrate to cortical region → form primary follicle

ACTIVATION

- On activation (antigen-binding), B cell forms germinal center → secondary lymphoid follicle
- Cross-linkage of two B cell receptors → Ig-alpha, Ig-beta, CD19 cluster
    - Blk, Fyn, Lyn phosphorylate tyrosine residues on immunoreceptor tyrosine based activation motif (ITAM) units → transcription factors nuclear factor kappa-light-chain-enhancer of activated B cells (NF-kB), nuclear factor of activated T cells (NFAT) → gene expression of cytokines, upregulation of antiapoptotic cell surface markers

DIFFERENTIATION

- B cells stimulated by cluster of differentiation 21 (CD21)/complement receptor Type II (CR2) (receptor for C3d complement fragment)
- Activated B cells differentiate into plasma cells, secrete antibodies
    - Plasma cells initially secrete IgM, remain mainly in bone marrow, safeguard against future encounters with same antigen

Activated CD4$^+$ T cell → class switching

- B cells: antigen-presenting cells; present antigens on major histocompatibility complex (MHC) class II to helper T cells
- CD40 ligand on T cell binds to CD40 on B cell → cytokines instruct B cell on type of antibody to produce (by activation-induced cytidine deaminase)
    - IL-4, IL-5 → IgE
    - Interferon (IFN) gamma → IgG

- Activation-induced deaminase removes constant regions during differentiation to leave desired antibody region

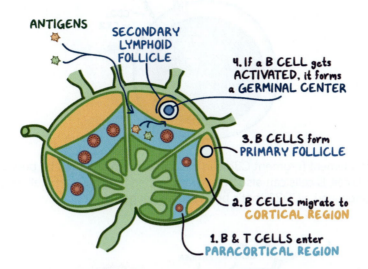

Figure 45.3 Mature, naive B cells form a primary follicle in the cortical region of a lymph node. When the B cell binds an antigen, it activates and forms a germinal center. The follicle is now called a secondary lymphoid follicle.

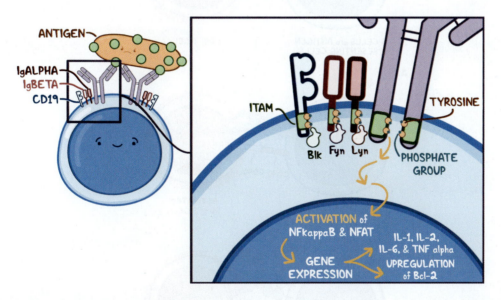

Figure 45.4 Series of events following antigen binding that lead to B cell activation. Ig-alpha, Ig-beta, and CD19 are intracellular side chains of the B cell receptors that cluster when two B cell receptors are cross-linked by an antigen.

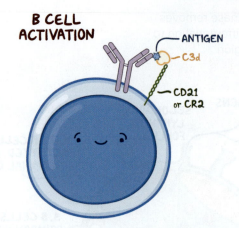

Figure 45.5 Complement fragment C3d can bind an antigen and then be bound by molecule CD21/CR2 on a B cell. B cells can also be activated when they have a B cell receptor that is bound to an antigen, and a CD21 that's bound to an antigen.

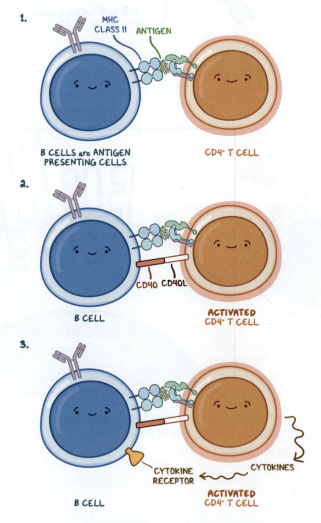

Figure 45.6 B cell differentiation. **1:** B cell presents an antigen to a CD4+ T cell. **2:** If the T cell activates, it expresses CD40L on its surface, which binds to CD40 on the B cell. **3:** CD40L and CD40 binding causes the B cell to express a cytokine receptor and the T cell to release cytokines. The type of cytokine determines what type of antibody the B cell will produce.

B CELL DEVELOPMENT

osms.it/b-cell-development

- **Lymphopoiesis**: development of diverse set of lymphocytes with unique antigen receptors

CREATION OF SUITABLE RECEPTOR
- B cell receptor contains two chains
  - Heavy, light
- Antigen-binding site made of variable (V), diversity (D), joining (J) protein segments coded by genes of same name
  - **Heavy chain**: all three segments
  - **Light chain**: V, J segments

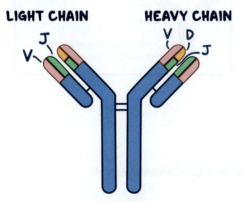

Figure 45.7 Antigen binding site on heavy chain is composed of V, D, and J segments, while antigen binding site on light chain has only V and J segments.

STAGES OF DEVELOPMENT
- **Six stages**: common lymphoid progenitor cell → early pro-B cell → late pro-B cell → large pre-B cell → small pre-B cell → immature B cell

Early pro-B cell
- Common lymphoid progenitor cell expresses recombination activating gene (RAG) 1, RAG2 → early pro-B cell

Late pro-B cell
- Heavy chain D, J gene segments spliced together (*allelic exclusion*: 1st chromosome to complete splicing suppresses 2nd) → late pro-B cell

Large pre-B cell
- Late pro-B-cell attaches D-J gene segment to V gene segment via V(D)J recombinase → binding site (heavy chain) recombined with mu gene → large pre-B cell
  - Mu gene codes for IgM constant region protein

Small pre-B cell
- Functionality of heavy chain tested by binding to surrogate light chain (VpreB, lambda 5) → if successful, cells proliferate → small pre-B cell

Immature B cell
- Light chain rearranged → functionality of light chain tested by autoimmune regulator (AIRE), identifies self-reactive cells by expressing bodily antigens in lymphoid organs → immature B cell
- *Central tolerance/negative selection*: elimination of self-reactive cells
  - Strong binding to self-antigen → cell undergoes apoptosis
  - Intermediate binding to self-antigen → light chain repeatedly rearranged with kappa gene on 1st, 2nd chromosomes, lambda gene 1st, 2nd chromosomes
  - Failure to eliminate self-reactive cells → autoimmunity
- Immature B cells finally undergo alternative splicing on constant region → IgD constant region replaces IgM constant region → cells released into blood

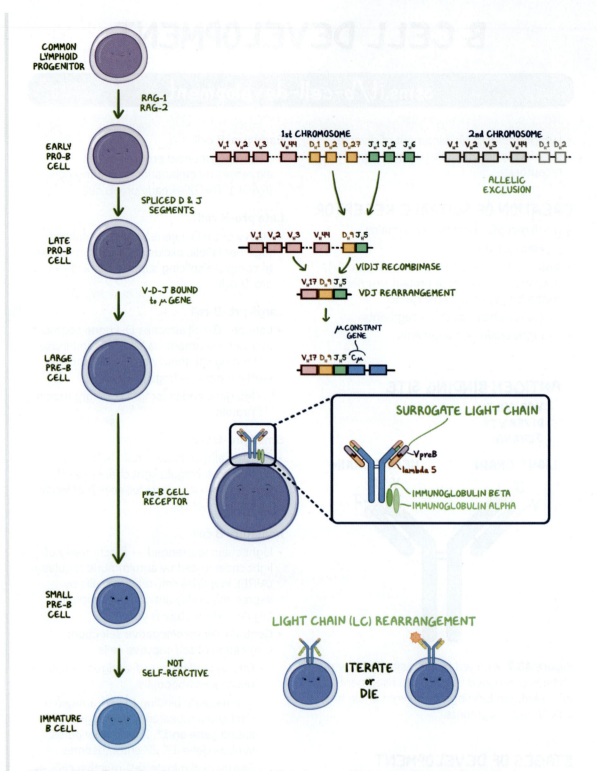

Figure 45.8 B cell development stages and the changes that move them to the next stage.

CELL MEDIATED IMMUNITY OF CD4 CELLS

osms.it/cell-mediated-immunity-CD4-cells

- CD4 cells = T helper cells (support other immune cells)
- T cells initially naive
- In response to antigen, T cell primed → effector T cell
  - Two signals: antigen (MHC molecule on antigen-presenting cell), costimulation (CD28 binds to B7 on antigen-presenting cells)
- Activated T helper cell → IL-2 → up-regulates IL-2 alpha receptor
- T helper cell binds to IL-2 (autocrine stimulation) → clonal expansion

FOUR TYPES OF T HELPER CELL

- Depends on cytokines in environment

T helper Type I (Th1)
- Fights intracellular infections
- Macrophages → IL-12, natural killer (NK) cells → IFN-γ, infected cells → IFNα, IFNβ → transcription factors signal transducer and activator of transcription 1 (STAT1), STAT2

T helper Type II
- Fights parasites
- Eosinophils, basophils, mast cells → IL-4, IL-4, IL-10 → transcription factors STAT6, GATA-binding protein 3 (GATA3)

T helper Type XVII
- Fights fungal, bacterial infections
- Fungi, bacteria → IL1, IL6, IL23, transforming growth factor (TGF)β → transcription factors ROR-γ, STAT3

T follicular helper (Tfh)
- Establishes memory B cells
- Antigen-presenting cells → IL6, IL21, IL27 → transcription factors B cell lymphoma protein 5 (BCL-5), cMaf

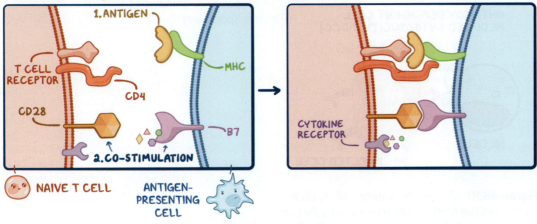

Figure 45.9 T helper cells require two signals to be primed and become effector T cells: presentation of an antigen and binding of CD28 on T cell to B7 on antigen-presenting cell.

CELL MEDIATED IMMUNITY OF NATURAL KILLER & CD8 CELLS

osms.it/cell-mediated-immunity-NK-CD8-cells

NATURAL KILLER (NK) CELLS

- Identify target cells; deliver perforin, granzymes
- Part of innate response → no need for specific antigen
- Activation receptors recognize surface molecules on infected cells; inhibitory receptors recognize molecules (e.g. native MHC class I molecules)
- Also activated by antibody-dependent cell-mediated cytotoxicity
  - IgG binds to virally-infected cell → CD16 on NK binds to antibody

CD8 CELLS

- CD8 cells = cytotoxic T cells
- T cells initially naive
- In response to antigen, T cell primed → effector T cell
  - **Two signals:** antigen (MHC molecule on antigen-presenting cell), costimulation (CD28 binds to B7 on antigen-presenting cells)
- Activated T helper cell → IL-2 → up-regulates IL-2 alpha receptor
- T helper cell binds to IL-2 (autocrine stimulation) → clonal expansion
- Needs to see antigen in context of MHC I to kill cell (doesn't need CD28)
- Binds nonspecifically to multiple cells with adhesion molecules → fails to bind to MHC I → disengages
- If antigen binds, cytoskeletal rearrangement → forms supramolecular activation cluster (SMAC)
  - Includes central SMAC (cSMAC) for antigen recognition, peripheral SMAC (pSMAC)
- Cytotoxic cell releases granules with perforin, granzymes (caspases → apoptosis)

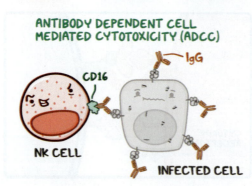

Figure 45.10 NK cells recognize cell surface molecules like MHC I to determine whether or not to kill a cell. They can also kill via ADCC. In this process, the NK cell is stimulated by binding to the constant chain of an IgG antibody attached to a virally infected cell.

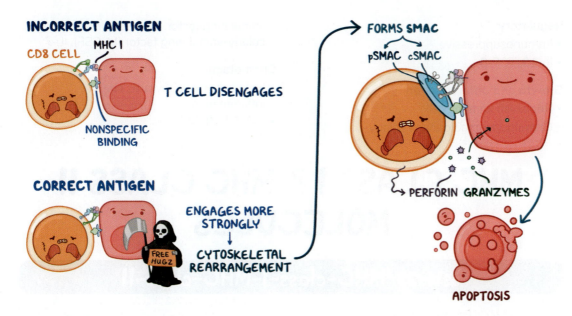

Figure 45.11 CD8 cells weakly bind a variety of cells with adhesion molecules. However, they only destroy cells with antigens on their MHC I molecules that allow the CD8 cells to bind tightly.

CYTOKINES

osms.it/cytokines

- Proteins secreted by all types of cells to communicate (bind to receptors, trigger response)

FIVE TYPES

Interleukins (ILs)
- Act as communication between leukocytes, nonleukocytes
- Promote development, differentiation of T, B cells
- Mostly synthesized by helper T cells

Tumor necrosis factors (TNFs)
- Bind to cell receptors, cause cells to die (induce apoptosis)
- Heavily involved in inflammatory response (up-regulate expression of adhesion molecules, increase vascular permeability, induce fever)

Interferons (IFNs)
- Type I
  ▫ Produced by virally infected cells → affect surrounding cells: degrade messenger RNA (mRNA), inhibit protein synthesis, express MHC
- Type II
  ▫ Interferon-gamma → promotes anti-viral state, activates macrophages, CD4⁺ helper T-cells

Colony stimulating factors (CSFs)
- Bind to surface receptors on hematopoietic stem cells → proliferation, differentiation

Transforming growth factors (TGFs)
- Control proliferation, differentiation of cells

MAIN FUNCTIONAL RESPONSES

Pro-inflammatory
- Enhance innate, adaptive immune responses
- IL-1, IL-12, IL-18, TNF, IFN-γ

Parasite/allergy
- Help immune system handle large parasites, induce allergic responses
- IL-4, IL-5, IL-10, IL13

Regulatory
- Immunosuppressive
- IL-10, TGF-β

Growth and differentiation
- Replenish immune cells
- Granulocyte-macrophage colony-stimulating factor (GM-CSF), macrophage colony-stimulating factor (M-CSF), IL-7

Chemotactic
- Help cells move towards site of inflammation
- IL-17, IL-8

MHC CLASS I & MHC CLASS II MOLECULES

osms.it/MHC-class-I-MHC-class-II

- Major histocompatibility complex (MHC), AKA "human leukocyte antigen"
    - Cell surface proteins, present antigens to T cells

MHC CLASS I
- Found on all nucleated cells, presents antigens from inside
- Bound by CD8 molecules on cytotoxic T cells
- Includes HLA-A, HLA-B, HLA-C

Structure
- Contains alpha, beta-2-microglobulin chains
- *Alpha chain:* peptide binding groove, transmembrane region
    - Binding groove binds peptides 8–10 amino acids long; hydrophobic peptide residues ↔ hydrophilic groove amino acids
- *Three extracellular domains:* alpha-1, alpha-2, alpha-3

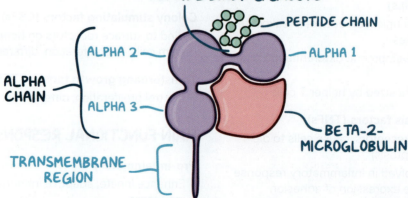

Figure 45.12 Structure of an MHC class I molecule.

Function
- Allows immune cells to sample cellular proteins (via endogenous pathway of antigen presentation)
  - Marked protein sent to proteasome
  - Proteasome degrades protein → short peptide chains
  - Transporters of antigenic peptides (TAP) move peptide chains to endoplasmic reticulum
  - TAP loads peptide onto MHC class I using tapasin
  - MHC class I loaded into exocytic vesicle, sent to cell surface
  - Cytotoxic T cells, NK cells interact with peptide (if necessary)

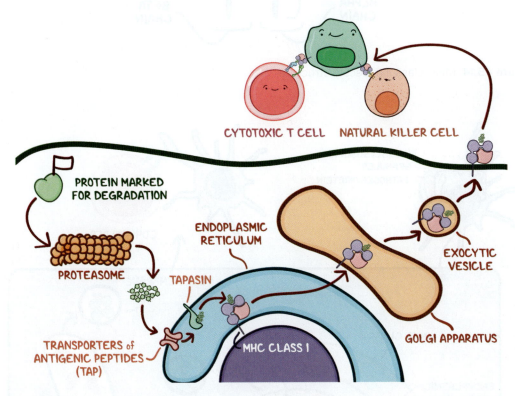

Figure 45.13 Endogenous pathway of antigen presentation.

MHC CLASS II
- Found on antigen-presenting cells, presents antigens from outside
- Bound by CD4 molecules on helper T cells
- Includes HLA-DP, HLA-DQ, HLA-DR

Structure
- Contains alpha, beta chains
  - Both penetrate cell membrane
  - Binding groove binds peptides 14–20 amino acids long

Function
- Engulfs, destroys pathogens; presents antigens to CD4+ T helper cells (via exogenous pathway of antigen presentation)
  - Antigen-presenting cell ingests antigen → endosome
  - Lysosome + endosome → phagolysosome; degrades protein → short peptide chains
  - MHC class II binding groove filled temporarily with invariant chain (degrades during vesicular transportation)
  - Vesicle fuses with phagolysosome
  - MHC class II binds peptide, sent to cell surface
  - CD4+ helper T cells interact with peptide (if necessary)

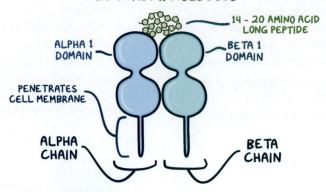

Figure 45.14 MHC class II molecule structure.

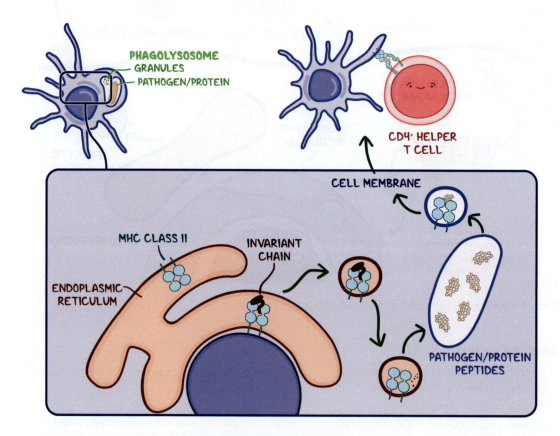

Figure 45.15 Exogenous pathway of antigen presentation.

SOMATIC HYPERMUTATION & AFFINITY MATURATION

osms.it/somatic-hypermutation-affinity-maturation

SOMATIC HYPERMUTATION

- Intentional mutation of antibody genes to create new antigen specificities → stronger, more specific response to antigen
- Occurs in activated B cells (germinal centers, spleen)
- CD40L on T cell binds to CD40 on B cell → cytokines instruct B cell to produce specific type of antibody
- Activation-induced cytidine deaminase (AID) turns cytidine into uridine (not usually found in DNA) → mismatch/base excision repair to remove uridine
  - Mismatch repair proteins MSH2, MSH6 use nucleases to remove uridine; DNA polymerase replaces nucleotides → mutations
  - Base excision: uracil-DNA glycosylase removes uracil from uridine → next round of replication, random nucleotide inserted → mutations
- Only some mutations increase affinity
  - Low affinity B cells die naturally with time
  - High affinity B cells live on (affinity maturation)

AFFINITY MATURATION

- Process by which B cells increase affinity for antigen during an immune response
- Somatic hypermutation, clonal selection (only high affinity cells activated → only high affinity cells replicate)

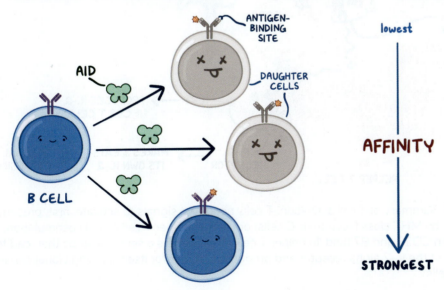

Figure 45.16 Somatic hypermutation only occurs in B cells which express enzyme AID. AID makes small mutations directly in antigen binding site of B cell receptor, which get expressed in daughter cells of a rapidly proliferating cell. These changes in the variable region change affinity (strength) that B cell receptor has for its antigen. As antigen becomes limited, B cells with lowest affinity will die off first, so only B cells with strongest affinity for their antigen remain.

T CELL ACTIVATION

osms.it/t-cell-activation

- **Priming:** T cell begins differentiation when exposed to antigen
  - **Two signals:** antigen (MHC molecule on antigen-presenting cell), **costimulation** (CD28 binds to B7 on antigen-presenting cells)
- Signal sent to nucleus by CD3 peptide chains
  - Lymphocyte-specific protein tyrosine kinase (LCK) phosphorylates tyrosine residues on immunoreceptor tyrosine based activation motif (ITAM) units
- Zeta-chain-associated protein kinase 70 (ZAP-70) phosphorylates LAT, SLP-76 → activation of transcription factors NF-kB, NFAT → gene expression of cytokines, upregulation of antiapoptotic cell surface markers
- Activated T cell → IL-2 → up-regulates IL-2 alpha receptor
- T helper cell binds to IL-2 (autocrine stimulation) → clonal expansion

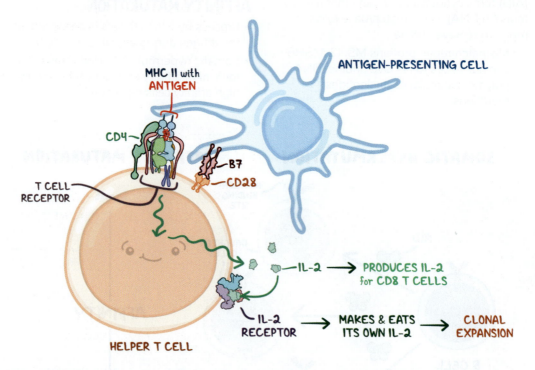

Figure 45.17 Summary of T cell activation. T cells need two signals to activate: first, presentation of its antigen by MHC class I (cytotoxic C cells) or class II (helper T cells), and costimulation, which is when CD28 and B7 bind. In helper T cells, this triggers a series of steps that lead to upregulation of the IL-2 alpha receptor and production of IL-2 for itself, causing clonal expansion, and CD8 T cells.

T CELL DEVELOPMENT

osms.it/t-cell-development

- **Lymphopoiesis:** hematopoietic stem cell → common lymphoid progenitor cell → immature B cell (bone marrow)

CREATION OF SUITABLE RECEPTOR

- T cell receptor contains two chains: alpha, beta
  - **Alpha:** comparable to B cell's light chain
  - **Beta:** comparable to B cell's heavy chain
- **Antigen-binding site:** V, D, J protein segments coded by genes of same name
  - **Beta chain:** all three segments
  - **Alpha chain:** V, J segments

STAGES OF REARRANGEMENT

- Tracked by CD3, CD4, CD8 cell surface markers

Double negative/DN stage

- Common lymphoid progenitor initially $CD3^-$, $CD4^-$, $CD8^-$ (double negative/DN stage; broken down into DN1, DN2, DN3, DN4)
  - DN1 cell expresses RAG1, RAG2 → DN2 cell
  - Beta chain D, J gene segments spliced together (allelic exclusion) → DN3 cell
  - V gene segment combines with DJ gene segment by V(D)J recombinase → V-D-J gene segment bound to μ gene segment → DN4 cell
  - Functionality of beta chain tested by binding to invariant pre-T alpha chain → if successful, cells proliferate

Double positive/DP stage

- Daughter cells express CD3, CD4, CD8 (double positive/DP stage)

Single positive/SP stage

- **Central tolerance:** eliminates potentially self-reactive cells by positive, negative selection
  - Self-reactive cell elimination failure → autoimmunity
- Positive selection
  - T cells recognize/bind to self-MHC molecules
  - Binding failure → apoptosis
- Negative selection
  - **Autoimmune regulator gene (AIRE):** allows primary lymphoid organs to express antigens normally found throughout body; aids in testing self-reactivity
  - Excessively strong binding to self-antigens → apoptosis

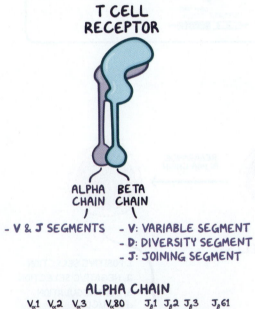

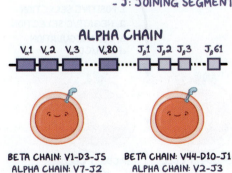

Figure 45.18 Structure of T cell receptor. Different combinations of V, D, and J segments provide T cell receptors with a wide variety of antigen specificities.

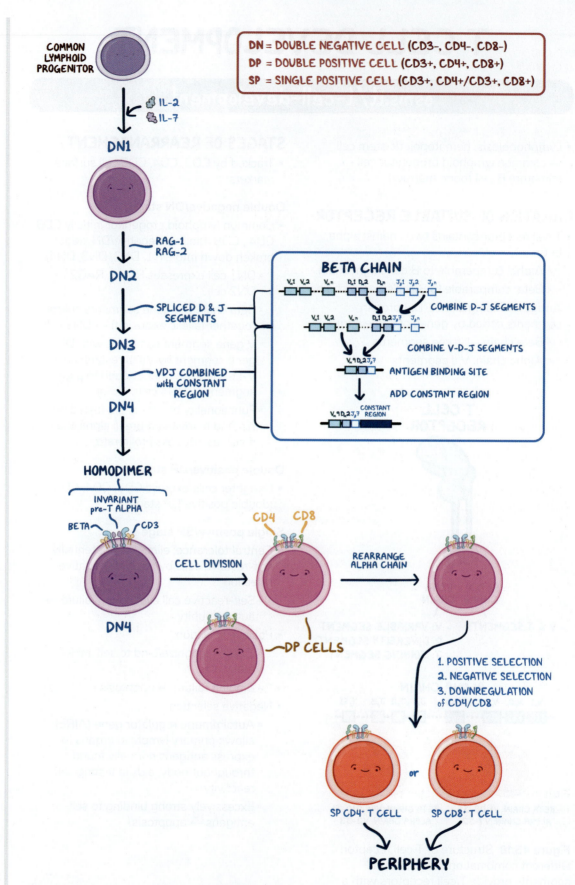

Figure 45.19 T cell development summary.

- DP cells recognize self-MHC but do not recognize self-antigen presented in MHC molecule → downregulate either CD4/CD8 receptor → further development into single positive (SP) cell
    - Strong binding to MHC → CD4 downregulated → SP CD8⁺ T cell
    - Weak binding to MHC → CD8 downregulated → SP CD4⁺ T cell

VDJ REARRANGEMENT

osms.it/VDJ-rearrangement

- Mechanism used to generate range of B, T cell receptors
- *Antigen-binding sites*: V, D, J protein segments coded by genes of same name
    - Each cell inherits multiple V, D, J segments → randomly recombine → recombinational inaccuracy, random assortment of two chains (heavy/beta chain rearranged first) → new specificities
- V(D)J rearrangement only affects V region (creates variability in hypervariable regions)

HEAVY/BETA CHAIN REARRANGEMENT

- Recombination signal sequence
    - Heptamer 5'-CACAGTC-3', 12, 23 nucleotides, nonamer 5'-ACAAAAACC-3'
    - DNA loops to bring together two recombination signal sequences
    - RAG1, RAG2 cut DNA at recombination signal sequence
    - Recombinases (e.g. ku, artemis) reattach, recombine DNA
- Error-prone process
    - Cut end placed onto terminal deoxynucleotide transferase (TdT) to add random nucleotides → alters antigen specificity
- Functionality of heavy chain tested → random assortment of chain

LIGHT CHAIN REARRANGEMENT

- Rearranged into kappa/lambda light chain (kappa rearranged before lambda)

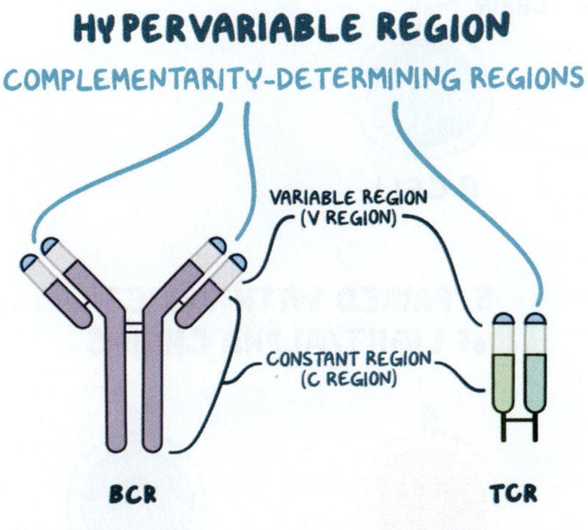

Figure 45.20 Locations of hypervariable regions on BCRs and TCRs affected by V(D)J rearrangement.

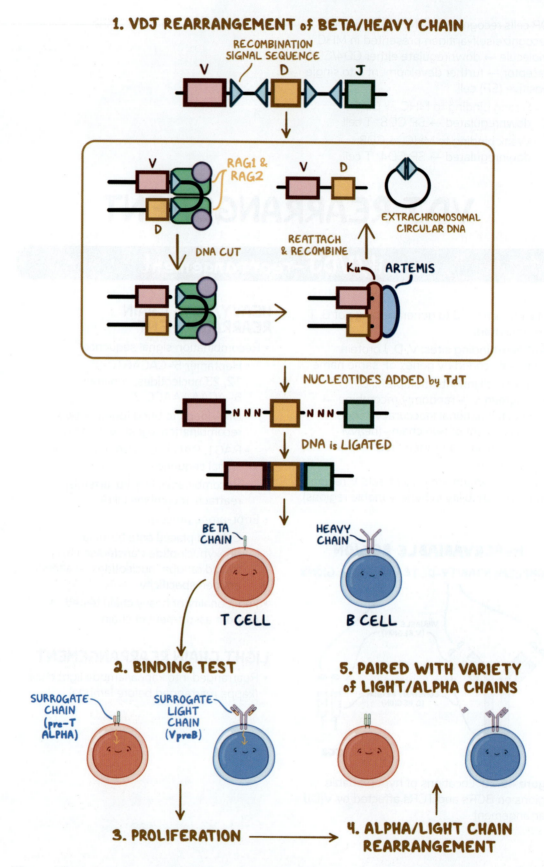

Figure 45.21 Summary of the process by which B and T cell receptors are made.

NOTES
CONTRACTION OF THE IMMUNE RESPONSE

ANERGY, EXHAUSTION, & CLONAL DELETION

osms.it/contracting-immune-response

CLONAL ANERGY

- Functional unresponsiveness to self antigens
- Lymphocytes can bind to antigens, without costimulation
- **T cells**: costimulation involves CD28 binding to B7 on antigen-presenting cells (APCs)
  - T regulatory cells reduce B7 expression on antigen presenting cells
  - Later in immune response, T cells begin to express cytotoxic T-lymphocyte associated protein 4 (CTLA-4) → binds to B7

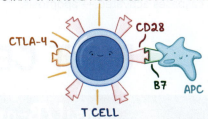

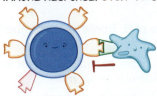

Figure 46.2 T cells express much more CTLA-4 later in immune response. B7 binds to CTLA-4 more strongly than it does to CD28 and inhibits T cell → T cell inactivation.

CLONAL EXHAUSTION

- Later in immune response, T cells begin to express program death 1 (PD-1)
- Program death ligand 1 (PD-L1) on antigen-presenting cells bind to PD-1 → T cells shut down

CLONAL DELETION

- Recognition of self antigens → T cell apoptosis (programmed cell death)
- Later in immune response, T cells express Fas
- Fas ligands on CD8+ T cells, NK cells bind to Fas → activate enzymes called caspases → apoptosis

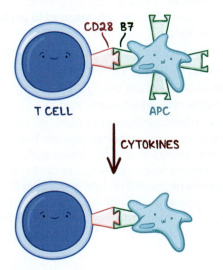

Figure 46.1 T regulatory cells reduce costimulation by releasing cytokines that reduce B7 expression on antigen-presenting cells (APCs).

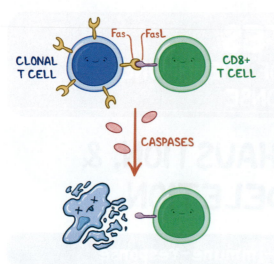

Figure 46.3 Clonal deletion. T cells express Fas → bind to Fas ligand on CD8+ T cell/NK cell → caspases activated → apoptosis.

B & T CELL MEMORY

osms.it/B-and-T-cell-memory

- Ability of B, T cells to "remember" particular antigen
  - B, T cells multiply when receptors detect particular antigen
  - After immune response mounted, excess cells undergo apoptosis
  - Memory B, T cells contain same receptors after immune response
- Immunologic memory → secondary (anamnestic) response
  - *Primary response*: naive B, T cells require activation before response to pathogen → high pathogen burden (response can take days, weeks)
  - *Secondary response*: memory B, T cells, antibodies needed to respond to pathogen already exist → low pathogen burden (response occurs right away)

MEMORY B CELLS
- Only B cells that have undergone class switching become memory B cells
  - Memory response limited to peptide antigens (not lipids/carbohydrates)—follicular T helper cells needed for class-switching only respond to peptide antigens
  - Memory B cells don't produce IgM/IgD
- Live up to 10 years in lymph nodes
- Often differentiate into IgG-producing plasma cells when reactivated
- Due to somatic hypermutation, IgG created late in immune response typically has higher affinity than IgM created early in immune response → IgG binds to Fc gamma receptor II on IgM-producing B cells, prevents differentiation into plasma cells → ↓ IgM production, ↑ IgG production

PRIMARY IMMUNE RESPONSE
B CELL ACTIVATION & CLASS SWITCHING

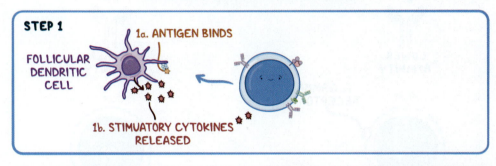

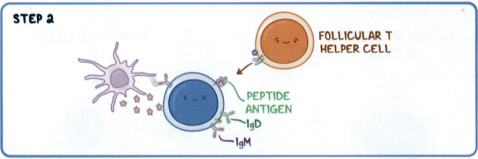

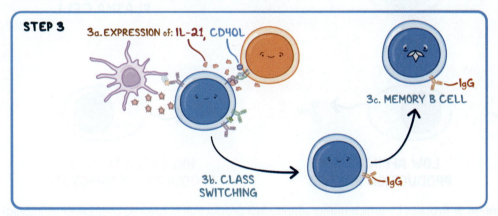

Figure 46.4 B cells are activated through interactions with other immune cells. **Step 1a:** follicular dendritic cell traps antigens and **1b:** sends out stimulatory cytokines. **Step 2:** the B cell presents the antigen to a follicular T helper cell. **Step 3a:** the follicular T helper cell expresses CD40L on its surface and produces IL-21. **3b:** together, they induce the B cell to undergo class switching (shift from expressing a B cell receptor with IgM and IgD to expressing IgG, IgE, or IgA. **3c:** some of these B cells become memory B cells.

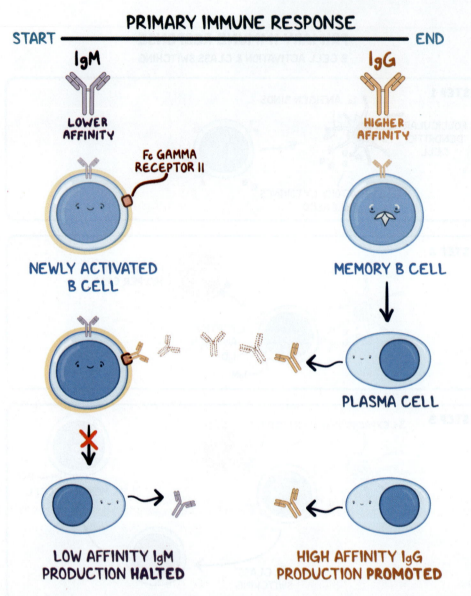

Figure 46.5 Process by which higher affinity IgG production is favored over lower affinity IgM production. Memory B cells differentiate into high affinity IgG-producing plasma cells. IgG binds to Fc gamma receptor II on newly activated B cells, which produce low affinity IgM. This prevents them from differentiating into low affinity IgM-producing plasma cells, allowing the proportion of high affinity IgG in the response to be greater.

MEMORY T CELLS
- Cell surface ligand CD45 used to identify T cells
  - Naive T cells express CD45A
  - Memory T cells express CD45O

Effector memory T cells
- Move around body looking for pathogens
- Respond as primary response (for CD4+ helper cells, secreting cytokines; for CD8+ cytotoxic cells, binding to, destroying target cells)
- IL-7 receptors replaced with IL-2 receptors during activation → cells die shortly after immune response

Central memory T cells
- Live up to 25 years
- Remain in lymphoid tissues
- High levels of IL-7 receptors maintained → cells live on after immune response

Chapter 46 Immunology: Contraction of the Immune Response

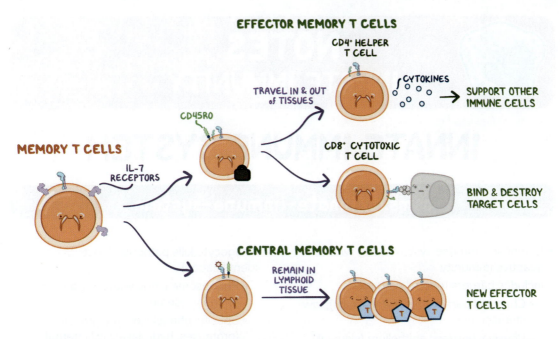

Figure 46.6 The two types of memory T cells (effector memory T cells and central memory T cells) and their functions.

CONTRACTING THE IMMUNE RESPONSE

osms.it/contracting-immune-response

- Immune response termination
- Peripheral tolerance to self antigens limits immune response (preventing autoimmune disease)
- Mechanisms directed primarily at T cells; includes use of T regulatory cells, clonal anergy, exhaustion, deletion

T REGULATORY CELLS

- Inhibit antigen-presenting cells by releasing specific molecules (e.g. indoleamine 2,3 dioxygenase)
- Release cytokines (e.g. IL-10, TGF-beta) → antigen-presenting cells express inhibitory ligand (e.g. PD-L1)
- Express high levels of IL-2, adenosine receptors (competing with other T cells)

B CELLS

- Similar mechanisms to T cells
- Later in immune response, reduced presence of antigens, T cells prevent B cell activation → anergy
- Surplus IgG binds to Fcγ II on B cells → prevent differentiation into plasma cells

NOTES
INNATE IMMUNITY

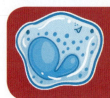

INNATE IMMUNE SYSTEM

osms.it/innate-immune-system

- Comprises immune system along with adaptive immunity
- Includes barriers to repel pathogens
    - *Chemical barriers*: lysozyme (tears), low stomach pH
    - *Physical barriers*: epithelium (skin/gut), cilia lining airways

Key features
- Nonspecific cells do not distinguish invaders
- Response occurs within minutes–hours
- No memory
    - Always responds to pathogen in same manner

Human microbiome
- Included in innate immunity
- Bacteria, fungi, viruses in/on humans
- May affect host response in own way

RESPONSE TO PATHOGENS

Phagocyte response to pathogens
- Phagocytes eat, kill pathogens
- Phagocyte consumes pathogen
    - Phagocytic pattern recognition receptors (PRRs) on phagocyte identify pathogen-associated molecular patterns (PAMPs) on pathogens (e.g. bacterial-wall components)
    - Phagocyte swallows pathogen, traps it in phagosome
- Phagocyte kills pathogen (post-identification)
    - Phagosome binds with lysosome, forms phagolysosome
    - Specific phagolysosome granules (proteases, hydrolases) kill internal microorganisms while decreasing pH
    - Azurophilic granules (hydrolases, oxidative enzymes) activate in acidic environment → more microorganisms killed
    - Nicotinamide adenine dinucleotide phosphate (NADPH) oxidases oxidize oxygen molecules → superoxide ion creation
    - Superoxide dismutase converts superoxide into hydrogen peroxide, killing remaining microorganisms

Signalling PRRs response to pathogens
- Large amount of pathogens enter → signalling pattern recognition receptors also activated
- Signalling PRRs → phagocytes to release cytokines
- Toll-like receptors (TLRs) especially important in signalling PRRs
    - PAMP activation → TLRs activate transcription factor NF-κB → proinflammatory cytokines (e.g. TNFα, IL-1β, IL-6) secreted → vasodilation, fever, recruiting leukocytes
    - *Intracellular pathogens*: interferon alpha, beta may be secreted (prevents pathogen multiplication)

Chapter 47 Immunology: Innate Immunity

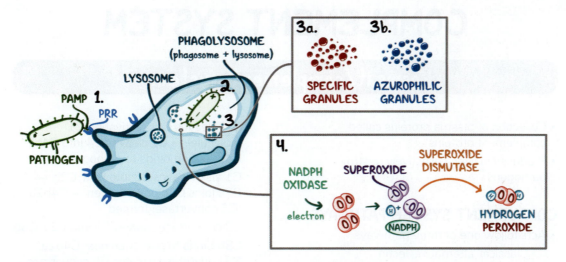

Figure 47.1 Overview of the phagocyte response to pathogens.
1. The phagocyte's pattern recognition receptors (PRRs) identify pathogen-associated molecular patterns (PAMPs) on the pathogen.
2. The pathogen is phagocytosed and trapped in a phagosome, which then
3. binds with lysosomes, forming a phagolysosome.
3a. Specific granules from the lysosomes act first to kill pathogens and decrease pH.
3b. After the pH is sufficiently lowered, azurophilic granules are activated and kill more pathogens.
4. NADPH oxidases oxidize oxygen molecules to create superoxide ions. The ions are then converted by superoxide dismutase into hydrogen peroxide, which kill the remaining pathogens.

COMPLEMENT SYSTEM

osms.it/complement-system

- Collection of plasma proteins called complement proteins
- Produced in liver, collectively destroy pathogens

COMPLEMENT SYSTEM PATHWAYS

- Acts follow one of three pathways
  - Classical, alternative, lectin

Classical pathway

- Features C1–C9 proteins
- C1
  - Component proteins C1q, C1r, C1s (latter two—serine proteases)

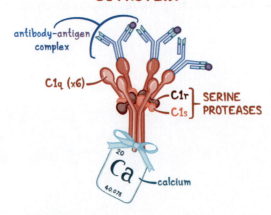

Figure 47.2 Structure of a C1 protein. Each of the six C1q proteins can bind to an antibody-antigen complex. Calcium ties the protein together.

- Proteins inactive until "cleaved" (portion of protein breaks off)
- Pathway steps
  - C1q proteins bind to Fc portion of antibody when bound to antigen
  - Two C1q proteins bind → C1 changes shapes (conformational change) exposing C1r, C1s
  - C1r cleaves C1s (activating C1 molecule) → C1 cleaves C4 into C4a, C4b → C4b binds to pathogen
  - C1 also cleaves C2 into C2a, C2b → C2a joins C4b on pathogen → C4b2a (C3 convertase) formed
  - C3 convertase cleaves C3 into C3a, C3b
  - C3b binds to pathogen near C4b2a/ C3 convertase, creates C5 convertase (C4b2a3b)
  - C5 convertase cleaves C5 into C5a, C5b
  - C5b binds to C6, C7, C8, many C9s → forms membrane attack complex (MAC) → penetrates pathogen cell membrane
- C1 consists of six C1q proteins
  - Binds to six antibody-antigen complexes
- Calcium ties together C1
  - Lack of calcium → lack of C1

Alternative pathway

- Factor B, factor D proteins
- C3 cleaved spontaneously (small amounts)
- Pathway steps
  - C3b binds to pathogen → factor B binds to pathogen
  - Factor D cleaves factor B → forms Ba, Bb → C3bBb formed (C3 convertase)
  - Follows classical pathway
- Constant activation prevention
  - C1-inhibitor protein dissociates C3bBb

Lectin pathway

- Features mannose-binding lectin protein (binds to bacterial mannose)
- Pathway steps
  - Mannose-binding lectin protein acts similar to C1 → cleaves C4, C2 to eventually establish C4b2a (C3 convertase)
  - Follows classical pathway

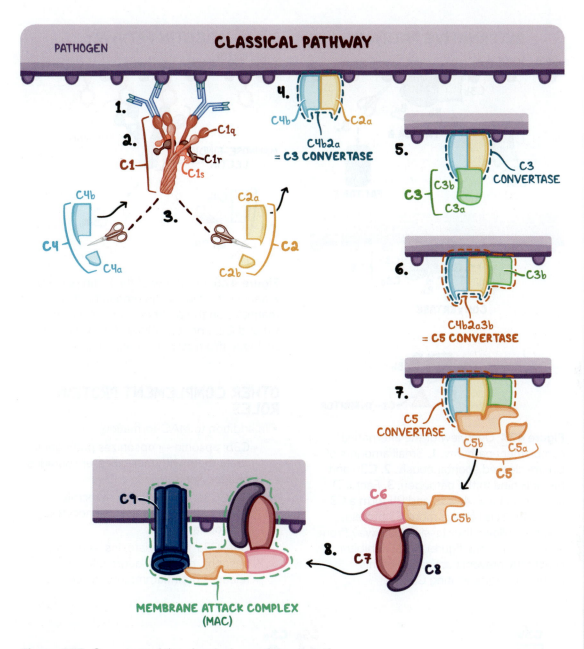

Figure 47.3 Overview of the classical complement pathway.
1. C1q binds to an antibody-antigen complex.
2. When two C1q proteins are bound, C1 undergoes a conformational change, exposing C1r and C1s. C1r then cleaves C1s to activate C1.
3. C1 cleaves C4 and C2.
4. C4 and C2 bind to the surface of the pathogen, forming C3 convertase.
5. C3 convertase cleaves C3.
6. C3b binds to the pathogen near the C3 convertase, forming C5 convertase.
7. C5 convertase cleaves C5.
8. C5b joins C6, C7, C8, and then multiple C9s to form the membrane attack complex, penetrating the pathogen cell membrane.

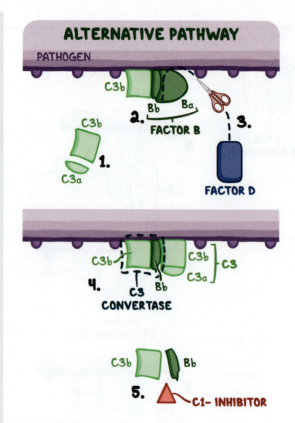
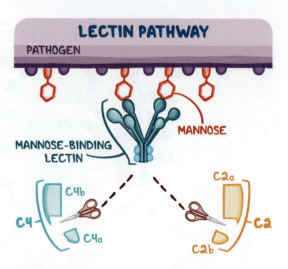

Figure 47.4 Overview of the alternative complement pathway. **1.** Small amounts of C3 are cleaved spontaneously. **2.** C3b and factor B bind to the pathogen. **3.** Factor D cleaves factor B. **4.** C3b and Bb form a C3 convertase and cleave more C3 proteins. The rest follows the classical pathway (from step 6 in previous figure). **5.** C1-inhibitor constantly prevents activation of this pathway by dissociating C3bBb.

Figure 47.5 Overview of the lectin pathway. Mannose-binding lectin protein binds to mannose on the pathogen, then cleaves C4 and C2. The rest follows the classical pathway (from step 4 in earlier figure).

OTHER COMPLEMENT PROTEIN ROLES

- In addition to MAC-formation
    - C3b: opsonin → opsonizes pathogens, coats them with molecules, encourages phagocytosis
    - C5a, C3a: chemotaxins → recruit neutrophils, eosinophils, monocytes, macrophages
    - C5a, C3a: anaphylatoxins → cause basophil, mast cell degranulation, releases proinflammatory molecules

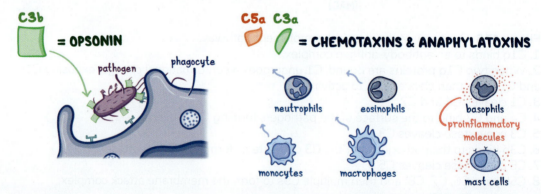

Figure 47.6 Other roles of complement proteins. C3b acts as an opsonin; it coats pathogens to facilitate phagocytosis. C5a and C3a act as chemotaxins; they recruit neutrophils, eosinophils, monocytes, and macrophages. C5a and C3a also act as anaphylatoxins; they cause basophils and mast cells to degranulate.

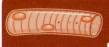

NOTES
BONES, JOINTS, & CARTILAGE

SKELETAL SYSTEM ANATOMY & PHYSIOLOGY

osms.it/skeletal-system-anatomy-physiology

SKELETAL BASICS
- 206 bones in skeleton
- Separated into axial, appendicular skeleton

Axial skeleton
- Vertical axis of body; 80 bones (22 in skull, 33 vertebrae, 24 ribs, 1 sternum)

Appendicular skeleton
- Supports limbs; pectoral girdle (clavicles, scapulae) holds humeri, pelvic girdle (hip bones) holds femora; 126 bones (4 in shoulders, 6 arms, 54 hands, 2 hips, 8 legs, 52 feet)

TYPES OF BONES

Long bones
- Length > width
- Humerus, radius, ulna (in arms); metacarpals, phalanges (hands, fingers); femur, tibia, fibula (legs); metatarsals, phalanges (feet, toes)
- Primarily responsible for height

Short bones
- Similar length, width
- Carpal bones (in wrists); tarsal bones (ankles)
- Support hands, feet

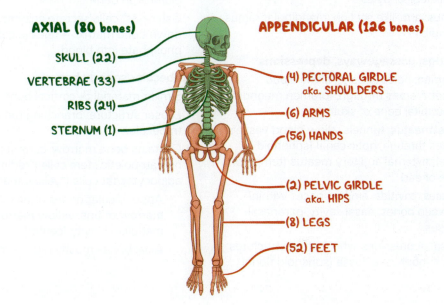

Figure 48.1 Overview of skeleton.

Flat bones
- Thin, sometimes curved
- Skull bones; scapulae, sternum, ribs
- Protect vital organs

Sesamoid bones
- Embedded in tendons, shaped like giant sesame seeds
- Pisiform bone (in wrists); patella (knees)
- Support, protect, give additional leverage to tendons

Irregular bones
- Facial bones; mandible; vertebrae; sacrum, coccyx

SURFACE FEATURES OF BONES

Sites of muscle, ligament attachment
- *Tubercle, tuberosity:* small bumps on bone, serve as attachment sites for muscles; large tubercle → tuberosity; deltoid tuberosity (on humerus)
- *Process:* bony prominence; xiphoid process (sternum)
- *Crest:* narrow ridge; iliac crest (ilium)

Projections
- Part of joints
- *Condyle:* rounded, articular projection; lateral, medial condyles (femur); epicondyle → raised portion on/above condyle (lateral, medial epicondyles)
- *Ramus:* arm-like section; mandibular ramus (mandible)

Openings, passageways, depressions
- *Foramen:* holes in bone, allow blood vessels/nerves through; foramen magnum (in occipital bone of skull)
- *Canal/meatus:* tunnels, allow blood vessels/nerves through; optic canal (sphenoid bone); external auditory meatus (temporal bone of ear)
- *Sinuses, cavities:* empty spaces within/between bones; nasal cavity, paranasal sinuses
- *Fossa:* depressions where other structures rest; hypophyseal fossa (sphenoid bone)

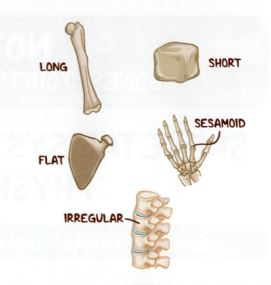

Figure 48.2 Types of bones.

STRUCTURE OF BONE

Cortical/compact bone
- Surrounded by periosteum
- Contains pipe-like structures called osteons
- Osteons contain hollow centers (Haversian canals) for nerves, blood cells; connected laterally by Volkmann's canals
- Osteon walls made of bone matrix (type I collagen reinforced with hydroxyapatite), produced by osteoblast cells
- Some osteoblasts get trapped in bone matrix → mature into osteocytes → repair old/broken bone
- Osteoclast cells secrete enzymes → break down bone matrix → release calcium, phosphate into blood

Trabecular/spongy bone
- Similar material to cortical bone
- Looser structure; branching rods called trabeculae
- Contains bone marrow, consists of hematopoietic stem cells ("red marrow"), adipocytes/fat cells ("yellow marrow")
  - Appendicular bones often contain red marrow at tips, yellow marrow in hollow medullary cavity (center)
  - Axial bones mostly red marrow

Chapter 48 Musculoskeletal Physiology: Bones, Joints, & Cartilage

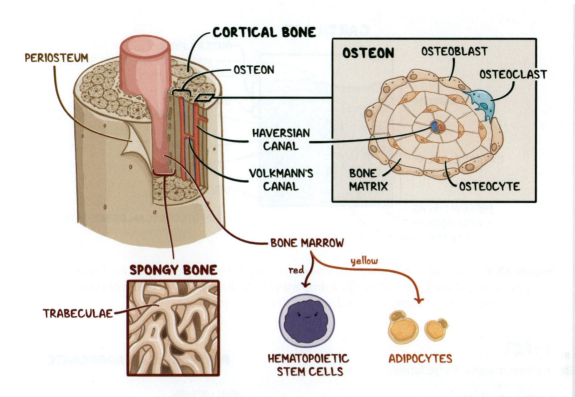

Figure 48.3 Bone cross-section showing structure which consists of cortical bone and spongy bone. Spongy bone contains two types of bone marrow, each made up of a different kind of cell.

CARTILAGE

osms.it/cartilage

WHAT IS CARTILAGE?
- Strong, flexible connective tissue
    - Comprises part of nose, ears
    - Provides cushioning between joints
    - Supports/connects body parts (e.g. costal cartilage connects ribs to sternum)
- **Perichondrium:** connective tissue that wraps around cartilage
    - Outer layer contains fibrous connective tissue, blood vessels
    - Inner layer contains chondroblasts → secrete proteins that make extracellular matrix
- **Extracellular matrix:** protein fibers (collagen for strength; elastin for flexibility) suspended in viscous gel (water, proteoglycan aggregates)
    - **Chondrocytes:** chondroblasts trapped in lacunae (small holes) of matrix; maintain, repair extracellular matrix
    - **Proteoglycan aggregates:** hyaluronan (long chain of hyaluronic acid molecules) with hundreds of proteoglycans (proteins + long chains of glycosaminoglycan sugars—GAGS) branching off

OSMOSIS.ORG 407

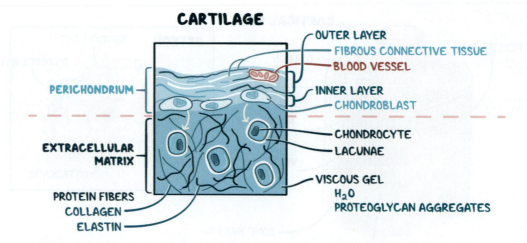

Figure 48.4 Cross-section through cartilage showing its histological structure. Perichondrium wraps around extracellular matrix. Chondroblasts originally in perichondrium become chondrocytes as they become trapped in the extracellular matrix.

TYPES
- Three main cartilage types

Elastic cartilage
- Least common type
- ↑ chondrocyte density; ↓ protein fiber density (mostly loose elastin fibers, some type II collagen fibers)
- Softest, most flexible cartilage
- Ear pinnae, throat epiglottis

Hyaline cartilage
- Most common type
- Medium chondrocyte density; medium protein fiber density (mostly type II collagen fibers, some loose elastin fibers)
- Stronger, but less flexible cartilage; ↓ friction surface
- Embryonic skeleton (eventually replaced by bone); nose; larynx walls; tracheal, costal cartilages; growth plates; articular cartilages

Fibrocartilage
- ↓ chondrocyte density; ↑ protein fiber density (mostly type I collagen fibers)
- Most tensile strength; resistant to compression, stretching; ↓ flexible
- Meniscus of knee, spinal intervertebral discs

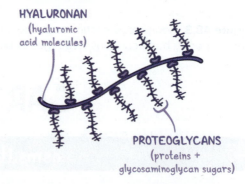

Figure 48.5 Proteoglycan aggregate, found in viscous gel of the extracellular matrix.

Chapter 48 Musculoskeletal Physiology: Bones, Joints, & Cartilage

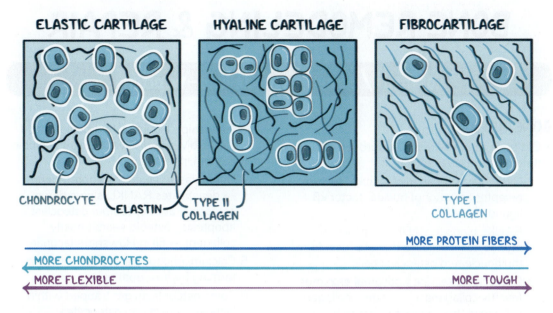

Figure 48.6 Histology, characteristics of the three main cartilage types.

GROWTH PATTERNS
- Two cartilage growth patterns
- Both growth patterns present in growing bones of children, teenagers (e.g. femur)
  - Chondrocytes in growth plate → interstitial growth → cartilage lengthens → **osteoblasts turn cartilage into bone**
  - Articular cartilage on tips of bone experience both appositional, interstitial growth

Appositional growth
- Chondroblasts secrete new matrix on existing surfaces → cartilage expands, widens

Interstitial growth
- Chondrocytes secrete new matrix within cartilage → cartilage grows in length

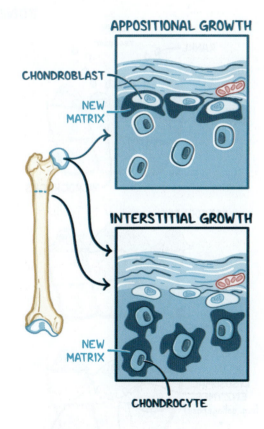

Figure 48.7 The two cartilage growth patterns. Both types of growth occur in articular cartilage. In the growth plate, only interstitial growth occurs.

BONE REMODELING & REPAIR

osms.it/bone-remodeling-repair

BONE REPAIR
- Old bone removed/resorbed (broken down) before new tissue replaces it
 1. **Osteoblasts** sense microcracks, secrete receptor activator of nuclear factor κβ ligand (RANKL)
 2. RANKL binds to RANK receptors on monocytes → causes them to fuse, form multinucleated **osteoclast cells**
 3. **Osteoclasts secrete** lysosomal enzymes (mostly **collagenase**) → digest collagen in bone matrix → create surface holes (Howship's lacunae), hydrochloric acid → dissolves hydroxyapatite into soluble calcium, phosphate
 4. Osteoblasts secrete **osteoprotegerin** → **deactivates RANKL, slows down** osteoclast activity (before osteoclast apoptosis), osteoid seam (mostly collagen) → fill in Howship's lacunae
 5. Calcium, phosphate deposit on seam forming hydroxyapatite
 6. Some osteoblasts get trapped within lacunae → turn into osteocytes

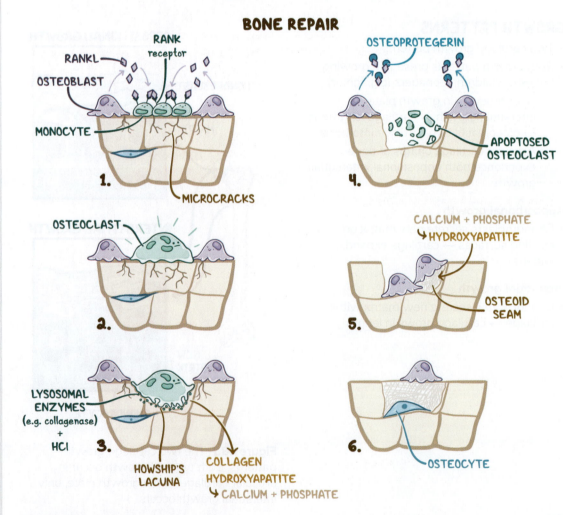

Figure 48.8 Summary of bone repair.

REMODELING FACTORS

- Hormonal
  - Parathyroid hormone enhances bone resorption
  - Calcitonin inhibits bone resorption
  - Vitamin D (→ ↓ calcitonin) enhances bone resorption
- Mechanical (physical stress)
  - Wolff's law: bones that bear more weight remodel more

FIBROUS, CARTILAGE, & SYNOVIAL JOINTS

osms.it/fibrous-cartilage-synovial-joints

TYPES

- Classification based on movement of three main groups
  - Fibrous joints: no movement
  - Cartilaginous joints: some movement
  - Synovial joints: freely movable

FIBROUS JOINTS

- Synarthrosis/fixed joints
- Bones are connected by ligaments

Three main categories (based on location)

- Sutures: junctions between adjacent skull bones; Sharpey's fibers connect bones; fixed (non-fused in babies → partially movable)
- Gomphoses: peg-and-socket joints for teeth; periodontal ligaments connect roots of teeth to sockets; slightly movable
- Syndesmoses: remaining fibrous joints; connected by interosseous membrane (e.g. between radius, ulna); slightly movable

FIBROUS JOINTS

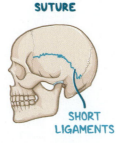
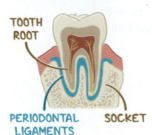
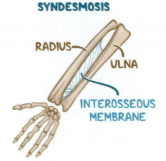

Figure 48.9 Three main categories of fibrous joints.

CARTILAGINOUS JOINTS

- Hyaline cartilage connects bones, stretches to allow some movement
- *Synchondrosis*: costochondral joint, where cartilage attaches rib to sternum; growth plates between bone diaphysis, epiphysis
- *Symphysis*: symphysis pubis in pelvic bone (fibrous cartilage)
    - ↑ strength, ↓ flexibility

SYNOVIAL JOINTS

- Joint capsule connects bones
    - Composed of outer fibrous capsule, inner synovial membrane
    - Filled with synovial fluid: lubricates joint, absorbs shock; made of hyaluronic acid, lubricin, proteinases, collagenases
    - Articular cartilage covers tips of bones (same function)
- Allow for abduction, adduction, rotation about axis

Six main categories (based on structure, movement)

- *Hinge joints*: allow movement only in one axis (e.g. between humerus, ulna)
- *Pivot joints*: allow for rotation (e.g. between head of radius, groove of ulna)
- *Plane (gliding) joints*: allow flat bones to glide across one another (e.g. in carpal, tarsal bones)
- *Ball and socket joints*: allow all movements (e.g. shoulder joint)
- *Condyloid (ellipsoid) joints*: allow most movements, but not rotation (e.g. metacarpophalangeal, metatarsophalangeal joints)
- *Saddle joints*: allow most movements, with limited rotation (e.g. carpometacarpal joint)

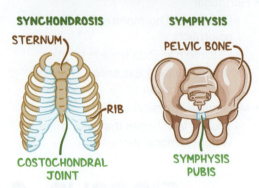

Figure 48.10 The two categories of cartilaginous joints (with examples).

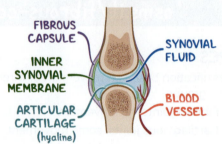

Figure 48.11 Synovial joint cross-section showing joint capsule.

Chapter 48 Musculoskeletal Physiology: Bones, Joints, & Cartilage

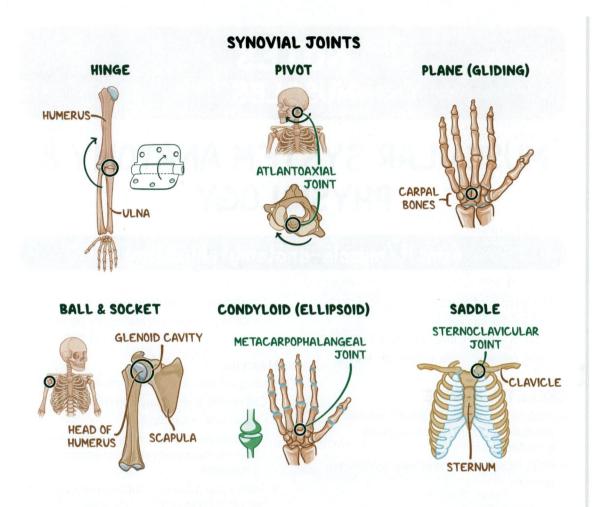

Figure 48.12 The six categories of synovial joints (with examples). Joints circled in green.

NOTES MUSCLES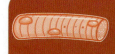

MUSCULAR SYSTEM ANATOMY & PHYSIOLOGY

osms.it/muscle-anatomy-physiology

- Three types of muscle cell/tissue
    - Skeletal, cardiac, smooth
- Differ in location, innervation, cell structure
    - All cells excitable, extensible, elastic

SKELETAL MUSCLE

- Attaches to bone/skin; mostly voluntary; maintains posture, stabilizes joints, generates heat
- Most muscles consist of belly (contracts), tendons

Connective tissue

- Layers of connective tissue separate muscle belly
    - *Epimysium:* wrapped around muscle
    - *Perimysium:* wrapped around fascicles in muscle
    - *Endomysium:* wrapped around muscle fibers/cells (e.g. myocytes in fascicles)

- Combine at end to form tendons
    - Origin attaches to stationary bone; insertion attaches to moving bone

Myocytes

- Long cylindrical cells with multiple nuclei
- Cell membrane → sarcolemma
- Cytoplasm → sarcoplasm
    - Contains smooth endoplasmic reticulum → sarcoplasmic reticulum (stores calcium)
- Transverse tubules (T tubules) project from sarcolemma to center of muscle
- Long filaments called myofibrils fill sarcoplasm, contain thin actin filaments, thick myosin filaments (arranged into sarcomeres)

Motor signals

- Brain's motor signals control skeletal system
- Motor neurons release acetylcholine receptors onto sarcolemma → rapid ion shifts across sarcolemma, down T tubules → calcium enters myocyte → sarcoplasmic reticulum releases calcium into sarcoplasm → actin, myosin bind → sarcomeres contract → myocyte contracts → sarcoplasmic reticulum grabs calcium → muscle relaxes

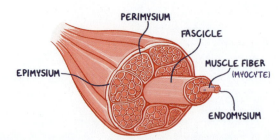

Figure 49.1 Cross section of skeletal muscle illustrating connective tissue layers, fascicles, muscle fibers.

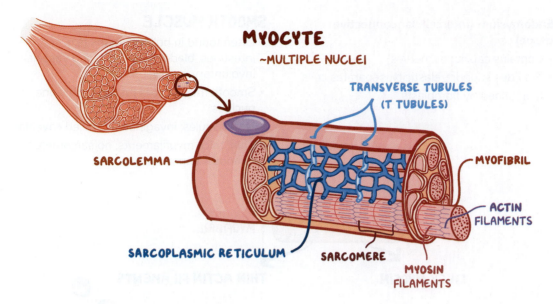

Figure 49.2 Composition of a myocyte.

CARDIAC MUSCLE

- Involuntary, striated muscle; found only in heart walls
- Shorter than skeletal muscle; branched and interconnected
- 1–2 central nuclei per fiber
- Numerous mitochondria provide resistance to fatigue
- Pacemaker cells demonstrate automaticity; generate action potentials

Intercalated discs

- Composed of gap junctions and desmosomes
    - *Gap junctions*: areas of low resistance, allows fast signal propagation between cardiomyocytes (coordinated contraction of cells)
    - *Desmosomes*: anchor the cells together; keeps cells from pulling apart during contraction
    - Allows heart to work as a unit (functional syncytium; syn = together, citos = cell)

T tubules/transverse tubules

- Invaginate from sarcolemma
- Also serve faster propagation
    - Help conduct signal deeper into cell, enabling more synchronized contraction
    - Run along Z bands, communicate with sarcoplasmic reticulum (Ca^{2+} storage)

Thick and thin filaments

- Like skeletal muscle, cardiac myofibrils contain sarcomeres bounded by Z bands
    - *Z bands*: perpendicular to myofibril, attached to thin filaments
    - Thick filaments lie between Z bands
    - All proteins involved are globular
- Thick, thin filaments slide over each other → contraction

Thick filaments

- *Myosin*: tail with two heads
    - Each head has ATPase, actin binding sites

Thin filaments

- *Actin*: globular/G-actin polymerizes into a strand of filamentous/F-actin
    - Two F-actins twist into strand with myosin binding site
- *Tropomyosin*: site blocker, prevents contraction by disabling attachment of myosin to actin
- *Troponin*: molecule composed of three subunits:
    - *C*: Ca^{2+} binding → stops troponin inhibition of actin
    - *I*: Inhibitory → inhibits ATPase
    - *T*: → relaxed state attachment of troponin complex to actin; myocardial infarction marker in blood

Endomysium (intercellular connective tissue)
- Contains capillaries, nerves
- Provides support, elasticity; separates cells
- Maintained by fibroblasts

SMOOTH MUSCLE
- Often found in hollow organs (e.g. intestines, bladder, uterus, blood vessels); involuntary muscle
- Smooth muscle cells fusiform, only one nucleus
- No T tubules; invaginations called caveolae
- Thin, thick myofilaments; no sarcomeres → "smooth" appearance

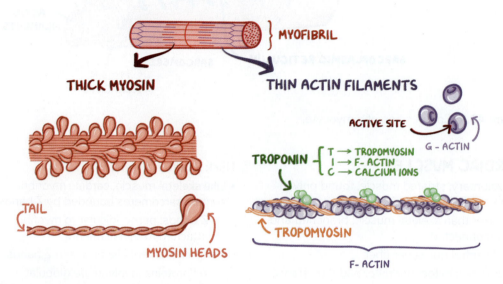

Figure 49.3 Appearance of myosin and actin filaments.

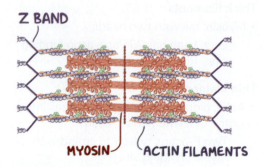

Figure 49.4 Z bands are the boundaries between sarcomeres in skeletal and cardiac muscles.

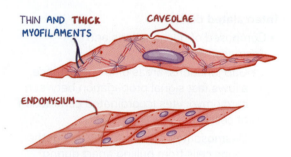

Figure 49.5 Features of smooth muscle cells.

TYPES OF MUSCLE

	SKELETAL	SMOOTH	CARDIAC
LOCATION	Attached to bones	Forms walls of hollow organs Lines blood vessels, glands	Heart
NEUROLOGICAL CONTROL	Voluntary Involuntary (reflexes, shivering) Innervation: somatic nervous system Neurotransmitter: ACh	Involuntary Innervation: autonomic nervous system Neurotransmitter: ACh, NE Also regulated by hormones (e.g. oxytocin), locally-produced substances (e.g. histamine) Autorhythmicity (e.g. visceral smooth muscle in digestive tract) Contracts in response to being stretched	Involuntary Innervation: autonomic nervous system Neurotransmitter: ACh Autorhythmicity: pacemaker cells
FUNCTIONS	Movement, posture, stabilization of body Shivering thermogenesis Voluntary control of micturition (external sphincter)	Wide distribution Digestive tract: movement of food Urinary: bladder emptying Vascular: vessel diameter Sensory: pupil size changes Endocrine: contraction of glands	Propulsion of blood
CELL CHARACTERISTICS	Long, cylindrical, striated	Spindle-shaped	Cylindrical, striated, branched
NUCLEUS	Multiple	One, centrally located	One, centrally located
SPECIAL CELL-TO-CELL CHARACTERISTICS	None	Gap junctions in some visceral cells	Intercalated discs Desmosomes Gap junctions

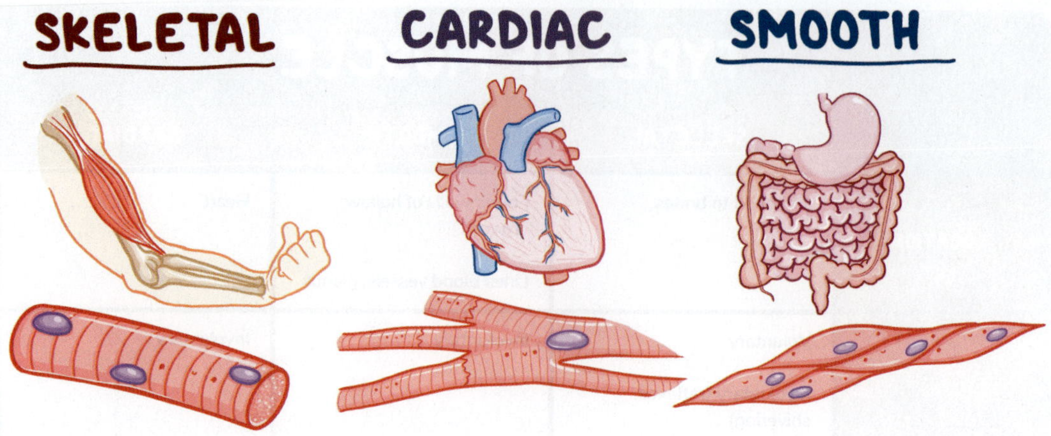

SKELETAL **CARDIAC** **SMOOTH**

Figure 49.6 An illustration of the three types of muscle: skeletal, cardiac, and smooth.

SLOW TWITCH & FAST TWITCH MUSCLE FIBERS

osms.it/slow-fast-twitch-muscle-fibers

- Each action potential generates brief muscle contraction (AKA twitch)
- Twitches overlap to create longer, smooth muscle contractions

Skeletal muscle fibers
- Slow twitch (AKA slow oxidative)
- Fast twitch (AKA fast oxidative, fast glycolytic)
- Slow twitch fibers → slow-functioning ATPases → slower individual twitches
- Fast twitch fibers → fast-functioning ATPases → longer individual twitches

SLOW OXIDATIVE FIBERS
- AKA Type I fibers
- Have aerobic respiration pathway for metabolizing glucose
- Relatively small → weakest contractions
- ↑ blood vessels, ↑ myoglobin → red color
  - AKA "slow red muscle fibers"
- ↑↑ mitochondria supports aerobic respiration
- Generate lots of ATP, use little; ↓ glycogen storage
- Sustain muscle ability for long time

FAST OXIDATIVE FIBERS
- AKA Type IIa fibers
- Have aerobic respiration pathway for metabolizing glucose
- Larger than slow fibers → stronger contractions
- ↑ blood vessels, ↑ myoglobin → red color
  - AKA "fast red muscle fibers"
- ↑↑ mitochondria supports aerobic respiration
- Generate lots of ATP, use more; ↑ glycogen storage
- Fatigue quickly

FAST GLYCOLYTIC FIBERS
- AKA Type IIx fibers
- Have anaerobic respiration pathway for metabolizing glucose
- Largest fibers → stronger contractions
- ↓ blood vessels, ↓ myoglobin → white color
  - AKA "white muscle fibers"
- ↓ mitochondria
- Generate little ATP, use lots; ↑↑ glycogen storage
- Fatigue fastest

SLIDING FILAMENT MODEL OF MUSCLE CONTRACTION

osms.it/sliding-filament-model

MECHANISM OF MUSCLE CONTRACTION AFTER POWER STROKE

- Thick myosin filaments pull thin actin filaments towards M-line → sarcomere shortens; A-band of the muscle does not change, but H-, I-bands shorten
- At max contraction, almost complete overlap of thick, thin filaments; H-, I- bands almost completely gone

FACTORS DETERMINING CONTRACTION FORCE

Size of muscle fibers
- Larger muscle fibers → ↑ filaments → ↑ cross-bridges → stronger contraction

Number of active muscle fibers
- ↑ muscle fibers → stronger contraction

Frequency of stimulation (force-frequency relationship)
- ↑ frequency of stimulation → ↑ calcium ions flow from sarcoplasmic reticulum into sarcoplasm → ↑ bind to troponin regulatory proteins on actin filaments → ↑ myosin binding → stronger contraction

Length of sarcomere
- AKA length-tension relationship
- Longer sarcomere → stronger contraction; directly proportional

Velocity of muscle shortening
- AKA force-velocity relationship
- Slower contraction → stronger contraction

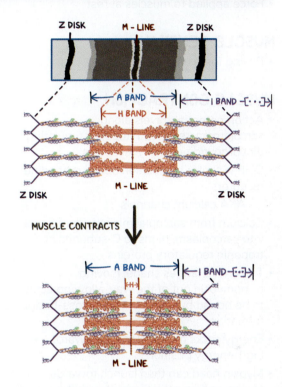

Figure 49.7 The changes that occur when muscle contracts.

ATP & MUSCLE CONTRACTION

osms.it/ATP-and-muscle-contraction

MUSCLE TONE
- Force applied to muscles at rest

MUSCLE TENSION
- Pulling force when muscles act

MUSCLE CONTRACTION
- Action potential travels along sarcolemma, reaches T-tubule, stimulating dihydropyridine (DHP) receptors
- DHP receptor stimulation opens ryanodine receptors
  - AKA calcium channels
- Calcium from sarcoplasmic reticulum flows into sarcoplasm, binds to C-subunits of troponin regulatory proteins
- Troponin changes shape, moving tropomyosin out of the way, allowing actin to be bound by myosin head's cross-bridge formation
- Energy cocks myosin head backwards → high-energy position
- Myosin head can then launch towards M-line, pulling actin filament with it
  - AKA power stroke
- Action potential ends → calcium ions pumped back into sarcoplasmic reticulum → C-subunit of troponin no longer bound → troponin, tropomyosin cover back up actin's active sites → no myosin binding (cross-bridge detaches) → muscle relaxes

ISOTONIC VS. ISOMETRIC CONTRACTIONS
- **Isotonic:** muscle length changes but tension stays same
- **Isometric:** muscle length stays same but tension increases

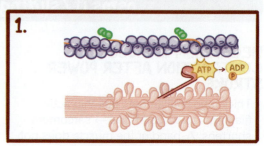
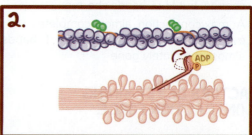
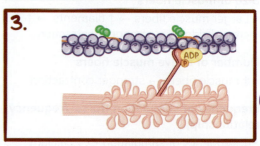
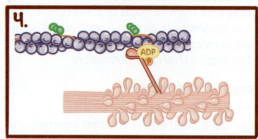

Figure 49.8 Muscle contraction.
1: Part of myosin head is an ATPase; it cleaves ATP into ADP and phosphate ion.
2: Myosin head uses this energy to tip back into its high-energy position.
3: Myosin head binds to active site on actin, triggering release of stored energy in myosin head.
4: Power stroke (myosin head launches, pulling actin with it).

NEUROMUSCULAR JUNCTION & MOTOR UNIT

osms.it/neuromuscular-junction-motor-unit

NEUROMUSCULAR JUNCTION
- Where axon terminal meets muscle fiber
- Presynaptic membrane
  - Membrane of axon terminal
- Postsynaptic membrane
  - AKA motor end plate
  - Membrane of skeletal muscle fiber
- Synaptic cleft
  - Gap between membranes

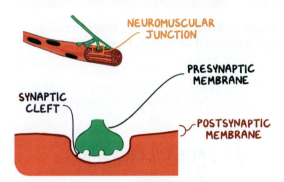

Figure 49.9 Illustration of the neuromuscular junction.

ACTION POTENTIAL GENERATION IN MUSCLE FIBER
- Action potentials in axon terminal stimulate voltage-gated calcium channels in presynaptic membrane → extracellular calcium ions flow into the axon terminal
- Calcium binds to acetylcholine-containing vesicles in axon terminal → vesicles fuse with presynaptic membrane, acetylcholine released into synaptic cleft
- Two acetylcholine molecules bind to one ligand gated ion channel
  - AKA nicotinic receptor
  - On motor end plate → sodium ions flow into muscle
- Positive charge builds up inside muscle fiber → creates end plate potential
  - AKA depolarization
- Resting potential of membrane: -100mV → -60mV
- Voltage-gated sodium channels open up → more sodium ions flow in, generating action potential in muscle fiber

ACTION POTENTIAL CESSATION IN MUSCLE FIBER
- Action potential in axon stops → voltage-gated calcium channels close → influx of calcium ions to axon terminal stops → synaptic vesicles stop fusing with membrane
- Remaining acetylcholine in cleft degraded by acetylcholinesterase into choline, acetate → choline taken back into axon terminal → acetylcholine transferase makes new acetylcholine → acetate diffuses away

MOTOR UNITS
- One lower motor neuron, fibers it innervates form single motor unit
- On average, one lower motor neuron innervates 150 skeletal muscle fibers
- More precise muscles → smaller motor units; e.g. 10–15 muscle fibers per neuron in eye
- Less precise muscles → larger motor units (e.g. ≤ 2000 muscle fibers per neuron in bicep)

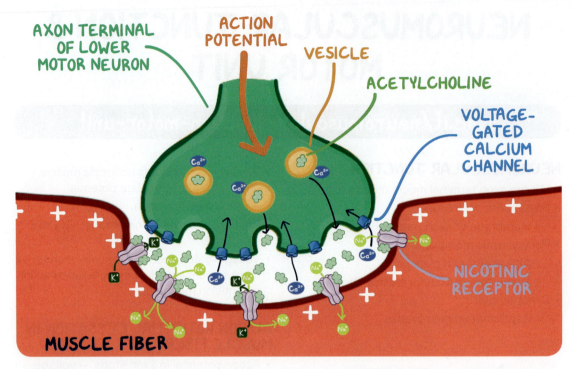

Figure 49.10 Action potential generation in muscle fiber. Influx of sodium ions leads to buildup of positive charge inside muscle fiber. Action potential generated → muscle fiber contracts.

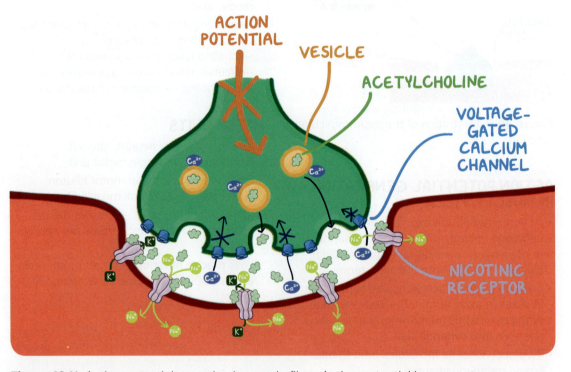

Figure 49.11 Action potential cessation in muscle fiber. Action potential in axons stops → voltage-gated calcium channels close → influx of calcium stops → synaptic vesicles stop fusing with membrane.

NERVOUS SYSTEM ANATOMY & PHYSIOLOGY

osms.it/nervous-system-anatomy-physiology

THE NERVOUS SYSTEM
- Network of brain, spinal cords, nerves
- Sensory/afferent, integrative, motor/efferent functions

Sensory/afferent
- Receptors monitor external, internal environment
  - Conscious stimuli (e.g. vision, hearing, touch)
  - Unconscious stimuli (e.g. pH, blood pressure)

Integrative
- Sensory/afferent input received by central nervous system → information processed → interpreted → response initiated

Motor/efferent
- Brings motor information from central nervous system to periphery
- Controls actions of effector organs (e.g. muscles, glands)

ORGANIZATION OF THE NERVOUS SYSTEM

Central nervous system (CNS)
- Brain, spinal cord

Peripheral nervous system (PNS)
- Nerves connect PNS with CNS
- Includes 12 pairs of cranial nerves, 31 pairs of spinal nerves
- Efferent (motor), afferent (sensory) divisions
  - Efferent divided into somatic (voluntary), autonomic (involuntary) nervous systems
  - Autonomic nervous system comprised of sympathetic, parasympathetic nervous systems
- *Sensory receptors*: structure at nerve ending; detects physical, environmental stimulus; e.g. pain, temperature
- *Ganglia/ganglion (plural/singular)*: collection of neuron cell bodies outside CNS
- *Plexuses/plexus (plural/singular)*: network of nerves outside CNS

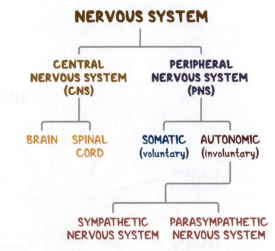

Figure 50.1 Organization of the nervous system.

CELLS OF THE NERVOUS SYSTEM: NEURON

- Specialized, excitable cell; receives, transmits signals, AKA action potentials
- Very long longevity; can last a lifetime with adequate nutrition
- Amitotic, except olfactory epithelium, some areas of hippocampus
- High metabolic rate; require steady supply of oxygen, glucose
  - Oxygen deprivation → death within minutes

Cell body/soma
- Contains endoplasmic reticulum (*ER*: chromatophilic substance, Nissl bodies), Golgi apparatus, mitochondria, neurofibrils, microtubules, pigments (e.g. melanin, lipofuscin); surrounds nucleus
- Site of protein synthesis, processing

Dendrite
- Short processes, project from cell body
- Receive information from adjacent neurons, contain receptors
- Brings information to cell body via graded potentials
- One neuron may have numerous dendrites

Axon
- Projection from specialized region of cell body, AKA axon hillock
  - *Axon hillock*: site of action potential generation
- Neuron's conducting region; forms synapses with dendrites
- Each neuron has only one axon
  - May be as long as 1m/3ft
  - *Nerve fiber*: one long axon
- *Axon collaterals*: axon branches
- Carries action potential from cell body to target cell (e.g. other neurons)
- Lacks rough ER, golgi apparatuses
- Cytoplasm contains numerous microtubules/microfilaments
  - Site of materials migration between cell body, axon terminus
- May be insulated with myelin sheath
- *Axolemma*: plasma membrane of axon
  - Responsible for maintaining neuron's membrane potential via ion channels
- *Axon terminals*: ends of axons, release neurotransmitters
- Clusters of axons
  - In PNS: nerves
  - In CNS: tracts

Myelin sheath
- Only axons are myelinated
- Functions
  - Protects fibers; ↑ transmission speed
- Produced by oligodendrocytes in CNS, by Schwann cells in PNS
- *Nodes of Ranvier*: gaps in myelin where action potential jumps from one node to next

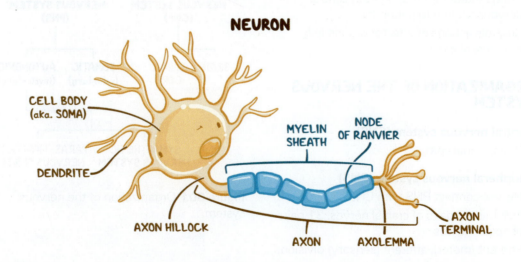

Figure 50.2 Structure of a neuron.

- Saltatory conduction → ↑ speed of propagation
- **Gray matter:** CNS regions containing nerve cell bodies, unmyelinated axons
- **White matter:** CNS regions containing myelinated axons

Structural and functional classification
- Unipolar neurons
    - One process, divides into two branches
    - Mostly function in PNS as first-order sensory neurons; conduct impulses along afferent pathways
- Bipolar neurons
    - Two processes (axon, dendrite) on opposite sides of cell body
    - Sensory neurons found in special sense organs (e.g. olfactory mucosa, retina)
- Multipolar neurons
    - ≥ three processes: one axon, rest are dendrites
    - *Primary functions:* interneurons within CNS; motor neurons (conduct impulses along efferent pathways)

CNS GLIAL CELLS (NEUROGLIA)

Astrocytes
- Most abundant; multiple functions
    - Provide structural, metabolic support for neurons
    - Determine capillary permeability (essential for blood-brain barrier via formation of tight junctions)
    - Control chemical environment (clean up spilled neurotransmitters, potassium ions)

Microglial cells
- Protective role
- Phagocytize microbes, debris

Oligodendrocytes
- Forms myelin sheath

Ependymal cells
- Line cavities of brain, spinal cord
- Form partially permeable barrier between cerebrospinal fluid (CSF), tissue
- Cilia assist in CSF circulation

PNS NEUROGLIA

Satellite cells
- Similar function as astrocytes

Schwann cells, AKA neurolemmocytes
- Form myelin sheath
- Involved in regeneration of damaged peripheral nerve fibers

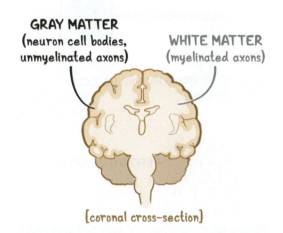

Figure 50.3 Coronal cross-section of the brain showing gray matter and white matter.

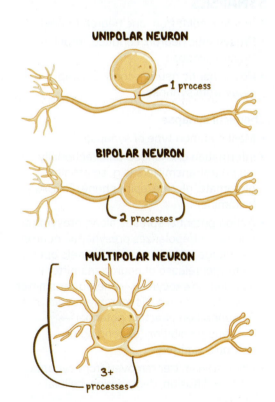

Figure 50.4 Structures of unipolar, bipolar, and multipolar neurons.

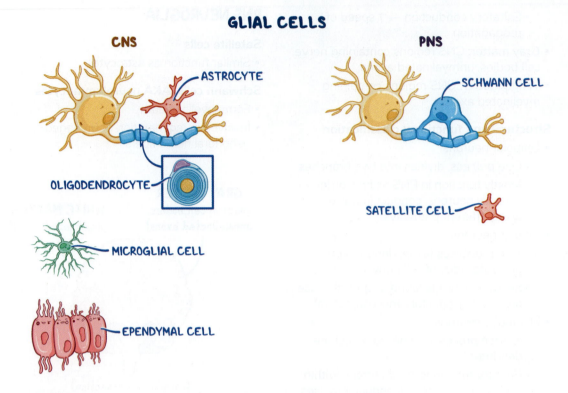

Figure 50.5 Glial cells of the CNS and PNS.

SYNAPSES

- Junction point from one neuron to next
- *Presynaptic neuron*: conducts impulse toward synapse
- *Postsynaptic neuron*: conducts impulse away from synapse

Chemical synapse

- Most common type of synapse
- Information exchanged unidirectionally via neurotransmitters (e.g. serotonin, glutamate, glycine, epinephrine, GABA, histamine)
- Action potential spreads along presynaptic neuron → depolarizes presynaptic neuron → voltage-gated calcium channels open → trigger release of neurotransmitter in vesicles via exocytosis → neurotransmitter binds to postsynaptic membrane receptor → generation of action potential → excitation/inhibition (depending on neurotransmitter)
- Neurotransmitter removed from synaptic cleft by diffusion, degradation, cellular uptake

Electrical synapse

- Open channels conduct electricity via gap junctions composed of connexons (protein channels); connecting cytoplasm of adjacent neurons
- Rapid, unidirectional or bidirectional transmission
- Examples
  - Cardiac muscles (promote synchronized activity)
  - Hypothalamic hormone-secreting neurons (creates burst of hormone release)

SPINAL CORD

- Long, tubular bundle of nervous tissue; protected by bony vertebral column, meninges, CSF
- Central canal continuous with fourth ventricle; carries CSF through spinal cord
- Extends from brainstem to lumbar region
  - Information travels up spinal cord via afferent (sensory) fibers, down via efferent (motor) fibers

- White matter: afferent, efferent fibers
- Gray matter: cell bodies
- Cell bodies arranged in three columns, AKA horns
  - Anterior (ventral) horns: receive information from brain's motor cortex → send it to skeletal muscles → trigger voluntary movement
  - Posterior (dorsal) horns: take sensory information → send it to brain's sensory cortex
  - Lateral horns: help regulate processes like urination, digestion, heart rate (mostly sympathetic activity)
- 31 pairs of nerves
  - Nerve pairs: 8 cervical, 12 thoracic, 5 lumbar, 5 sacral, 1 coccygeal
  - Cauda equina: nerve roots at end of vertebral canal
- Nerves arising from spinal column innervate specific bodily regions
  - Each spinal nerve (except C1) provides cutaneous sensory perception
  - Dermatome: section of skin supplied by pair of spinal nerves

STRUCTURES OF THE BRAIN

Brainstem: medulla, pons, midbrain

- Posterior part of brain continuous with spinal cord
- Responsible for basic life-sustaining body functions; e.g. breathing, blood pressure, consciousness, swallowing
- 10/12 cranial nerves (cranial nerves III-XII) arise in brainstem
- Medulla
  - Vasomotor (cardiovascular) center, respiratory center, swallowing/coughing/vomiting centers
  - All ascending sensory, descending motor tracts connecting spinal cord with other parts of brain
  - Pyramids on anterior surface of medulla: descending corticospinal tracts cross (decussate) to opposite side
- Pons
  - Controls facial expressions, sensations
  - Controls body equilibrium, posture
  - Works with medulla to regulate breathing (pneumotaxic center), relay information between cerebellum, cerebral hemispheres
- Midbrain (mesencephalon)
  - Participates in vision, hearing, motor control, sleep-wake cycle, consciousness
- Reticular formation (RF) scattered throughout brainstem
  - Responsible for consciousness; maintaining posture, general muscle tone, major visceral functions; interpretation, processing of noxious stimuli

Cerebellum

- AKA "little brain"
- Responsible for coordinating, planning, executing movements; balance, posture, spatial perception
- Integrates sensory information; fine-tunes motor activity (e.g. learned motor skills), stores it as muscle memory

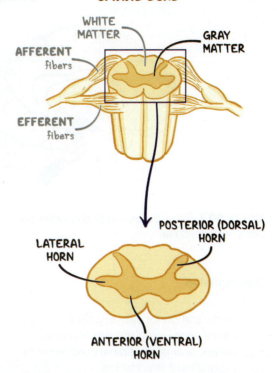

Figure 50.6 Cross-section of the spinal cord showing its structure.

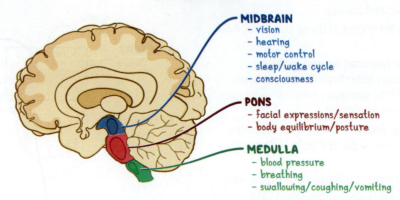

Figure 50.7 Sagittal section of the brain showing the brainstem, which includes the midbrain, pons, and medulla.

Diencephalon

- Thalamus
  - Relay station for sensory, motor information going to/from cerebral cortex, brainstem, spinal cord; screens insignificant information
- Hypothalamus
  - Major homeostatic control system
  - Links nervous system to endocrine system via pituitary gland
  - Thermostatic control of body temperature
  - Along with limbic system, participates in emotions such as anger, emotional response to pain, sexual arousal-related behaviors
  - Regulates circadian rhythms
  - Plays role in regulating eating, drinking; contains thirst center, which senses osmotic pressure of extracellular fluid
- Pineal gland
  - Produces melatonin

Cerebrum

- Divided into right, left hemispheres
- Separated by corpus callosum: connects left side to right side
- Contain folds (gyri): increase surface area
- Sulci: grooves between gyri
- Four lobes: frontal, parietal, temporal, occipital
- Frontal
  - *Primary motor cortex*: voluntary movement (motor homunculus)
  - *Premotor cortex*: orientation of body
  - *Supplementary motor area*: planning sequence of movement
- Parietal
  - Somatosensory processing
  - Has homunculus pattern similar to motor cortex
- Temporal
  - Functions in hearing, olfaction, visual recognition
- Occipital
  - Responsible for analyzing, interpreting visual information

Cerebral cortex

- Gray matter (cell bodies, dendrites) on outer surface of cerebrum: information processing
  - *Motor association area*: determines appropriate movements for specific tasks
  - *Primary somatosensory*: receives sensory input; somatosensory association area provides discrete interpretation
- Language processing
  - *Broca's area*: generation of spoken word (moving muscles to speak)
  - *Wernicke's area*: comprehension of speech
- White matter: axons; carry information to other parts of brain

Chapter 50 Neurology: Anatomy & Physiology

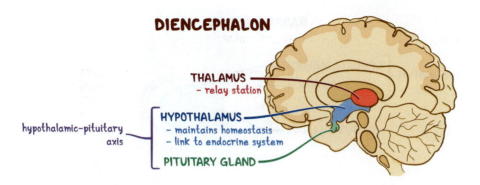

Figure 50.8 Sagittal section of the brain showing the diencephalon, which includes the thalamus, hypothalamus, and pituitary gland.

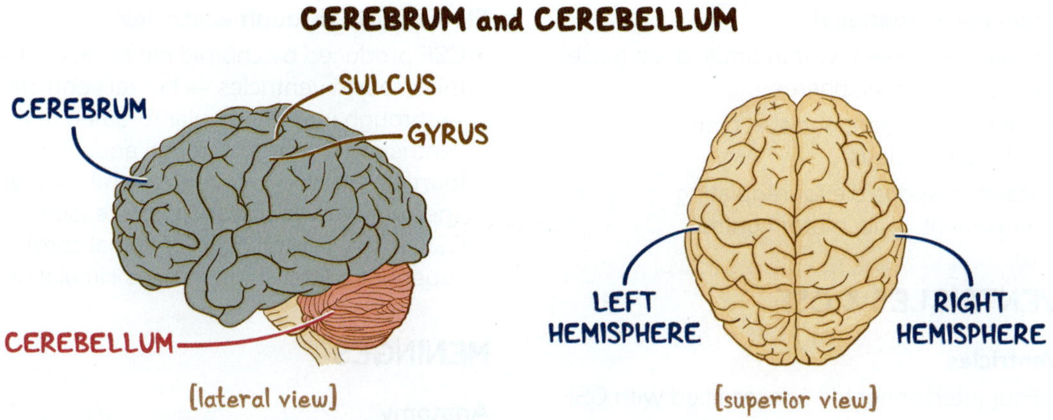

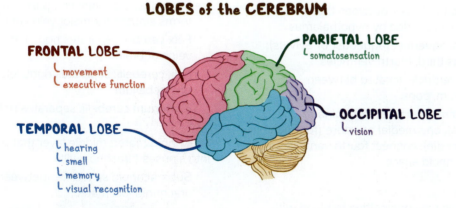

Figure 50.9 The structure of the cerebrum and cerebellum. The cerebrum contains gyri (which are the folds) and sulci (which are the grooves between the folds).

Figure 50.10 The four lobes of the cerebrum and some of their functions.

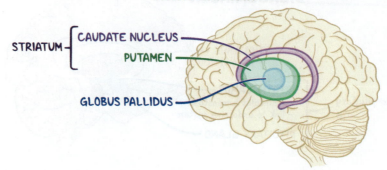

Figure 50.11 The structures of the basal ganglia.

Basal nuclei (ganglia)
- Gray matter deep within brain; deep nuclei of cerebral hemispheres
- Contains caudate nucleus, globus pallidus, putamen nucleus
- Mainly responsible for regulating movement, tone, motor control

VENTRICLES & CSF

Ventricles
- Four interconnected spaces filled with CSF
- *Two lateral ventricles*: located in frontal lobes, extend posteriorly into parietal lobes
- *Interventricular foramen (foramen of Munro)*: connects lateral ventricles to each other, to third ventricle
- *Third ventricle*: lies between thalamic bodies, surrounded by hypothalamus
- *Cerebral aqueduct (aqueduct of Sylvius)*: connects third, fourth ventricles
- *Fourth ventricle*: located between cerebellum, pons
- *Two lateral apertures (foramina of Luschka), one medial aperture (foramen of Magendie)*: connect fourth ventricle to subarachnoid space

CSF
- CSF similar in composition to blood with most proteins removed
- Made by ependymal cells of choroid plexuses
- Circulates throughout ventricles, central canal; also covers brain, meninges
- Protects brain (brain "floats" in cushioning fluid), provides nutrients to tissues in CNS

Flow of CSF through ventricles
- CSF produced by choroid plexus in lateral, third, fourth ventricles → lateral ventricle → through interventricular foramen to third ventricle → through cerebral aqueduct to fourth ventricle → through lateral, median apertures to subarachnoid space (some CSF enters central canal of spinal cord) → superior sagittal sinus, venous circulation

MENINGES

Anatomy
- Made up of three layers
- *From superficial to deep*: dura mater, arachnoid mater, pia mater
- *Dura mater*: tough, inflexible layer
  - Separates brain into compartments, forms sinuses for major veins of brain
  - *Falx cerebri*: separates right, left major veins of brain
  - *Falx cerebelli*: separates right, left lobes of cerebellum
  - *Tentorium cerebelli*: separates right, left lobes
- *Arachnoid mater*: middle layer that projects into sinuses (arachnoid villi)
  - *Subarachnoid space*: lies between arachnoid, pia mater
  - Contains CSF
  - Contains all blood vessels, cranial nerve of brain
- *Pia mater*: innermost layer
  - Adheres to brain
  - Fuses with empyema, forming choroid plexus, which produce CSF

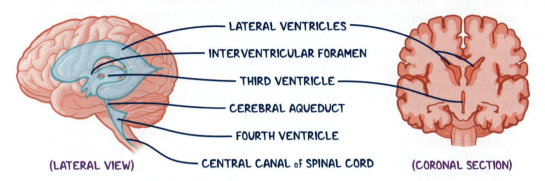

Figure 50.12 Ventricular system of the brain.

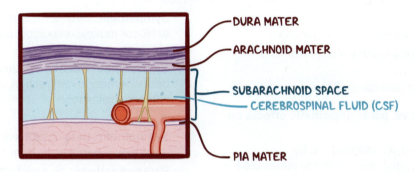

Figure 50.13 The meninges: three tissue layers which protect the brain and spinal cord.

AUTONOMIC NERVOUS SYSTEM
- Involuntary branch of PNS
- Extends from CNS to target organ via two-neuron chain; interact at autonomic ganglion
    - Preganglionic fiber: synapses with cell body of second neuron
    - Postganglionic fiber: innervates effector organ
- Both systems are active; one dominates other depending on situation
- Dual innervation of organs by both sympathetic and parasympathetic divisions
    - Exceptions: most arterioles, veins, sweat glands only innervated by sympathetic nerve fibers

Sympathetic
- "Fight or flight" functions: activated when individual exposed to stressful situation
- Originates in thoracic, lumbar region of spinal cord (T1-L2)
- Preganglionic axon length: short
- Postganglionic axon length: long
- Neurotransmitters, receptors
    - Preganglionic fibers release acetylcholine → binds to nicotinic receptor in postganglionic neuron → releases norepinephrine → binds to alpha/beta receptors on effector organs → releases acetylcholine → binds to muscarinic receptors on sweat glands
    - Preganglionic fibers release acetylcholine → binds to nicotinic receptor on adrenal medulla → epinephrine released → binds to alpha/beta receptors on effector organs

Parasympathetic
- *"Rest and digest" functions*: conserves, stores energy; maintains "housekeeping" functions
- Originates in craniosacral areas of spinal cord (CN III, VII, IX, X; S2-S4)
- *Preganglionic axon length*: long
- *Postganglionic axon length*: short
- Neurotransmitters, receptors
  - Preganglionic fiber releases acetylcholine → binds to nicotinic receptor in postganglionic neuron → releases acetylcholine → binds to muscarinic receptor on effector organ

Enteric nervous system (GI)
- *"Second brain:"* autonomous function independently from autonomic nervous system
- Neurons collected into two ganglia
  - Myenteric (Auerbach's), Meissner's plexus
- Coordinates peristalsis, GI tract secretions

Sympathetic vs. parasympathetic effects on organs
- Some organs only innervated by sympathetic division, but many innervated by both sympathetic, parasympathetic divisions → work cooperatively to regulate normal function
- Heart
  - *Sympathetic*: beta-1 receptors → ↑ heart rate, contractility → ↑ cardiac output
  - *Parasympathetic*: muscarinic (M) receptors → ↓ heart rate, contractility (atria only) → ↓ cardiac output
- Vascular smooth muscle
  - *Sympathetic*: skin/splanchnic alpha-1 receptors → constriction; skeletal muscle vascular beta-2 receptors → dilation; skeletal muscle vascular alpha-1 receptors → constriction
  - *Parasympathetic*: no direct effect
- Bronchial tree
  - *Sympathetic*: beta-2 receptors → dilation
  - *Parasympathetic*: M receptors → constriction
- Eye
  - *Sympathetic*: beta-2 receptors → ciliary muscle relaxation for far vision; alpha-1 → radial muscle contraction → pupil dilation
  - *Parasympathetic*: M receptors → ciliary muscle contraction for near vision + sphincter muscle constriction → pupil constriction
- GI tract
  - *Sympathetic*: alpha-2, beta-2 receptors → GI tract smooth muscle wall relaxation, ↓ GI motility; alpha-1 → ↑ sphincter tone
  - *Parasympathetic*: M receptors → ↑ GI smooth muscle wall contraction and motility, ↓ sphincter tone; ↑ gastric secretion
- Bladder
  - *Sympathetic*: beta-2 receptors → detrusor muscle relaxation, urinary sphincter contraction
  - *Parasympathetic*: M receptors → detrusor muscle contraction, urinary sphincter relaxation
- Liver
  - *Sympathetic*: beta-2, alpha-1 receptors → gluconeogenesis, glycogenolysis
  - *Parasympathetic*: no direct effect
- Adrenals
  - *Sympathetic*: nicotinic receptors → release of epinephrine, norepinephrine
  - *Parasympathetic*: no direct effect

NEURON ACTION POTENTIAL

osms.it/neuron-action-potential

- Electric signals sent down axons
- Generated by rapid rising, falling of membrane potential
- Resting membrane potential (approx. -65mV) determined by intra, extracellular ion concentrations
  - Ion channels open → depolarization of neuron (net influx of positive charge/ excitatory postsynaptic potential)
  - Depolarization to approx. -55mV → voltage-gated sodium channels open at axon hillock → sodium rushes into cell → action potential (neuron is positively charged to approx. +40mV)
  - Sodium channel becomes inactivated (absolute refractory period)
  - Voltage-gated potassium channels then act → potassium flows out
  - Sodium/potassium pump moves sodium out of cell, potassium in → hyperpolarization
  - Sodium channels remain closed but can be activated (relative refractory period); hyperpolarization → stronger stimulus needed
- In myelinated areas, electrical force of moving ions pushes subsequent ions along (saltatory conduction)

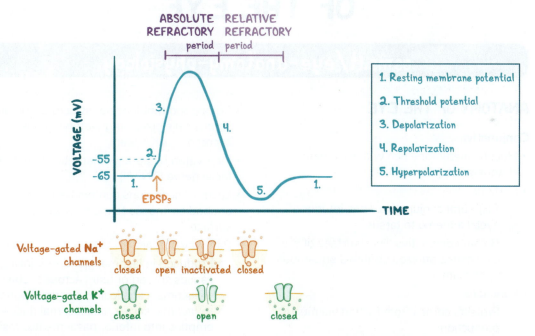

Figure 50.14 Graphical summary of the voltage changes that occur during a neuron action potential and the accompanying states of voltage-gated sodium and potassium channels. The action potential is initiated by a net influx of excitatory postsynaptic potentials (EPSPs). Not shown above are sodium/potassium pumps, which help to maintain the resting membrane potential, as well as help to return to that resting potential through repolarization.

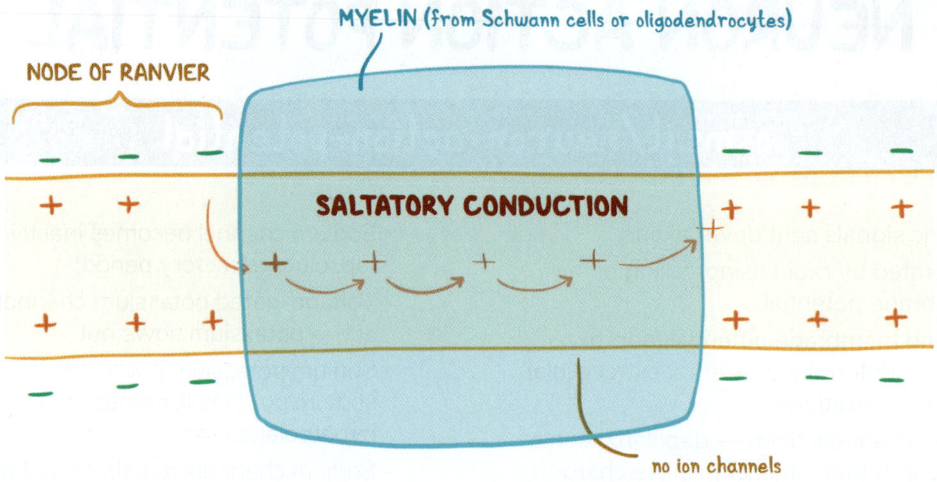

Figure 50.15 Saltatory conduction through myelinated areas of an axon increases the speed of signal conduction down the axon.

ANATOMY & PHYSIOLOGY OF THE EYE

osms.it/eye-anatomy-physiology

ANATOMY OF THE EYE

Conjunctiva
- Mucous membrane rich with lymphatic channels
- Portions
    - *Palpebral conjunctiva*: lines interior of eyelid adhered to tarsus
    - *Bulbar conjunctiva*: lines surface of the eye; nonkeratinized stratified squamous epithelium
- Functions
    - Protects cornea from friction via mucus production
    - Contributes to immune surveillance by preventing microbes from entering eye

Lacrimal apparatus
- Consists of lacrimal gland, draining ducts

Lacrimal gland
- Paired, almond-shaped exocrine glands located at upper lateral portion of each orbit
- Compound tubuloacinar structure, contains serous cells producing watery serous secretions, AKA tears
- Innervated by parasympathetic fibers from facial nerve (CN VII)
- Lacrimal secretions contain lysosomes, antibodies, mucus to moisten, protect eye surface
- Pathway of tears
    - Produced in lacrimal gland → blinking causes spread of tears across eyeball → lacrimal canaliculi via lacrimal puncta → lacrimal sac → nasolacrimal duct → empties into inferior nasal meatus inside nasal cavity

CHAMBERS & FLUIDS
- Anterior, posterior segments separated by lens

Posterior segment
- Largest segment
- Filled with gel-like vitreous humor

- Transmits light
- Holds neural layer of retina against retinal pigmented layer
- Maintains shape of eyeball
- Contributes to intraocular pressure

Anterior segment
- Divided into anterior and posterior chambers
- Filled with aqueous humor

Anterior chamber
- Larger chamber
- Bounded by cornea anteriorly, trabecular meshwork laterally, iris posteriorly

Posterior chamber
- Smaller chamber; irregularly shaped; size changes during accommodation
- Bounded by iris anteriorly, lens posteriorly
- Base formed by the ciliary processes

Aqueous humor
- Continually produced by ciliary processes
- Composed of filtered plasma
- Transports needed metabolites to avascular cornea, lens; removes metabolic wastes
- Pathway of flow: enters posterior chamber → passes through pupil → anterior chamber → trabecular network → scleral venous sinus (canal of Schlemm) → venous blood
  - Small amount diffuses into vitreous humor
  - Intraocular pressure primarily depends on balance between production and drainage

LAYERS OF EYE WALL
- Divided into fibrous layer, vascular layer, innermost layer (retina)
  - Superficial → deep

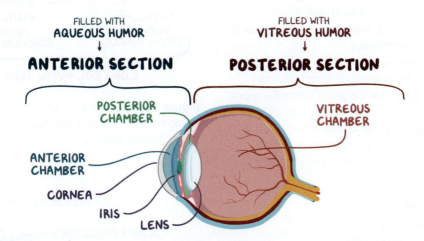

Figure 50.16 Three eye chambers. Anterior and posterior chambers are filled with aqueous humor. Vitreous chamber is filled with vitreous humor.

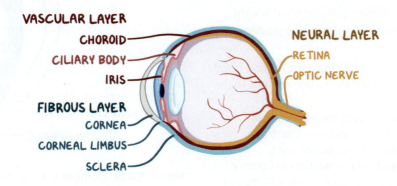

Figure 50.17 The three layers of the eye.

Fibrous layer
- Sclera
  - "White" of eye
  - Composed mainly of collagen, elastic fibers
  - Attachment point for extrinsic eye muscles
  - Continuous with cornea, dura mater of brain
- Limbus
  - Intersection between sclera, cornea
- Cornea
  - Anterior, transparent avascular portion of fibrous layer
  - Makes up major refractive surface of eye
  - Layers: anterior → posterior
- Corneal (sub) layers
  - *Stratified squamous epithelium*: derived from neural crest cells
  - *Bowman layer*: acellular; serves as barrier, protecting underlying stroma from malignant cells in epithelium
  - *Stroma*: transparent due to lack of blood vessels, lymphatics
  - *Descemet membrane*: basement layer separating epithelium from Bowman layer; protective function; epithelial stem cells located in this layer
- *Simple squamous epithelium*: AKA corneal endothelium; contains sodium pumps to pump water out of cornea, preserving its clarity

Vascular layer
- AKA uvea
- Choroid, iris, ciliary body
- Pigmented middle layer
- Choroid
  - Richly vascularized
  - Contains melanocytes to absorb light
  - Discontinued by optic nerve posteriorly
- Iris
  - Visible colored portion surrounding pupil (central opening in iris; allows light to enter eye)
  - Composed of two smooth muscle layers: sphincter pupillae (contracts during close vision, bright light, parasympathetic activation to constrict pupil), dilator pupillae (contracts during distance vision, dim light, sympathetic activation to dilate pupil)
- Ciliary body
  - *Ciliary muscles*: smooth muscles that control shape of lens
  - *Ciliary processes*: secrete aqueous humor
  - *Ciliary zonule/suspensory ligament*: fibers extending from ciliary processes to lens (secures lens in place)

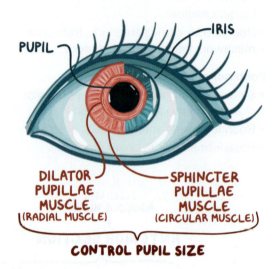

Figure 50.18 The iris is composed of two smooth muscle layers, the dilator pupillae and the sphincter pupillae.

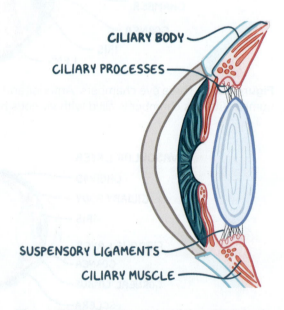

Figure 50.19 Components of the ciliary body.

Retina
- Innermost layer
  - Further divided into outer pigmented layer, inner neural layer
- *Sub-layers:* superficial → deep
  - Pigment cell → photoreceptor → outer nuclear → outer plexiform → inner nuclear → inner plexiform → ganglion cell → optic nerve layer

Retina: outer pigmented layer
- Pigmented epithelial cells absorb light, store vitamin A for photoreceptor cells to use
- *Function:* photoreceptor maintenance

Retina: inner neural layer
- Extends anteriorly to ciliary body
- *Three types of neurons:* photoreceptors, bipolar cells, ganglion cells
  - *Night-vision photoreceptors (rods):* dim-light, non-color vision; more numerous, more sensitive to light than cones; not present on fovea; do not create sharp, clear images/low acuity
  - *Day-vision photoreceptors (cones):* bright-light, color vision; present on fovea; high resolution/high acuity
  - *Bipolar cells:* synapse with ganglion cells
  - *Ganglion cells:* where action potentials are generated; leave eye as optic nerve

- Optic disc
  - Spot where optic nerve (CN II) exits eye
  - AKA "blind spot"
  - Not noticeable since each blind spot is compensated by other eye
- Macula lutea
  - Area of greatest visual acuity
  - Contains mainly cones
  - Only portion of eye with enough cone density to allow detailed color vision, hard focus
  - Lateral to blind spots
- Fovea centralis
  - Center of macula lutea
  - Contains only cones
  - Region of greatest visual acuity in macula
- Optic nerve
  - Composed of retinal ganglion cell axons
  - Exits retina via optic disc
- Optic chiasm
  - X-shaped structure where optic nerves meet
  - Axons from nasal retina cross over to opposite sides → optic tracts
- Optic tract
  - Synapses with cells in lateral geniculate nucleus in both sides of thalamus

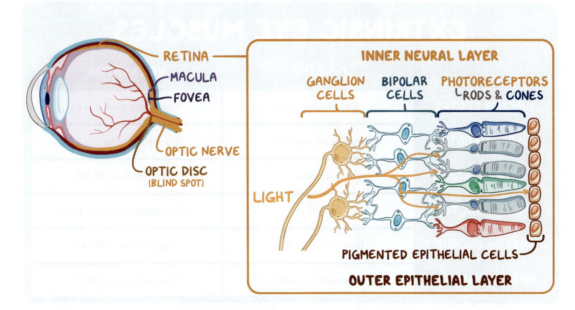

Figure 50.20 Components of the neural layer of the eye.

- Sharpens contrasts, enhances depth perception
- Optic radiations sent to primary visual cortex, AKA occipital lobe

VASCULAR SUPPLY
- Choroidal vessels supply external ⅓ of eye
- Retinal central artery and central vein supply internal ⅔ of the eye

EXTRAOCULAR MUSCLES
- Orbicularis oculi
  - Circular muscle that encircles eye
  - Closes eyelid when contracted
- Levator palpebrae superioris
  - Located inside eyelid
  - Raises eyelid
- Extrinsic eye muscles
  - Control eye movement
  - Originate from walls of orbit (common tendinous/annular ring), insert onto surface of eye

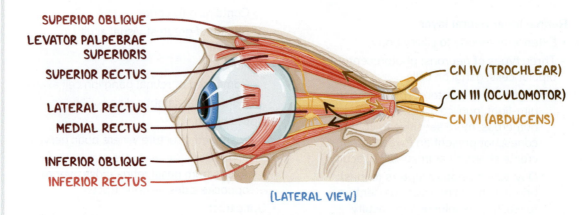

Figure 50.21 Lateral view of the left eye showing the extraocular muscles. Not shown: orbicularis oculi.

EXTRINSIC EYE MUSCLES

	FUNCTION	INNERVATION
SUPERIOR RECTUS	Elevation, intorsion	Oculomotor nerve (CN III)
INFERIOR RECTUS	Depression, extorsion	Oculomotor nerve (CN III)
LATERAL RECTUS	Abduction	Abducens nerve (CN VI)
MEDIAL RECTUS	Adduction	Oculomotor nerve (CN III)
SUPERIOR OBLIQUE	Depression, intorsion	Trochlear nerve (CN IV)
INFERIOR OBLIQUE	Elevation, extorsion	Oculomotor nerve (CN III)

PHYSIOLOGY OF VISION: PHOTORECEPTION & PHOTOTRANSDUCTION

- Photoreceptors, ganglion cells, bipolar cells generate excitatory (EPSPs), inhibitory postsynaptic potentials (IPSPs) instead of action potentials
- Light hits retina, 11-*cis* retinal converted to all-*trans* retinal → production of metarhodopsin II → activation of transducin → activation of phosphodiesterase, converting cGMP to 5-GMP → ↓ cGMP → closure of sodium channels → hyperpolarization of photoreceptor membrane → ↓ glutamate release (excitatory neurotransmitter) from photoreceptors → either inhibition or excitation
  - Depends on which type of glutamate receptor activated

Glutamate receptors

- *Ionotropic receptor*: excitatory/depolarizing
  - ↓ excitatory glutamate response → hyperpolarization of bipolar, horizontal cells → inhibition
- *Metabotropic receptor*: inhibitory/hyperpolarizing
  - ↓ inhibitory glutamate response → depolarization of bipolar, horizontal cells → excitation
- Establish on-off patterns of visual fields

LIGHT VS. DARKNESS

Light

- Photoreceptors hyperpolarize → ↓ glutamate release
  - *Glutamate*: inhibitory
- → Lack of IPSPs causes bipolar cells to depolarize, release neurotransmitter onto ganglion cells → ganglion cells propagates EPSPs → action potential transmitted to brain via optic nerve

Darkness

- Photoreceptors depolarize → increased glutamate release → glutamate causes IPSPs → IPSPs cause bipolar cells to hyperpolarize, inhibits release of neurotransmitters onto ganglion cells → ganglion cells do not propagate EPSPs → no action potentials carried along optic nerve to brain

Focusing light on retina

- Light → cornea → aqueous humor → lens → vitreous humor → neural layer of retina
  - Excites photoreceptors of pigmented layer → photoreception, AKA conversion of light into electrical impulses
- Light bent three times:
  - Entering cornea, AKA major refractive step; entering lens; exiting lens
  - Refractive power of cornea is constant, whereas lens' refractive power can be changed

Distant vision

- Normal resting status of human eye: preset for distant vision
- Ciliary muscles relaxed → ciliary zonule fibers taut → lens is flat (lowest refractive power) → parallel rays focus on retina
- Sympathetic activation causes ciliary muscle relaxation, pupillary dilation
- *Far point of vision*: distance beyond which no accommodation/change in lens shape required for focusing

Near vision

- Involves accommodation, pupillary constriction, convergence
- Lens accommodation
  - Ciliary muscles contract → ciliary zonule fibers relaxed → lens becomes spherical (increases refractory power of lens)
  - Parasympathetic activation → ciliary muscle contraction
- Pupil constriction
  - Mediated by sphincter pupillae muscles of iris
  - Parasympathetic activation
  - ↑ depth of focus
- Convergence of eyes
  - Eyes rotate medially as object moves closer
  - Mediated by extrinsic eye muscles via oculomotor nerve (CN III)

Visual field

- Everything seen by single eye
  - Overlap → central "binocular" visual field

- Split into two parts
  - *Nasal visual field:* projected onto temporal retina, axons stay on that side of brain
  - *Temporal visual field:* projected onto nasal retina, axons cross to opposite side of brain at optic chiasm
- Information from left visual fields of both eyes travel to right half of brain, vice versa
  - *Cause:* axons from nasal retina crossing over
- Some nerve fibers synapse at superior colliculi instead of lateral geniculate body, ascend to midbrain

ANATOMY & PHYSIOLOGY OF THE EAR

osms.it/ear-anatomy-physiology

EXTERNAL EAR ANATOMY

Pinna/auricle
- Composed of elastic cartilage covered with thick skin
- Function
  - Captures sound waves, guides them into auditory canal

External auditory meatus
- AKA auditory canal
- Contains ceruminous glands
  - Secretes cerumen (ear wax); with small hairs, traps foreign objects
- Function
  - Guides sound waves to tympanic membrane

Tympanic membrane
- AKA eardrum
- Thin, connective tissue membrane covered by skin (external), mucous membrane (internal)
- Separates external, middle ear
- Vibrates when hit by sound waves → vibrates ossicles

MIDDLE EAR ANATOMY

Auditory ossicles
- Linked by synovial joints in chain; transmit vibration of tympanic membrane to oval window
- *Malleus/"hammer":* connected to tympanic membrane, incus
- *Incus/"anvil":* connects malleus, stapes
- *Stapes/"stirrup":* footplate inserts onto oval window; connects middle, inner ear
- *Stapedius, tensor tympani:* two skeletal muscles attached to auditory ossicles; protect ears from prolonged, loud noises; not brief explosive, noise (e.g. gunshot)

Oval window
- Membrane-covered opening connecting middle, inner ear; transforms vibrations into fluid waves

Round window
- Membrane-covered opening relieves pressure created by fluid waves

Mastoid antrum
- Canal in posterior wall of tympanic cavity, communicates with mastoid air cells

Pharyngotympanic/eustachian tube
- Canal links middle ear, nasopharynx
- Swallowing/yawning opens tube to equalize middle ear cavity, atmospheric air pressure
- Pathogens may travel through tube → otitis media

INNER EAR ANATOMY
- *Bony labyrinth:* system of channels/cavities, houses membranous labyrinth, fluid filled
- *Three semicircular canals:* rotational acceleration in three planes of movement (lateral, superior, posterior)

Chapter 50 Neurology: Anatomy & Physiology

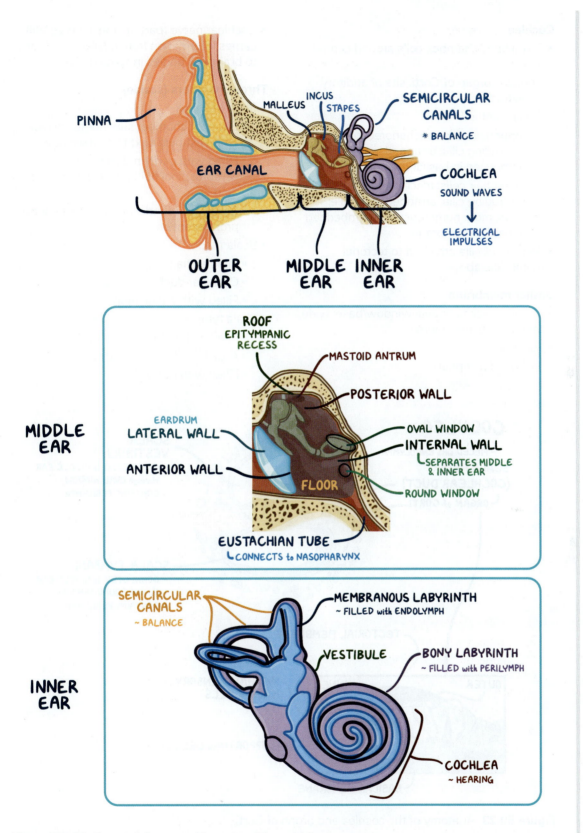

Figure 50.22 Parts of the ear with parts of the middle, inner ear.

Cochlea

- Spiral bony chamber, coils around central axis
- Contains **organ of Corti**: site of auditory transduction
- Two receptors
  - *Inner hair cells*: mechanoreceptors with protruding cilia; arranged in single rows embedded in basilar membrane
  - *Outer hair cells*: mechanoreceptors with protruding cilia; arranged in parallel rows; more numerous; body embedded in basilar membrane
- All hair cell cilia attached to tectorial membrane above

Basilar membrane

- Narrow, thick near oval window/base; wide, thin near cochlea (apex)
- Function
  - Sound reception
- Cochlear nerve (part of cranial nerve VIII) carries information from basilar membrane to brain; cell bodies in spiral ganglia

Three chambers (scalae)

- Scala vestibuli
  - Superior chamber superior to cochlea; with vestibule next to oval window
  - Filled with **perilymph**: similar to cerebrospinal fluid (CSF), extracellular fluid
  - Conducts sound vibrations for hearing, proprioception
- Scala media
  - Middle chamber
  - Cochlear duct
  - Filled with endolymph
- Scala tympani
  - Inferior chamber in cochlea
  - Attaches to round window
  - Filled with perilymph

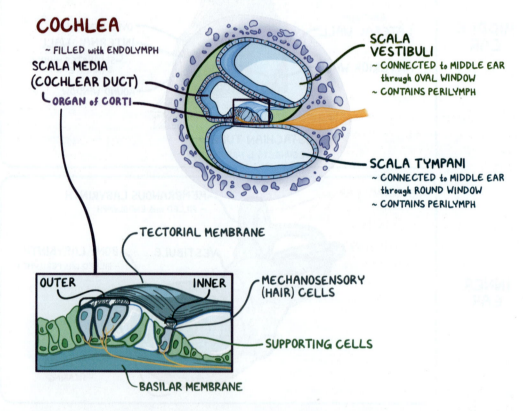

Figure 50.23 Anatomy of the cochlea and organ of Corti.

Chapter 50 Neurology: Anatomy & Physiology

AUDITORY SYSTEM

Pathway of sound waves

- Sound waves travel through external ear → vibrate tympanic membrane
- Tympanic membrane vibrates ossicles → ossicles amplify sound → stapes vibrates oval window
- Perilymph in scala vestibuli moves → pressure waves travel through perilymph towards helicotrema → cochlear duct → vibrates basilar membrane
- Hair cells bend by shearing force, cilia pushes against tectorial membrane → cilia bend in one direction → ↑ potassium conduction → depolarization (cilia bends in other direction → ↓ potassium → hyperpolarization) → action potential generated in cochlear nerve → sends signals to brain
- Sounds waves > 20Hz
    - Pressure waves → cochlear duct → perilymph of scala tympani → cochlear duct → vibrates basilar membrane → sound waves converted to electrical signal → hearing sensation
- ↑ intensity of sound = ↑ distal membrane displaced in vibratory motion

Amplification of sound waves

- Pressure exerted on oval window > pressure exerted on tympanic membrane (due to smaller size of oval window)
- Ossicles

Frequency mapping (tonotopic map)

- Sound frequencies displace basilar membrane at different locations
- *Base (short, stiff fibers)*: 20,000Hz; nearest to stapes, responds best to high frequencies
- *Apex (long, floppy fibers)*: 20Hz; responds best to low frequencies

Central connections

- Hair cell receptors in organ of Corti → primary cell bodies located in spiral/auditory ganglion (bipolar cells in spiral of cochlea) → axon carries signal → dorsal, ventral cochlear nuclei in pons → secondary axons project via lateral lemniscus → inferior colliculus in midbrain → medial geniculate nucleus in thalamus → projects to primary auditory cortex located at transverse gyrus of Heschl in temporal lobe
- Accessory auditory nuclei
- Superior olivary nucleus: sound localization; integration, interpretation of sound received in both ears at slightly different times

VESTIBULAR SYSTEM

- Sensory information from vestibular system → generates visual images for retina → posture adjustments to maintain balance
- Vestibular organ located within temporal bone adjacent to cochlea; three semicircular canals, otolith organs (utricle, saccule)

Semicircular ducts

- Function
    - Rotational/angular acceleration to maintain balance
- Three canals at right angles to one another in each plane of space (anterior, posterior, lateral)
- Filled with *endolymph*: similar to intracellular fluid (↑ potassium; ↓ sodium)
- *Ampulla*: dilated portion at one end; contains hair cells, protrudes into gelatinous substance, cupula
- *Hair cells*: tonic rate of electrical firing
    - Fire constantly when head not moving
- Head rotation → endolymph deflects hair cells in certain direction in semicircular canals → change in baseline electrical firing rate → propagation down vestibular nerve → brainstem

Otolith organs: utricle, saccule

- Function
    - Linear acceleration
- Contain
    - Hair cells with calcium carbonate crystals
    - Maculae (balance receptor, responds to changes in head position)
- Moving head in any direction → gravity deflects calcium carbonate crystals, attached hair cells → stereocilia bends toward/away from kinocilium → depolarization/hyperpolarization respectively → excitation/inhibition respectively
- *Head upright*: macula horizontal, saccule vertical

- *Tilting head forward/laterally:* ipsilateral utricle excited
- *Tilting head backward/medially:* ipsilateral utricle inhibited
- *Forward movement of head:* saccule excited
- *Lateral, medial movement of head:* saccule excited

Pathway of signal centrally
- Hair cells receptor → propagation of signal → vestibular/Scarpa's ganglion (primary sensory cell bodies of vestibular system; bipolar cell type) → vestibular nuclei in pons (superior, inferior, lateral) → secondary sensory axons project to five areas in central nervous system (CNS)
- Spinal cord via medial, lateral vestibulospinal tracts
- Cerebellum via vermis, flocculonodular lobe
- Extraocular muscles via medial longitudinal fasciculus (MLF), CN nuclei III, IV, VI
- Reticular formation in medulla (vomiting center)
- *Medial geniculate body/cortex:* provides orientation of body in space

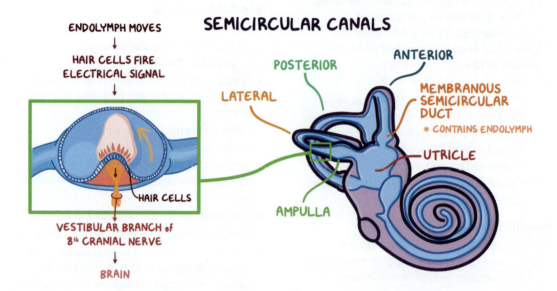

Figure 50.24 The semicircular canals measure rotational/angular acceleration to maintain balance. Movement of endolymph displaces hair cells in the ampulla. Hair cells then transmit this information as an electrical signal along the vestibular branch of CN VIII to the brain.

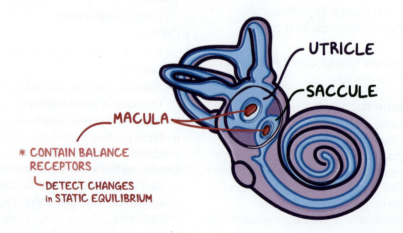

Figure 50.25 The otolith organs, the utricle and saccule, measure linear acceleration using balance receptors in the macula.

NOTES
AUTONOMIC NERVOUS SYSTEM

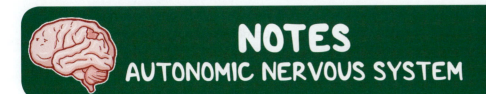

- Part of peripheral nervous system (PNS); regulates basic visceral processes necessary to homeostasis
- Autonomic nervous system (ANS) affects visceral organs, glands, involuntary muscles → regulates heart rate, respiration rate, digestion, urination, salivation, sexual arousal, etc.
- Divided into two systems
  - Sympathetic, parasympathetic
- Unlike somatic nervous system, in ANS
  - Neurotransmitters synthesized, stored, released in varicosities (analogous to presynaptic nerve terminals in somatic nervous system)
  - Target organ's tissue can be innervated by multiple postganglionic neurons
  - Postsynaptic receptors widely scattered on target organ

NEURONS

- Two neuron types in both sympathetic, parasympathetic systems
  - Preganglionic, postganglionic
- Preganglionic neurons → preganglionic fibers → synapse with autonomic ganglia (postganglionic neurons) → postganglionic fibers → target organ

Preganglionic neurons
- General visceral efferent (GVE) neurons
- Located in central nervous system (CNS) (spinal cord)
- Release acetylcholine (ACh)

Postganglionic neurons
- GVE, general visceral afferent (GVA) neurons
- Located outside central nervous system
- Release acetylcholine/norepinephrine/neuropeptides

Autonomic ganglia
- Contain neuron cell body clusters (postganglionic neurons)
- Synapse points between preganglionic fibers, postganglionic fibers

SYMPATHETIC NERVOUS SYSTEM

osms.it/sympathetic-nervous-system

- ANS component; controls visceral functions requiring fast response (i.e. "fight or flight")
- Ganglia close to spinal cord → short preganglionic fibers, long postganglionic fibers

Preganglionic neurons
- **Located:** thoracolumbar spinal cord's intermediate horn (T1–L2)
- Cholinergic neurons → release ACh

Postganglionic neurons
- Located close to spinal cord
  - Paravertebral ganglia (cervical, thoracic, rostral lumbar, caudal lumbar, pelvic ganglia)
  - Prevertebral ganglia (celiac, aorticorenal, superior mesenteric, inferior mesenteric ganglion)
  - Chromaffin cells of adrenal medulla (modified sympathetic ganglion)

- Either adrenergic/cholinergic
  - Adrenergic neurons → release norepinephrine/epinephrine (adrenal medulla)
  - Cholinergic → release ACh
- Effector organ receptors: $α_1$, $α_2$, $β_1$, $β_2$, $β_3$

Sympathetic nervous system effects
- **Cardiovascular:** ↑ heart rate, ↑ cardiac output, vasoconstriction
- **Respiratory:** bronchodilation
- **Gastrointestinal:** ↓ motility, ↓ secretions
- **Genitourinary:** ↓ bladder's detrusor muscle activity, ejaculation
- **Metabolic:** ↑ gluconeogenesis
- **Glands:** ↓ salivation, ↑ sweating
- **Pupils:** mydriasis

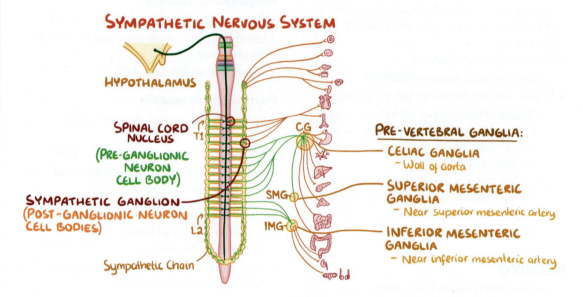

Figure 51.1 Neurons originating in the hypothalamus synapse with sympathetic pre-ganglionic cells bodies in spinal cord nuclei. Some pre-ganglionic neurons synapse in the paravertebral ganglia of the sympathetic chain; others synapse in the pre-vertebral ganglia.

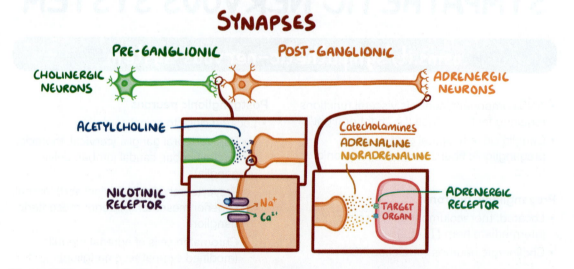

Figure 51.2 Sympathetic preganglionic neurons release acetylcholine, which bind to nicotinic receptors on postganglionic neurons. Postganglionic neurons release catecholamines, which are received by adrenergic receptors on target organs.

PARASYMPATHETIC NERVOUS SYSTEM

osms.it/parasympathetic-nervous-system

- ANS component controls visceral functions not requiring fast response (i.e. "rest and digest")
- Ganglia close to target organ → long preganglionic fibers, short postganglionic fibers

Preganglionic neurons
- Located in brainstem (nuclei of cranial nerves II, VII, IX, X), sacral spinal cord (S2–S4)
- Cholinergic neurons → release ACh

Postganglionic neurons
- Located close to target organs
  - Ciliary ganglion (cranial nerve III)
  - Submandibular ganglion (cranial nerve VII)
  - Otic ganglion (cranial nerve IX)
  - Near/inside target organ (cranial nerve X, sacral nerves)

- Mostly cholinergic, but some non-adrenergic, non-cholinergic → release neuropeptides
- Effector organ receptors are muscarinic

Parasympathetic nervous system effects
- *Cardiovascular:* ↓ heart rate, ↓ cardiac output
- *Respiratory:* bronchoconstriction
- *Gastrointestinal:* ↑ motility, ↑ secretions
- *Genitourinary:* ↑ bladder's detrusor muscle activity, erection
- *Metabolic:* ↓ glycogenesis
- *Glands:* ↑ salivation
- *Pupils:* miosis

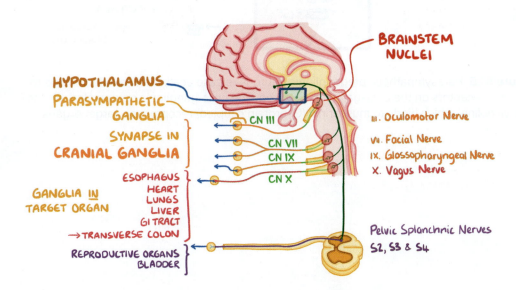

Figure 51.3 Neurons originating in the hypothalamus synapse with parasympathetic pre-ganglionic cells bodies in brainstem, spinal cord at levels S2, S3, and S4. Pre-ganglionic neurons synapse in cranial ganglia and near/in target organ.

NERVE	GANGLIA	LOCATION	INNERVATION
OCULOMOTOR NERVE	CILIARY GANGLIA	BEHIND EYE	PUPIL
FACIAL NERVE	PTERYGOPALATINE GANGLION	PTERYGOPALATINE FOSSA, BEHIND MAXILLA	SUBLINGUAL & SUBMANDIBULAR SALIVARY GLANDS
	SUBMANDIBULAR GANGLION	ABOVE SUBMANDIBULAR SALIVARY GLANDS, in NASAL CAVITY	LACRIMAL GLANDS; GLANDS in NASAL CAVITY
GLOSSOPHARYNGEAL NERVE	OTIC GANGLIA	INFRATEMPORAL FOSSA, BELOW & MEDIAL TO ZYGOMATIC ARCH	PAROTID SALIVARY GLAND

Figure 51.4 Summary of parasympathetic components of cranial nerves III (oculomotor), VII (facial), and IX (glossopharyngeal).

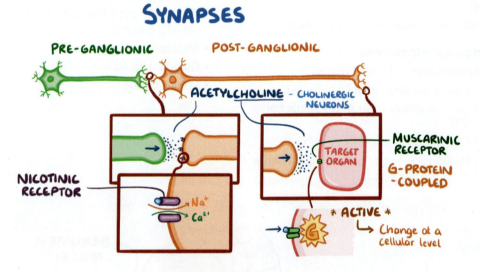

Figure 51.5 Parasympathetic preganglionic neurons release acetylcholine, which binds to nicotinic receptors on the post-ganglionic neuron. The post-ganglionic neuron also releases acetylcholine, which binds to muscarinic (G-protein coupled) receptors on target organs.

SYMPATHETIC & PARASYMPATHETIC NERVOUS SYSTEMS OVERVIEW

	NEURONS	FIBER LENGTH	NEURO-TRANSMITTERS	RECEPTORS
SYMPATHETIC NERVOUS SYSTEM	Preganglionic	Short	ACh	Muscarinic
	Postganglionic	Long	Norepinephrine, ATP, neuropeptide Y	Adrenergic (α_1, α_2, β_1, β_2)
PARASYMPATHETIC NERVOUS SYSTEM	Preganglionic	Long	ACh	Nicotinic (N_n, N_m)
	Postganglionic	Short	ACh	Muscarinic (M_1, M_2, M_3, M_4, M_5)

SYMPATHETIC VS. PARASYMPATHETIC: EFFECTS ON EFFECTORS

EFFECTOR	SYMPATHETIC NERVOUS SYSTEM		PARASYMPATHETIC NERVOUS SYSTEM	
	RECEPTOR	EFFECT	RECEPTOR	EFFECT
PUPILS	α_1	Dilation	M_3	Constriction
HEART	β_1	Positive inotropic, chronotropic, dromotropic effect	M_2	Negative inotropic, chronotropic, dromotropic effect
LUNGS	β_2	Bronchodilation	M_3	Bronchoconstriction, ↑ gland secretion
GI TRACT	α_1	Vasoconstriction, sphincter contraction	M_3	↑ motility, sphincter relaxation, ↑ gland secretion
URINARY TRACT	α_1, β_1	Bladder sphincter contraction, ↑ renin secretion	M_3	Bladder sphincter relaxation
SKELETAL MUSCLE	β_2	Vasodilatation	-	None
SKIN	α_1	Vasoconstriction	-	None
GLANDS	α_1	↑ sweating, ↓ pancreatic activity	M_1, M_3	↑ salivation, ↑ lacrimation, ↑ pancreatic activity

ADRENERGIC RECEPTORS

osms.it/adrenergic-receptors

- **Metabotropic receptors:** respond to catecholamines (norepinephrine, epinephrine)
- Located on sympathetic effector organs → stimulated → sympathetic/sympathomimetic response
- Types
  - α, β adrenergic receptors: $α_1$, $α_2$, $β_1$, $β_2$, $β_3$

$α_1$ Adrenergic receptors (stimulatory effect)

- Gastrointestinal tract blood vessels, skin blood vessels → vasoconstriction
- Bladder, gastrointestinal (GI) tract sphincters → contraction
- Radial (dilator) muscle of iris → contraction
- Pancreas → ↓ secretion
- Liver → ↑ glycogenolysis

$α_2$ Adrenergic receptors (inhibitory effect)

- Presynaptic nerve terminals (autoreceptors) → presynaptic inhibition of neurotransmitter release
- Postganglionic parasympathetic nerve terminals in GI tract (heteroreceptors) → ↓ insulin secretion
- ↓ platelet aggregation

$β_1$ Adrenergic receptors (stimulatory effect)

- Heart
  - Sinoatrial (SA) node → ↑ heart rate (positive chronotropic effect)
  - Atrioventricular (AV) node → ↑ conduction (positive dromotropic effect)
  - Ventricular muscle → ↑ contractility (positive inotropic effect)
- Salivary glands → ↓ salivation
- Adipose tissue → lipolysis
- Kidney → ↑ renin secretion

$β_2$ adrenergic receptors (stimulatory effect)

- Skeletal muscle blood vessels → vasodilation
- Bronchioles → relaxation
- Pancreas → ↑ secretion
- Liver → ↑ glycogenolysis, ↑ gluconeogenesis

$β_3$ adrenergic receptors (stimulatory effects)

- Adipose tissue → lipolysis, thermogenesis
- Detrusor muscle → relaxation

Adrenergic receptor mechanism

- Catecholamines binding → G_q (stimulatory) or G_i (inhibitory) protein activation → second messenger cascade → ↑ phospholipase C or ↓ adenylate cyclase → effect
- $α_1$ adrenergic receptors
  - G_q protein activation → second messenger cascade → ↑ phospholipase C → ↑ IP_3, DAG, Ca^{2+} → stimulatory effect
- $α_2$ adrenergic receptors
  - G_i protein activation → ↓ adenylate cyclase → ↓ cAMP → inhibitory effect
- $β_1$ adrenergic receptors
  - G_s protein activation → ↑ adenylate cyclase → ↑ cAMP → stimulatory effect
- $β_1$ adrenergic receptors
  - G_s protein activation → ↑ adenylate cyclase → ↑ cAMP → stimulatory effect

CATECHOLAMINES

- Neurotransmitters synthesized, released by adrenergic neurons
- Include epinephrine (adrenaline), norepinephrine (noradrenaline), dopamine

Synthesis

- Tyrosine → L-dopa; catalyzed by tyrosine hydroxylase
- L-dopa → dopamine; catalyzed by dopa decarboxylase
- Dopamine → norepinephrine; catalyzed by β hydroxylase
- Norepinephrine → epinephrine; catalyzed by phenylethanolamine-N-methyltransferase (PNMT); only in adrenal medulla

Degradation

- All catecholamines can be degraded by deamination by monoamine oxidase (MAO)/methylation by catechol-O-methyltransferase (COMT)/both
- Norepinephrine
  - MAO: dihydroxymandelic acid
  - COMT: normetanephrine
  - Both: 3-methoxy-4-hydroxymandelic acid (VMA)
- Epinephrine
  - MAO: dihydroxymandelic acid
  - COMT: metanephrine
  - Both: 3-methoxy-4-hydroxymandelic acid (VMA)
- Dopamine
  - MAO: dihydroxyphenylacetic acid
  - COMT: 3-methoxytyramine
  - Both: homovanillic acid (HVA)

Adrenergic transmission

- Present in
  - Most postganglionic sympathetic neurons (norepinephrine)
  - Adrenal medulla's chromaffin cells (epinephrine)
  - Ventral tegmental area, substantia nigra (dopamine)

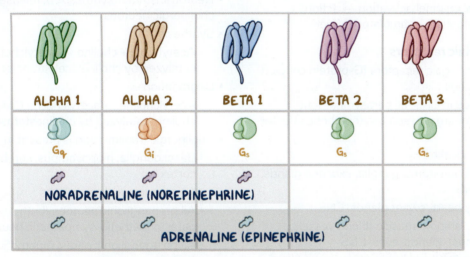

Figure 51.6 Types of adrenergic receptors, the G-proteins with which they can be coupled, and the catecholamines that bind with them.

CHOLINERGIC RECEPTORS

osms.it/cholinergic-receptors

- Receptors respond to neurotransmitter acetylcholine
- Located on parasympathetic effector organs, CNS → stimulated → parasympathetic/parasympathomimetic response

Nicotinic receptors
- Ionotropic receptors
- Type: location
  - Nm: neuromuscular junction (non autonomic)
  - Nn: autonomic ganglia and adrenal medulla
- Mechanism
  - Acetylcholine binding → Na^+, K^+ diffusion → depolarization → voltage Na^+ channel activation → action potential → stimulatory effect

Muscarinic receptors
- Metabotropic receptors (G-protein coupled receptors)
- Located in CNS, all parasympathetic effector organs, some sympathetic effector organs
- Type: location
  - M_1: autonomic ganglia, exocrine glands, CNS
  - M_2: heart, sweat glands, CNS
  - M_3: smooth muscle (blood vessels, lungs), glands, eyes, CNS
  - M_4: CNS, sweat glands
  - M_5: CNS
- Mechanism
  - Acetylcholine binding → G_q (stimulatory) or G_i (inhibitory) protein activation → second messenger cascade → ↑ phospholipase C/↓ adenylate cyclase → stimulatory/inhibitory effect
  - M_1, M_3, M_5 → G_q protein activation → ↑ phospholipase C → ↑ IP_3, DAG, Ca^{2+} → stimulatory effect
  - M_4 → G_i protein activation → ↓ adenylate cyclase → ↓ cAMP → inhibitory effect
  - M_2 → G_i protein activation → K^+ channel activation → inhibitory effect

ACETYLCHOLINE (ACh)

- Neurotransmitter synthesized, released by cholinergic neurons
- Synthesis
  - Acetyl CoA + choline → acetylcholine; catalyzed by choline acetyltransferase
- Degradation
  - Acetylcholine → acetylcholine CoA + choline; catalyzed by cholinesterase
- Cholinergic transmission is present in
  - Basal ganglia, hippocampus, cerebral cortex
  - All neuromuscular junctions
  - All preganglionic neurons (both parasympathetic, sympathetic neurons)
  - All postganglionic parasympathetic neurons
  - Some postganglionic sympathetic neurons (sweat glands)

Chapter 51 Neurology: Autonomic Nervous System

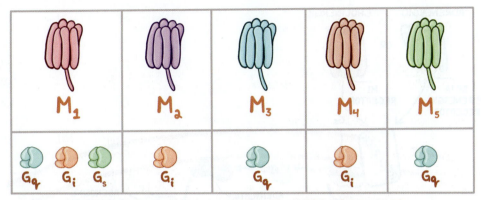

Figure 51.7 Types of muscarinic receptors and the G-proteins with which they can be coupled.

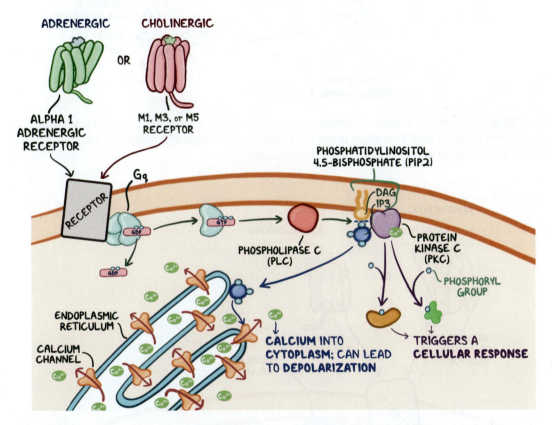

Figure 51.8 Mechanism of action of receptors coupled with G_q protein. The type of adrenergic receptor that couples with G_q protein is the alpha 1 receptor. The types of cholinergic muscarinic receptors that couple with G_q protein are the M_1, M_3, and M_5 receptors.

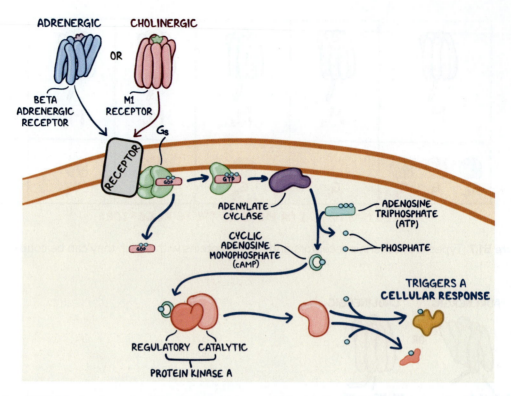

Figure 51.9 Mechanism of action of receptors coupled with G_s protein. The type of adrenergic receptor that couples with G_s protein is the beta receptor. The type of cholinergic muscarinic receptor that couples with G_s protein is the M_3 receptor.

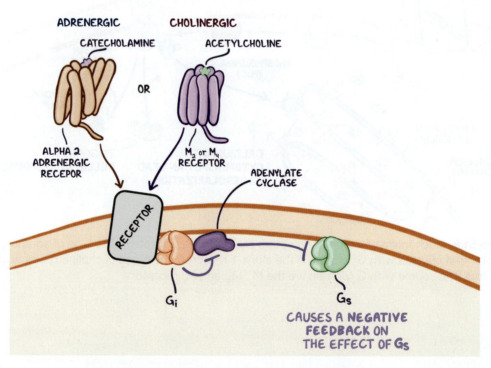

Figure 51.10 Mechanism of action of receptors coupled with G_i protein. The type of adrenergic receptor that couples with G_i protein is the alpha 2 receptor. The types of cholinergic muscarinic receptors that couple with G_i protein are the M_2 and M_4 receptors.

NOTES
BLOOD BRAIN BARRIER & CSF

BLOOD BRAIN BARRIER (BBB)

osms.it/blood-brain_barrier

- Selective barrier separating blood, interstitial liquid in central nervous system (CNS)
- Molecular transport keeps harmful substances out, allows metabolic waste products to diffuse from brain → plasma
- Formed by
  - Tight junctions between endothelial cells of brain capillaries
  - Astrocyte projection ("feet") supporting, maintaining structure
  - Basal (basement) membrane
- *Passive transport:* no energy needed (e.g. passive diffusion of lipid-soluble molecules)
- *Active transport:* energy needed (e.g. facilitated diffusion of glucose, amino acids)
- *Primary function:* CNS homeostasis
  - Providing selective nutrient passage
  - Controlling fluid movement
  - Protecting from toxins, microbes

BBB PERMEABILITY
- May change due to inflammation, irradiation, tumors
- Permeant molecules (lipid-soluble molecules)
  - Steroid hormones; oxygen; carbon dioxide; water; glucose, essential amino acids; certain electrolytes
- Impermeant molecules
  - Non-essential amino acids; waste products; microbes, toxins; proteins; certain electrolytes (e.g. potassium); water-soluble drugs

BBB IN CIRCUMVENTRICULAR ORGANS
- Absent in circumventricular organs → connection between CNS, blood
- Includes sensory, secretory organs

Sensory organs
- Sense plasma molecules, coordinate response to them
  - Area postrema/vomiting center (senses harmful substances in blood → vomiting reflex)
  - Subfornical organ
  - Vascular organ of lamina terminalis

Secretory organs
- Receive stimuli, secrete substances directly in plasma
  - Posterior pituitary gland
  - Median eminence of hypothalamus
  - Pineal gland

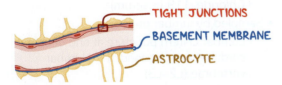

Figure 52.1 Components of the blood brain barrier.

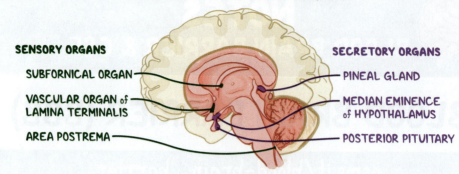

Figure 52.2 Sensory and secretory circumventricular organs.

CEREBROSPINAL FLUID (CSF)

osms.it/cerebrospinal-fluid

- Body fluid found within CNS
- Fills, circulates through
  - Ventricular system (lateral ventricles, third ventricle, fourth ventricle, central canal of spinal cord)
  - Subarachnoid space surrounding brain, spinal cord

CIRCULATION

- Lateral ventricles → interventricular foramina → third ventricle → cerebral aqueduct → fourth ventricle → lateral, median apertures → subarachnoid space, cisterns (some enters spinal column) → arachnoid granulations (arachnoid mater outpouching) → venous system circulation
- Kept in motion by cilia of ependymal cells lining ventricle system

PRODUCTION

- Mostly produced by choroid plexuses
  - Network of capillaries, modified ependymal cells in ventricles
  - Also functions as blood-CSF barrier
- Rate
  - 500mL/day
- Regulated by
  - Hormones, blood pressure, autonomic nervous system

CHARACTERISTICS

- *Quantity*: 125mL in total
- *Color*: limpid
- *Pressure*: range from 8–15mmHg (supine) to 16–24mmHg (sitting)
- *pH*: 7.33
- *Protein content*: 35mg/dL (< serum)
- *Glucose*: 60mg/dL (< serum)
- Electrolytes (mEq/L)
  - *Sodium*: 138
  - *Potassium*: 2.8
  - *Calcium*: 2.1
  - *Magnesium*: 2.0
  - *Chloride*: 119 (> serum)
- Sampled by lumbar puncture
  - Lumbar cistern puncture at end of spinal cord; between second, third lumbar vertebrae (L2–L3)

FUNCTIONS

- CNS protection
  - Trauma → absorbs mechanical energy
  - Own weight → provides buoyancy
  - Ischemia → decreases quantity, relieves intracranial pressure
  - Toxic metabolites → clears them out
- Transportation medium for chemical signals, nutrients

Chapter 52 Neurology: Blood Brain Barrier & CSF

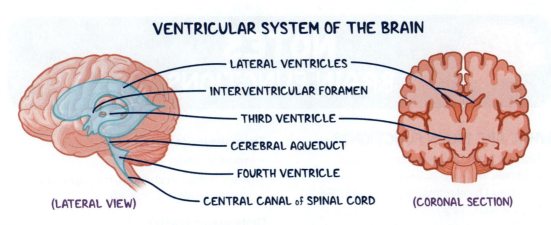

Figure 52.3 Ventricular system of the brain through which CSF flows.

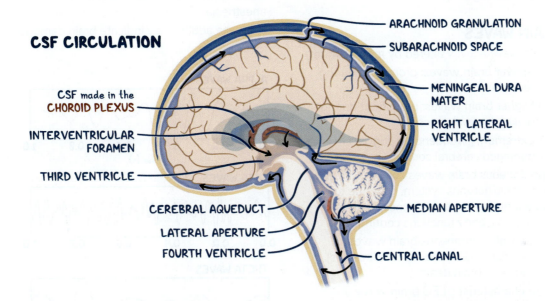

Figure 52.4 CSF circulation. CSF is produced by the choroid plexuses of the ventricles and is reabsorbed through the arachnoid granulations.

NOTES: BRAIN FUNCTIONS

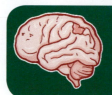

WHAT ARE BRAIN FUNCTIONS?

- *Normal brain functions*: continuous neuronal electrical activity
- Measured by electroencephalogram (EEG) for research, diagnostics
    - Electrodes on scalp record brain activity (measure voltage differences between cortical regions)

BRAIN WAVES

- Brain wave activity altered by mental state
    - *Slower brain waves*: prominent during relaxation
    - *Higher brain waves*: prominent during wakefulness/alertness
    - *Extreme ↑/↓ frequencies*: suggest damaged cerebral cortex
- Spontaneous brain waves controlled by autonomic nervous system, continue to appear during unconsciousness, coma (if some brain, body functions continue)
    - Lack of spontaneous brain waves (i.e. "flat EEG" without peaks/troughs) suggests brain death
- *Four characteristic EEG brain wave patterns*: different consciousness/sleep stages
    - *Appearance*: continuous peaks/troughs
    - *Wave frequency*: number of peaks/second (hertz (Hz))
    - *Wave amplitude/intensity*: indicates synchronicity of many neurons

Alpha waves (8–13Hz)
- Low amplitude, rhythmic, regular, synchronous waves
- Appear during relaxed consciousness states

Beta waves (14–30Hz)
- Rhythmic, but ↑ frequency, ↓ regularity compared to alpha waves
- Appear during alert consciousness states

Theta waves (4–7Hz)
- Irregular waves
- Often appear in children, may appear in conscious, alert-stage adults

Delta waves (<4Hz)
- ↑ amplitude waves
- Often appear during deep sleep stages, anesthesia
- In awake adults, may indicate brain damage

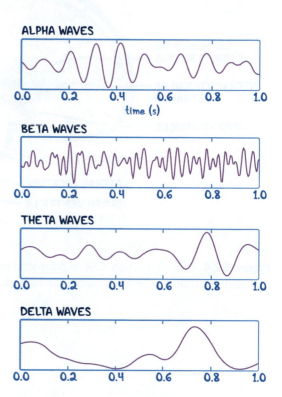

Figure 53.1 Four types of brain waves. From top to bottom: alpha waves (awake but relaxed), beta waves (awake and alert), theta waves (common in children), delta waves (deep sleep).

SLEEP

osms.it/sleep

WHAT IS SLEEP?

- Naturally recurring partially-unconscious state (inhibited response to external stimuli)
  - Coma: unconscious state (no response to external stimuli)
- Depressed cortical, continued brain stem activity → continued autonomic nervous system functions (e.g. controlling heart rate, respiration, blood pressure)
- Alternating stages based on EEG patterns

SLEEP STAGES

Non-rapid eye movement (NREM) sleep

- Little/no eye movement, thought-like brain activity, less voluntary muscle inhibition
- Stage 1
  - Immediately after falling asleep
  - EEG: irregular waveforms: slow frequencies, ↑ amplitudes
- Stage 2
  - First 30–45 minutes of sleep; occurs with deeper sleep
  - EEG: theta waves present
- Stages 3/4
  - Slow-wave sleep (SWS)
  - 90 minutes into sleep
  - EEG: activity slows down progressively
  - Decreased heart rate, blood pressure
  - Important for restorative functions

Rapid eye movement (REM) sleep

- Characterized by irregular brain waves → alpha waves (typically seen when awake)
- ↑ heart rate, blood pressure, respiratory rate; ↓ gastrointestinal function
  - Paradoxical sleep: although most body function activity increases/mimics wakefulness, individual is asleep
- Brain oxygen use: REM sleep > awake
- Spinal cord interneurons inhibit motor neurons → temporary skeletal muscle paralysis
- Most dreaming occurs
- Associated with memory consolidation; important for learning, cognitive performance

SLEEP PATTERNS

- Hypothalamus controls sleep cycle timing
  - Retina directly connected to hypothalamus, controls pineal gland (produces melatonin)
  - Decreasing light → melatonin release → sleepiness
- Alternating sleep/wake cycles = body's natural circadian rhythm
- Young/middle-aged adults: sleep starts in 4-stage NREM sleep → alternating REM, NREM cycles
- REM occurs approximately every 90 minutes; each cycle ↑ time
  - First REM: 5–10 minutes
  - Last REM: 20–50 minutes
  - Early in the night: deep sleep → awake periods (SWS sleep dominant)
  - Later in the night: REM sleep dominant
- Sleep patterns change over lifetime; ↑ age = ↓ sleep needs
  - Infants: 16 hours
  - Adults: 7.5–8.5 hours
  - ↑ age = ↑ length of each sleep cycle
  - Children spend more time in SWS than adults

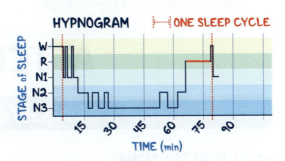

Figure 53.2 Hypongram illustrating progression through one sleep cycle. W = wakefulness, R = REM sleep, N1 = stage 1 NREM, N2 = stage 2 NREM, N3 = stage 3 NREM.

CONSCIOUSNESS

osms.it/consciousness

WHAT IS CONSCIOUSNESS?
- Awake, responsive state; simultaneous cerebral cortex electrical activity
- Associated with stimuli perception, voluntary movement control, high mental processing levels
- Superimposed by different neuron activities
    - E.g. same neurons involved in cognition, motor control
- Holistic, interconnected (e.g. memories can be triggered by smells, locations, people, etc.)
- Clinically, consciousness used to assess response (range: conscious → coma)
- Commonly assessed based on response to stimuli (movements, sounds, touch, etc.)

CONSCIOUSNESS STAGES
- *Alertness*: information processing, physical arousal
- *Sleep*: partially unconscious state (reduced sensory activity)
- *Dreaming*: mental experiences during sleep
- *Altered*: hypnosis, meditation, drug-induced, brain diseases, age → brain wave activity changes

LEARNING

osms.it/learning

WHAT IS LEARNING?
- Respond to stimulus → acquire new/adjust existing knowledge/skills/information/behaviors
- Influenced by single/repeated events
- Active process
    - Absorb knowledge by experiencing, exploring, interacting with world
- Begins at birth, ends at death
- Can occur in different forms
- Affected by internal, external factors
    - *External*: genetics, environment
    - *Internal*: attention, attitude, goals, values, behavior, emotions

ATTENTION

osms.it/attention

WHAT IS ATTENTION?
- Behavioral, cognitive process
    - Selective concentration on information
- Attention placed on subset of all perceived stimuli (e.g. one person in a crowd)
- Limited by capacity, duration
- Involves allocating processing resources (e.g. while multitasking)
- Integral component of cognitive system for environmental responses

MEMORY

osms.it/memory

WHAT IS ATTENTION?
- Information storage, retrieval
  - Important for learning, behavior, consciousness

MEMORY STAGES
- Sensory memory
  - Visual, auditory memory
  - Generally lasts 1 second without rehearsal, but recalled information very detailed
- Short-term memory (STM) (AKA working memory)
  - Generally fades over 30 seconds without rehearsal
  - Limited capacity
- Working memory
  - Information kept in consciousness for manipulation, integration
- Long-term memory (LTM)
  - Vast information amounts stored, recalled on demand
  - Short-term → long-term memory transfer influenced by emotional states; repetition; new, old information association; automatic memory

MEMORY TYPES
- Declarative (explicit/fact) memory
  - Explicit information learned, requires conscious recall
- Non-declarative memory
  - Procedural (skills) memory; motor memory; emotional memory; conditioned responses from repetition, experience

LANGUAGE

osms.it/language

WHAT IS LANGUAGE?
- System that communicates ideas, feelings through words

COMPONENTS OF LANGUAGE
- *Phonology*: language's auditory sound
- *Morphology*: word structure
- *Semantics*: word meaning
- *Syntax*: words combined into sentences
- *Pragmatics*: language depends on context, pre-existing knowledge, audience

BRAIN'S LANGUAGE PROCESSING
- Processed in dominant left hemisphere, especially Broca's area, Wernicke's area (connected by arcuate fasciculus)
  - *Broca's area*: controls speech's motor functions
  - *Wernicke's area*: language comprehension
- *Non-dominant right hemisphere*: body language (language's nonverbal component)
- *Aphasia*: inability to produce/comprehend language

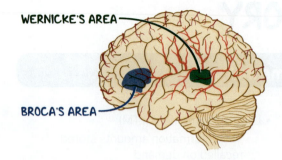

Figure 53.3 Lateral view of the left side of the brain showing the locations of Wernicke and Broca's areas. These areas are responsible for language comprehension and production, respectively.

EMOTION

osms.it/emotion

WHAT IS EMOTION?
- Conscious experience involving mental activity, pleasure/displeasure levels
- Associated with mood, motivation, behavior
- Involves experience, processing, behavior, psychological changes, behavioral changes

EMOTIONAL RESPONSE
- *Physiological response*: arousal → heart rate, body temperature, blood pressure changes
- *Behavioral response*: facial expressions, body language
- *Cognitive response*: interpretation depends on past experience

STRESS

osms.it/stress

WHAT IS STRESS?
- Body's physical, mental, emotional response to change requiring adaptation
- *Positive stress (eustress)*: motivation, alertness
- *Negative stress (distress)*: decreased performance, anxiety
- *Stress level severity*: dependent on individual's skills, abilities, coping mechanisms

STRESSORS
- Biological elements, external stimuli, causal events
  - *Environment*: uncomfortable temperature, loud noises
  - *Daily events*: losing keys, forgetting items
  - *Work/academic events*: assignments, time management
  - *Social events*: family-, friend-, society-related demands

462 OSMOSIS.ORG

- **Chemical/biological:** diet, alcohol, drugs
- **Psychological:** pressure, lack of control, unpredictability, frustration, conflict

STRESS RESPONSES
- Physiological
    - *Alarm stage:* initial reaction activates sympathetic nervous system (to maintain body functions enabling response)
    - *Resistance stage:* continuous hormone release (e.g. cortisol to maintain blood sugar levels; epinephrine to stimulate sympathetic nervous system) to continue engaging body
    - *Exhaustion stage:* body unable to maintain increased sympathetic nervous system activity
- Emotional
    - Individual may feel irritable, tense, helpless
    - May affect concentration, memory
- Behavioral
    - Individual may withdraw, abuse substances, become aggressive, suicidal
    - Chronic stress may lead to mental health disorders

NOTES: MOTOR NERVOUS SYSTEM

MOTOR CORTEX

osms.it/motor-cortex

MOTOR CORTEX BASICS
- Cerebral cortex region dedicated to voluntary movement planning, control, execution
- Location: posterior precentral gyrus, anterior to central sulcus

THREE INTERCONNECTED REGIONS

Premotor cortex
- Movement preparation, sensory guidance
- Emphasis on control of proximal, trunk muscles

Supplementary motor cortex
- Internally generates movement planning sequences
- Programs complex motor sequences
  - Active during mental movement rehearsal (even without physical execution)
- Coordinates two sides of body, bilateral movement

Primary motor cortex (area four)
- Topographically organized into motor homunculus
- Origin of programmed motor neuron activation patterns → movement execution
- Upper motor neurons in motor cortex become excited → transmit to brain stem, spinal cord → activate lower motor neurons → coordinated appropriate muscle contraction (voluntary movement)

MOTOR ACTIVATION PATTERN
- Supplementary motor, premotor cortices develop motor plan (specific muscles to contract, extent, sequence) → upper motor neurons in primary motor cortex → descending nerve tracts → lower motor neurons in spinal cord
- Basal ganglia, cerebellum provide additional fine tuning of motor output

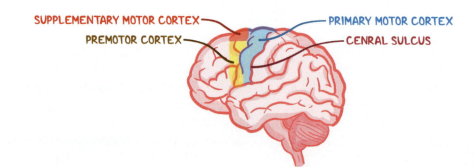

Figure 54.1 The three regions of the motor cortex.

MOTOR NEURONS & MUSCLE SPINDLES

osms.it/motor-neurons-and-muscle-spindles

MOTOR NEURONS

Motor unit
- Single motor neuron, muscle fibers it innervates
- All muscle fibers in motor unit are same fiber type (slow vs. fast twitch)
- *Fine control:* few muscle fibers per neuron (e.g. eye muscles)
- *Coarse control:* thousands of muscle fibers per neuron (e.g. postural muscles)
- *Motor neuron pool:* motor neuron collection innervating muscle fibers in same muscle

Force of contraction
- Graded action; determined by number of motor units recruited
- *Small motor neurons:* innervate few muscle fibers (generate relatively small amounts of force) → low threshold to activation → typically fire first
- *Large motor neurons:* innervate many muscle fibers (generate relatively large amounts of force) → require large action potentials to activate → typically fire last
- *Size principle:* more motor units recruited → larger motor neurons involved → greater tension developed

MUSCLE SPINDLE FIBERS

Extrafusal fibers
- Majority of skeletal muscle
- Innervated by α motor neurons
    - Large, myelinated multipolar (one axon, many dendrites) neurons that innervate extrafusal muscle fibers of skeletal muscles
    - Directly responsible for muscle contraction
    - Generate force

Intrafusal fibers
- Innervated by γ motor neurons
    - Small myelinated neurons that don't directly innervate muscle
    - Innervate intrafusal fibers → keep muscle spindles tight → allows for accurate detection of degree of stretch
- Too small to generate significant force
- Encapsulated in sheaths → form muscle spindles
    - Run parallel to extrafusal fibers
    - Abundant in muscles used for fine movements
    - Spindle-shaped organs composed of intrafusal muscle fibers
    - Innervated by sensory, motor nerve fibers
    - Attached to connective tissue

Intrafusal muscle spindle types
- Both subtypes present in every spindle
- Nuclear bag fibers
    - Larger, nuclei accumulate in central "bag" region
- Nuclear chain fibers
    - Smaller, nuclei arranged in rows (chains), more common

MUSCLE SPINDLES INNERVATION

Sensory (afferent) nerves
- Group Ia afferent nerves
    - Innervates central region of both intrafusal muscle spindle subtypes
    - Relatively large nerves → fast conduction velocity
    - Form primary endings in spiral-shaped terminal around central region of muscle spindle fibers

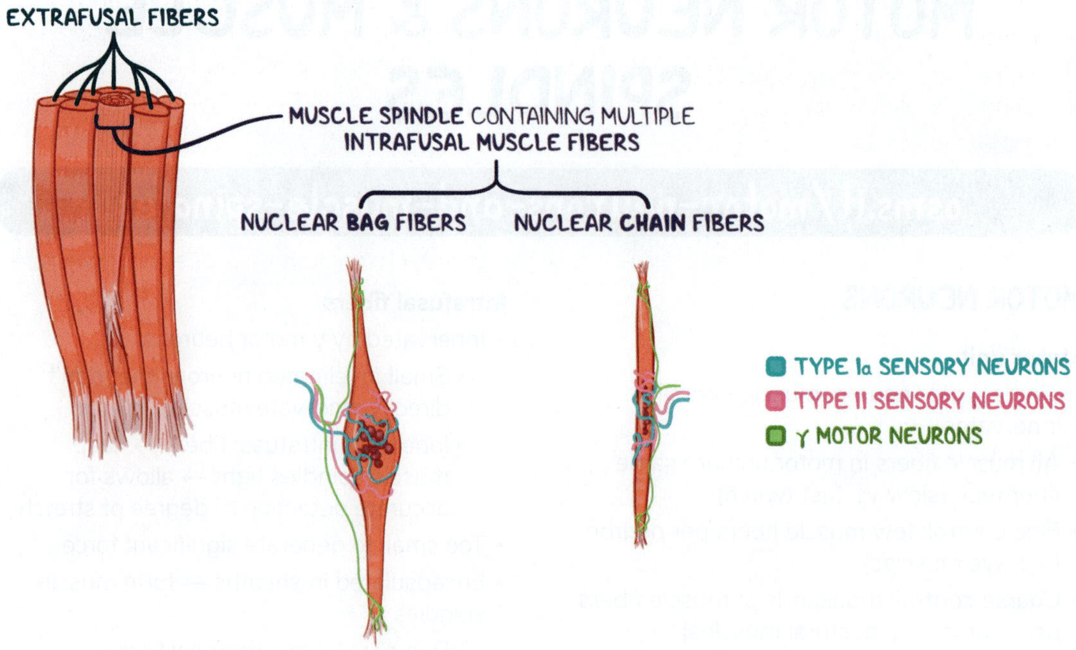

Figure 54.2 Muscles are composed of muscle fibers bundles with extrafusal muscle fibers on the outside and intrafusal fibers on the inside. There are two intrafusal fiber subtypes: nuclear bag fibers and nuclear chain fibers, determined by the nuclei arrangement within.

- Group II afferent nerves
  - Primarily innervate nuclear chain fibers
  - Intermediate diameter → intermediate conduction velocity
  - Form secondary endings on nuclear chain fibers (primarily)

Motor (efferent) nerves
- Two types
  - Dynamic γ motor neurons → synapse on nuclear bag fibers → "plate endings"
  - Static γ motor neurons → synapse on nuclear chain fibers → form "trail endings" → spread out over longer distances

MUSCLE SPINDLES FUNCTION
- Stretch receptors
- Extrafusal muscle fibers contract/stretch → muscle spindles correct for changes in muscle length → return muscle to resting length after shortening/lengthening

- Muscle stretch → extrafusal muscle fibers lengthen, parallel intrafusal fibers stretch
- Increased length of intrafusal fibers detected by sensory afferent fibers innervating them; increase in length of intrafusal fibers activates group Ia, group II sensory afferent fibers (group Ia afferent fibers detect velocity of length change; group II afferent fibers detect length of muscle fibers)
- Activation of group Ia afferent fibers stimulates α motor neurons in spinal cord → innervation of extrafusal fibers in same muscle → muscle contraction → original stretch is opposed when reflex causes muscle to contract
- γ motor neurons coactivated with α motor neurons → muscle spindle remains sensitive to muscle length changes (even during contraction)

Chapter 54 Neurology: Motor Nervous System

MOTOR NEURONS CLASSIFICATION
- α motor neurons
  - Innervate extrafusal skeletal muscle fibers → contraction
- γ motor neurons
  - Smaller, slower
  - Regulate sensitivity of intrafusal muscle fibers
  - Innervate specialized intrafusal muscle fibers (part of muscle spindles that sense muscle length) → adjust sensitivity of muscle spindles → ensures appropriate response as extrafusal fibers contract
- α, γ motor neurons are co-activated → muscle spindles remain sensitive to muscle length changes as muscle contracts

STRETCH REFLEX

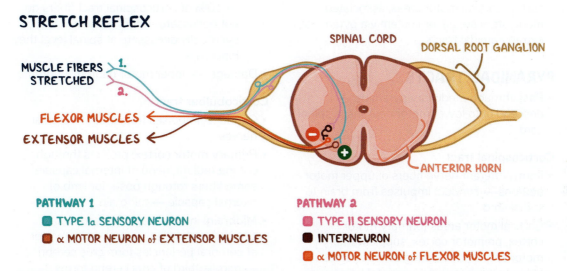

Figure 54.3 Stretch reflex when extensor muscles are stretched. Type Ia sensory neurons synapse with α motor neurons of extensor muscles, causing extensor muscle contraction. Type II sensory neurons synapse with an interneuron, which inhibits the α motor neurons to the flexor muscles → flexor muscles relax. These actions together oppose the original stretch.

α-γ COACTIVATION

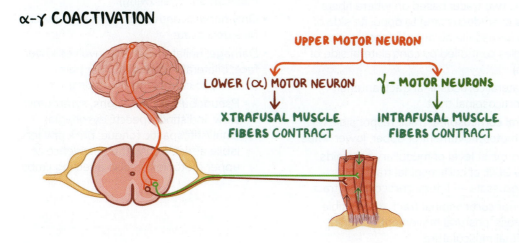

Figure 54.4 Coactivation of lower motor neurons and gamma motor neurons by upper motor neurons ensures that muscle spindle remains sensitive to muscle length changes (even during contraction).

PYRAMIDAL & EXTRAPYRAMIDAL TRACTS

osms.it/pyramidal-and-extrapyramidal-tracts

- Motor neurons descend from cerebral cortex (cortical motor areas, associated modulatory areas), brainstem via pyramidal, extrapyramidal tracts

PYRAMIDAL TRACTS

- Pass through medullary pyramids → descend onto lower motor neurons in spinal cord

Corticospinal tract

- Forms efferent nerve fibers of upper motor neurons → conduct impulses from brain to spinal cord
- Cortical motor areas (primary motor cortex, premotor cortex, supplementary motor areas), modulating sensory areas (somatosensory cortex, parietal lobe, cingulate gyrus) → posterior limb of internal capsule → cerebral peduncle (base of midbrain) → pons → medulla → spinal cord → synapse directly onto alpha motor neurons → control voluntary movement
- Forms two tracts based on where fibers cross over (decussate) to opposite side of body in medulla oblongata (decussation → muscles controlled by contralateral side of brain)
    - Lateral corticospinal tract, anterior corticospinal tract
- *Lateral corticospinal tract:* responsible for fine-motor movement of upper, lower limbs
    - Forms at level of medullary pyramids → 90% of corticospinal tract fibers decussate → lateral corticospinal tract
- *Anterior corticospinal tract:* responsible for gross, postural movement of trunk, proximal musculature
    - Forms at level of medullary pyramids → 10% of corticospinal tract fibers do not decussate → forms anterior tract; eventually decussate at spinal level they innervate
- Damage → upper motor neuron syndrome

Corticobulbar tract

- Conducts impulses from brain → cranial nerves
- *Primary motor cortex:* projects through corona radiata, genu of internal capsule/ some fibers through posterior limb of internal capsule → midbrain
- *Midbrain:* internal capsule becomes cerebral peduncles, ventral white matter of cerebral peduncles form crus cerebri → middle third of crus cerebri forms corticobulbar (and corticospinal fibres) → corticobulbar fibers exit brainstem at appropriate level to synapse on lower motor neurons of cranial nerves
- Controls facial, neck muscles (expression, mastication, swallowing)
- Only nerves controlling muscles of lower face decussate
- *Damage:* unilateral → only involves lower face; bilateral → pseudobulbar palsy (inability to control facial muscles)
    - *Pseudobulbar palsy signs, symptoms:* slow, indistinct speech; dysphagia; small/stiff/spastic tongue; brisk jaw jerk, labile affect with/without evidence of upper motor lesion also affecting limbs

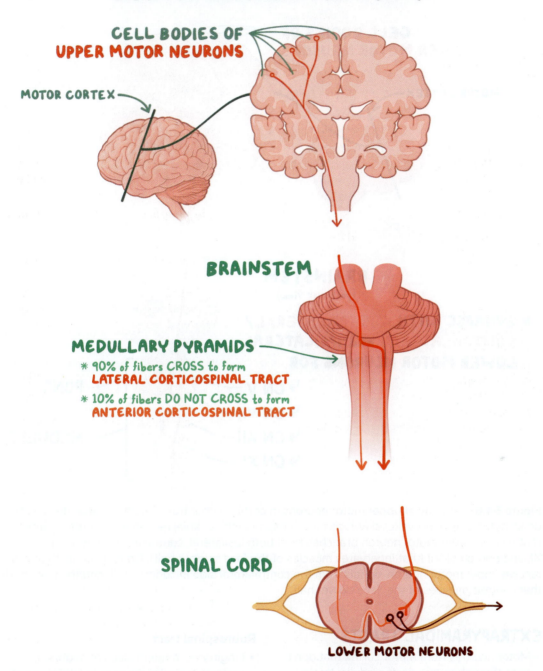

Figure 54.5 Upper motor neuron pathway in corticospinal tract. Lateral corticospinal tract fibers decussate in medulla, while anterior corticospinal tract fibers decussate at the level of the lower motor neuron (which they synapse with).

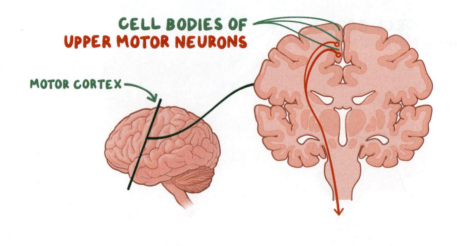
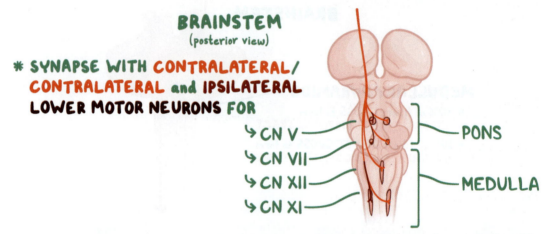

Figure 54.6 Pathway of upper motor neurons in corticobulbar tract. The fibers that decussate do so at the cranial nerve level (which they synapse with). Cranial nerve lower motor neurons that receive upper motor neuron branches from both ipsilateral, contralateral sides include: CN V, XI, and portion of VII (that innervates muscles of the face's upper half). Cranial nerves that only receive upper motor neuron signals from the contralateral side include: CN XII and the part of VII that controls muscles of the face's lower half.

EXTRAPYRAMIDAL TRACTS

- Motor neurons from motor cortex that don't pass through pyramids of medulla; tracts run through pons, medulla, target lower motor neurons in spinal cord
- Control reflexes, locomotion, complex movements, posture
- Modulated by nigrostriatal pathway, basal ganglia, cerebellum, vestibular nuclei, sensory areas of cerebral cortex
- *Extrapyramidal tract damage:* various types of dyskinesias (involuntary movement disorders)

Rubrospinal tract

- Originates in red nucleus of midbrain, projects to motor neurons in lateral spinal cord (runs adjacent to lateral corticospinal tract), terminates in cervical spinal cord
- Mediates voluntary movement (primarily upper limbs)
- Activates flexor muscles
- Inhibits extensor muscles
- Can assume function of corticospinal tract if corticospinal tract is injured
- *Damage:* temporary slowness of movement

Lateral vestibulospinal tract
- Originates in lateral vestibular nucleus (Deiters nucleus), projects to ipsilateral motor neurons in spinal cord
- Activates extensors; inhibits flexors
- Maintains upright balance, posture through action on muscles of trunk, legs
- Receives input from cerebellum

Reticulospinal tract
- Coordinates automatic locomotion, posture movements
- Facilitates, inhibits voluntary movement
- Mediates autonomic function
- Modulates pain
- Damage at/just below level of red nucleus
  - *Decerebration:* unopposed extension of head, limbs
- *Pontine (medial) reticulospinal tract:* originates in nuclei of pons, projects to ventromedial spinal cord; activates anti-gravity extensor muscles
- *Medullary (lateral) reticulospinal tract:* originates in medullary reticular formation, projects to spinal cord; inhibits excitatory axial extensors

Tectospinal tract (colliculospinal tract)
- Originates in superior colliculus, projects to cervical spinal cord
- *Controls neck muscles:* mediates reflex, postural movements of head in response to visual, auditory stimuli

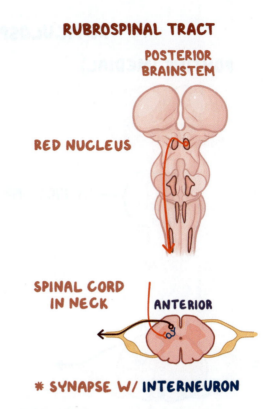

Figure 54.7 Rubrospinal tract.

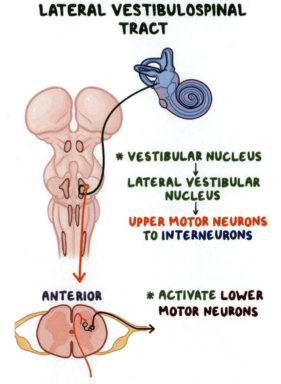

Figure 54.8 Lateral vestibulospinal tract.

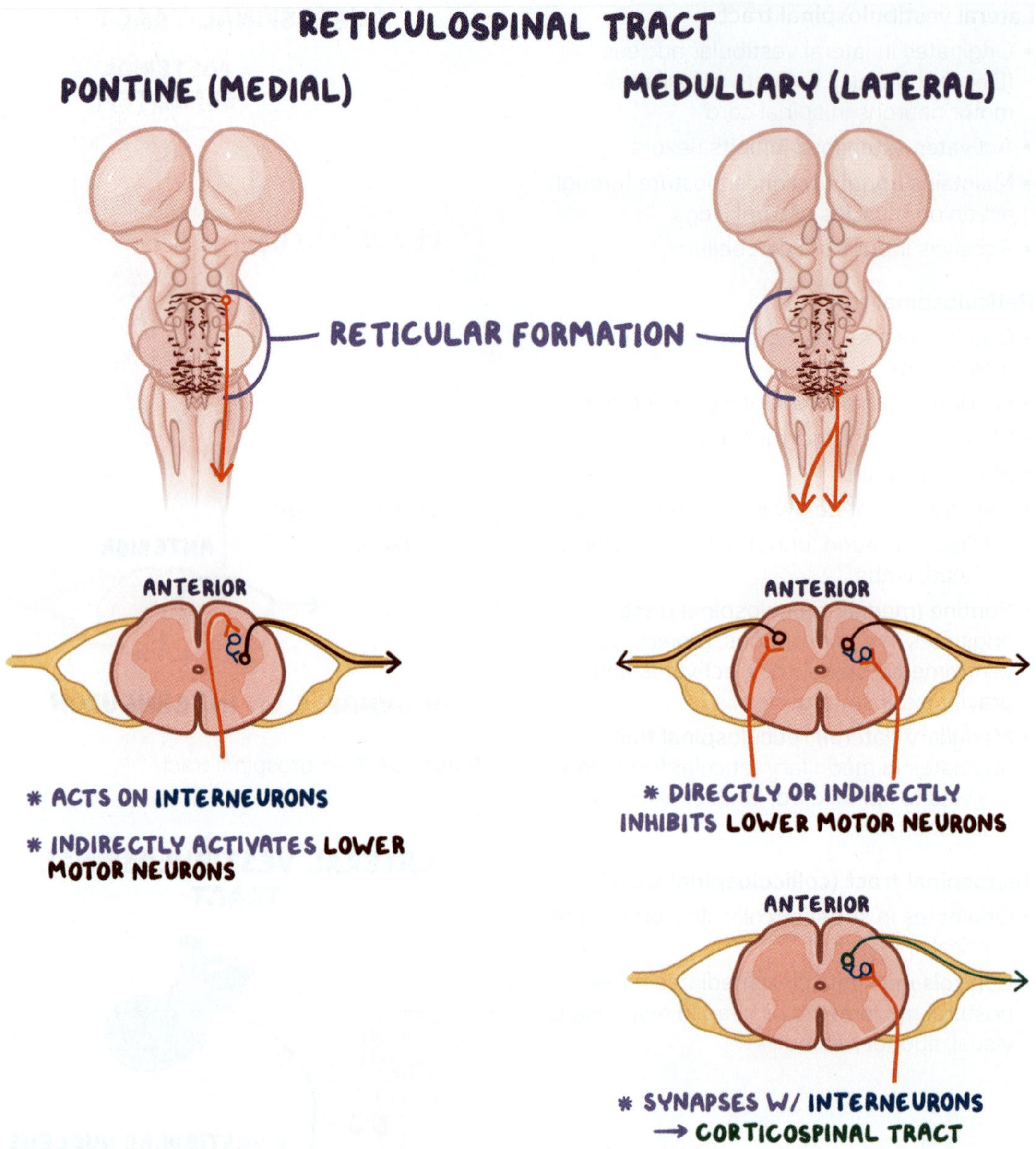

RETICULOSPINAL TRACT

PONTINE (MEDIAL)

RETICULAR FORMATION

ANTERIOR

* ACTS ON INTERNEURONS
* INDIRECTLY ACTIVATES LOWER MOTOR NEURONS

MEDULLARY (LATERAL)

ANTERIOR

* DIRECTLY OR INDIRECTLY INHIBITS LOWER MOTOR NEURONS

ANTERIOR

* SYNAPSES W/ INTERNEURONS → CORTICOSPINAL TRACT

Figure 54.9 Pontine and medullary reticulospinal tracts.

SIGNS OF UPPER VS. LOWER MOTOR NEURON LESIONS

	UPPER MOTOR NEURON LESION	LOWER MOTOR NEURON LESION
LESION	Lesion anywhere in motor tract above anterior horn cell of spinal cord	Lesion affects nerve fibers travelling from anterior horn of spinal cord to relevant muscle
TONE	↑ Spasticity: (↑, involuntary, velocity-dependent muscle tone, causes resistance to movement) Clonus: (involuntary, rhythmic, muscular contractions, relaxation) Clasp-knife response: initial higher resistance to movement followed by lesser resistance	↓
POWER	Upper limb → primarily extensor weakness Lower limb → primarily flexor weakness	Distal > proximal distribution Flexors, extensors equally affected
DEEP TENDON REFLEXES	↑	↓/absent
BABINSKI REFLEX*	Babinski sign present	Absent
MUSCLE WASTING	Not notably wasted	Present
MUSCLE FASCICULATION	Absent	Present

*Babinski reflex: sole of the foot is stimulated with a pointed instrument → hallux flexion (normal) or extension (sign of pathology)

CEREBELLUM

osms.it/cerebellum

CEREBELLUM

- **Location:** posterior fossa below occipital lobe
- Connected to brain stem by three **cerebellar peduncles** containing afferent, efferent fibers
- **Regulates movement, posture:** controls movement synergy (rate, range, force, direction)

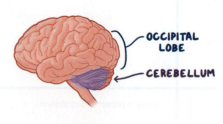

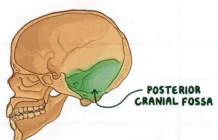

Figure 54.10 Cerebellum location relative to brain and skull.

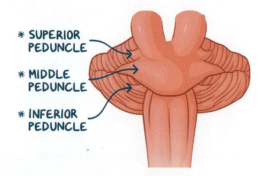

Figure 54.11 Superior, middle, inferior peduncles attach cerebellum to brain stem.

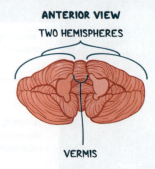

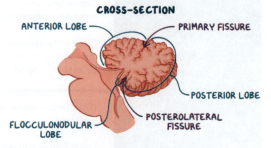

Figure 54.12 Cerebellum divisions from anterior, lateral views. The vermis is the narrow ridge separating the two hemispheres, fissures separate the lobes.

FUNCTIONAL DIVISIONS

Vestibulocerebellum
- Anatomical components: flocculonodular lobe (plus immediately adjacent vermis)
- Vestibular input: balance, eye movement

Spinocerebellum
- Anatomical components: vermis, intermediate parts of hemispheres
- Spinal cord input (proprioception): regulation of movement synergy

Pontocerebellum
- Anatomical components: lateral part of cerebellar hemispheres
- Cerebral input (via pontine nuclei): controls planning, movement initiation

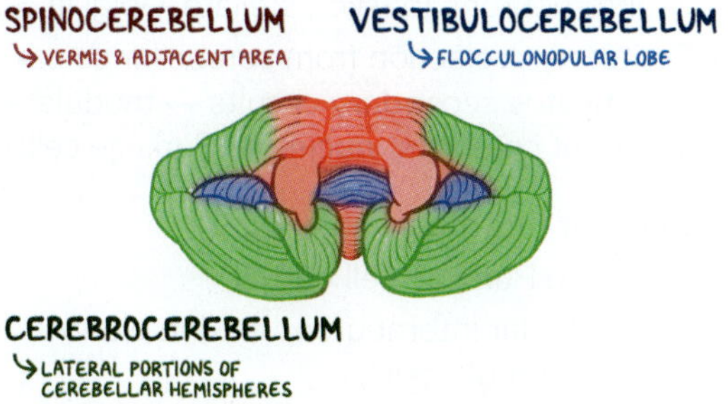

Chapter 54 Neurology: Motor Nervous System

Figure 54.13 Functional cerebellum divisions (anterior view).

CEREBELLAR CORTEX

Three layers

- Molecular layer
  - *Outermost layer:* contains outer stellate cells, basket cells, dendrites of Purkinje, Golgi II cells, axons of granule cells
  - *Two inhibitory interneuron types:* stellate cells, basket cells (inhibit Purkinje cells, basket cells, outer stellate cells, Golgi type II cells)
- Purkinje cell layer
  - *Middle layer:* contains Purkinje cells
  - Primary integrative neurons of cerebellar cortex
  - Provides sole output of cerebellar cortex
  - Exclusively inhibitory output onto deep cerebellar neurons, vestibular nuclei of brainstem
- Granular layer
  - *Innermost layer:* contains granule cells, Golgi II cells, glomeruli
  - Excitatory mossy fibers from pontine nuclei enter granular layer, deep cerebellar nuclei; in glomeruli axons of mossy fibers from spinocerebellar, pontocerebellar tracts synapse on dendrites of granules, Golgi type II cells

Cerebellar cortex output

- Purkinje cell axons → always inhibitory (GABAergic)
- Purkinje cells axons project topographically to deep cerebellar nuclei, lateral vestibular nuclei
- Regulates movement synergy

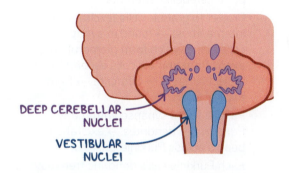

Figure 54.15 Deep cerebellar and vestibular nuclei, to which Purkinje cells project. The lateral vestibular nuclei are in the medulla.

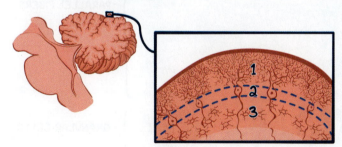

Figure 54.14 The three layers of the cerebellar cortex, from superficial to deep.

Excitatory input to cerebellar cortex
- *Arises from two systems:* climbing fibers, mossy fiber system (both project to deep cerebellar nuclei)
- *Climbing fibers:* originate in inferior olive of medulla, project directly to Purkinje cells in 1:1 ratio
    - Single action potential → multiple excitatory bursts of descending amplitude (complex spikes) in Purkinje dendrites
    - Modulate Purkinje cell response to mossy fiber input
    - May be involved in cerebellar learning
- *Mossy fiber system:* majority of cerebellar input
    - Vestibulocerebellar, spinocerebellar pontocerebellar afferents
    - Project to granule cells (excitatory interneurons) → found in synapse collections which form glomeruli → axons from granule cells ascend to molecular layer → bifurcate → form parallel fibers
    - Parallel fibers synapse with many Purkinje cell dendrites → excitation beams across Purkinje cell row
    - Each Purkinje cell's dendritic tree may receive input from up to 250,000 parallel fibers (contrast with climbing fiber input to Purkinje dendrites → 1:1)
    - Mossy fiber input produces single action potential (AKA simple spikes)
    - Parallel fibers also synapse on cerebellar interneurons (basket, stellate, Golgi II)
- Excitatory projection from cerebellar cortex → activates secondary circuits → modulate output of cerebellar nuclei via Purkinje cells

Cerebellar interneurons
- Modulate Purkinje cell output
- All cerebellar interneurons are inhibitory (except granule cells)
    - Granule cells offer excitatory input for basket cells, stellate cells, Golgi II cells, Purkinje cells
    - Basket, stellate cells inhibit Purkinje cells (parallel fibers)
    - Golgi II cells inhibit granule cells → reduce excitatory effect on Purkinje cells

LESION DISORDERS
- Lesions → lack of voluntary coordination of muscle movements, limbs, posture, gait (ataxia)

General signs and symptoms
- Lack of coordination → errors in fine movement control
- Delayed onset of movement/poor execution of sequences
- Overshoot target, stop before reaching
- *Dysdiadochokinesia:* unable to perform rapid alternating movements
- *Intention tremor:* tremor perpendicular to direction of voluntary movement, increases near end of movement

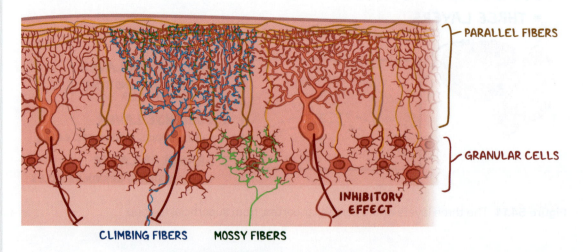

Figure 54.16 Projection destinations for climbing and mossy fibers.

- **Rebound phenomenon:** inability to stop movement

Specific signs and symptoms
- According to affected portion of cerebellum
  - *Posterior (flocculonodular lobe):* nystagmus, poor postural control, gait dysfunction
  - *Midline (vermis):* truncal, gait ataxia
  - *Lateral (hemispheric):* limb ataxia, dysmetria, dysdiadochokinesia, intention tremor, dysarthria, hypotonia

BASAL GANGLIA: DIRECT & INDIRECT PATHWAY OF MOVEMENT

osms.it/basal-ganglia-direct-indirect-pathways

BASAL GANGLIA
- Collection of subcortical nuclei
- Consists of globus pallidus, striatum (caudate nucleus, putamen, amygdala)
- Associated nuclei: ventral anterior, ventral lateral nuclei of thalamus; subthalamic nucleus of diencephalon; substantia nigra of midbrain
- **Function:** influence motor cortex via pathways through thalamus
  - Aid in planning, execution of smooth movements; contribute to affective, cognitive function

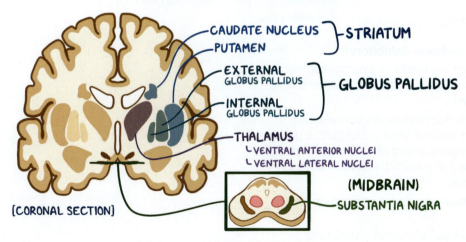

Figure 54.17 Location of basal ganglia and associated structures in coronal slice of the brain.

COMPLEX AFFERENT & EFFERENT PATHWAYS

- Excitatory pathways use glutamate as neurotransmitter
- Inhibitory pathways use GABA (γ-aminobutyric acid) as neurotransmitter
- Almost all cerebral cortex areas project topographically onto striatum, input from motor cortex → striatum → thalamus → back to the cortex via indirect/direct pathways
- Outputs of indirect, direct pathways from basal ganglia to motor cortex are opposed, balanced
    - Disturbance of output → upsets balance of motor control → activity increases/decreases
- Back-and-forth connection between striatum, pars compacta of substantia nigra are dopaminergic
    - Dopaminergic pathway is inhibitory via D2 receptors on indirect pathway; excitatory effect via D1 receptors on direct pathway

Direct pathway (excitatory)

- Striatum → inhibits → internal segment of globus pallidus, pars reticulata of substantia nigra (structures that would inhibit otherwise excitatory structures)
- Substantia nigra → inhibitory input to thalamus
- Thalamus → excitatory input to motor cortex
- Overall input is excitatory

Indirect pathway (inhibitory)

- Striatum → inhibits → external segment of globus pallidus → inhibits → subthalamic nucleus
- Subthalamic nucleus projects excitatory input to internal segment of globus pallidus → internal segment of globus pallidus, pars reticulata of substantia nigra → inhibits → thalamus
- Thalamus → excitatory input to motor cortex
- Overall input of indirect pathway is inhibitory

BASAL GANGLIA DISEASES

Parkinson's disease

- Cellular damage → cells of pars compacta of substantia nigra degenerate → reduce inhibition via indirect pathway, reduce excitation via direct pathway
- Initial accumulation in olfactory bulb, medulla oblongata, pontine tegmentum; early non-motor symptoms (loss of smell, sleep disturbances, autonomic dysfunction)
- **Progression:** affects midbrain, basal forebrain, neocortex, typical Parkinson's symptoms (resting tremor; movement slowness, delay; shuffling gait)
- **Treatment:** aim to ↑ dopamine level in brain/mimic its action with dopaminergic drugs
    - L-DOPA (dopamine precursor) → remaining dopamine neurons produce, secrete more dopamine
    - Dopamine agonists (e.g. bromocriptine) → bind to postsynaptic dopaminergic receptors
    - MAO-B inhibitors → impede dopamine breakdown

Huntington's disease

- Hereditary disorder caused by destruction of striatal, cortical cholinergic neurons, inhibitory GABAergic neurons
- Presents with chorea (writhing movements), dementia
- No known cure

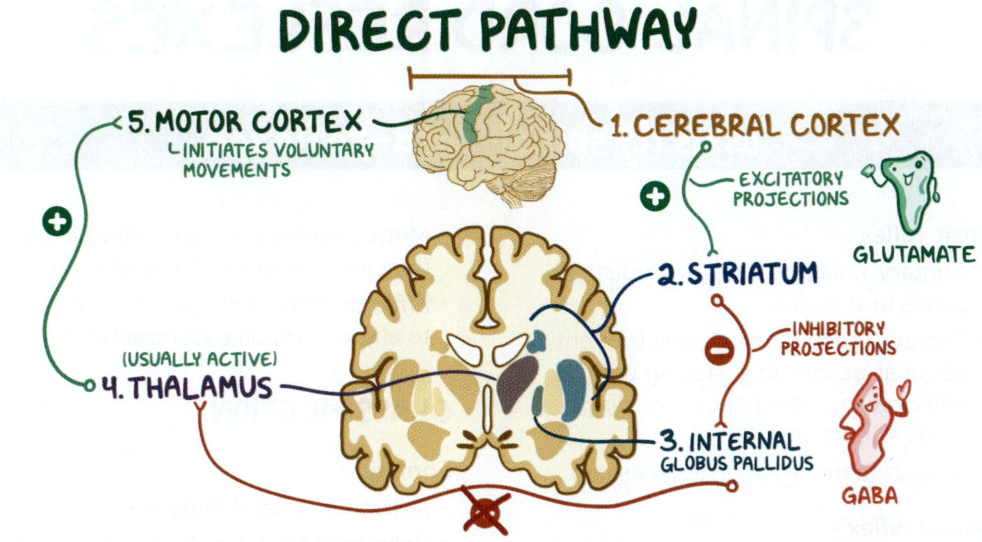

Chapter 54 Neurology: Motor Nervous System

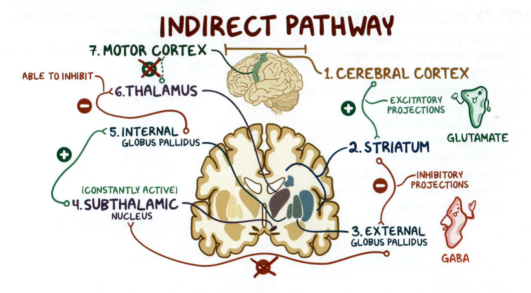

Figure 54.18 Direct pathway. Cerebral cortex sends excitatory projections to striatum → sends inhibitory projections to internal globus pallidus → sends inhibitory projections to thalamus. When striatum inhibits internal globus pallidus, internal globus pallidus can't inhibit thalamus → thalamus is free to send excitatory signals to motor cortex.

Figure 54.19 Indirect pathway. Cerebral cortex sends excitatory projections to striatum → sends inhibitory projections to external globus pallidus → sends inhibitory projections to subthalamic nucleus. When striatum inhibits external globus pallidus, external globus pallidus can't inhibit subthalamic nucleus → subthalamic nucleus is free to send excitatory signals to internal globus pallidus. Internal globus pallidus inhibits thalamus, preventing it from sending excitatory signals to the motor cortex.

SPINAL CORD REFLEXES

osms.it/spinal-cord-reflexes

Intrinsic reflex
- Involuntary, unlearned, rapid, predictable response to stimulus
    - Prevents need for conscious thought about all actions (e.g. staying upright, withdrawing from pain, controlling visceral reactions)
    - Subject to modification if necessary

Acquired reflex
- Acquired after sufficient repetition (e.g. complex sequence of reactions that occur while driving a car)
    - Process is automatic, but had to be learned initially

REFLEX ARC COMPONENTS
- *Receptor:* detects stimulus
- *Sensory neuron:* transmits afferent impulse to central nervous system (CNS)
- *Integration center:* processes information, dictates response
    - *Simple reflex arcs:* single synapse between sensory neuron, motor neurons (monosynaptic reflex)
    - *Complex reflex arcs:* multiple synapses with chains of interneurons (polysynaptic reflex)
- *Motor neuron:* conducts efferent impulse from integration center to effector
- *Effector:* muscle fiber/gland that responds to efferent impulse (contracts/secretes)

CLASSIFICATION

Somatic
- Activates skeletal muscle
- Voluntary; occasionally non-voluntary (reflexes)

Autonomic (visceral)
- Activates visceral organ effectors
    - *Smooth muscle:* involuntary; forms walls of hollow organs, glands, blood vessels, tracts of respiratory, urinary, reproductive systems
    - *Cardiac muscle:* involuntary; forms heart walls

NOTES
SENSORY NERVOUS SYSTEM

SENSORY RECEPTOR FUNCTION

osms.it/sensory-receptor-function

- 1st order neurons carry information from somatosensory receptors
    - *Pseudounipolar*: no separate dendrites, axons
    - Single axon splits into central branch, peripheral branch
    - Peripheral branch goes from cell body in dorsal root ganglia to receptive field on peripheral tissue
    - Small receptive field = ↑ resolution
    - Large receptive field = ↓ resolution
    - Ion channels open, close in response to stimulus → membrane depolarizes → voltage gated channels open → triggers action potential
    - To prevent multiple neurons firing, neurons have inhibitory interneurons, AKA lateral inhibition
    - Stimulus strength, duration determined by frequency of nerve firing
- *Adaption*: fewer signals sent in response to same stimulus over time
    - *Fast adapting/phasic*: high sensitivity; falls off quickly
    - *Slow adapting/tonic*: constant sensitivity

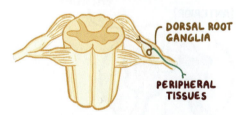
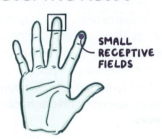
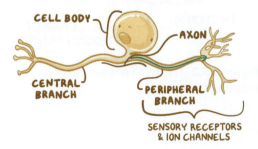
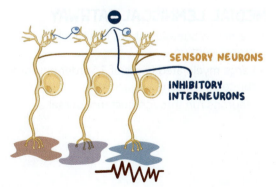

Figure 55.1 Features of 1st order neurons and lateral inhibition. Interneurons suppress activity of the neurons next to one that has received a stimulus (lateral inhibition) → pin points stimulus by defining its boundaries.

SOMATOSENSORY PATHWAYS

osms.it/somatosensory-pathways

- **Somatic senses**: touch, proprioception, pain, temperature
- Types of somatosensory fibers
  - **Non-myelinated fibers (type C)**: slowest; sense burning pain, hot temperature
  - **Small myelinated fibers (type Aδ)**: faster; sense sharp pain, gross touch, cold temperature
  - **Large myelinated fibers (type A-α; A-β)**: fastest; sense proprioception, vibration, fine touch

SOMATOSENSORY PATHWAYS

- Carry somatosensory input up spinal cord to brain
- Consist of 4-neuron relay
  - **1st order neuron/afferent sensory neuron**: has sensory receptors, converts stimuli into impulse
  - **2nd order neuron**: cell body in spinal cord or brainstem, synapses with 3rd-order neuron
  - **3rd order neuron**: cell body in thalamus, sends signal to somatosensory cortex
  - **4th order neuron/cortical neuron**: cell body in sensory cortex
- Includes medial lemniscal/posterior pathway, spinothalamic/anterolateral pathway

MEDIAL LEMNISCAL PATHWAY

- Carries information about fine touch, proprioception
- Large myelinated fibers of 1st order neurons run to spinal cord
- Neurons run through posterior/dorsal funiculus of spinal cord
  - Via cuneate fascicle for arms, chest
  - Via gracilis fascicle for trunk, legs
- 1st, 2nd order neurons synapse in medulla
  - 1st synapse
- 2nd order neurons run to medial lemniscus, decussate; run through pons, midbrain to the thalamus
- 2nd, 3rd order neurons synapse in thalamus
  - 2nd synapse
- 3rd order neurons run to sensory cortex in parietal lobe
- 3rd, 4th order neurons synapse in sensory cortex
  - 3rd synapse
- Some 1st order neurons synapse with interneurons at posterior horn
  - Axons run to anterior horn, synapse directly with motor neuron
  - Important for reflexes

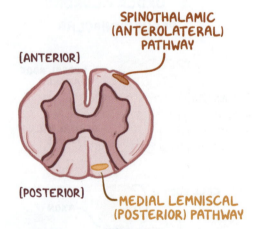

Figure 55.2 The two somatosensory pathways.

Chapter 55 Neurology: Sensory Nervous System

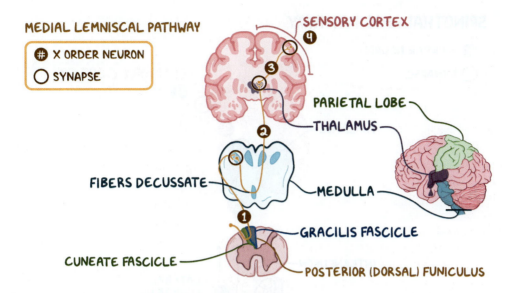

Figure 55.3 The medial lemniscal pathway carries information about fine touch and proprioception. It includes three synapses between four neurons.

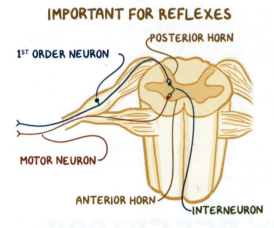

Figure 55.4 Reflex pathway occurs at the level of the spinal cord: 1st order neuron synapses with an interneuron, which synapses with a motor neuron.

SPINOTHALAMIC PATHWAY

- Carries information about pain, temperature, crude touch
- Small/non-myelinated fibers of 1st order neurons run to spinal cord
  - *Small myelinated fibers*: sharp pain, cold temperature
  - *Non-myelinated fibers*: hot temperature, burning pain, crude touch

- 1st, 2nd order neurons synapse in posterior horn of spinal cord/1st synapse
  - *Small myelinated fibers*: enter through dorsal root, bend upwards, travel through two vertebral segments
  - *Non-myelinated fibers*: follow same pathway but synapse with interneurons first, AKA before reaching posterior horn
- 2nd order neurons decussate, cross to anterior horn through central canal
- Neurons then carried through one of two tracts to thalamus
  - *Lateral tract*: carries information for pain, pressure, temperature through lateral funiculus
  - *Anterior tract*: carries information for crude touch through anterior funiculus
- 2nd, 3rd order neurons synapse in thalamus/2nd synapse
- 3rd order neurons run to sensory cortex in parietal lobe
- 3rd, 4th order neurons synapse in sensory cortex/3rd synapse

OSMOSIS.ORG 483

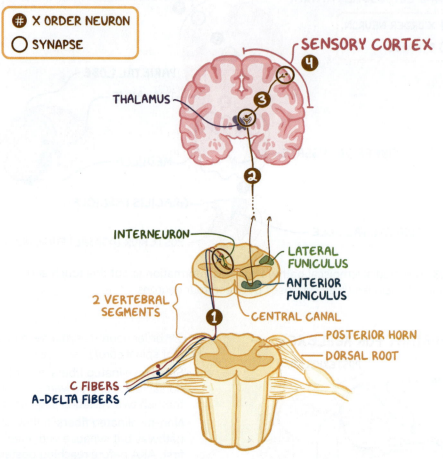

Figure 55.5 The spinothalamic pathway carries information about pain, temperature, and crude touch. It includes three synapses between four neurons. The 1st order C fibers synapse with an interneuron, which then synapses with the 2nd order neuron.

SOMATOSENSORY RECEPTORS

osms.it/somatosensory-receptors

- Perceive general somatic senses
- Include mechanoreceptors, AKA both mechanosensors and proprioceptors, thermoreceptors, nociceptors

MECHANOSENSORS

- Used for touch; several types

Meissner/tactile corpuscles
- Sensitive to light touch
- Encapsulated; located in dermis of hairless skin
- Fast adapting; small receptive fields

Merkel (tactile) discs
- Sensitive to pressure
- Non-encapsulated; located in epidermis of hairless skin
- Slow adapting; small receptive fields

Ruffini (bulbous) corpuscles
- Sensitive to skin stretching
- Encapsulated; located in dermis of all skin
- Slow adapting; big receptive fields

Pacinian (lamellar) corpuscles
- Sensitive to vibration
- Encapsulated; located deep in dermis/subcutaneous tissue of all skin
- Fast adapting; big receptive fields

PROPRIOCEPTORS
- Used for proprioception; several types

Muscle spindle
- Detect when muscle stretched
- Located throughout perimysium, AKA connective tissue around muscle cells

Golgi tendon organ
- Detect when tendon stretched
- Located in tendons close to muscle insertion

Joint receptors
- Detect joint position, motion
- Located in joint

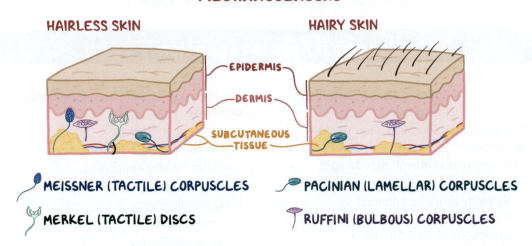

Figure 55.6 The four types of mechanosensors. Only Pacinian and Ruffini corpuscles are present in all kinds of skin (hairless and hairy).

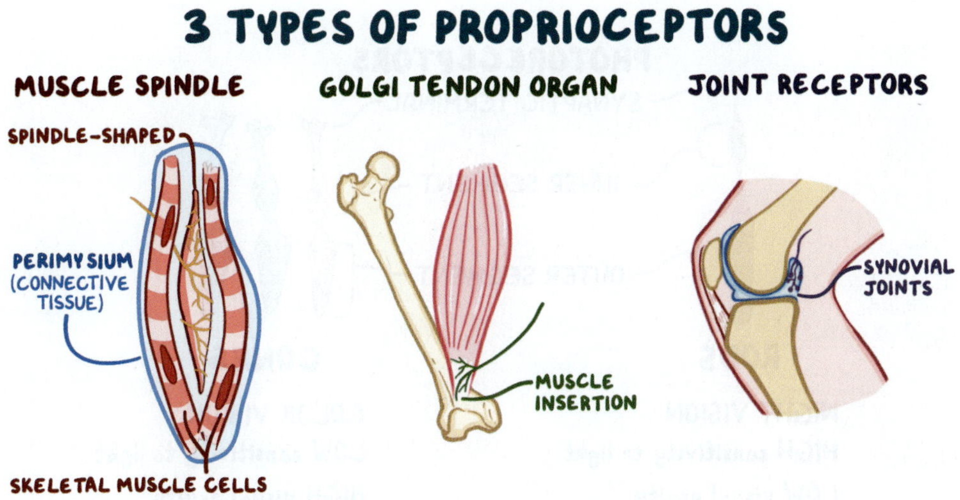

Figure 55.7 The three types of proprioceptors.

THERMORECEPTORS

- Used for temperature
- Transient receptor potential channels mediate sensations
    - Transduction of heat involves TRPV channels; activated at 32–48°C/90–118°F
    - Transduction of cold involves TRPM8; activated at 10–40°C/ 50–104°F
- At extremely cold/hot temperatures, nociceptors take over

NOCICEPTORS

- Used for pain; several types
    - *Thermals*: sense extremely cold/hot temperatures
    - *Mechanical*: sense excess pressure/deformation
    - *Polymodal*: Sense combination of both

PHOTORECEPTION

osms.it/photoreception

- Process by which rods, cones convert light waves into electrical signals
- **Photoreceptors**: modified neurons, AKA rods/cones
    - **Have outer segment**: detects light
    - Inner segment: cell body
    - **Synaptic terminal**: connects to interneurons
- Photoreceptors located in retina

- 10 retina layers; numbered from deepest outwards
    - Pigment epithelium
    - Photoreceptor
    - Outer limiting membrane
    - Outer nuclear
    - Outer plexiform
    - Inner nuclear
    - Inner plexiform
    - Ganglion cell
    - Nerve fiber
    - Inner limiting membrane

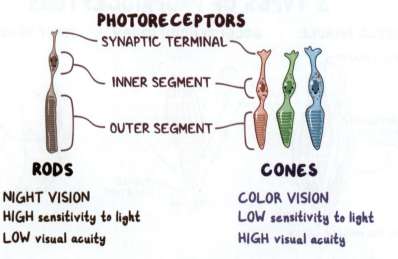

Figure 55.8 The two types of photoreceptors (rods and cones) and their main features.

Chapter 55 Neurology: Sensory Nervous System

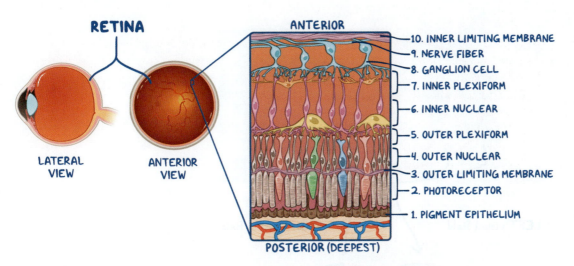

Figure 55.9 Retina = light-sensitive neural layer of tissue at back of eye, composed of 10 layers. Axons of ganglion cells exit eye through optic disc, form optic nerve (CN II).

OPTIC PATHWAYS

osms.it/optic-pathways-and-visual-fields

- Visual phototransduction: light waves on retina → electrical signals
- Rods, cones send electrical signal through optic nerve (cranial nerve II)
    - Exits via the optic disc on the retina
- Optic nerves meet at optic chiasm
- Axons from nasal retina cross over to opposite sides → optic tract (synapses with cells in lateral geniculate nucleus in both sides of thalamus) → primary visual cortex/ occipital lobe

VISUAL FIELD
- Everything seen by single eye
- Split into two parts
    - Nasal visual field: projected onto temporal retina, axons stays on that side of brain
    - Temporal visual field: projected onto nasal retina, axons cross to opposite side of brain at optic chiasm
- Information from left visual fields of both eyes goes to right half of brain, vice versa
    - Due to axons from nasal retina crossing over

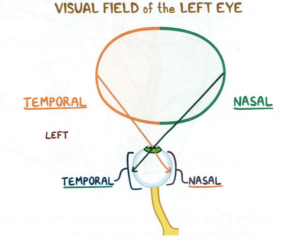

Figure 55.10 The nasal portion of the eye's visual field is projected onto the temporal retina, and the temporal portion of the eye's visual field is projected onto the nasal retina. Axons from the nasal retina cross to the opposite side of the brain at the optic chiasm so that all the information from the left and right visual fields stay together.

OSMOSIS.ORG **487**

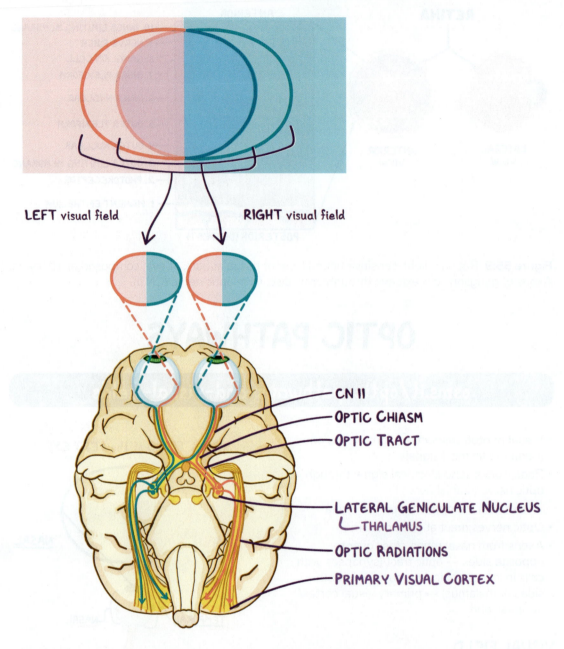

Figure 55.11 Visual field projections onto the retinas and the primary optic pathway, which carries information from the retina to the primary visual cortex in the occipital lobe of the brain.

AUDITORY TRANSDUCTION & PATHWAYS

osms.it/auditory-transduction-and-pathways

- Process by which ear converts sound waves into electrical pulses

OUTER EAR
- Amplifies sound, directs sound waves
  - Pinna → external auditory canal → eardrum vibrates

MIDDLE EAR
- Transmits airborne sound waves to inner ear
  - Malleus (attached to eardrum) → incus → stapes → oval window → cochlea/inner ear

COCHLEA
- Coils around the modiolus/bone
- Base is contiguous with middle ear through vestibule
- Has bony outer shell
  - Contains perilymph
- Cochlear duct is inside bony shell
  - Contains endolymph
  - Above is scala vestibuli, below is scala tympani
- Cochlear duct, scala vestibuli, scala tympani communicate through helicotrema
- Oval window amplifies, transfers sounds waves to scala vestibuli → perilymph → helicotrema → cochlear duct → displaces basilar membrane towards scala tympani
  - Higher frequencies: early membrane
  - Lower frequencies: late membrane

ORGAN OF CORTI
- Stimulated by vibration of basilar membrane
- Made up of mechanosensory/hair cells
- Project out 30–300 stereocilia, AKA sensory organelles
  - Tips of stereocilia embedded in tectorial membrane
- Inner hair cells closer to medialis
  - Innervated by sensory nerve fibers

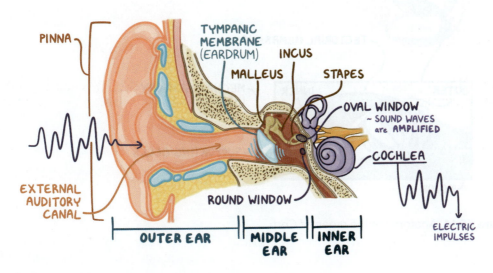

Figure 55.12 Anatomy of the ear.

- Outer hair cells closer to spiral ligament
    - Innervated by motor nerve fibers
    - Changes stiffness of membrane to adjust auditory signal
- Vibration of basilar membrane pushes organ of Corti, hair cells against tectorial membrane
- Pressure on basilar membrane allows protein filaments/tip links to reach, open potassium channels
- Potassium flows in → membrane depolarizes → voltage-gated calcium channels open → glutamate vesicles released into synaptic space → sends electrical impulse to auditory cortex, AKA Brodmann's areas 41 and 42, via auditory nerve

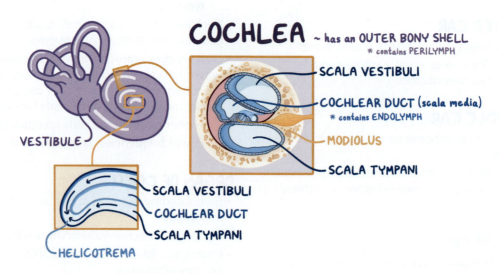

Figure 55.13 Anatomy of the cochlea.

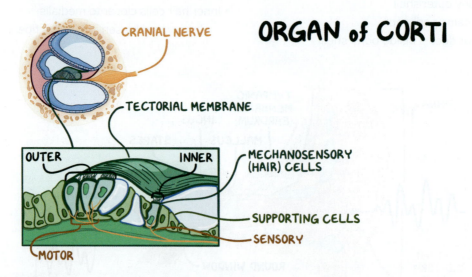

Figure 55.14 Anatomy of the organ of Corti.

Chapter 55 Neurology: Sensory Nervous System

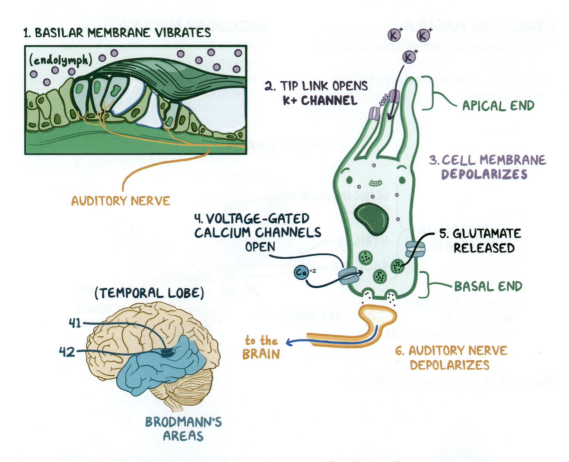

Figure 55.15 Electrical impulse production via organ of Corti hair cells.

VESTIBULAR TRANSDUCTION

osms.it/vestibular-transduction

- Process by which the ear determines spatial equilibrium and converts it into electrical signals
  - Signals are sent to brain via vestibular branch of vestibulocochlear nerve
- Vestibular apparatus located in inner ear
  - Includes semicircular canals (dynamic equilibrium), utricle, saccule (static equilibrium)

STATIC EQUILIBRIUM
- Managed by otolith organs (utricle, saccule)
  - Both contain round macula
- Contains balance receptors/hair cells with stereocilia, kinocilium

- Tips of cilia embedded in otolithic membrane
- Bottom of each cell connected to sensory neurons
- Striola divides hair cells into two sections
  - Receptors arranged to face striola
- Movement pushes protein filaments/tip links on cilia on one side of striola to reach, open potassium channels on kinocilium
  - Potassium flows in → membrane depolarizes → voltage-gated calcium channels open → glutamate vesicles are released into the synaptic space → sends electrical impulse to brain

OSMOSIS.ORG 491

UTRICULAR MACULA

- *Horizontally oriented*: detects horizontal movement
- *Receptors arrangement*: kinocilia face towards striola

SACCULAR MACULA

- *Vertically oriented*: detects vertical movement
- *Receptor arrangement*: kinocilia face away from striola

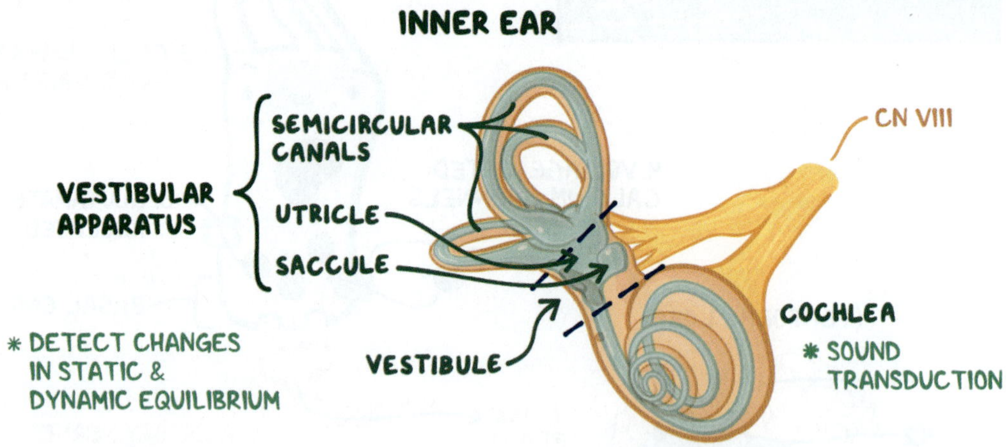

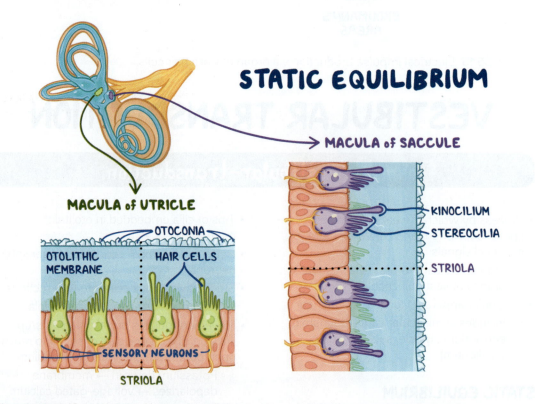

Figure 55.16 Anatomy of the inner ear.

Figure 55.17 Orientation of hair cells relative to the striola in the macula and saccule.

Chapter 55 Neurology: Sensory Nervous System

DYNAMIC EQUILIBRIUM

- Managed by semicircular canals
    - U-shaped ducts containing endolymph; oriented at 90° to each other
- Ampulla
    - Houses crista ampullaris
    - Contains balance receptors/hair cells with stereocilia, surrounded by cupula
    - Bottom of each cell connected to sensory neurons
    - Axial rotation in plane of a semicircular canal drags cupula in opposite direction due to inertia → depolarization/hyperpolarization of hair cells → sends electrical impulse to brain
- Brain uses combination of signals from both ears to determine equilibrium

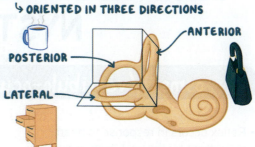

Figure 55.18 Orientation of the three semicircular canals.

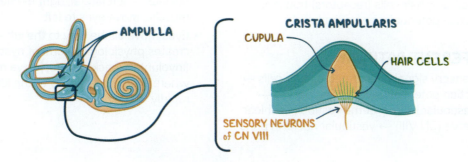

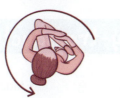
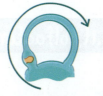

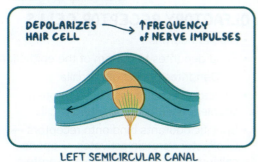

Figure 55.19 Simultaneous depolarization, hyperpolarization of hair cells in left, right ears allows brain to determine direction of movement.

VESTIBULO-OCULAR REFLEX & NYSTAGMUS

osms.it/vestibulo-ocular_reflex_nystagmus

- Reflex occurs in response to head movement by the vestibular apparatus; results in eye movement in the opposite direction of the head
    - Stabilizes position of the eye in the line of sight during head movement
- Semicircular canals within the vestibular apparatus respond to rotation and angular acceleration/deceleration of the head
- Contains hair cells (receptors) that create action potential when stimulated

AFFERENT PATHWAY
- Sensory signals generated by hair cells → action potential travels along nerves → vestibular branch of the vestibulocochlear nerve (CN VIII) → vestibular nuclei in pons

EFFERENT PATHWAY
- From the right vestibular nucleus, nerves cross over to contralateral (left) abducens nucleus → lateral rectus muscle stimulated via abducens nerve/CN VI → left lateral rectus muscle contracts → left eye moves to left
- Other fibers from left abducens act as interneurons → travel to right oculomotor nucleus → left lateral, right medial rectus muscles move eyes to left
- Eyes move all the way to the left → creates physiological form of nystagmus (involuntary back-and-forth eye movement) where eyes move slowly to the left, then rapidly to the right

OLFACTORY TRANSDUCTION & PATHWAYS

osms.it/olfactory-transduction-and-pathways

OLFACTION
- Process by which nose converts smells into electrical signals
- Perceived by sensory neurons in roof of nasal cavity, AKA olfactory region
- Carried by olfactory nerve (CN I)

OLFACTORY REGION
- Lined by olfactory epithelium
- Consists of olfactory receptor cells
    - AKA chemoreceptors; respond to odorants
- Supported by columnar epithelial cells
- Mucus produced in Bowman's glands in connective tissue below, AKA lamina propria

OLFACTORY RECEPTOR CELLS
- Bipolar neurons
- Send dendrites to bottom of the epithelium
    - Dendrites project out as cilia
- Olfactory receptor proteins/G-protein coupled receptors embedded in cilia
- Specific odorants bind onto receptors → G-olfactory protein activates → opens calcium, sodium channels via G-protein coupled receptor pathway

Chapter 55 Neurology: Sensory Nervous System

- Calcium-activated chloride channels open → chloride ions flow out → cell membrane depolarizes → neuron fires
- Neuron sends axons that join up to form olfactory nerves (collectively called CN1)
- CN1 passes through olfactory foramina to olfactory bulb
    - Second order neurons send signals to olfactory cortex via olfactory tract

OLFACTORY TRACT

- Lateral tract runs to ipsilateral piriform complex
    - Some fibers go to limbic system
- Medial tract crosses to contralateral piriform complex
- **Adaption**: fewer signals sent in response to same odorants over time

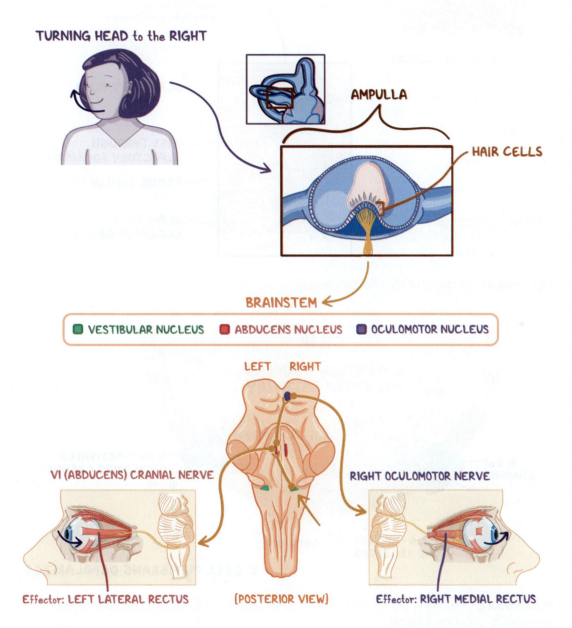

Figure 55.20 Vestibulo-ocular reflex pathway at work when an individual turns their head to the right.

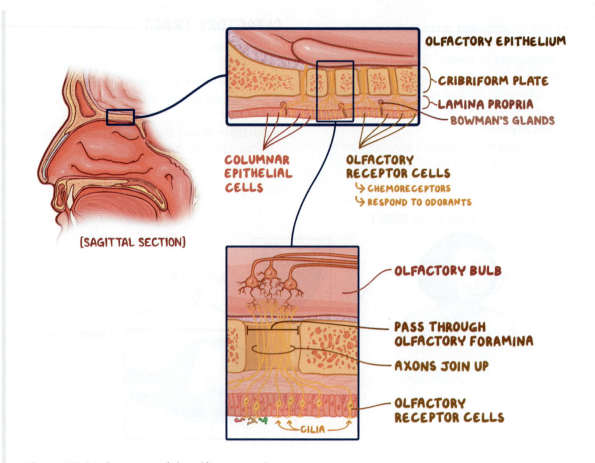

Figure 55.21 Anatomy of the olfactory region.

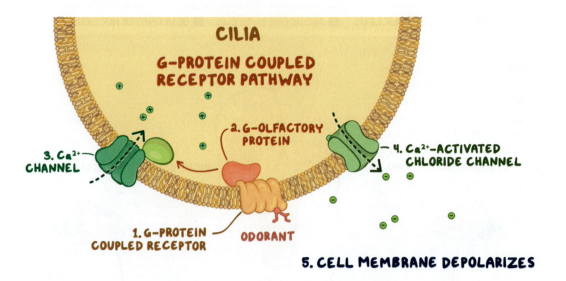

Figure 55.22 The cilia of bipolar olfactory receptor cells use a G-protein coupled receptor pathway to generate a signal.

Chapter 55 Neurology: Sensory Nervous System

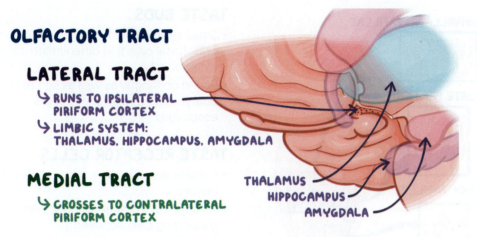

OLFACTORY TRACT

LATERAL TRACT
- RUNS TO IPSILATERAL PIRIFORM CORTEX
- LIMBIC SYSTEM: THALAMUS, HIPPOCAMPUS, AMYGDALA

MEDIAL TRACT
- CROSSES TO CONTRALATERAL PIRIFORM CORTEX

Figure 55.23 Destinations of the olfactory tract.

TASTE & THE TONGUE

osms.it/taste-and-the-tongue

- Taste: sensation produced when substances react with taste receptor cells, AKA gustation
    - Five primary tastes of bitter, salty, sour, sweet, umami/savory

TONGUE
- Surface is covered by mucosa
- Contains both intrinsic, extrinsic muscles
    - *Intrinsic muscles*: start, end within tongue; help change shape
    - *Extrinsic muscles*: attach to structures outside tongue; help guide movement
- Divided by a V-shaped group, AKA sulcus terminalis, into posterior third, an anterior two-thirds
- Covered with papillae
    - Small bumps/projections

TYPES OF PAPILLAE

Filiform papillae
- On anterior two-thirds
- Used for sensation of touch

Fungiform papillae
- On tip of tongue

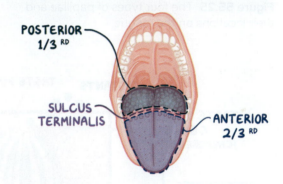

Figure 55.24 Sulcus terminalis divides tongue into posterior third and anterior two thirds.

- Contain taste buds
    - More sensitive to sweet, umami

Foliate papillae
- On sides of tongue
- Contain taste buds
    - More sensitive to salty, sour

Circumvallate papillae
- On back of anterior two-thirds
- Contain taste buds
    - More sensitive to bitter

OSMOSIS.ORG 497

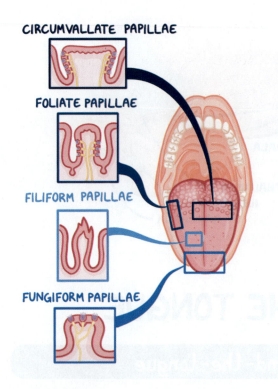

TASTE BUDS

- Small structures housing taste receptor cells, basal cells that differentiate into taste receptor cells
- Found on tongue as well as soft palate, pharynx, epiglottis, larynx, upper esophagus

TASTE RECEPTOR CELLS

- Used to perceive taste, AKA respond to tastants
- Arranged like orange wedges with supporting cells between
- Have thin, hair-like microvilli/gustatory hair protruding out of taste pore
- Send signals to brain via axons
  - Anterior two-thirds innervated by facial nerve
  - Posterior third, oral cavity innervated by glossopharyngeal nerve
  - Back of throat, esophagus innervated by vagus nerve

Figure 55.25 The four types of papillae and their locations on the tongue.

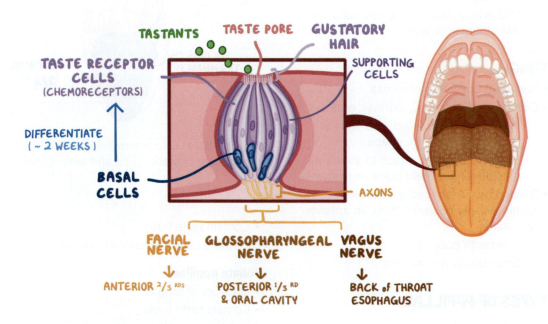

Figure 55.26 Anatomy of a taste bud.

PERCEPTION OF TASTE

- Chewed up particles → mix with saliva → travel to papillae → make contact with gustatory hairs
- For salty/sour tastes
  - Na^+, H^+ ions make contact with gustatory hair
  - Ion channels allow these ions into cell
  - Membrane depolarizes
  - Voltage gated channels open
  - Extracellular calcium flows inside
  - Neurotransmitters fuse with cell membrane
  - Nerves tell brain
- For sweet, bitter, umami tastes
  - Tastants bind to G-protein coupled receptors
  - Triggers G-protein coupled pathway
  - Calcium channels on endoplasmic reticulum open
  - Intracellular calcium ions flow into cell
  - Neurotransmitters fuse with cell membrane
  - Nerves tell brain
- **Complex tastes**: combination of taste receptors
- **Adaption**: fewer signals sent in response to same tastants over time
- Factors affecting taste
  - **Hunger**: ↑ sensitivity to sweet, salty tastes
  - **Infections, allergies**: ↓ sensitivity
  - **Age**: ↓ sensitivity; because receptor cells not replaced as quickly

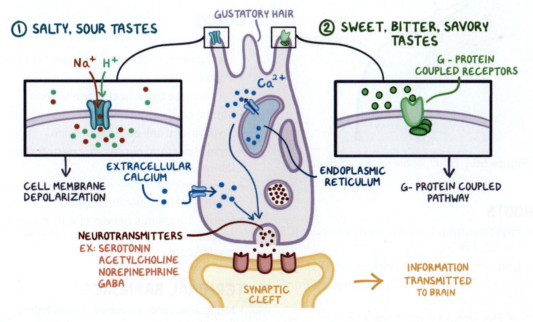

Figure 55.27 The two taste perception methods.

NOTES
SPINAL CORD & NERVES

BRACHIAL PLEXUS

osms.it/brachial-plexus

- Network of nerves innervating shoulder, arm, hand (supply afferent/sensory, efferent/motor nerve fibers); one on each side of body
- Begins as five roots → combine to three trunks → split into six divisions (three anterior, three posterior) → combine into three cords → end in five terminal branches; also preterminal (collateral) branches

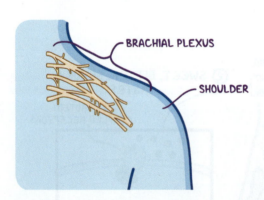

Figure 56.1 Brachial plexus location in body.

ROOTS

- *First four*: from last four cervical nerves (C5, C6, C7, C8)
- *Last one*: from first thoracic nerve (T1)
- Long thoracic nerve (LT) branches off from C5, C6, C7
    - Innervates serratus anterior
- Dorsal scapular (DS) nerve branches off from C5
    - Innervates rhomboid muscles
- Phrenic nerve contributed to by C5
    - Innervates diaphragm

TRUNKS

- C5, C6 form superior trunk
- C7 remains as middle trunk
- C8, T1 form inferior trunk
- Suprascapular nerve branches off from superior trunk
    - Innervates supraspinatus, infraspinatus, acromioclavicular, glenohumeral joints

DIVISIONS

- Each trunk splits into anterior, posterior division

CORDS

- Lateral cord
    - Superior, middle trunk anterior divisions
- Posterior cord
    - All three trunk posterior divisions
- Medial cord
    - Inferior trunk anterior division
- Lateral pectoral nerve branches off from lateral cord
- Upper, middle, lower subscapular nerves branch off from posterior cord
- Medial cutaneous nerves of arm, forearm, medial pectoral nerve branch off from medial cord

TERMINAL BRANCHES

- Musculocutaneous nerve comes from lateral cord
    - Innervates biceps brachii, brachialis, coracobrachialis
- Median nerve formed from lateral, medial cords
    - Innervates flexors of forearm, hand

Chapter 56 Neurology: Spinal Cord & Nerves

- Axillary, radial nerves split out from posterior cord
  - Axillary nerve innervates deltoid, teres minor
- Radial nerve innervates triceps brachii, brachioradialis, forearm extensors
- Ulnar nerve off from medial cord
  - Innervates wrist, fingers

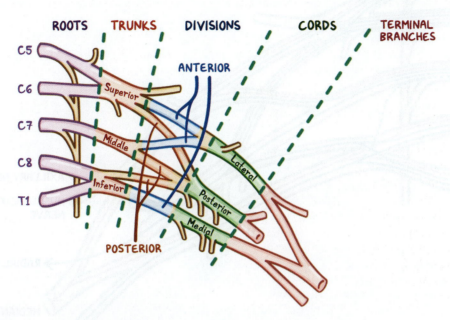

Figure 56.2 Divisions of the brachial plexus.

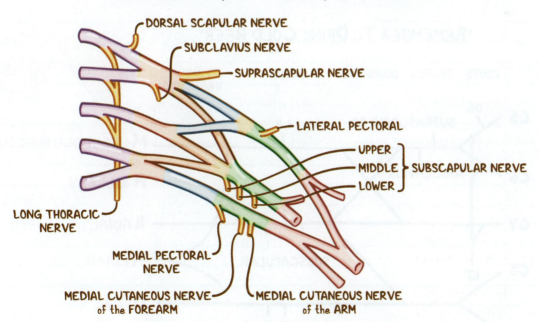

Figure 56.3 Names and locations of brachial plexus' collateral branches.

OSMOSIS.ORG **501**

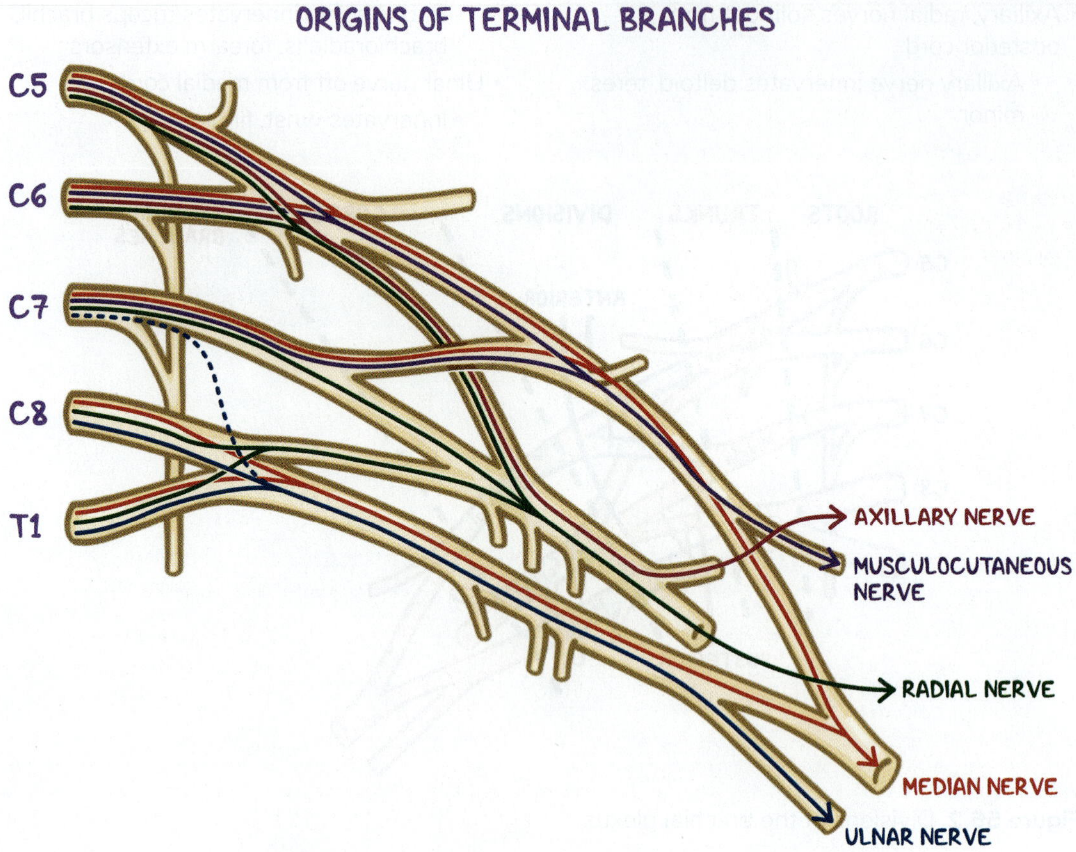

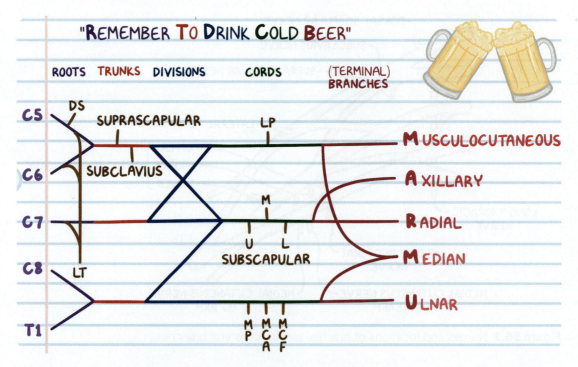

Figure 56.4 Contributions of the spinal nerves to the brachial plexus' terminal branches.

Figure 56.5 A simplified diagram of the brachial plexus with mnemonics for names and order of divisions (Remember To Drink Cold Beer) and the terminal branches (MARMU).

Chapter 56 Neurology: Spinal Cord & Nerves

CRANIAL NERVES

osms.it/cranial-nerves

- 12 nerve pairs originating in brain, brainstem
  - Supply body (primarily head, neck) with motor, sensory information
- Includes olfactory, optic, oculomotor, trochlear, trigeminal, abducens, facial, vestibulocochlear, glossopharyngeal, vagus, accessory, hypoglossal nerves

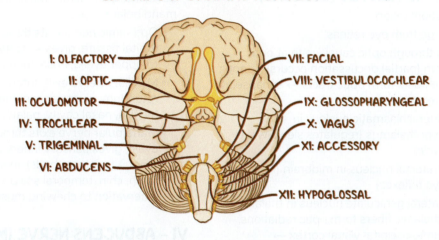

Figure 56.6 The cranial nerves originate from the brain (including brainstem).

MNEMONIC:
Cranial Nerve Names
On
Old
Olympus
Towering
Top,
A
Fine
Victorian
Gentleman
Viewed
A
Hawk

MNEMONIC:
Cranial Nerve Functions
(S = sensory, M = motor)
Some
Say
Marry
Money
But
My
Brother
Says
Big
Brains
Matter
More

OSMOSIS.ORG 503

I - OLFACTORY NERVE (SENSORY)
- **Function**: smell
- Arises from primary olfactory cortex (temporal lobe)
- Neurons form olfactory tracts → run to olfactory bulb (above cribriform plate of ethmoid bone)
- Receives information from sensory nerve fibers (axons from nasal cavity's olfactory neurons) which synapse with olfactory bulb's neurons

II - OPTIC NERVES (SENSORY)
- **Function**: vision
- Emerge from eye retinas
- Pass through optic canal, unite at optic chiasm (partial decussation occurs) → optic nerve fibers form optic tracts → synapse at different nuclei
    - Suprachiasmatic nucleus in hypothalamus (regulates sleep-wake cycle)
    - Pretectal nucleus in midbrain (regulates eye reflexes)
    - Lateral geniculate nucleus in thalamus (thalamic fibers form optic radiations, run to occipital visual cortex → determines sight)

III - OCULOMOTOR NERVE (MOTOR)
- **Function**: eye movement
- Arises from ventral midbrain; runs through superior orbital fissure to eye
- Splits into superior, inferior branch
    - Superior branch innervates levator palpebrae superioris (raises upper eyelid), superior rectus (elevates eye)
    - Inferior branch innervates inferior oblique (abducts eyeball), inferior rectus (depresses, adducts eyeball), medial rectus (adducts eyeball) with proprioception; controls pupil constriction (sphincter pupillae), visual focusing (ciliaris) via ciliary ganglion

IV - TROCHLEAR NERVE (PRIMARILY MOTOR/SOME SENSORY)
- **Function**: eyeball movement
- Arises from dorsal midbrain; runs around midbrain, follows oculomotor nerve through superior orbital fissure
- Innervates superior oblique muscles (abducts, depresses, internally rotates eyeball)

V - TRIGEMINAL NERVE (SENSORY/MOTOR)
- **Function**: facial movement, chewing, temperature, touch, pain
- Emerges from pons; travels to trigeminal ganglion
- Splits into ophthalmic, maxillary, mandibular nerves
    - Opthalmic nerve exits through superior orbital fissure, gives sensory innervation to upper eyelid, nose, forehead, scalp
    - Maxillary nerve exits through foramen rotundum, gives sensory innervation to maxilla, nasal cavity, palate, cheeks' skin
    - Mandibular nerve exits through foramen ovale, gives sensory innervation to tongue (not taste buds), lower lip, lower teeth, chin, temporal scalp. Gives motor innervation to chewing muscles

VI - ABDUCENS NERVE (MOTOR)
- **Function**: eyeball movement
- Emerges from pons; runs through superior orbital fissure
- Innervates lateral rectus muscle (abducts eye)

VII - FACIAL NERVE (SENSORY/MOTOR)
- **Function**: taste, saliva, tears, facial movement (i.e. facial expressions)
- Emerges from pons; enters temporal bone through internal acoustic meatus
- Runs within bone to geniculate ganglion
- Splits into greater petrosal nerve, stapedius nerve, chorda tympani
    - Greater petrosal nerve provides autonomic fibers to lacrimal, nasal, palatine, pharyngeal glands
    - Stapedius nerve sends motor fibers to middle ear's stapedius
    - Chorda tympani gives sensory innervation to taste buds of tongue's anterior two thirds

- Remaining nerve exits skull through stylomastoid foramen
- Splits again into temporal, zygomatic, buccal, mandibular, cervical branches (innervating forehead, nose, cheeks, around eyes/lips, chin)

VIII – VESTIBULOCOCHLEAR NERVE (SENSORY)

- *Function*: hearing, equilibrium
- Emerges from pons; runs through internal acoustic meatus
- Splits into cochlear, vestibular nerves
  - Cochlear nerve supplies cochlea's hearing receptors
  - Vestibular nerve supplies vestibule's equilibrium receptors

IX – GLOSSOPHARYNGEAL NERVE (SENSORY/MOTOR)

- *Function*: swallowing, monitoring blood pressure/oxygen/carbon dioxide
- Arises from medulla; runs through jugular foramen
- Innervates tongue, pharynx
- Sends motor fibers to stylopharyngeus (elevates pharynx in swallowing), parasympathetic motor fibers to parotid salivary glands, sensory fibers to tongue's posterior third
- Conveys information from carotid bodies' chemoreceptors (blood oxygen, carbon dioxide levels), carotid sinus' baroreceptors (blood pressure)

X – VAGUS NERVE (SENSORY/MOTOR)

- *Function*: smooth muscle control, digestive enzyme secretion
- Arises from medulla; runs through jugular foramen
- Dips down into thorax, abdomen
- Sends somatic motor innervation to pharynx, larynx (swallowing), parasympathetic fibers to heart, lungs, abdominal organs (heart rate, breathing, digestion)
- Brings in sensory information from thoracic, abdominal organs; aortic arch's baroreceptors; chemoreceptors in carotid, aortic bodies; epiglottis' taste buds

XI – ACCESSORY NERVE

- *Function*: swallowing; head, shoulder movement
- Considered vagus nerve accessory
- Forms from rootlets emerging from spinal cord; enters skull via foramen magnum, emerges from medulla, runs through jugular foramen
- Innervates trapezius, sternocleidomastoid muscles (head, neck movement); carries sensory proprioceptive information from larynx, pharynx

XII – HYPOGLOSSAL NERVE

- *Function*: tongue movement, speech, swallowing
- Arises from medulla; runs through hypoglossal foramen
- Sends motor fibers to tongue muscles, carries sensory proprioceptive information

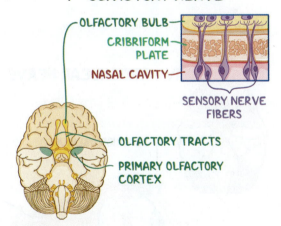

Figure 56.7 CN I: olfactory nerve.

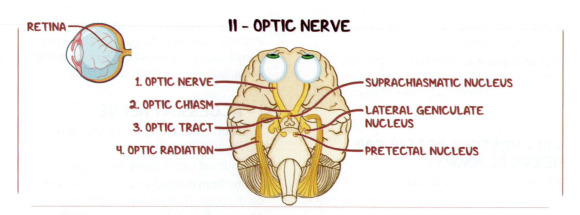

Figure 56.8 CN II: optic nerve.

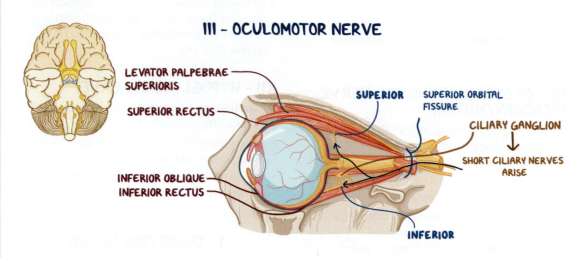

Figure 56.9 CN III: oculomotor nerve.

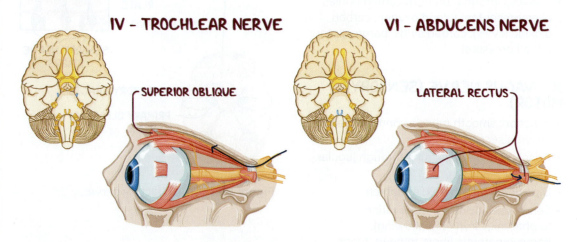

Figure 56.10 CN IV: trochlear nerve and CN VI: abducens nerve. Together, CN III, IV, and VI control eye movement.

Chapter 56 Neurology: Spinal Cord & Nerves

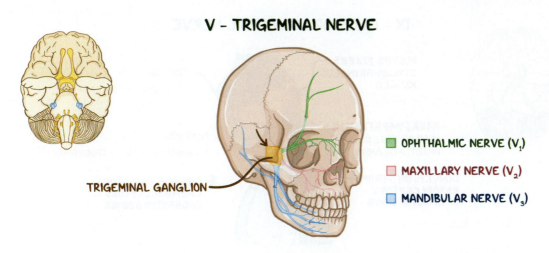

Figure 56.11 CN V: trigeminal nerve. The three branches include the ophthalmic nerve (V_1), maxillary nerve (V_2), and mandibular nerve (V_3).

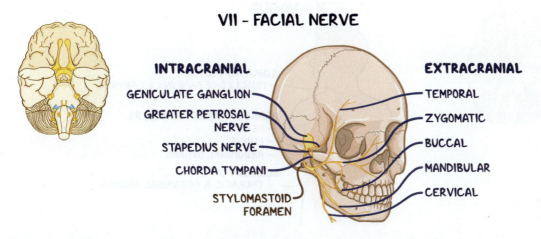

Figure 56.12 CN VII: facial nerve, including the intracranial and extracranial branches.

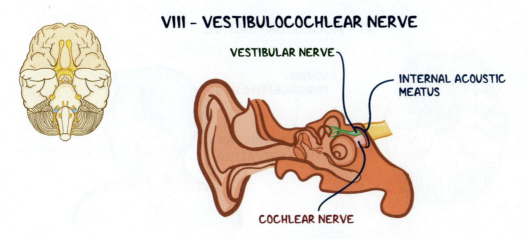

Figure 56.13 CN VIII: vestibulocochlear nerve, which splits into the vestibular and cochlear nerves once it passes through the internal acoustic meatus.

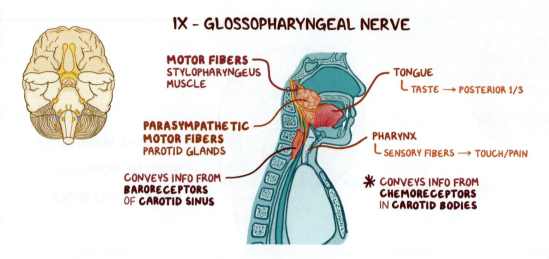

Figure 56.14 CN IX: glossopharyngeal nerve has sensory and motor functions.

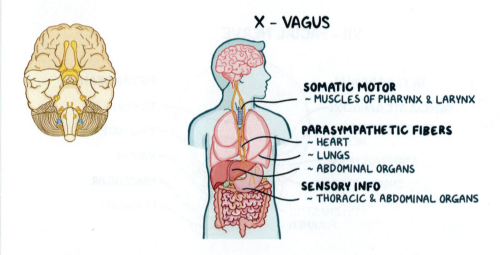

Figure 56.15 CN X: vagus nerve also has sensory and motor functions.

XI - ACCESSORY NERVE

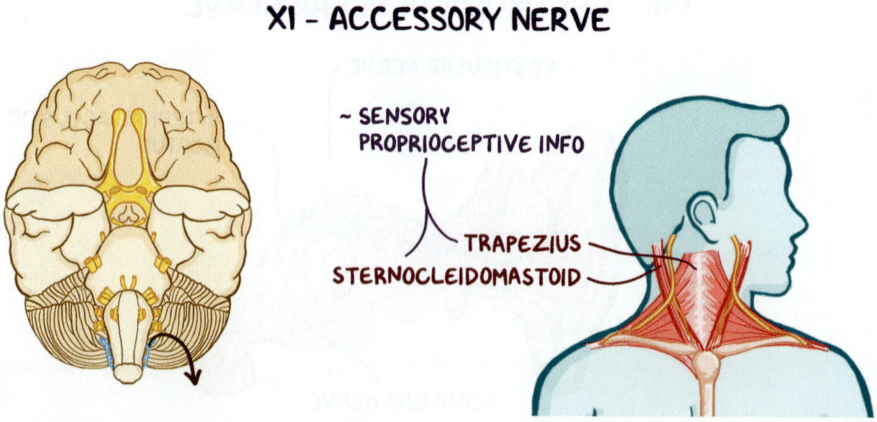

Figure 56.16 CN XI: accessory nerve enters the skull through foramen magnum, then exits again through the jugular foramen. It innervates the trapezius and sternocleidomastoid muscles.

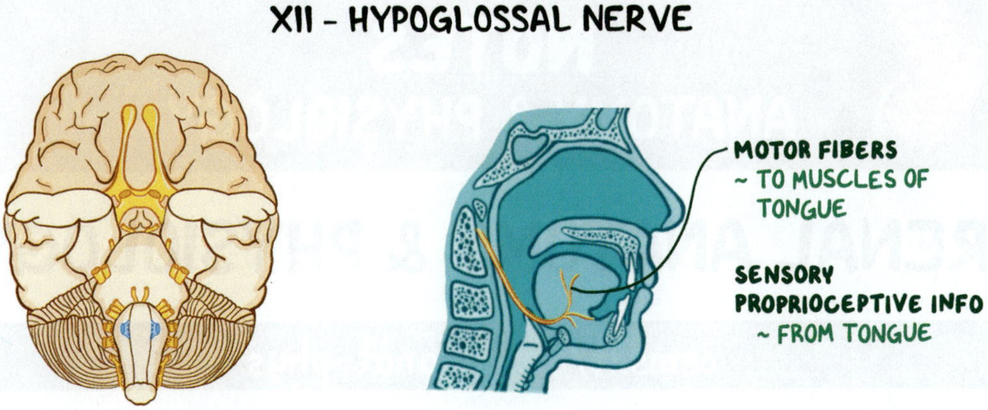

Figure 56.17 CN XII: hypoglossal nerve innervates the tongue and has both motor and sensory function.

NOTES
ANATOMY & PHYSIOLOGY

RENAL ANATOMY & PHYSIOLOGY

osms.it/renal-anat-phys

RENAL SYSTEM
- Two kidneys
  - Filter the blood from harmful substances
  - Regulate blood pH, volume, pressure, osmolality
  - Produce hormones
- Located between T12, L3 vertebrae; partially protected by ribs 11, 12; behind peritoneal membrane (retroperitoneal)
- Right kidney slightly lower due to larger portion of the liver on right side
- Filter 150 liters of blood everyday; receive ¼ of cardiac output from renal arteries (from aorta)
  - Renal arteries divide → segmental arteries → interlobar arteries (between renal columns) → arcuate arteries (cover bases of renal pyramids) → cortical radiate arteries (supply the cortex) → afferent arterioles (supply nephrons)

MORPHOLOGY

Renal hilum
- Indentation in the middle of each kidney
- Entry/exit point for ureter, arteries, veins, lymphatics, nerves

Surrounding tissue (three layers)
- Renal fascia (outer)
  - Dense connective tissue
  - Anchors kidney
- Adipose capsule (middle)
  - Fatty tissue
  - Protects kidney from trauma
- Renal capsule (inner)
  - Dense connective tissue
  - Gives kidney shape

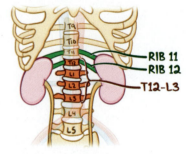

Figure 57.1 Kidney placement in relation to ribs and vertebrae.

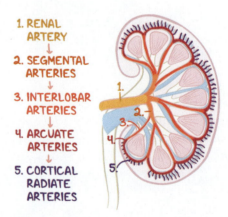

Figure 57.2 Arterial bloodflow in the kidney.

Chapter 57 Renal Physiology: Anatomy & Physiology

Renal cortex (outer portion)
- Outer cortical zone
- Inner juxtamedullary zone
- Renal columns project into the kidney, separating medulla

Renal medulla (inner portion)
- 10-18 renal pyramids with pointy ends (renal papilla/nipples) towards center of kidney
- *Renal lobes:* renal pyramids including cortex above them
- Renal papilla → minor calyces → major calyces → renal pelvis → ureter

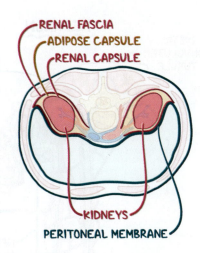

Figure 57.3 Transverse cross-section showing retroperitoneal position of kidneys, surrounding tissue layers.

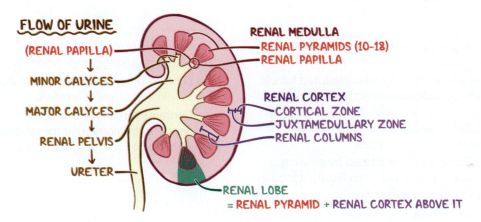

Figure 57.4 Cross-section through kidney showing renal medulla, renal cortex, and urine flow through kidney.

Nephron
- Functional unit of kidney (about one million in each kidney)
- Composed of renal corpuscle, renal tubule
- Blood filtration starts in renal corpuscle
    - Includes glomerulus, a tuft of capillaries supplied by afferent arteriole, and Bowman's capsule
    - Blood flows into glomerulus → water, solutes (e.g. sodium) pass through capillary endothelium → through basement membrane → through epithelium → into Bowman's space (becoming filtrate)
    - Epithelium comprises podocytes wrapped around basement membrane; gaps called filtration slits allow small solutes through but block large proteins, red blood cells
    - Blood leaving glomerulus enters efferent arteriole → divides into peritubular capillaries → these reunite into cortical radiate veins → arcuate veins → interlobar veins → renal veins → inferior vena cava

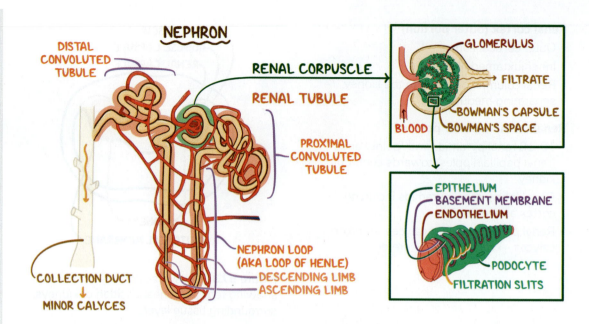

Figure 57.5 Nephron anatomy.

- Filtrate from Bowman's capsule enters renal tubule
  - Made up of proximal convoluted tubule, descending/ascending limbs of nephron loop (loop of Henle), distal convoluted tubule, collection ducts (which send urine to minor calyces)
  - Filtrate is further filtered by passing water, solutes between filtrate, blood in peritubular capillaries

- Blood pressure, glomerular filtration rate regulated by juxtaglomerular complex
  - Located between distal convoluted tubule and afferent arteriole
  - **Contains three types of cells:** macula densa, extraglomerular mesangial, juxtaglomerular (granular) cells

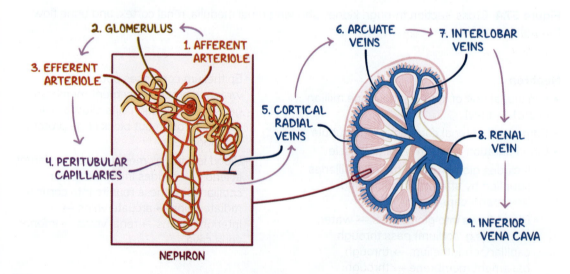

Figure 57.6 Blood flow through nephron and venial bloodflow in kidney.

Chapter 57 Renal Physiology: Anatomy & Physiology

- Macula densa cells in distal convoluted tubule sense ↓ sodium/blood pressure → juxtaglomerular cells secrete renin → ↑ sodium reabsorption, constricting blood vessels → ↑ blood pressure via the renin–angiotensin–aldosterone system (RAAS)
- Urine from renal tubules enters minor calyces → major calyces → renal pelvis → ureter

Bladder

- Bladder receives urine from ureter
  - Urine enters at ureterovesical junctions
  - Muscular walls fold into rugae as bladder empties
- Bladder wall contains multiple layers
  - *Transitional epithelium*: allows bladder to distend while maintaining a barrier
  - *Detrusor muscle*: helps with bladder contraction
  - *Fibrous adventitia*: holds bladder loosely in place
- Located in front of rectum in biologically-male individuals; in front of vagina, uterus, and rectum in biologically-female individuals
- Holds 750mL of urine
  - *Biologically-female individuals*: slightly less due to crowding from uterus
- Contains smooth triangular region (trigone region) on bladder floor
  - Bounded by two ureterovesical junctions and internal urethral orifice
  - Highly sensitive to expansion → signals brain as bladder fills

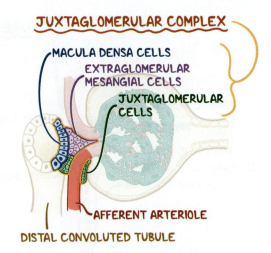

Figure 57.7 Cross-section through renal capsule showing juxtaglomerular complex.

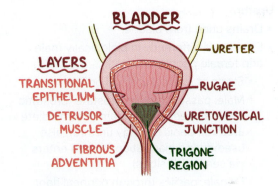

Figure 57.8 Bladder anatomy.

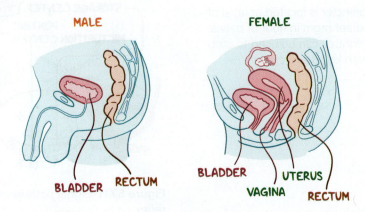

Figure 57.9 Sagittal cross-section showing placement of bladder in relation to other organs.

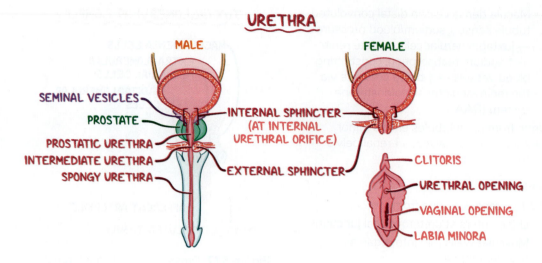

Figure 57.10 Coronal cross-section through bladder showing urethra anatomy.

Urethra

- Drains urine from bladder
- Structured differently in biologically male and female people
  - Starts at internal urethral orifice
  - *Male:* passes through prostate (prostatic urethra), deep peritoneum (intermediate urethra), penis (spongy urethra); also used during ejaculation (semen enters via seminal vesicles)
  - *Female:* passes through perineal floor of pelvis, exits between labia minora (above vaginal opening but below clitoris)
  - Detrusor muscle thickens at internal urethral orifice forming internal sphincter (involuntary control; controlled by autonomic nervous system; keeps urethra closed when bladder isn't full)
  - External sphincter is located at level of urogenital diaphragm in floor of pelvis (voluntary control; can be used to stop urination with kegel exercises)

Urination

- Involves close coordination between nervous system and bladder muscles
- Bladder volume of > 300–400mL, sends signals to micturition center in spinal cord (located at S2 and S3) → micturition reflex causes contraction of bladder and relaxation of both sphincters
  - Pontine storage center in pons of brain can be activated to stop micturition reflex
  - Pontine micturition center can be activated to allow micturition reflex

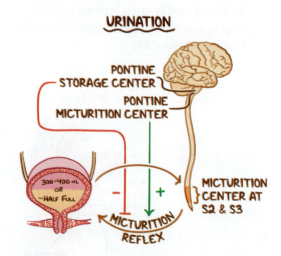

Figure 57.11 Signal pathways of micturition reflex.

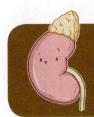

NOTES
ACID-BASE PHYSIOLOGY

ACID-BASE MAP & COMPENSATORY MECHANISMS

osms.it/acid-base_map_compensatory_mechs

ACID-BASE MAP
- Main physiologic pH factors
    - HCO_3^-, CO_2
- Acid-base map
    - HCO_3^- concentration (x-axis)/CO_2 partial pressure (y-axis) diagram
- Henderson–Hasselbalch equation
    - pH = 6.1+log ($[HCO_3^-]/0.03P_{CO_2}$)
    - P_{CO_2} is partial pressure of CO_2
- Diagonal lines
    - Drawn where each point on graph has same pH (isohydric lines)
- Drawing lines for pH = 7.35, pH = 7.45
    - Comprises area where all HCO_3^-, CO_2 combinations correspond to "normal" pH

pH out of normal range
- One of two ways
    - **Acidosis**: pH ↓ 7.35, enters top-left portion of map
    - **Alkalosis**: pH ↑ 7.45, enters bottom-right portion of map
- One of two reasons
    - **Respiratory**: P_{CO_2} too ↑/↓
    - **Metabolic**: $[HCO_3^-]$ too ↑/↓

COMPENSATORY MECHANISMS
- Simple acid-base disorder
    - Single problem changing pH
- Mixed acid-base disorder
    - Multiple problems compounding/cancelling out

Multiple compensatory mechanisms
- Respiratory acidosis
    - Kidneys retain more HCO_3^-
- Respiratory alkalosis
    - Kidneys excrete more HCO_3^-
- Metabolic acidosis
    - Lungs blow off CO_2 (deeper, more frequent breaths)
- Metabolic alkalosis
    - Lungs retain CO_2 (shallower, less frequent breaths)

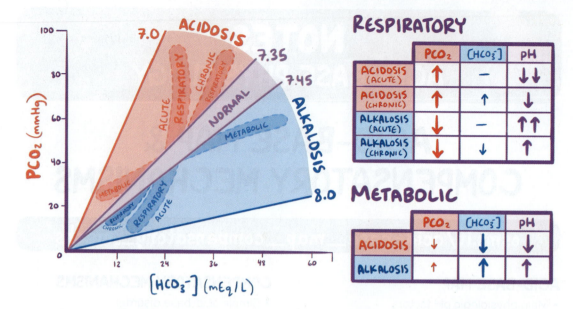

Figure 58.1 An acid-base map shows the relationship between pH, bicarbonate concentration, and partial pressure of carbon dioxide in respiratory and metabolic acidosis/alkalosis, and how these values are adjusted when there is renal or respiratory compensation. The accompanying tables depict the changes in PCO_2, $[HCO_3^-]$, and pH associated with respiratory/metabolic acidosis/alkalosis.

BUFFERING & HENDERSON–HASSELBALCH EQUATION

osms.it/buffering_henderson-hasselbalch

BUFFERING

- **Buffers**: pH change-resisting solutions
- Can comprise
  - *Acidic buffer*: weak acid, conjugate base
  - *Basic buffer*: weak base, conjugate acid
- Weak acids, bases do not dissociate fully → equilibrium formation (e.g. $HA \rightleftharpoons H^+ + A$ or $B + H_2O \rightleftharpoons BH^+ + OH^-$)
  - *Le Chatelier's principle*: equilibriums move forward/backward, balance products/reactants' gain/loss

Resisting pH change

- Acidic, basic buffers resist all pH changes
- Strong base added to acidic buffer
  - OH^- ions react with H^+ ions → ↑ pH
  - H^+ ion loss shifts acid's equilibrium → more H^+ ions created, resists pH change
- Strong acid added to acidic buffer
  - H^+ ions would ↓ pH
  - Shifts acid equilibrium in opposite direction → conjugate base reacts with H^+ ions → resists pH change
- Strong acid added to basic buffer
  - H^+ ions would ↓ pH, also reacts with excess OH^- ions
  - OH^- loss ions shifts base's equilibrium → ↑ OH ion creation → resists pH change
- Strong base added to basic buffer
  - OH^- ions would react with H^+ ions to ↑ pH
  - Shifts base's equilibrium in opposite direction → conjugate acid reacting with OH^- ions → resists pH change

HENDERSON-HASSELBALCH EQUATION

- Henderson–Hasselbalch equation determines buffer's pH
  - pH = pK + log([A⁻]/[HA])
- This is derived
  - **Weak acid equilibrium**: equilibrium constant K → K = [H⁺][A⁻]/[HA]
  - Solving for H⁺ → [H⁺] = K([HA]/[A⁻])
  - Negative log of both sides → pH = pK + log([A⁻]/[HA])
- Note
  - If [A⁻] = [HA], then pH = pK

PHYSIOLOGIC pH & BUFFERS

osms.it/physiologic-pH-and-buffers

PHYSIOLOGIC pH

- Measures balance between acids, bases in body
- **pH**: -log[H⁺]
  - **[H⁺]**: hydrogen ion concentration
- **Ideal**: [H⁺] = 40 × 10⁻⁹ Eq/L = 40 nEq/L → pH = 7.4 (slightly alkaline)
  - **Acidemia**: pH < 7.4
  - **Alkalemia**: pH > 7.4
- ↑ [H⁺] → ↓ pH (negative sign in equation)
- pH, [H⁺] has logarithmic (not linear) relationship

PHYSIOLOGIC BUFFERS

- Physiologic buffers occur naturally in body
  - Maintains stable pH between 7.35–7.45

Bicarbonate buffer system

- Extracellular, most important
- **Acidic buffer**: carbonic acid (H_2CO_3)
- **Conjugate base**: bicarbonate ion (HCO_3^-)
- Carbonic acid can be formed from H_2O, CO_2 (carbonic anhydrase catalyzes reaction)
- Equilibrium reaction
  - $H_2O + CO_2 \rightleftharpoons H_2CO_3 \rightleftharpoons H^+ + HCO_3^-$
- Excess
  - CO_2 blown off by lungs
  - HCO_3^- eliminated by kidneys

Phosphate buffer system (extracellular)

- **Acidic buffer**: dihydrogen phosphate ($H_2PO_4^-$)
- **Conjugate base**: monohydrogen phosphate (HPO_4^{2-})
- Equilibrium reaction
  - $H_2PO_4^- \rightleftharpoons H^+ + HPO_4^{2-}$

Protein buffer system (extracellular)

- Protein amino acids may have exposed carboxyl (-COOH), amine (NH_2) groups
- Results in separate acidic (-COOH $\rightleftharpoons$ -COO⁻ + H⁺), basic (-NH_2 + H⁺ $\rightleftharpoons$ -NH_3^+) buffers

Intracellular buffer systems

- **Hemoglobin**: buffer in red blood cells (selectively binds H⁺ ions)
- Organic phosphates (e.g. ATP) can buffer similarly

PLASMA ANION GAP

osms.it/plasma-anion-gap

PLASMA ANION GAP
- Cations, anions coexist within plasma
    - To keep plasma electrically neutral sum of cation charges must equal sum of anion charges
- Not all cation, anion concentrations can be measured
    - Often gap ("plasma anion gap") between measured cation charges (mainly Na^+), smaller measured anion charges sum (mainly Cl^-, HCO_3^-)
- *Plasma anion gap range*: 3–11 mEq/L
    - High gap → high unmeasured anion number
    - Low gap → low unmeasured anion number
- Unmeasured anions include anion component of several organic acids, negatively charged plasma proteins (e.g. albumin)

DIAGNOSTIC TOOL
- Plasma anion gap serves as useful diagnostic tool

Metabolic acidosis
- Organic acids' H^+ ions convert HCO_3^- into H_2CO_3
    - Organic anions aren't measured → plasma anion gap ↑
    - Organic acids include lactic acid, ketoacids, oxalic acid, formic acid, hippuric acid
- Some cases (e.g. diarrhea/renal tubular acidosis)
    - Kidneys reabsorb more $Cl-$ ions → plasma anion gap remains normal (hyperchloremic metabolic acidosis)

High gap may suggest
- Unmeasured anion buildup (e.g. hyperphosphatemia, hyperalbuminemia)
- Metabolic alkalosis (high pH triggers albumin to release H^+ ions → negative charge ↑ on unmeasured albumin molecules)

Low gap may suggest
- Unmeasured anion ↓ (e.g. hypoalbuminemia)
- Unmeasured cation ↑ (rarely)
    - E.g. hyperkalemia, hypercalcemia, hypermagnesemia

THE ROLE OF THE KIDNEY IN ACID-BASE BALANCE

osms.it/kidney_acid-base_balance

KIDNEY FUNCTION
- Kidneys maintain acid-base balance in two ways
    - HCO_3^- *reabsorption*: urine into blood
    - H^+ *secretion*: blood into urine
- Kidneys consist of nephrons
    - Each has glomerulus (capillaries clump)
- During filtration, plasma leaves glomerulus entering renal tubule (consists of proximal convoluted tubule, loop of Henle, distal convoluted tubule)

- Tubules lined with brush border cells (apical surface facing tubular lumen, basolateral surface facing peritubular capillaries)

HCO_3^- reabsorption

- Primarily in proximal convoluted tubule
    - Na^+ ions exchanged for H^+ ions through apical surface → bind with HCO_3^- → form H_2CO_3
    - Carbonic anhydrase type 4 splits H_2CO_3 into H_2O, CO_2
    - H_2O, CO_2 diffuse across membrane
    - Carbonic anhydrase type 2 recombines them into H_2CO_3
    - H_2CO_3 dissolve into H^+, HCO_3^-
    - Sodium/chloride bicarbonate cotransporters on basolateral surface snatch up HCO_3^-, nearby sodium/chloride ion, moving both into blood

H^+ secretion

- Primarily in proximal convoluted tubule
    - **Sodium-hydrogen countertransport**: H^+ ions exchanged for Na^+ ions through apical surface
    - Another mechanism in distal convoluted tubule, collecting ducts involving alpha-intercalated cells
    - Chemical buffers (ammonia, phosphate) prevent urine pH from dropping too low in tubules (< 4.5)

METABOLIC ACIDOSIS

osms.it/metabolic-acidosis

METABOLIC ACIDOSIS

- HCO_3^- ion reduction → blood pH ↓ to < 7.35

TYPES

- Distinguished by high/normal anion gap
    - Measured cation concentration
    - E.g. Na^+ ions, minus measured anion concentration (e.g. Cl^-, HCO_3^- ions)

High anion gap

- H^+ ions from organic acids convert HCO_3^- to H_2CO_3
    - ↓ HCO_3^- ion concentration (measured in anion gap), ↑ organic anion concentration (not measured)
    - **Naturally-occurring organic acids**: e.g. lactic acid production (lactic acidosis), ketoacid production (diabetic ketoacidosis), excessive uric, sulfur-containing acid retention (chronic renal failure)
    - **Ingestible organic acids**: e.g. oxalic acid (antifreeze), formic acid (methanol), hippuric acid (toluene)

Normal anion gap

- HCO_3^- lost in various ways, Cl^- ↑ prevents anion gap change (hyperchloremic metabolic acidosis)
- Possible causes
    - Diarrhea, renal tubular acidosis

REGULATORY MECHANISMS

- Body has several regulatory mechanisms to reverse ↓ pH
    - H^+ ions moved from blood into cells, exchanged for K^+ ions (may cause hyperkalemia); if organic anions present, can enter cells with H^+ ions → K^+ ions are not released
    - Chemoreceptors fire more in low pH → ↑ respiratory rate, breath depth → ↑ ventilation, CO_2 movement out of body
    - H^+ ions excreted by kidneys → HCO_3^- reabsorbed (with normal renal function)

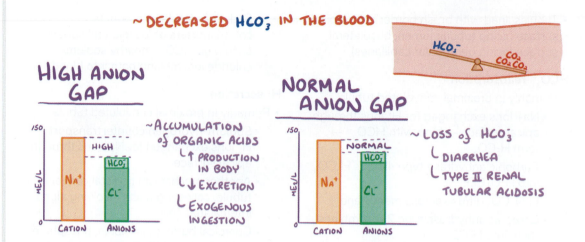

Figure 58.2 Illustration depicting the two kinds of metabolic acidosis: high anion gap (where H+ from organic acids converts HCO_3^- to H_2CO_3), and normal anion gap (where Cl- increase maintains normal anion gap).

METABOLIC ALKALOSIS

osms.it/metabolic-alkalosis

METABOLIC ALKALOSIS
- HCO_3^- ion gain → blood pH ↑ > 7.45

CAUSES
- Associated with direct HCO_3^- ion gain/ loss of H+ ion loss (thus → HCO_3^- ion gain), usually both
- Hypokalemia
  - Metabolic alkalosis cause
  - May also be result of other root causes

Excessive H+ ion loss causes
- Vomiting (gastric secretions acidic)
  - Also causes HCO_3^- ion buildup in pancreas (would normally neutralize gastric secretions)
- Abnormal renal function
  - E.g. adrenal tumors secrete aldosterone → distal convoluted tubule dumps H+ ions, reabsorbs HCO_3^- ions

Excessive HCO_3^- ion gain causes
- ↑ kidney reabsorption
  - Volume contraction with loop/thiazide diuretics/severe dehydration cases (contraction alkalosis)
- Hypokalemia
  - Diarrhea/diuretic use, triggering renin-angiotensin-aldosterone mechanism → distal convoluted tubule dumps H+ ions, reabsorbs HCO_3^- ions
- HCO_3^- ion ingestion
  - E.g. excessive antacid use ($NaHCO_3$)

REGULATORY MECHANISMS
- Body has regulatory mechanisms to reverse ↑ pH
  - K+ ions move from blood into cells → exchanged for H+ ions (may contribute to hypokalemia)
  - Chemoreceptors fire less in high pH → ↓ respiratory rate, breathing depth → ↓ ventilation, CO_2 retention
  - HCO_3^- ions excreted by kidneys → H+ reabsorbed (normal renal function)

Chapter 58 Renal Physiology: Acid-base Physiology

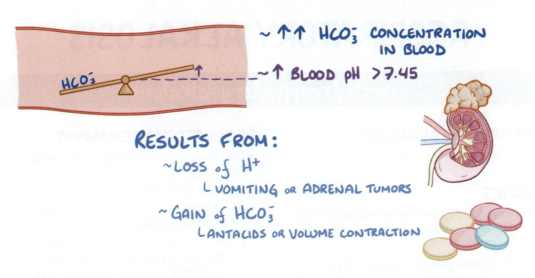

Figure 58.3 Illustration summarizing the definition and causes of metabolic alkalosis.

RESPIRATORY ACIDOSIS

osms.it/respiratory-acidosis

RESPIRATORY ACIDOSIS
- CO_2 gain → blood pH ↓ < 7.35

CAUSES
- Ventilation ↓ (frequency, breath depth) for variety of reasons → lungs blow off too little CO_2
  - Stroke/medication overdose/etc. → respiratory-center abnormality in brainstem
  - Obesity, trauma, neuromuscular disorders (myasthenia gravis), etc. → respiratory muscle-contraction failure
  - Airway obstruction
  - Alveoli damage (chronic obstructive pulmonary disease); alveoli fluid buildup (pneumonia); fluid buildup between alveoli, capillary walls (pulmonary edema) → impaired gas exchange between alveoli, capillary

REGULATORY MECHANISMS
- Body has several regulatory mechanisms to reverse pH ↓
  - Low pH → chemoreceptors fire more → attempted ↑ in respiratory rate, breathing depth → ↑ ventilation
  - H^+ ions bind to basic protein molecules (mainly exposed hemoglobin $-NH_2$ groups), although in small amounts
  - H^+ ions excreted by kidneys, HCO_3^- reabsorbed

RESPIRATORY ALKALOSIS

osms.it/respiratory-alkalosis

RESPIRATORY ALKALOSIS
- CO_2 loss → blood pH ↑ > 7.45

CAUSES
- Ventilation ↑ (frequency, breath depth) for variety of reasons → lungs blowing off too much CO_2
  - Respiratory-center abnormality in brainstem
  - Pneumonia, pulmonary embolism, etc. → low oxygen levels (hypoxia)
  - Anxiety, panic attacks, sepsis, salicylates overdose
  - Incorrectly-set ventilator → medical intervention

REGULATORY MECHANISMS
- Body has several regulatory mechanisms to reverse pH ↑
  - High pH → chemoreceptors fire less → attempted ↓ in respiratory rate, breathing depth → ↓ ventilation
  - H^+ ions released from acidic protein molecules (mainly exposed hemoglobin -COOH groups), although in small amounts
  - HCO_3^- ions excreted by kidneys, H^+ are reabsorbed

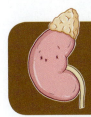

NOTES

FLUIDS IN THE BODY

BODY FLUID COMPARTMENTS

osms.it/body-fluid-compartments

GENERAL CHARACTERISTICS
- Fluid divisions in body
  - Includes intracellular fluid, extracellular fluid
- "60-40-20 rule"
  - Total body water is 60% of body weight, of which two thirds is intracellular → total intracellular fluid is 40% of body weight, total extracellular fluid is 20% of body weight
- Due to macroscopic electroneutrality principle, fluid compartments have same concentration of positive charges as negative charges

INTRACELLULAR & EXTRACELLULAR FLUID
- Large difference between intracellular fluid and extracellular fluid (e.g. Na^+K^+ ATPases establish high concentration of K^+ inside cell and high concentration of Na^+ outside cell)

Intracellular fluid
- Dissolves cations (esp. K^+ and Mg^{2+}) and anions (esp. proteins and organic phosphates e.g. ATP)

Extracellular fluid
- Includes interstitial fluid (around cells) and plasma (aqueous part of blood, containing about 10% proteins e.g. albumin)
  - Both dissolve cations (esp. Na^+) and anions (esp. Cl^- and HCO_3^-)
  - Solutes and water travel between the interstitial fluid and plasma through pores in endothelial cells of capillaries
  - Negative plasma proteins are too big to travel through pores; electroneutrality is maintained by repelling small anions into interstitial fluid and attracting small cations into plasma (Gibbs–Donnan effect) → interstitial fluid has ↑ small anion concentration (e.g. Cl^-) and ↓ small cation concentration (e.g. Na^+)

VOLUMES OF BODY FLUID COMPARTMENTS
- Determined by administering and measuring concentration of substances that are known to settle in specific compartments (dilution method)
  - Radiolabeled albumin for plasma (cannot pass into interstitial fluid)
  - Smaller molecules like mannitol and inulin for interstitial fluid (cannot pass through cell membranes)
  - Heavy water (D_2O) for total body water (knowing this and above, intracellular fluid can be calculated too)
  - Measuring concentration of these substances in their respective body fluid compartments allows us to calculate volume $\left(= \frac{AmountGiven}{Concentration}\right)$
  - To account for loss of these substances in urine, subtract amount lost from amount given and use this value in formula

DILUTION METHOD SAMPLE PROBLEM

A 70 kg man is injected with 150mCi of D_2O and 650mg of mannitol. During a two hour equilibration period, he excretes 10% of the D_2O and 10% of the mannitol in his urine. After that, the concentration of D_2O in the plasma is 0.32mCi/100 mL, and the concentration of mannitol is 4.6 mg/100mL. Calculate the total body water (TBW), extracellular fluid (ECF), and intracellular fluid (ICF) volumes.

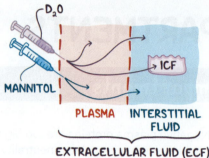

	INJECTED	EXCRETED	CONCENTRATION
D_2O	150 mCi	10%	0.32 mCi/100 mL
MANNITOL	650 mg	10%	4.6 mg/100 mL

STEP 1: CALCULATE VOLUME$_{TBW}$ (D_2O) & VOLUME$_{ECF}$ (MANNITOL)

STEP 1a: Determine amount remaining in body after excretion

Amount remaining = amount injected - amount excreted

$Amount_{D2O}$ = 150mCi - (10% × 150mCi)
= 150mCi - 15mCi
= 135mCi

$Amount_{mannitol}$ = 650mg - (10% × 650mg)
= 650mg - 65mg
= 585mg

STEP 1b: Divide remaining amount by concentration

$Volume_{TBW}$ = $Volume_{D2O}$

= 135mCi × $\frac{100mL}{0.32mCi}$

= 42.2L

$Volume_{ECF}$ = $Volume_{mannitol}$

= 585mg × $\frac{100mL}{4.6mg}$

= 12.7L

STEP 2: CALCULATE VOLUME$_{ICF}$

$Volume_{ICF}$ = $Volume_{TBW}$ - $Volume_{ECF}$

= 42.2 L - 12.7 L
= 29.5 L

Figure 59.1 A sample problem demonstrating how to solve for total body water, extracellular fluid, and intracellular fluid volumes using information gained from D_2O and mannitol.

WATER SHIFTS BETWEEN BODY FLUID COMPARTMENTS

osms.it/water-shifts-between-body-fluid-compartments

Key features
- Movement of water between body fluid compartments to maintain constant osmolarity
- Shifts are characterized by change in volume and concentration of extracellular fluid
  - ECF volume: ↑ = expansion; ↓ = contraction
  - ECF osmolarity: ↑ = hyperosmotic; ↓ = hyposmotic; no change = isosmotic
- Six possible combinations

VOLUME CONTRACTION

Isosmotic volume contraction
- Loss of isosmotic fluid from ECF
- Volume ↓ but osmolarity is constant → no water shift
- ↓ plasma volume and arterial pressure; ↑ plasma protein concentration and hematocrit
- E.g. diarrhea

Hyperosmotic volume contraction
- Loss of hyposmotic fluid from ECF
- Volume ↓ and osmolarity ↑ → water shifts from ICF (net effect is still volume contraction)
- ↓ plasma volume and arterial pressure; ↑ plasma protein concentration but hematocrit is unchanged (since red blood cells lose volume too)
- E.g. heavy sweating (sweat is hyposmotic relative to ECF)

Hyposmotic volume contraction
- Loss of solutes/hyperosmotic fluid from ECF
- Volume ↓ and osmolarity ↓ → water shifts to ICF
- ↓ plasma volume and arterial pressure; ↑ plasma protein concentration and hematocrit
- E.g. adrenal insufficiency (deficiency in several hormones, including aldosterone). Aldosterone important for sodium reabsorption from kidneys; ↓ aldosterone = ↑ sodium loss in urine

VOLUME EXPANSION

Isosmotic volume expansion
- Gain of isosmotic fluid in ECF
- Volume ↑ but osmolarity is constant → no water shift
- ↑ plasma volume and arterial pressure; ↓ plasma protein concentration and hematocrit
- E.g. receiving an infusion of isotonic NaCl solution

Hyperosmotic volume expansion
- Gain of solutes or hyperosmotic fluid in ECF
- Volume ↑ and osmolarity ↑ → water shifts from ICF
- ↑ plasma volume and arterial pressure; ↓ plasma protein concentration and hematocrit
- E.g. eating salty chips

Hyposmotic volume expansion
- Gain of hyposmotic fluid in ECF
- Volume ↑ and osmolarity ↓ → water shifts to ICF (net effect is still volume expansion)
- ↑ plasma volume and arterial pressure; ↓ plasma protein concentration but hematocrit is unchanged
- E.g. too much antidiuretic hormone causing excessive water reabsorption

TYPES of VOLUME CONTRACTION

ISOSMOTIC VOLUME CONTRACTION (Example: Diarrhea)

1. ISOSMOTIC FLUID LOST FROM ECF

   → ECF VOLUME ↓   PLASMA VOLUME ↓ → PLASMA PROTEIN [ ] ↑
                            HEMATOCRIT ↑

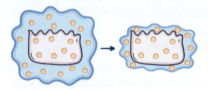

2. ECF OSMOLARITY = ICF OSMOLARITY → NO ICF WATER MOVEMENT

HYPEROSMOTIC VOLUME CONTRACTION (Example: Running a marathon)

1. HYPOOSMOTIC FLUID LOST FROM ECF → ECF VOLUME ↓, ECF OSMOLARITY ↑

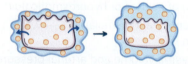

2. ECF OSMOLARITY > ICF OSMOLARITY → WATER MOVES FROM ICF TO ECF

   → ECF & ICF VOLUME ↓   PLASMA VOLUME ↓ → PLASMA PROTEIN [ ] ↑
   ECF & ICF OSMOLARITY ↑   HEMATOCRIT UNCHANGED

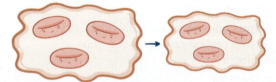

HYPOOSMOTIC VOLUME CONTRACTION (Example: Adrenal insufficiency)

1. ↓ ECF SOLUTES → ECF OSMOLARITY ↓

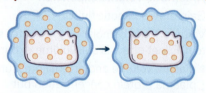

2. ECF OSMOLARITY < ICF OSMOLARITY → WATER MOVES FROM ECF TO ICF

   → ECF VOLUME ↓, ICF VOLUME ↑   PLASMA VOLUME ↓ → PLASMA PROTEIN [ ] ↑
   ECF & ICF OSMOLARITY ↓   HEMATOCRIT ↑

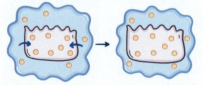
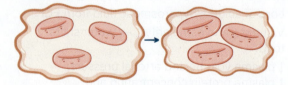

Figure 59.2 Visualization of the types of volume contraction.

Chapter 59 Renal Physiology: Fluids in the Body

TYPES of VOLUME EXPANSION

ISOSMOTIC VOLUME EXPANSION (Example: Isotonic NaCl infusion)

1. ISOSMOTIC FLUID ADDED TO ECF
   → ECF VOLUME ↑
   OSMOLARITY UNCHANGED
   PLASMA VOLUME ↑ → PLASMA PROTEIN [ ] ↓
   HEMATOCRIT ↓

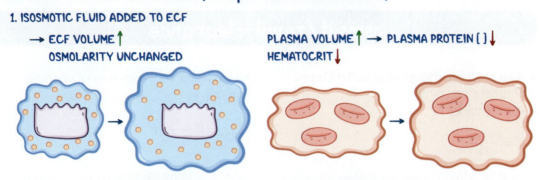

2. ECF OSMOLARITY = ICF OSMOLARITY → NO ICF WATER MOVEMENT

HYPEROSMOTIC VOLUME EXPANSION (Example: Eating salty chips)

1. ECF SOLUTES ↑ → ECF OSMOLARITY ↑

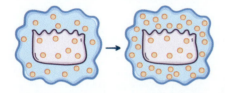

2. ECF OSMOLARITY > ICF OSMOLARITY → WATER MOVES FROM ICF TO ECF
   → ECF VOLUME ↑, ICF VOLUME ↓
   ECF & ICF OSMOLARITY ↑
   PLASMA VOLUME ↑ → PLASMA PROTEIN [ ] ↓
   HEMATOCRIT ↓

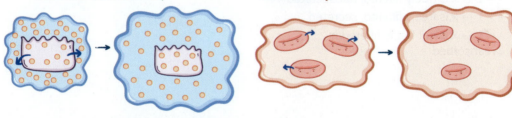

HYPOOSMOTIC VOLUME EXPANSION (Example: SIADH)

1. ↑↑ WATER REABSORPTION, EXCESS WATER DISTRIBUTED THROUGHOUT TOTAL BODY WATER
   → ECF & ICF VOLUME ↑
   ECF & ICF OSMOLARITY ↓
   PLASMA VOLUME ↑ → PLASMA PROTEIN [ ] ↓
   HEMATOCRIT UNCHANGED

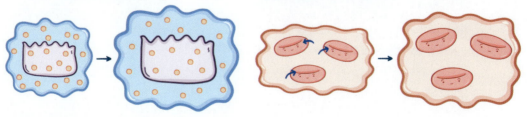

Figure 59.3 Visualization of the types of volume expansion.

RENAL CLEARANCE

osms.it/renal-clearance

- Rate at which kidneys clear blood plasma of substance
- For substance "x", renal clearance

$$C = \frac{[U]_x \times V}{[P]_x}$$

  - $[U]_x$: urine concentration of x
  - $[P]_x$: plasma concentration of x
  - V: urine flow rate

- To measure reabsorption/secretion of substance in kidneys, **inulin** can be used as reference point
  - Inulin is **freely filtered**
  - Inulin is **not reabsorbed/secreted**
- Clearance ratio for substance x is

$$\frac{C_x}{C_{inulin}}$$

  - = 1 → x is freely filtered, not secreted
  - > 1 → x is freely filtered, secreted
  - < 1 → x is not freely filtered/is reabsorbed

- Free water clearance is renal clearance of pure water

$$C_{H_2O} = V - \frac{U_{osm}}{P_{osm}} V$$

  - U_{osm}: urine osmolarity
  - P_{osm}: plasma osmolarity

RENAL CLEARANCE SAMPLE PROBLEM

PART 1

In a 24 hour period, a man has 2 liters of urine. His plasma Na⁺ concentration is 145mEq/L, whereas his urine Na⁺ concentration is 190mEq/L. What is the man's renal clearance for sodium?

$$C = \frac{[U]_x \times \dot{V}}{[P]_x}$$

STEP 1: CALCULATE $\dot{V}$

$$\dot{V} = \frac{\text{URINE VOLUME}}{\text{TIME}} = \frac{2000mL}{1440min} = 1.39mL/min$$

STEP 2: CALCULATE C_{Na^+}

$$C_{Na^+} = \frac{[U]_x \times \dot{V}}{[P]_x} = \frac{190mEq/L \times 1.39\ mL/min}{145mEq/L} = 1.43mL/min$$

→ 1.43mL of plasma is cleared of Na⁺ per minute.

PART 2

Returning to the scenario in Part 1, let's assume we gave that man an infusion of inulin over 2 hours. The urine concentration of inulin is 140mg/mL, and the plasma concentration of inulin is 1mg/mL. The urine flow rate is 1.39mL/min (the value calculated in Part 1). What is the man's clearance of inulin? What is the clearance ratio for Na⁺?

$$C = \frac{[U]_x \times \dot{V}}{[P]_x}$$

STEP 1: CALCULATE C_{INULIN}

$$C_{INULIN} = \frac{[U]_x \times \dot{V}}{[P]_x} = \frac{140mg/mL \times 1.39\ mL/min}{1mg/mL} = 194.6mL/min$$

→ 194.6mL of plasma is cleared of inulin per minute.

STEP 2: CALCULATE CLEARANCE RATIO FOR Na⁺

$$C_{Na^+} = \frac{C_{Na^+}}{C_{INULIN}} = \frac{1.43mL/min}{194.6mL/min} = 0.007$$

→ 0.007 << 1, so very little Na⁺ is excreted in the urine. Since it is freely filtered, it must be extensively reabsorbed by the nephron to have such a low clearance ratio.

FREE WATER CLEARANCE SAMPLE PROBLEM

A woman has a urine flow rate of 1.5mL/min, a urine osmolarity of 130mOsm/L, and a plasma osmolarity of 280mOsm/L. What is her free water clearance?

$$CH_2O = \dot{V} - C_{OSM}$$

$$CH_2O = \dot{V} - \frac{[U]_{OSM} \times \dot{V}}{[P]_{OSM}}$$

$$= 1.5mL/min - \frac{130mOsm/L \times 1.5mL/min}{180mOsm/L}$$

$$= 1.5mL/min - 0.7mL/min$$

$$= 0.8mL/min$$

→ 0.8mL of plasma is cleared of solute-free water every minute by the kidneys.

Figure 59.4 Sample questions solving for renal clearance of a solute and free water clearance.

NOTES
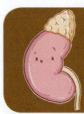
RENAL BLOOD FLOW REGULATION

RENAL BLOOD FLOW REGULATION

osms.it/renal-blood-flow-regulation

- Blood enters kidney via renal artery, leaves via renal vein
    - Blood enters glomerulus via afferent arteriole, leaves via efferent arteriole
- *Renal blood flow*: volume of blood that reaches kidneys in unit time; determined by pressure gradient (pressure in renal artery - pressure in renal vein) divided by arteriolar resistance
    - ↑ blood pressure → ↑ pressure in renal artery → ↑ renal blood flow
    - ↓ arteriolar resistance → ↑ renal blood flow
- Renal blood flow determines glomerular filtration rate (GFR)
    - ↑ renal blood flow → ↑ GFR
- *Regulation of renal blood flow*: increasing/decreasing arteriolar resistance

Key hormones: increasing arteriolar resistance (decreasing renal blood flow)
- Adrenaline (epinephrine)
    - Secreted by adrenal gland in response to sympathetic stimulation
    - Binds to alpha-1 adrenergic receptors along afferent, efferent arterioles → smooth muscle cells contract
- Angiotensin II
    - Renin produced by juxtaglomerular cells in afferent arteriole → released into blood, becomes angiotensin I in response to low blood pressure → converted into angiotensin II by angiotensin-converting enzyme (ACE), synthesized in endothelial cells (esp. in lungs)
    - Binds to angiotensin receptors along afferent, efferent arterioles → smooth muscle cells contract
    - Efferent arterioles more sensitive to angiotensin II → constrict more → blood builds up in glomerulus → GFR constant
    - High levels of angiotensin II → afferent arterioles constrict equally → ↓ GFR

Key hormones: decreasing arteriolar resistance (increasing renal blood flow)
- Atrial natriuretic peptide
    - Secreted by atria of heart in response to increased cardiac workload
    - Binds to natriuretic peptide receptors along afferent, efferent arterioles → smooth muscle cells relax
- Brain natriuretic peptide
    - Secreted by ventricles of heart in response to increased cardiac workload
    - Binds to natriuretic peptide receptors along afferent, efferent arterioles → smooth muscle cells relax
- Prostaglandins (e.g. prostaglandin E2, I2)
    - Produced by kidneys in response to sympathetic stimulation
    - Binds to prostaglandin receptors along afferent, efferent arterioles → smooth muscle cells relax
    - Prevents kidney damage during sympathetic stimulation
- Dopamine
    - Synthesized in brain, kidneys
    - Binds to dopaminergic along afferent, efferent arterioles → smooth muscle cells relax

Chapter 60 Renal Physiology: Renal Blood Flow Regulation

AUTOREGULATION OF RENAL BLOOD FLOW

- Keeps renal blood flow, GFR constant over range of systemic blood pressures (80–200mmHg)
  - **80mmHg:** smooth blood cells in arterioles completely relaxed, renal blood flow optimal
  - Systemic blood pressure increases → smooth blood cells contract to maintain optimal renal blood flow

Mechanisms for autoregulation

- *Myogenic mechanism:* smooth muscle cells in arterioles automatically contract when stretched by high blood pressure (related to increased renal blood flow)
- *Tubuloglomerular mechanism:* macula densa cells release adenosine → increases resistance in afferent arteriole when more sodium, chloride ions detected in distal convoluted tubule (related to increased GFR, renal blood flow)

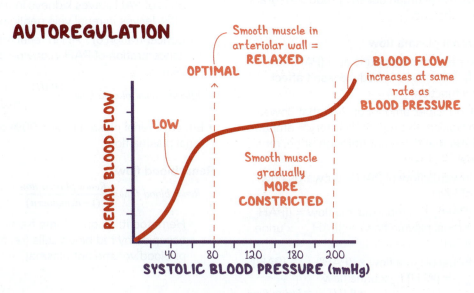

Figure 60.1 Graph displaying the relationship between systolic blood pressure and renal blood flow. The kidneys achieve consistency between 80–200mmHg by adjusting their own arteriole resistance.

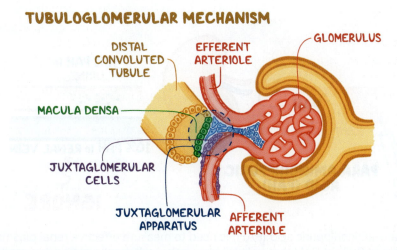

Figure 60.2 The region where the distal convoluted tubule and the afferent arteriole are close to one another is called the juxtaglomerular apparatus. This proximity allows adenosine from the macula densa cells to diffuse over to the juxtaglomerular cells of the afferent arteriole, alerting them to ↑ GFR. This increases arteriolar resistance → ↓ GFR.

MEASURING RENAL PLASMA FLOW & RENAL BLOOD FLOW

osms.it/measuring-renal-plasma-blood-flow

- **Fick principle**: amount of substance in blood that flows into organ = amount that flows out (if organ doesn't produce/degrade that substance)

True renal plasma flow

- Add para-aminohippuric acid (PAH) to body (isn't made in body, doesn't affect renal function)
- **Fick principle**: amount of PAH that flows into kidneys through renal artery = amount of PAH that flows out (through urine, renal veins)
  - Inwards flow of PAH = outwards flow of PAH
  - $[PAH]_{artery}$ × renal plasma flow = ($[PAH]_{vein}$ × renal plasma flow) + ($[PAH]_{urine}$ × urine flow)
  - Renal plasma flow × ($[PAH]_{artery}$ - $[PAH]_{vein}$) = $[PAH]_{urine}$ × urine flow
  - $$Renal\ plasma\ flow = \frac{[PAH]_{urine} \times Urine\ flow}{[PAH]_{artery} - [PAH]_{vein}}$$
- Measure concentration of PAH in renal artery/vein, urine; measure urine flow

Effective renal plasma flow

- Two assumptions
  - 90% of PAH leaves kidneys in urine → 10% leaves in renal vein negligible
  - Concentration of PAH in renal artery = concentration of PAH in any peripheral vein
- $$Effective\ renal\ plasma\ flow = \frac{[PAH]_{urine} \times Urine\ flow}{[PAH]}$$
- Effective renal plasma flow = 90% of true renal plasma flow

Renal blood flow

- $$Renal\ blood\ flow = \frac{Renal\ plasma\ flow}{(1 - hematocrit)}$$
  - **Hematocrit**: blood volume fraction occupied by red blood cells (i.e. fraction of blood volume not plasma)

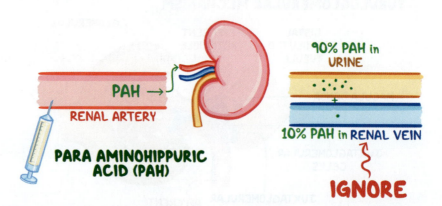

Figure 60.3 Para-aminohippuric acid (PAH) is used to measure effective renal plasma flow. It is assumed that about 90% of PAH that enters kidneys through renal artery is excreted in urine, and only 10% enters the renal vein → ignore this, assume that effective renal plasma flow = 90% of true renal plasma flow.

NOTES

RENAL ELECTROLYTE REGULATION

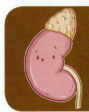

GLOMERULAR FILTRATION

osms.it/glomerular-filtration

- Fluid passage through glomerular filtration barrier; approx. 125mL/min
- **Glomerular filtrate:** fluid that passes through all glomerular filtration barriers
  - Blood minus red blood cells, plasma proteins
- Anything remaining in glomerulus carried away by efferent arteriole
- Starling forces → glomerular filtration
  - Different pressures of fluids, proteins in glomerular capillaries, Bowman's space
- Most filtration occurs at beginning of glomerulus, nearer afferent arteriole

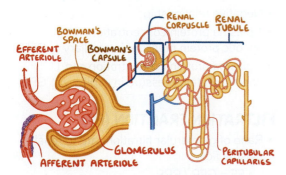

Figure 61.1 An illustration depicting the glomerulus and its relationship to the rest of the nephron.

GLOMERULAR FILTRATION BARRIER

- Capillary walls of glomerulus
  - **Glomerulus:** tuft of capillaries in nephron's renal corpuscle
  - Blood enters glomerulus through afferent arteriole → leaves through efferent arteriole → divides into peritubular capillaries
- Separates blood in capillaries from Bowman's space, Bowman's capsule
- Allows only water, some solutes to pass into Bowman's space
- **Three layers:** endothelium, basement membrane, epithelium
- **Juxtaglomerular apparatus:** secretes renin

Endothelium
- Comprised of glomerular capillary endothelial cells featuring pores (AKA fenestrations)
- Allows passage of solutes, proteins
- Blocks red blood cell passage

Basement membrane
- Gel-like layer with tiny pores
- Blocks plasma protein passage
  - Due to pore size, negative membrane charge

Epithelium
- Comprised of podocytes (wrap around basement membrane)
- Also blocks plasma protein passage

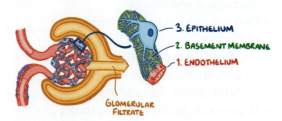

Figure 61.2 The three layers of the glomerular filtration barrier.

STARLING FORCES

- Determine fluid movement through capillary wall
- Includes hydrostatic/fluid pressures, oncotic/protein pressures
- Three Starling forces at play in glomerular filtration barrier
    - Hydrostatic pressure of blood in capillary (P_{gc})
    - Hydrostatic pressure of filtrate in Bowman's space (P_{bs})
    - Oncotic pressure of proteins in capillary (π_{gc})
- Determines net ultrafiltration pressure of glomerulus: $P_{uf} = P_{gc} - (P_{bs} + \pi_{gc})$
    - Net ultrafiltration pressure ↓ along each glomerular capillary—as fluid removed, proteins remain (↑ π_{gc})
    - At filtration equilibrium, net ultrafiltration pressure equals 0 (no fluid filtered)

Hydrostatic blood pressure in capillary
- Positive relationship
- Afferent arteriole vasoconstriction → ↓ renal blood flow
    - ↓ hydrostatic blood pressure in capillary (↓ GFR)
- Afferent arteriole vasodilation → ↑ renal blood flow
    - ↑ hydrostatic blood pressure in capillary (↑ GFR)
- Efferent arteriole vasoconstriction → ↑ fluid in glomerular capillary
    - ↑ hydrostatic blood pressure in capillary (↑ GFR)
- Efferent arteriole vasodilation → ↓ fluid in glomerular capillary
    - ↓ hydrostatic blood pressure in capillary (↓ GFR)

Hydrostatic filtrate pressure in Bowman's space
- Negative relationship
- Doesn't normally occur
- Urine flow blockage → urine backup (e.g. stone lodged in ureter)
    - ↑ hydrostatic filtrate pressure in Bowman's space (↓ GFR)

Oncotic protein pressure in capillary
- Negative relationship
- ↑ plasma protein concentration can ↑ oncotic protein pressure in capillary (↓ GFR)
- ↓ plasma protein concentration can ↓ oncotic protein pressure in capillary (↑ GFR)

FILTRATION FRACTION (FF)
- Ratio of glomerular filtration rate to renal plasma flow
    - FF = GFR / RPF
- Indicates how much fluid reaching kidneys is filtered into renal tubules

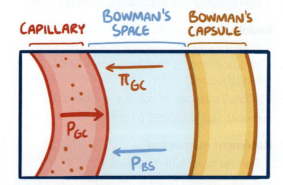

Figure 61.3 Illustration depicting the three Starling forces at play in the glomerular filtration barrier.

GLOMERULAR FILTRATION RATE (GFR)
- Filtrate volume produced by all of body's glomeruli in one minute
- GFR = $P_{uf} \times K_f$ where K_f is filtration coefficient
    - K_f: indicates capillary's fluid permeability
    - Fenestrations, large surface area → high K_f for glomerular capillaries
- Depends on all three Starling forces

Chapter 61 Renal Physiology: Renal Electrolyte Regulation

PROXIMAL CONVOLUTED TUBULE

osms.it/proximal-convoluted-tubule

- First renal tubule segment
- Receives filtrate from renal corpuscle
- Passes filtrate to loop of Henle
- Lined by brush border cells
  - Apical surface faces lumen; lined with microvilli
  - Basolateral surface faces interstitium
- Surrounded by peritubular capillaries → reabsorption, secretion of solutes to/from blood via interstitium
- Reabsorbs Na^+, K^+, Ca^{2+}, Cl^-, Mg^{2+} into bloodstream

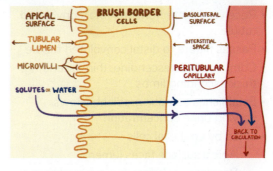

Figure 61.4 The relationship between the proximal convoluted tubule's brush border cells and a peritubular capillary.

NA⁺ MOVEMENT

Natural concentration gradient from lumen into cells

- **Cotransporters:** use this energy to move other solutes (e.g. Na^+-glucose cotransporter)
- **Na^+/K^+ ATPase:** pumps $3Na^+$ from cell into interstitium, $2K^+$ from interstitium into cell
  - Movement against two concentration gradients → ATP required
- **Na^+/H^+ exchanger:** pumps Na^+ from cell into cell, H^+ from cell into lumen
  - Assists HCO_3^- reabsorption by creating $H_2CO_3 \rightarrow H_2O + CO_2$

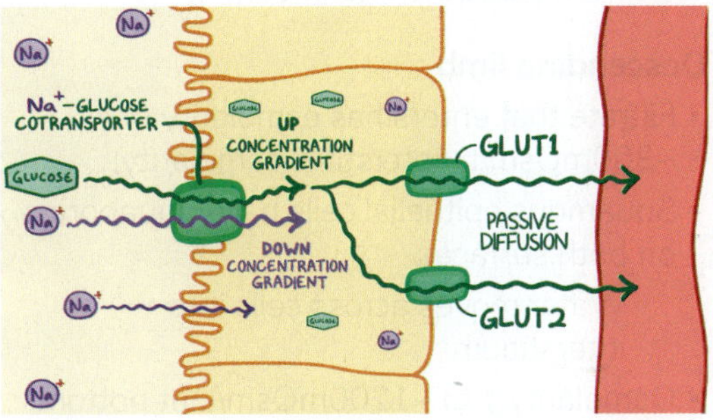

Paracellular route

- Leaky tight junctions → some Na^+ movement between cells
  - ↓ claudin proteins → ↑ permeability
- Urea, water diffuse straight across cells → interstitium
- Glutamine breakdown inside cell → NH_4^+ (cell → lumen) + HCO_3^- (cell → interstitium)
- Organic acids, some medications diffuse directly from capillaries into lumen (e.g. penicillin)

Figure 61.5 The Na^+-glucose cotransporter uses the concentration gradient of Na^+ to transport glucose against its concentration gradient.

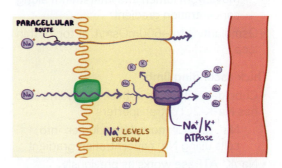

Figure 61.6 Na^+/K^+ ATPase and the paracellular route of Na^+ movement.

LOOP OF HENLE

osms.it/loop-of-henle

- Receives filtrate from proximal convoluted tubule
- Passes filtrate to distal convoluted tubule
- Composed of descending, thin ascending, thick ascending limbs
- Establishes osmotic gradient; allows varying urine concentration
- Lined by epithelial cells
    - Apical surface faces lumen
    - Basolateral surface faces interstitium
- Surrounded by peritubular capillaries
    - AKA vasa recta
    - Reabsorption, secretion of solutes to/from blood via interstitium

Descending limb
- Filtrate that enters has osmolarity of ~300mOsm/L (interstitial osmolarity)
- Squamous epithelial cells have aquaporins on both surfaces
    - Water moves across cells into interstitium
- Osmolarity ↑ to ~1200mOsm/L at bottom of loop

Thin ascending limb
- No aquaporins on thin ascending limb; Na^+, Cl^- channels instead
    - Move from lumen into interstitium along concentration gradient
- Osmolarity ↓ to ~600mOsm/L at top of thin loop

Thick ascending limb
- Cuboidal epithelium in thick ascending limb has Na-K-2Cl cotransporters
    - Na^+, K^+, $2Cl^-$ moved from lumen into cells using Na^+ concentration gradient
- Na^+/K^+ ATPase works as previously
- K^+, Cl^- channels → move from cell into interstitium along concentration gradient
- Osmolarity ↓ to ~325mOsm/L at top of thick loop
- **Countercurrent multiplication:** process of creating concentration gradient along loop

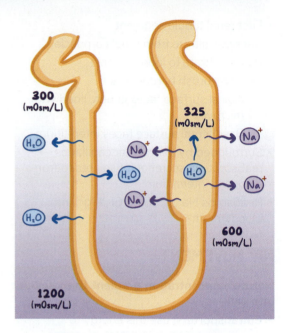

Figure 61.7 Countercurrent multiplication is the process of creating the concentration gradient along the loop of Henle. It uses ATP.

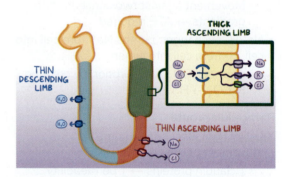

Figure 61.8 Aquaporins transport H_2O out of the thin descending limb; channel proteins transport Na^+ and Cl^- out of the thin ascending limb; Na-K-2Cl cotransporters and channels transport Na^+, K^+, and Cl^- out of the thick ascending limb.

DISTAL CONVOLUTED TUBULE

osms.it/distal-convoluted-tubule

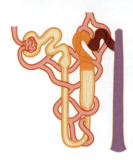

* EARLY DISTAL CONVOLUTED TUBULE
* LATE DISTAL CONVOLUTED TUBULE
* COLLECTING DUCT

Figure 61.9 Filtrate passes through the early and late portions of the distal convoluted tubule, then reaches the collecting duct.

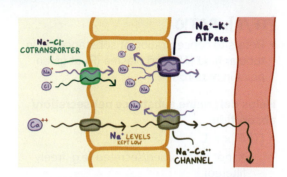

Figure 61.10 Illustration of transporters present in the early distal convoluted tubule.

- Receives filtrate from loop of Henle
- Passes filtrate to collecting ducts
- Composed of early, late distal convoluted tubules
- Lined by brush border cells
    - Apical surface faces lumen; not lined with microvilli
    - Basolateral surface faces interstitium
- Surrounded by peritubular capillaries → reabsorption, secretion of solutes to/from blood via interstitium

Early distal convoluted tubule

- Impermeable to water
- Na^+: natural concentration gradient from lumen → cells
- Cotransporters use this energy to move other solutes (e.g. Na^+-Cl^- cotransporter)
- Cl^- moves from cells → interstitium through direct channels
- Ca^{2+} moves across cells → interstitium through direct channels
    - On basolateral surface: Na^+-Ca^{2+} channel pumps Na^+ from interstitium → cell, Ca^{2+} from cell → interstitium
- Ca^{2+} reabsorption regulated by parathyroid hormone
    - Creates more Na^+-Ca^{2+} channels
- Na^+/K^+ ATPase works as previously

Late distal convoluted tubule

- → collecting ducts
- Principal cells, α-intercalated cells dispersed among brush border cells
- Aldosterone upregulates pump synthesis
- Principal cells have
    - K^+ pumps (cell → lumen; uses ATP)
    - Na^+ pumps ("ENaC"; lumen → cell)
    - Na^+/K^+ ATPases
- Aquaporin 2 in principal cells allows for water reabsorption in response to antidiuretic hormone
- α-intercalated cells have
    - H^+ ATPases, H^+-K^+ ATPases (movement against concentration gradients → ATP required)
    - Na^+/K^+ ATPases

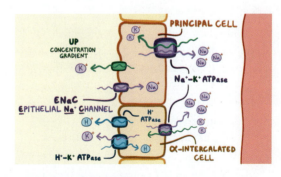

Figure 61.11 Illustration of transporters present in the late distal convoluted tubule.

TF/P$_x$ RATIO & TF/P$_{INULIN}$

osms.it/TF_Px-ratio-TF_Pinulin

[TF/P]$_x$ RATIO

- Refers to concentration of substance (X) in tubular fluid (TF) and plasma (P) at given point in nephron

Helps determine substance net secretion/absorption

- [TF/P]$_x$ = 1
  - X: not reabsorbed/secreted (e.g. freely filtered)
  - X: reabsorbed in proportion to water
  - E.g. [TF/P]$_{glucose}$ = 1 when glucose, water reabsorbed equally in Bowman's space
- [TF/P]$_x$ < 1
  - X: reabsorbed more than water
  - E.g. [TF/P]$_{glucose}$ < 1 when glucose reabsorbed more than water along proximal tubule
- [TF/P]$_x$ > 1
  - X: reabsorbed less than water/X secreted into tubular fluid
  - E.g. [TF/P]$_{urea}$ > 1 in presence of antidiuretic hormone (ADH) at collecting ducts (water reabsorbed, not urea)

[TF/P]$_{INULIN}$

- Inulin (inert substance—neither reabsorbed nor secreted) concentration throughout nephron helps determine how much is reabsorbed
- Inulin concentration will ↑ as water is reabsorbed
- Determined using this formula:

$$\text{Fraction of filtered water reabsorbed} = 1 - \frac{1}{[TF/P]_{inulin}}$$

  - Fraction of filtered water reabsorbed = 1 - 1/2 = 0.5 (50%)
  - [TF/P]$_{inulin}$ = 2 when 50% of water is reabsorbed (inulin concentration doubles)
- Double ratio formula determines fraction of filtered load of substance in nephron at any point

$$\frac{[TF/P]x}{[TF/P]_{inulin}}$$

- If [TF/P]$_{Na+}$ divided by [TF/P]inulin = 0.3, then 30% sodium remains in tubule, 70% reabsorbed

Chapter 61 Renal Physiology: Renal Electrolyte Regulation

CALCIUM HOMEOSTASIS

osms.it/calcium-homeostasis

- 1% Ca^{2+} found in intracellular fluid (ICF), extracellular fluid (ECF); 99% in bones, teeth
- *Functions*: cell membrane permeability, blood clotting, muscle contraction
- 40% plasma Ca^{2+} bound to protein
    - Unbound is physiologically active
    - Regulated by parathyroid hormone (PTH)

Ca^{2+} HANDLING

Filtration
- Only unbound Ca^{2+} (60%) is filtered
- Calculation of Ca^{2+} filtered load if total plasma Ca^{2+} = 5mEq/L and GFR = 180L/day
    - 180 X 5 X 0.6 = 540mEq/day

Filtered load reabsorption
- Coupled with Na^+ reabsorption in proximal tubule, loop of Henle (passively reabsorbed via electrochemical gradient created by Na^+, water)
    - 67% reabsorbed by proximal tubule
    - 25% reabsorbed in thick ascending limb of loop of Henle (paracellular route); loop diuretics ↓ reabsorption/↑ secretion
- 8% reabsorbed in distal tubule
    - Reabsorptive Ca^{2+} regulation site: only nephron segment not coupled with Na^+ reabsorption; PTH, thiazide diuretics → ↑ Ca^{2+} reabsorption (hypocalciuric action)

Excretion
- < 1%

MAGNESIUM HOMEOSTASIS

osms.it/magnesium-homeostasis

- < 1% Mg^{2+} found in ECF; 60% in bones, 20% in skeletal muscle, 19% in soft tissues, remainder found in ICF
- *Functions*: neuromuscular activity; enzymatic reactions within cells; ATP production; Na^+, Ca^{2+} transport across cell membranes
- 20% plasma Mg^{2+} bound to protein
    - Unbound is physiologically active

Mg^{2+} HANDLING

Filtration
- Only unbound Mg^{2+} (80%) is filtered

Filtered load reabsorption
- 30% reabsorbed by proximal tubule
- 60% reabsorbed by thick ascending limb of loop of Henle
    - Loop diuretics ↓ Mg^{2+} reabsorption (↑ excretion)
- 5% reabsorbed by distal tubule

Excretion
- 5%

PHOSPHATE HOMEOSTASIS

osms.it/phosphate-homeostasis

- ICF phosphate (15%) used for DNA, ATP synthesis, other metabolic processes
  - ECF phosphate (<0.5%) serves as buffer for H^+
  - 85% in bones

PHOSPHATE HANDLING

Filtration
- Freely filtered across glomerular capillaries

Filtered load reabsorption
- 70% reabsorbed by proximal tubule; 15% by proximal straight tubule via Na^+-phosphate cotransporter in luminal membrane
- Excess phosphate excreted when T_m (transport maximum) is reached
- PTH inhibits Na^+-phosphate cotransporter → ↓ phosphate T_m → phosphaturia

Excretion
- 15%

POTASSIUM HOMEOSTASIS

osms.it/potassium-homeostasis

- *Potassium (K^+)*: primary intracellular cation
  - Regulates intracellular osmolarity
  - Concentration gradient across cell membrane establishes resting membrane potential, essential for excitable cell function (e.g. myocardium)

INTERNAL K^+ BALANCE

- Difference between intracellular K^+ concentration (98% of total K^+), extracellular K^+ concentration (2% of total K^+) maintained by Na^+-K^+ ATPase
- K^+ shifts in/out of cells
  - Potentially causes hypo-/hyperkalemia

Outward K^+ shifts
- ↓ insulin
  - ↓ Na^+-K^+ ATPase activity → ↓ cellular K^+ uptake
- Cell lysis
  - K^+ released from ICF
- H^+-K^+ exchange in acidosis
  - ↑ blood H^+ → H^+ enters cell → K^+ moves from ICF to ECF
- ↑ ECF osmolarity
  - Osmotic gradient causes H_2O movement out of cells → ↑ intracellular K^+ → diffusion of K^+ from ICF to ECF (H_2O brings K^+ with it)
- Exercise
  - Cellular ATP stores depleted → K^+ channels open in muscle cell membrane → K^+ moves down concentration gradient to ECF
- α-adrenergic receptor activation
  - Hepatic Ca^{2+}-dependent-K^+-channel activation → K^+ moves from ICF to ECF

Inward K^+ shifts
- Insulin
  - ↑ Na^+-K^+ ATPase activity → ↑ cellular K^+ uptake
- H^+-K^+ exchange in alkalosis
  - ↓ blood H^+ → H^+ leaves cell → K^+ enters cell
- ↓ ECF osmolality
  - Osmotic gradient causes H_2O movement into cells → ↓ ICF K^+ concentration → diffusion of K^+ from

ECF to ICF
- β_2-adrenergic receptor activation
  - ↑ Na^+-K^+ ATPase activity → K^+ enters cell

EXTERNAL K^+ BALANCE
- Dietary K^+ intake = renal excretion of K^+ via renal mechanisms

K^+ HANDLING

Filtration
- Freely filtered across glomerular capillaries

Filtered load reabsorption
- 67% reabsorbed by proximal tubule (isosmotic fluid reabsorption along with water, Na^+)
- 20% reabsorbed by thick ascending limb
  - K^+ reabsorbed without water (impermeable to water) via Na^+-K^+-$2Cl^-$ cotransporter
  - K^+ diffuses through K^+ channels across basolateral membrane (reabsorption)/K^+ diffuses into lumen (no reabsorption)
- Fine-tuning of K^+ balance at distal tubule, collecting duct depending on current physiological requirements
- Reabsorbed by α-intercalated cells/ secreted by principal cells
  - *Dietary K^+*: high K^+ diet—K^+ enters cells (via insulin) → ↑ intracellular K^+ → ↑ K^+ in principal cells → ↑ K^+ secretion across luminal membrane → ↑ K^+ excretion; low K^+ diet—↓ K^+ secretion by principal cell, ↑ K^+ reabsorption by α-intercalated cells
  - *Aldosterone effects on principal cells*: presence of aldosterone/ hyperaldosteronism (↑ K^+ secretion); hypoaldosteronism (↓ K^+ secretion)
- *Acid-base imbalance effects on principal cells*: alkalosis (↑ K^+ secretion); acidosis (↓ K^+ secretion)
- *Diuretic effects on principal cells*: loop, thiazide (↑ K^+ secretion); K^+ sparing (inhibit aldosterone effects → ↓ K^+ secretion)
- Luminal anions (e.g. sulfate, HCO_3^-) in distal tubule, collecting duct (↑ lumen electronegativity by non-reabsorbable anions → ↑ K^+ secretion)

Excretion
- Varies from 1–110% of filtered load

SODIUM HOMEOSTASIS

osms.it/sodium-homeostasis

- *Sodium (Na^+)*: primary cation in ECF
  - Determines ECF osmolarity

Na^+ BALANCE REGULATION
- Na^+ balance (Na^+ excretion = Na^+ intake) determines ECF volume, blood volume, blood pressure (BP)
  - *Positive Na^+ balance*: ↑ Na^+ retained → ↑ Na^+ in ECF → ECF expansion → ↑ blood volume, ↑ blood pressure
  - *Negative Na^+ balance*: ↑ excreted, lost in urine → ↓ Na^+ in ECF → ECF contraction → ↓ blood volume, ↓ blood pressure

Effective arterial blood volume (EABV)
- ECF volume with arterial system perfuses tissue
- Normal ECF changes → parallel EABV changes (e.g. ↑ ECF = ↑ EABF)
- *Edema*: fluid filtered into interstitial space → ↑ ECF → ↓ EABV (↓ BP) → Na^+ excretion altered by kidneys (attempts to restore normal EABF, BP)

Na^+ excretion regulation (↑/↓) mechanisms
- Sympathetic nervous system activity
  - Baroreceptors detect ↓ BP → sympathetic nervous system activation → afferent arteriole vasoconstriction, ↑

Na⁺ reabsorption by proximal tubule
- **Natriuretic hormones**: respond to ↑ ECF volume → ↑ GFR, natriuresis (renal Na⁺, water excretion) → ↓ ECF
  - *Atrial natriuretic peptide (ANP)*: volume receptors detect atrial wall stretching → ANP secreted by cells in atria
  - *Brain natriuretic peptide (BNP)*: volume receptors in ventricles detect stretching → BNP secreted by cells in ventricles
  - *Urodilatin*: synthesized in distal tubular cells → paracrine actions on kidney
- **Peritubular Starling forces**
  - ↑ ECF volume → ECF dilution, ↓ π_c (capillary oncotic pressure); ↓ proximal tubule Na⁺ reabsorption
  - ↓ ECF volume → ↑ ECF concentration, ↑ π_c; ↑ proximal tubule Na⁺ reabsorption
- **Renin-angiotensin-aldosterone system (RAAS)**: ↓ arterial blood pressure (BP) → ↓ renal perfusion → juxtaglomerular apparatus secretes renin → angiotensinogen (plasma protein) converted to angiotensin I → angiotensin I converted to angiotensin II → adrenal cortex secretes aldosterone, vasoconstriction → ↑ Na⁺, Cl⁻, water reabsorption → ↑ ECF volume, ↑ BP

Excess Na⁺ intake response
- → Na⁺ ECF distribution → ↑ ECF, ↑ EABV, ↓ π_c → ↓ sympathetic activity, ↑ ANP (and other natriuretic hormones), ↓ RAAS → ↑ Na⁺ excretion

Decreased Na⁺ intake response
- → ↓ ECF, ↓ EABV, ↑ π_c → ↑ sympathetic activity, ↓ ANP (and other natriuretic hormones), ↑ RAAS → ↓ Na⁺ excretion

Na⁺ HANDLING

Filtration
- Freely filtered across glomerular capillaries

Filtered load reabsorption
- 67% reabsorbed by proximal tubule
  - Isosmotic reabsorption of water, Na⁺
  - Water reabsorption coupled with Na⁺ reabsorption ($[TF/P]_{Na+} = 1$)
- 25% reabsorbed by thick ascending limb
  - Na⁺ reabsorbed without water (impermeable to water) via Na⁺-K⁺-2Cl⁻ cotransporter
  - Influenced by ADH, loop diuretics
- 5% reabsorbed by early distal convoluted tubule
  - Na⁺ reabsorbed without water (impermeable to water) via Na⁺-2Cl⁻ cotransporter
  - Influenced by thiazide diuretics
- 3% reabsorbed by late distal convoluted tubule
  - Influenced by aldosterone

Excretion
- < 1% excreted (99% net Na⁺ reabsorption)

NOTES
RENAL REABSORPTION & SECRETION

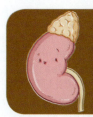

TUBULAR REABSORPTION & SECRETION

osms.it/tubular-reabsorption-secretion

- Blood chemistry balanced, urine formed through glomerular filtration, tubular reabsorption, secretion
  - Filtered blood continues through glomerulus, substances reabsorbed/secreted according to body's needs
  - Entire plasma volume filtered approx. 60 times/day

REABSORPTION
- Retention of substances contained in filtrate back into peritubular capillary blood

Filtration only/no reabsorption
- *Occurs with:* products of metabolism (e.g. urea, creatinine), foreign substances (e.g. drugs)

Filtration with partial reabsorption
- Electrolytes (e.g. sodium, bicarbonate) easily reabsorbed, may be partially reabsorbed, secreted

Filtration with complete reabsorption
- Nutritional substances (e.g. glucose, amino acids) completely reabsorbed

SECRETION
- Substances not reabsorbed (e.g. organic acids), secreted into tubular fluid to become urine

TUBULAR REABSORPTION OF GLUCOSE

osms.it/tubular-reabsorption-glucose

- *Filtration rate of glucose:* mass of glucose filtered through kidneys per day (depends on plasma glucose concentration)
- Kidney filtrate passes through renal tubules in nephron before becoming urine
  - Tubules lined by brush border cells with apical surface (lined with microvilli), basolateral surface; peritubular capillaries surround tubules

GLUCOSE REABSORPTION
- Occurs primarily in proximal convoluted tubule

OSMOSIS.ORG 543

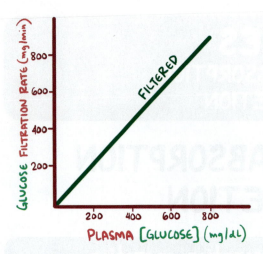

Figure 62.1 Graph showing glucose filtration rate as a function of plasma glucose. As the plasma glucose concentration increases, the filtered load of glucose increases linearly.

Two steps

1. Glucose moves across apical membrane into brush border cells
   - Glucose concentration inside cells typically higher than outside → sodium-glucose linked transporters use energy from existing sodium concentration gradient to move glucose against concentration gradient
2. Glucose diffuses across basolateral membrane into peritubular capillaries (facilitated diffusion with GLUT1/GLUT2)
   - *Normal plasma glucose levels (< 200mg/dL)*: glucose reabsorption matches filtration
   - *High plasma glucose levels (> 200mg/dL)*: limited number of glucose transporter proteins prevents reabsorption from keeping up with filtration
   - *Higher glucose levels (> 350mg/dL)*: glucose transporter proteins fully saturated, reabsorption cannot go faster; transport maximum (T_m)

GLUCOSE EXCRETION

- Excess glucose excreted in urine
  - *Threshold*: plasma glucose level at which glucose excretion starts
  - *Splay*: initial, nonlinear increase in urine excretion
- Glycosuria (glucose excreted in urine) may be caused by diabetes mellitus (↓ insulin → ↑ plasma glucose)/hormonal changes during pregnancy (↑ renal blood flow → ↑ glucose filtration)

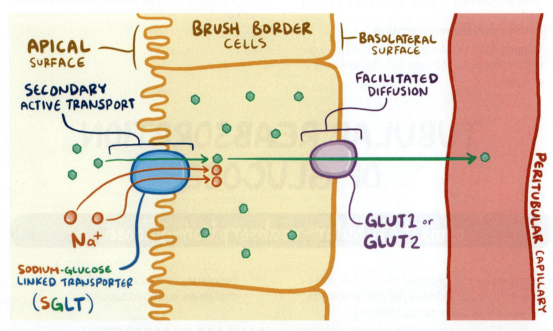

Figure 62.12 An illustration depicting the two steps of glucose reabsorption that occur in the proximal convoluted tubule: transport across the apical membrane of the brush border cells, followed by transport across the basolateral membrane of the brush border cells by GLUT1 or GLUT2.

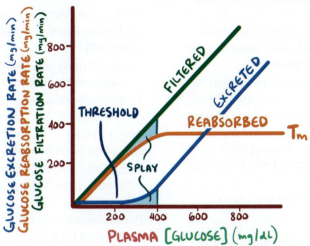

Figure 62.2 A graph showing glucose reabsorption and secretion rates as a function of plasma glucose. The glucose reabsorption line plateaus because the plasma [glucose] has been reached where all the GLUT1/GLUT2 transporters in virtually all the nephrons are occupied by glucose molecules.

TUBULAR SECRETION OF PARA-ANIMOHIPPURIC ACID (PAH)

osms.it/tubular-secretion-PAH

- Body's entire plasma volume, including some para-aminohippuric acid (PAH), filtered approx. 60 times/day
  - *PAH*: organic acid; approx. 90% bound to plasma proteins, cannot be filtered
  - *Filtration rate of PAH*: mass of PAH filtered through kidneys per day (depends on plasma concentration of unbound PAH)
- Kidney filtrate passes through renal tubules in nephron before becoming urine
  - Tubules lined by brush border cells with apical surface (lined with microvilli), basolateral surface; peritubular capillaries surround tubules

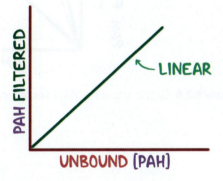

Figure 62.3 Graph showing PAH filtration rate as a function of unbound plasma PAH.

- No renal reabsorption of PAH
- PAH secretion occurs primarily in proximal convoluted tubule
  - Special carrier proteins on basolateral membrane transport PAH, other organic anions directly into tubules
- *Low plasma PAH levels:* PAH secretion increases linearly with PAH concentration
- *Higher plasma PAH levels:* limited number of carrier proteins prevents secretion from increasing, even with increasing PAH concentration (T_m) → some PAH left behind in peritubular capillaries
- Both filtered, secreted PAH excreted in urine

Using PAH to estimate renal plasma flow (RPF)

- *Fick's principle:* $PAH_{entering} = PAH_{leaving}$
- PAH enters kidney via renal artery; leaves via renal vein/urine
- *Low PAH concentrations* ($< T_m$): all PAH leaves via urine
- $PAH_{entering} = PAH_{excreted}$
- $[PAH]_{R.A.} \times RPF = [PAH]_{urine} \times$ urine flow rate (UFR)
  - Renal, urine concentrations of PAH both measured in milligrams per millilitre
  - RPF, urine flow rate (UFR) both measured in liters per minute
- $RPF = ([PAH]_{urine} \times UFR)/[PAH]_{R.A.}$ (milliliters of plasma per minute)
- Some PAH may remain in renal vein → estimate usually accurate to 10% of true RPF
- Renal plasma flow can be used to calculate renal blood flow (RBF)
  - $RBF = RPF/(1-Hct)$
  - *Hematocrit (Hct):* volume of blood occupied by red blood cells (RBCs)

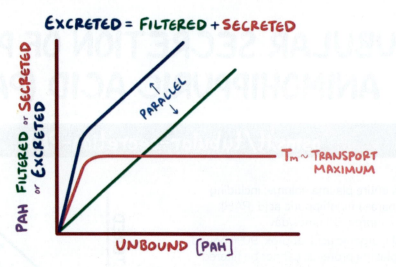

Figure 62.4 Graph showing PAH secretion and excretion rates as a function of plasma PAH.

UREA RECYCLING

osms.it/urea-recycling

- **Urea:** one of body's waste products (byproduct of amino acid breakdown)
- Freely filtered across kidneys' glomerular capillaries, travels through renal tubule
- Part of reabsorbed urea secreted back into loop of Henle → "urea recycling"
  - Helps establish corticopapillary gradient (reabsorbs water from kidneys back into blood)

Four steps to urea recycling

- 50% of urea reabsorbed by simple diffusion in proximal convoluted tubule (leaving behind 50% of initial urea), together with water
- Urea from medullary interstitium secreted back into tubule in descending limb of loop of Henle (resulting in 110% of initial urea in bottom of loop of Henle)
  - Occurs due to higher urea concentration in medullary interstitium
- Ascending limb of loop of Henle, early distal convoluted tubule impenetrable to urea, water (urea levels stay same)
- 70% of initial urea reabsorbed into interstitium in late distal convoluted tubule, cortical, outer medullary collecting ducts (leaving behind 40% of initial urea to be excreted in urine)
  - Occurs due to antidiuretic hormone (ADH)-induced water reabsorption through aquaporins → concentration gradient of urea towards interstitium

WEAK ACIDS & BASES – NON-IONIC DIFFUSION

osms.it/non-ionic_diffusion

- Many substances secreted by proximal tubule weak acids/bases
- Exist in uncharged (nonionic)/charged (ionized) forms; amount depends on pH of tubular fluid
  - **Urine with low pH:** nonionic forms dominate
  - **Urine with higher pH:** ionized forms dominate
- Nonionic weak acids, bases lipid soluble, able to passively diffuse back into blood from urine
- Ionized weak acids, bases not lipid soluble, remain in tubular fluid to be excreted
- Excretion of unwanted substances, toxins accomplished by manipulating urine pH, promoting ionization

NOTES

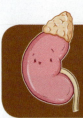

NOTES
WATER REGULATION

OSMOREGULATION

osms.it/osmoregulation

- Regulation of body fluid solute concentrations
  - Concentrations measured in osmolarity (mOsm/L)
  - **Osmole**: single ion in solution

BLOOD PLASMA OSMOLARITY
- 290–300 mOsm/L
- Main components
  - Sodium, glucose, urea
- Osmolarity = $2[Na^+] + [Glucose]/18 + [BUN]/2.8$
  - Glucose, blood urea nitrogen (BUN) measured in mg/dL

HYDRATION
- Changes in hydration affect plasma osmolarity, blood pressure
  - Osmoreceptors in supraoptic nuclei of anterior hypothalamus detect changes in plasma osmolarity
  - Baroreceptors in cardiovascular system detect changes in blood pressure
- Osmoreceptors, baroreceptors regulate production of ADH in hypothalamus

Overhydration
- Plasma osmolarity decreases, blood pressure increases
- Osmoreceptors, baroreceptors fire less, stimulating less ADH production
- Less/no water reabsorbed from kidneys

Dehydration
- Plasma osmolarity increases, blood pressure decreases
- Osmoreceptors, baroreceptors fire more, stimulating greater ADH production
- More water reabsorbed from kidneys

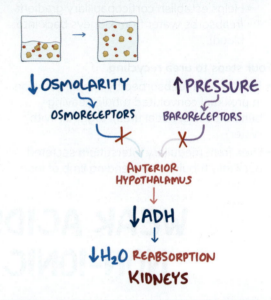

Figure 63.1 Body response to overhydration.

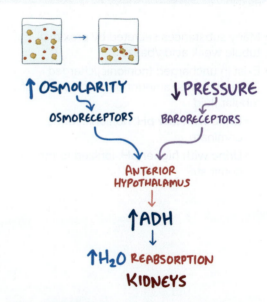

Figure 63.2 Body response to dehydration.

KIDNEY COUNTERCURRENT MULTIPLICATION

osms.it/kidney-countercurrent-multiplication

- Concentration gradient (corticopapillary gradient) established in medulla of kidney

TWO STEPS
- In nephron loop of Henle

Single effect
- Takes advantage of ascending limb being impermeable to water
- Sodium, potassium, chloride ions enter tubule cells along ascending limb via $Na^+K^+2Cl^-$ cotransporters on apical surface
- Na/K ATPase pumps sodium ions through basolateral surface into interstitium in exchange for potassium ions
- Potassium, chloride ions enter interstitium
- Osmosis → ions in interstitium diffuse into descending limb → fluid concentration

Flow of fluid
- Uses new fluid to distribute ions
- New fluid pushes existing fluid around loop
- Concentrated fluid (previously in descending limb) enters ascending limb

- Single effect recurs, fluid more concentrated at bottom of ascending limb → more ions enter interstitium at bottom

Two steps repeat
- Form concentration gradient of 1200mOsm/L at inner medulla, 300mOsm/L at outer cortex

COUNTERCURRENT EXCHANGE
- Important process for corticopapillary gradient
- Peritubular capillaries permeable to water, solutes
- Osmosis would destroy corticopapillary gradient if capillaries only ran along descending limb → peritubular capillaries run down descending limb, up ascending limb → allow extra solutes pulled from interstitium near descending limb to return to interstitium near ascending limb (as corticopapillary gradient decreases) → water diffused from capillary into interstitium returns

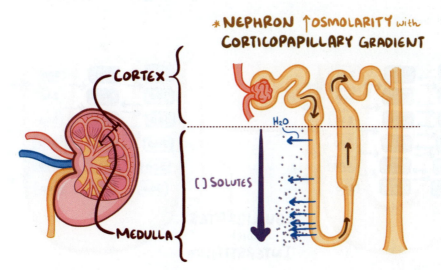

Figure 63.3 To increase urine osmolarity, nephrons rely on the corticopapillary gradient. The interstitium becomes increasingly hypertonic relative to the lumen of the tubule.

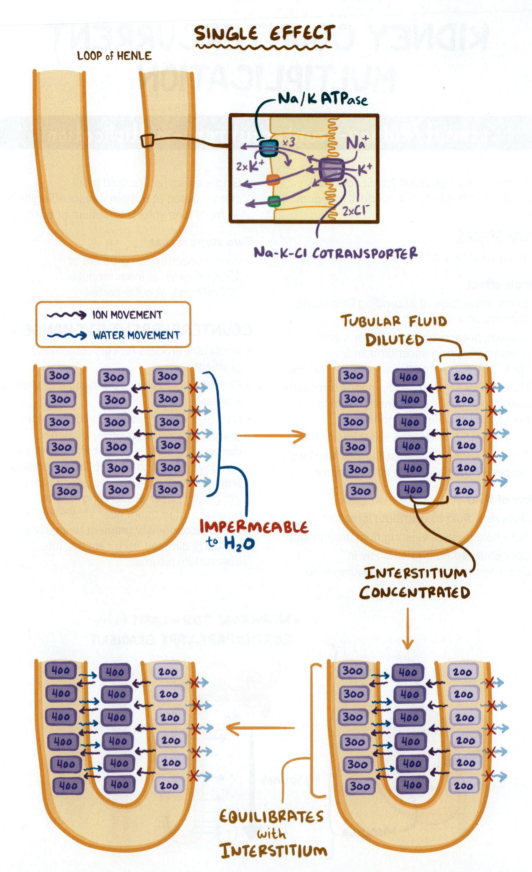

Figure 63.4 *Single effect*: ions leave ascending limb, but water can't follow → urine osmolarity in ascending limb decreases. Water can pass through descending limb → descending limb equilibrates with the interstitium. Numeric values = number of mOsm/L (e.g. 300 = 300mOsm/L).

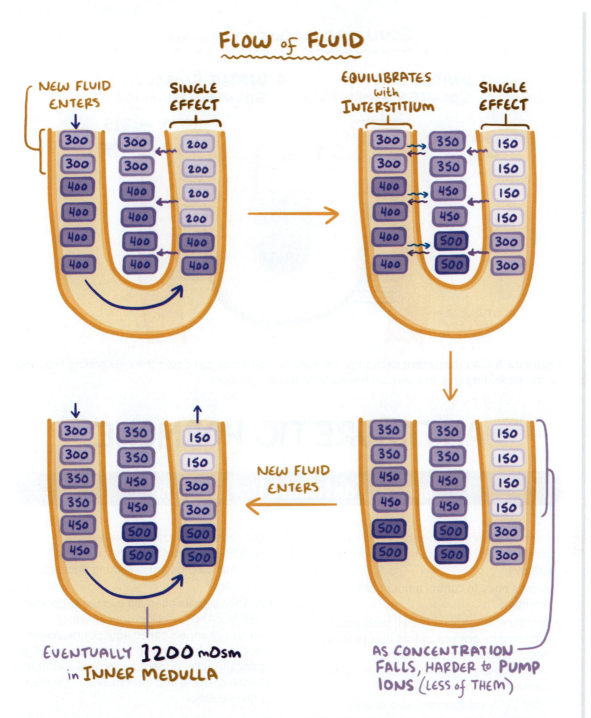

Figure 63.5 Flow of new fluid into the loop of Henle + single effect = corticopapillary gradient. Numeric values = number of mOsm/L (e.g. 300 = 300mOsm/L).

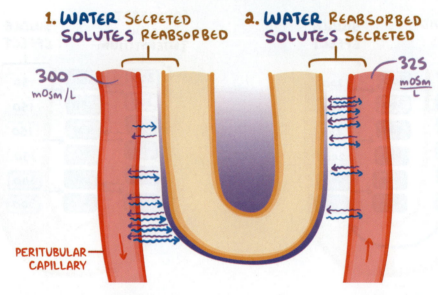

Figure 63.6 *Countercurrent exchange:* peritubular capillaries run down the descending limb and up the ascending limb to maintain the corticopapillary gradient.

ANTIDIURETIC HORMONE

osms.it/antidiuretic-hormone

- Peptide hormone prevents excessive urine production by reabsorbing water from kidneys
- Allows body to control amount of fluid retention
- Antidiuretic hormone (ADH) production triggered by osmoreceptors in supraoptic nuclei of anterior hypothalamus, baroreceptors in cardiovascular system; stimulated by angiotensin II
- ADH (AKA vasopressin) also causes smooth muscles cells in arteries to constrict

ADH PATHWAY

- Produced in paraventricular, supraoptic neurons of hypothalamus → travels down axons through infundibulum → stored in posterior pituitary gland
- When needed, released into blood, travels to kidneys
- In kidneys, travels through peritubular capillaries → binds to V2 receptors (AVPR2) on basolateral membrane of principal cells (along collecting ducts of nephrons)
- AVPR2 signals adenylyl cyclase to convert ATP to cAMP → cell produces water protein channels called aquaporins, opens existing aquaporins (in apical membrane) of principal cells → osmosis pulls water from lumen of ducts into interstitium, reabsorbed into circulation

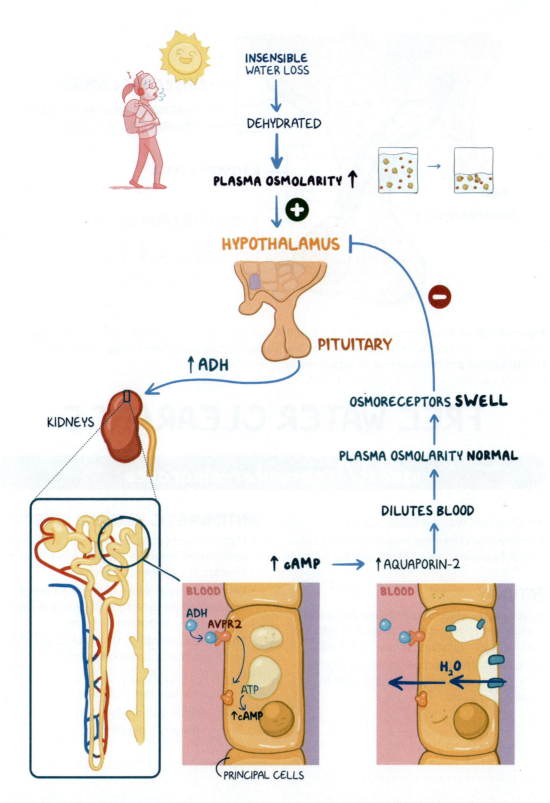

Figure 63.7 The ADH pathway. Increased plasma osmolarity triggers ADH release from the posterior pituitary. ADH acts on the principal cells of the distal convoluted tubule, collecting ducts → ↑ aquaporins in the cell membranes → ↑ water reabsorption → ↓ plasma osmolarity.

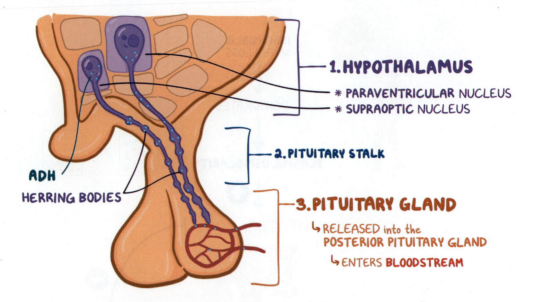

Figure 63.8 ADH is produced in the paraventricular and supraoptic nuclei in the hypothalamus, stored in Herring bodies in paraventricular and supraoptic neurons, and released into the bloodstream from the posterior pituitary gland.

FREE WATER CLEARANCE

osms.it/free-water-clearance

- Free water: water without solutes
- Free water clearance: rate at which kidneys filter free water out of blood plasma

PATHWAY
- Free water filtered out of blood plasma in ascending limbs, distal convoluted tubules of kidneys' nephrons, solutes removed
- Free water reabsorbed into circulation through aquaporin protein channels in collecting ducts

ANTIDIURETIC HORMONE EFFECTS
- High amounts of ADH → lots of free water reabsorbed, retained (negative free water clearance) → hyperosmotic urine
- Low amounts of ADH → little free water reabsorbed, excreted (positive free water clearance) → hypoosmotic urine
- Free water clearance, 0: excreted urine has same osmolarity as blood plasma
- $C_{H2O} = V - (U_{osm}/P_{osm})V$
  - V: urine flow rate (mL/min)
  - U_{osm}: urine osmolarity
  - P_{osm}: plasma osmolarity

NOTES
FEMALE REPRODUCTIVE SYSTEM

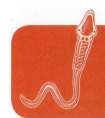

ANATOMY & PHYSIOLOGY OF THE FEMALE REPRODUCTIVE SYSTEM

osms.it/female-reproductive-system

EXTERNAL ORGANS

- Labia minora, labia majora, clitoris (erectile tissue), mons pubis
    - *Vulvar vestibule*: space between labia minora; includes vaginal, urethral opening

INTERNAL ORGANS

Ovaries (female gonads)

- Epithelial, follicular, granulosa, theca, oocyte cells
- Secrete estrogen, progesterone
- Located superior, lateral to uterus
- Held in place by ovarian, broad, suspensory ligaments
    - Suspensory ligaments contain ovarian artery, vein, nerve plexus
- Made up of outer cortex, inner medulla
    - Cortex contains ovarian follicles (oocytes surrounded by granulosa cells); medulla contains blood vessels, nerves

Fallopian tubes (uterine tubes)

- Two tubes, each associated with one ovary, on side of uterus
- Flattened mesothelial, epithelial, secretory, intercalary cells
- Fimbriae around ovary → infundibulum → ampulla (where fertilization most commonly occurs) → isthmus region opens into uterine cavity
- Covered by peritoneum, supported by mesosalpinx
- Lined with smooth muscle, cilia to sweep zygote towards uterus; inner mucosa provides nutrients for oocyte

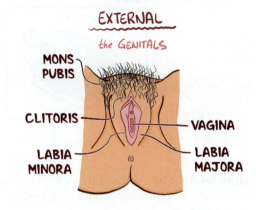

Figure 64.1 External organs of the female reproductive system.

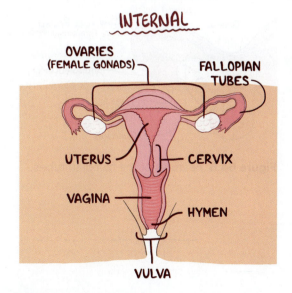

Figure 64.2 Internal organs of the female reproductive system.

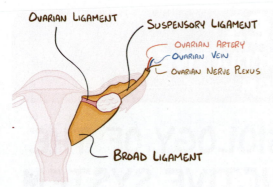

Figure 64.3 The locations of the ovarian, suspensory, and broad ligaments.

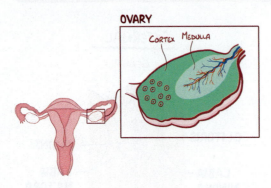

Figure 64.4 Outer cortex of ovary containing follicles and inner medulla containing blood vessels, nerves.

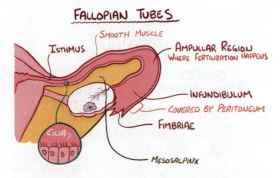

Figure 64.5 Features of the fallopian tubes.

Uterus

- Located posterior to bladder, anterior to rectum
- Fundus (top) → uterine body → uterine isthmus → cervix (neck of uterus)
  - **Cervical opening to vagina**: external os; thins, dilates during childbirth
  - **Cervical opening into uterine cavity**: internal os
- Anchored to sacrum (uterosacral ligaments) → anterior body wall (round ligaments)
- Supported by cardinal ligaments, mesometrium
- Three layers of uterine wall
  - Perimetrium, myometrium (smooth muscle), endometrium (highly vascular mucosal layer)

Vagina

- Extends from uterus, opens into vulva (covered by hymen in childhood)
- Outer muscular wall containing rugae; inner mucous membrane of stratified squamous epithelium
- Fornix (superior, domed area) connects to sides of cervix

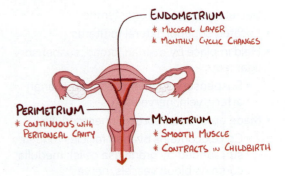

Figure 64.6 The three layers of the uterine wall. External to internal: perimetrium → myometrium → endometrium.

Chapter 64 Reproductive Physiology: Female Reproductive System

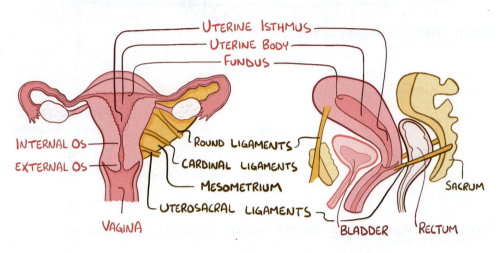

Figure 64.7 Anterior view of the uterus and lateral view of the uterus in relationship to surrounding structures.

OOGENESIS

Fetal development
- Oogonia (primordial oocyte cell) undergo mitotic division → ↑ oogonia (diploid cells)
- Seven months
  - Oogonia begin meiotic division, become primary oocytes (diploid cells)

Follicular development
- Infancy to puberty
  - Primary oocyte surrounded by granulosa cells form primary (primordial) follicle
- Menstrual cycle (approx. every 28 days)
  - Primary follicle → secondary follicle → tertiary (Graafian) follicle
- Antrum (fluid-filled cavity) forms in Graafian follicles; granulosa cells secrete nourishing fluid for primary oocyte
- Theca cells produce androstenedione (sex hormone precursor) → converted into estradiol in granulosa cells
- *Follicular phase of menstrual cycle*: Graafian follicles grow
  - Follicle with most follicle-stimulating hormone (FSH) receptors becomes dominant follicle; primary oocyte → meiosis I completed, secondary oocyte (haploid cell with 23 chromosomes) formed
- **Ovulation**: dominant follicle ruptures → secondary oocyte released → peritoneal cavity → pulled inside fallopian tube
- **Luteal phase**: follicle remains → corpus luteum (luteinized granulosa, theca cells)
  - Luteinized granulosa cells secrete inhibin → ↓ FSH → ↓ estrogen → ↓ luteinizing hormone (LH)
  - **Luteinized theca cells**: ↑ progesterone → dominant hormone

Fertilization
- If fertilization occurs → oocyte becomes mature ovum → progesterone produced until placenta forms
- If fertilization does not occur → corpus luteum → corpus albicans

FOLLICULAR DEVELOPMENT

First Stage: Infancy to Puberty

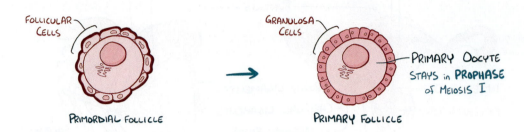

Second Stage: a few Primary Follicles enter each Menstrual Cycle

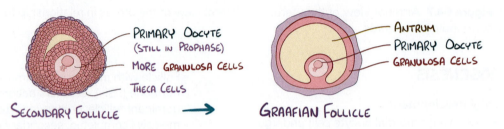

Third Stage: Begins when Graafian Follicles are Ready. Occurs during Follicular Phase

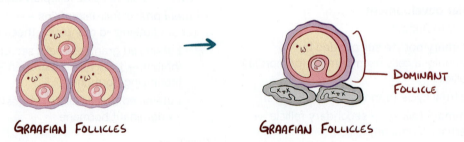

Ovulation

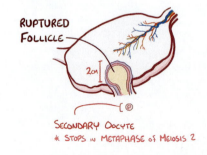

Luteal Phase (Weeks 3 & 4)

Figure 64.8 Stages of follicular development. **Stage one:** primordial follicles → primary follicles, meaning that the follicular cells surrounding the primary oocyte develop into granulosa cells. **Stage two:** primary follicles → secondary follicles → tertiary (Graafian) follicles. This stage results in a few fast-growing Graafian follicles. **Stage three:** dominant follicle is established. **Ovulation:** dominant follicle ruptures, releases secondary oocyte into fallopian tube. The secondary oocyte stops in metaphase of meiosis II. **Luteal phase:** weeks 3–4 of menstrual cycle. The remains of the follicle turn into the corpus luteum. If fertilization occurs, the corpus luteum keeps making progesterone until the placenta forms. If not, the corpus luteum stops making hormones after about ten days, becomes fibrotic → corpus albicans.

OXYTOCIN & PROLACTIN

osms.it/oxytocin-prolactin

- Peptide hormones involved in production, release of milk

→ stored in Herring bodies → released into blood → target tissues (e.g. breasts, uterus)

OXYTOCIN

- Essential for progression of labor, control of postpartum bleeding, return of uterus to pre-pregnancy state (involution)
- Synthesized, secreted by hypothalamus → travels down axons to posterior pituitary

PROLACTIN (PL)

- Synthesized by lactotrophs in anterior pituitary → target tissue (breasts)
- Synthesis inhibited by dopamine during non-pregnant/non-breastfeeding state

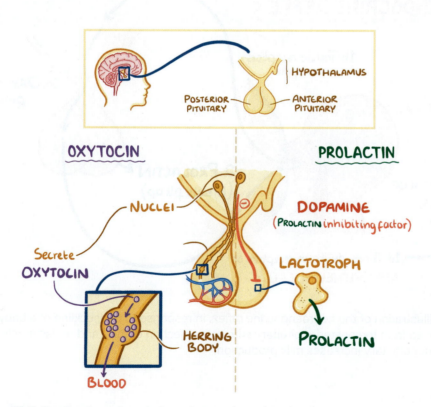

Figure 64.9 Synthesis and secretion of oxytocin and prolactin.

FUNCTIONS DURING LACTATION

- **Neuroendocrine reflex:** suckling by infant at breast → stimulates mechanoreceptors in nipple, areola → action potential travels up spinal cord to hypothalamus
- First, burst of oxytocin released from posterior pituitary → enters bloodstream → breasts, uterus
  - Myoepithelial cells surrounding alveoli in breasts contract → milk ejection from alveolus (let-down reflex)
  - Stimulates contractile activity of uterine myometrium → ↓ postpartum bleeding; promotes uterine involution
- Second, thyrotropin-releasing hormone (TRH) from hypothalamus → PL released from anterior pituitary → enters bloodstream → breasts → ↑ milk production, secretion by alveolar epithelial cells
- ↑ PL inhibits release of GnRH from hypothalamus → ↓ LH, FSH from anterior pituitary → ↓ development of ovarian follicles, ovulation, menstrual periods

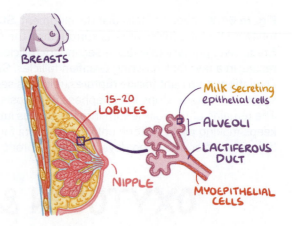

Figure 64.10 Anatomy of the breast.

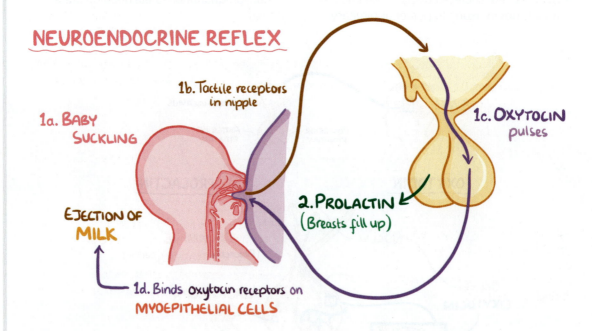

Figure 64.11 Illustration of the neuroendocrine reflex. In response to the suckling of a baby, oxytocin released from the posterior pituitary stimulates ejection of milk, and prolactin released from the anterior pituitary increases milk production.

FUNCTIONS DURING & AFTER LABOR

- Oxytocin (powerful uterine muscle stimulant) produced during pregnancy, does not stimulate uterine contractions due to
  - Rapid degradation by placental oxytocinase
  - Progesterone-induced inhibition of oxytocin receptors on myometrium
- Estrogen-induced oxytocin receptor expression + ↑ myometrial sensitivity to oxytocin promotes uterine contractions during labor
- Positive feedback loop: ↑ uterine contractions → fetal head pushes against cervix → neural signal travels to spinal cord → hypothalamus → ↑ oxytocin release from posterior pituitary → ↑ uterine contractions → cycle continues until delivery (baby, placenta)
- After labor, milder contractions continue
  - Clamp down on placental arteries at placental attachment site → ↓ bleeding
  - Gradually ↓ size of uterus (involution)
  - Additional oxytocin released during breastfeeding → speeds involution

MENSTRUAL CYCLE

osms.it/menstrual-cycle

- Menstruation (menses): shedding of uterine functional endometrium
- Occurs approx. every 28 days

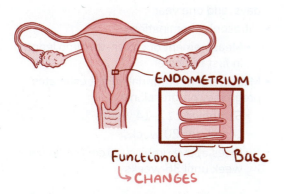

Figure 64.12 The uterine endometrium consists of a thin base layer and a functional layer. The functional layer is subject to the changes (thickening and shedding) that occur during the menstrual cycle.

FOLLICULAR PHASE

- Ovulation (days 1–14): maturing follicles, proliferation of uterine mucosa, dominated by estrogen

Day 1

- Hypothalamus releases gonadotropin-releasing hormone (GnRH) → anterior pituitary releases FSH, LH → one oocyte dominates → develops within primary follicle
- Primary (primordial) follicle: oocyte surrounded by single layer of granulosa cells (nourish oocyte)

Days 1–13

- Granulosa cells proliferate → follicle grows → develops outer layer of cells (theca layer) → respond to LH by producing estrogen → mature follicle
  - Estrogen acts on uterine endometrium to prepare for fertilized egg → initiates uterine proliferative phase → endometrial lining grows
  - Estrogen also feeds back to hypothalamus, pituitary → turns off GnRH, FSH, LH

Day 14

- Brief LH surge stimulates ovulation → follicle ruptures → oocyte ejected out of follicle

LUTEAL PHASE

- After ovulation, empty follicle collapses → turns into corpus luteum → produces progesterone (approx. 14 days)
  - Endometrium becomes highly vascularized, glycogen-filled tissue (secretory phase)

Days 15–24

- Egg travels through fallopian tube

Day 25

- If fertilization does not occur → corpus luteum undergoes apoptosis → progesterone levels fall
- If fertilization does occur → embryonic tissue secretes human chorionic gonadotropin (hCG) → signals corpus luteum to continue production of estrogen, progesterone to support pregnancy

PREGNANCY

osms.it/pregnancy

- Obstetric history (GTPAL)
  - G (gravida): number of pregnancies, regardless of duration (including current pregnancy)
  - T: number of term infants born
  - P: number of preterm infants born
  - A: number of spontaneous/induced abortions
  - L: number of currently living children
  - Example: G3P1202 (3 pregnancies, 1 term birth, 2 preterm births, 0 abortions, 2 living children)
- Pregnancy lasts approx. 280 days (40 weeks); divided into three trimesters

SIGNS & SYMPTOMS

Presumptive

- Amenorrhea; breast fullness, tenderness; nausea/vomiting ("morning sickness"); urinary frequency; fatigue; fetal movement (16–20 weeks of gestation)

Probable

- Uterine enlargement; softening of uterine isthmus (Hegar sign); vaginal, cervical purplish-blue discoloration (Chadwick sign); positive urine/serum hCG

Positive

- Auscultation of fetal heart tones (7–8 weeks of gestation); "quickening" (fetal movements); fetal sac visualized by ultrasound (5–6 weeks); fetal cardiac activity (6–8 weeks)

ESTIMATED DATE OF DELIVERY (EDD)

- Calculated from last menstrual period (LMP) to estimated date of delivery (EDD)
- Naegele's rule: add seven days to first day of LMP, subtract thee months, add seven days, add one year
- Ultrasonic examination
  - Measurement of crown-to-rump length in first trimester
- Measurement of fundal height estimates pregnancy progression
  - Symphysis: 12–14 weeks
  - Umbilicus: 20 weeks
  - Rises above umbilicus 1cm/0.39in per week until 36 weeks

PHYSIOLOGICAL CHANGES IN THE REPRODUCTIVE SYSTEM

Uterus

- ↑ size, capacity due to hypertrophy, hyperplasia, mechanical stretching
- 20 times larger
- ↑ strength, distensibility, contractile proteins, number of mitochondria
- ↑ volume capacity (10mL–5 L)
- Softening of uterine isthmus (Hegar's sign)

Chapter 64 Reproductive Physiology: Female Reproductive System

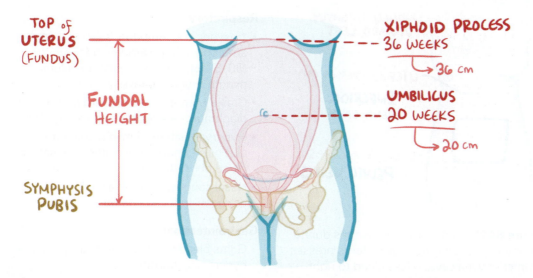

Figure 64.13 Fundal height = distance from symphysis pubis to top of uterus (fundus). Fundal height is a good estimate of gestational age.

Cervix
- Formation of mucus plug; seals endocervical canal
- ↑ vascularity → purplish-blue color
- Mild softening due to edema, hyperplasia (Goodell's sign); ↑ softening in third trimester

Placenta
- Develops where embryo attaches to uterine wall
- Expands to cover 50% internal uterine surface
- Functions as maternal-fetal organ for metabolic, nutrient exchange
- Secretes estrogen, progesterone, relaxin, hCG

Vagina
- ↑ vascularity → bluish-purple color
- Loosening of connective tissue → ↑ distensibility
- Leukorrhea
  - pH of 3.5–6.0 → protects against bacterial infections

Breasts
- ↑ size, weight, nodularity, blood flow, vascular prominence
- Areola, nipples are a darker pigmentation due to ↑ melanocyte activity
- ↑ activity of Montgomery's tubercles (sebaceous glands)
- Progesterone
  - ↑ alveolar-lobular development; prevents milk production during pregnancy (inhibits prolactin)
- Estrogen
  - ↑ growth of lactiferous ducts
- Secretion of colostrum begins week 16

PHYSIOLOGICAL CHANGES IN OTHER BODY SYSTEMS

Cardiovascular
- Mild hypertrophy
- S2, S3 more easily auscultated, split exaggerated
- Heart displaced upward, forward, slightly to left
- ↑ heart rate by 15–20 beats/minute
- Stroke volume ↑ 30%, cardiac output (CO) ↑ 30-50% (by term); ↓ blood pressure (BP) despite ↑ CO due to progesterone-induced vasodilation; BP = CO × systemic vascular resistance (SVR)
- Supine hypotensive syndrome caused by gravid uterus pressing on inferior vena cava (left lateral recumbent position optimal for CO, uterine perfusion)
- Gravid uterus elevates pressure veins draining legs, pelvic organs → slowed venous return, dependent edema, varicose veins, hemorrhoids

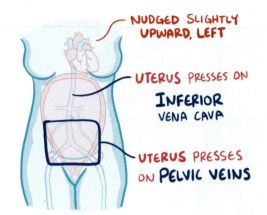

Figure 64.14 Cardiovascular changes during pregnancy. When lying down, uterus presses on inferior vena cava → less blood to right atrium → hypotension. The uterus also presses on pelvic veins → varicose veins, swelling in lower legs, ankles.

Hematologic

- ↑ blood volume (approx. 1500mL)
  - Related to sodium, water retention due to changes in osmoregulation, secretion of vasopressin by anterior pituitary, renin-angiotensin-aldosterone system (RAAS)
- ↑ total red blood cell (RBC) volume (approx. 30%), with iron supplementation
  - ↑ volume, oxygen-carrying capacity needed for ↑ basal metabolic rate (BMR), needs of uterine-placental unit (offsets blood loss at delivery)
  - Plasma > RBC volume → hemodilution, ↓ hematocrit (physiologic anemia)
- ↑ white blood cell (WBC) count (approx. 5,000–12,000/mm3)
- ↑ clotting factors (fibrin, fibrinogen): hypercoagulable state of pregnancy

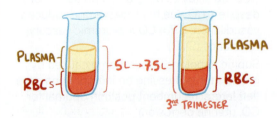

Figure 64.15 Pregnancy is a high volume state. Plasma volume ↑ > RBC volume ↑ → ↓ hematocrit (physiologic anemia).

Respiratory

- ↑ oxygen consumption, subcostal angle, anteroposterior diameter, tidal volume (30–50%), minute ventilatory volume, minute oxygen uptake
- Gravid uterus places upward pressure on diaphragm → elevates approx. 4cm/1.57in
- Hyperventilation → mild respiratory alkalosis (renal compensation → maternal blood pH 7.40–7.45)
- Nasal congestion, epistaxis due to estrogen-induced edema

Gastrointestinal

- Gums bleed easily due to estrogen-induced hyperemia, friability
- Progesterone-induced smooth muscle relaxation, delayed gastric emptying, ↓ peristalsis → nausea, vomiting (AKA "morning sickness"); constipation; heartburn (pyrosis), esophageal reflux; intrahepatic cholestasis of pregnancy due to ↓ gallbladder emptying time → ↑ risk of cholelithias
- ↑ saliva production (ptyalism)

Urinary & renal

- Bladder
  - *First trimester*: gravid uterus presses on bladder → urinary frequency, nocturia, stress incontinence
  - *Second trimester*: uterus occupies abdominal space → ↓ urinary frequency
  - *Third trimester*: presenting part descends into pelvis → urinary frequency, nocturia, stress incontinence
- ↑ glomerular filtration rate (GFR)
  - 40–50% by second trimester; ↑ urinary output (25%)
- ↑ size of kidneys (1–1.5cm/0.39–0.59in)
- Dilation of urinary collecting system → physiologic hydronephrosis
- Urinalysis
  - Glycosuria (due to ↑ glucose load), ↑ protein excretion (due to altered proximal tubule function + ↑ GFR)

Integumentary

- Hyperpigmentation (due to estrogen, ↑ melanocyte activity) → melasma (chloasma) brownish "mask of pregnancy"; linea nigra formation on abdomen; darkening of

Chapter 64 Reproductive Physiology: Female Reproductive System

- nipples, areolae, vulva
- ↑ cutaneous blood flow → ↑ heat dissipation → pregnancy "glow"
- ↓ connective tissue strength secondary to ↑ adrenal steroid levels → stretch marks (striae gravidarum) in breasts, abdomen, thighs, inguinal area
- Estrogen-induced vascular permeability → spider nevi, angiomas, palmar erythema

Musculoskeletal
- Abdominal distension + shift in center of gravity → lordosis
- Enlarging uterus → separation of abdominal rectus muscles (diastasis recti)
- ↑ progesterone, relaxin → ↑ joint mobility, "waddling" gait
  - Widening of symphysis pubis
  - Facilitates accommodation of fetus into pelvis
- High bone turnover, remodeling

Endocrine
- ↑ size of pituitary gland; mostly due to proliferation of lactotroph cells
  - ↑ intrasellar pressure → ↑ risk of postpartum infarction (Sheehan syndrome) in setting of postpartum hemorrhage
- ↑ parathyroid hormone (meets calcium need of developing fetal skeleton)
- Physiologic hypercortisolism
  - ↑ need for estrogen, cortisol → ↑ glucocorticoids from adrenal glands → supports fetal somatic, reproductive growth
- "Diabetogenic state" of pregnancy
  - ↑ need for glucose, insulin production → hypertrophy, hyperplasia of pancreatic beta cells
- ↓ thyroid-stimulating hormone (TSH); thyroid gland enlarges; ↑ total T3, T4
- Reproductive hormones
  - hCG from placenta; estrogen, progesterone from corpus luteum (first, second trimesters), placenta (second, third trimesters)
  - Suppressed FSH, LH due to feedback from estrogen, progesterone, inhibin
  - ↓ oxytocin levels throughout pregnancy → ↑ labor onset → ↑↑ second stage of labor

NUTRITIONAL NEEDS
- Recommendation of additional 300 kcal/day, weight gain of 25–35lbs/11.5–16kg
  - 5kg/11lbs: placenta, amniotic fluid, fetus
  - 0.9kg/2lbs: uterus
  - 1.8kg/4lbs: ↑ blood volume
  - 1.4kg/3lbs: breast tissue
  - 2.3–4.5kg/5–10lbs: maternal reserves
- 600mcg folic acid/day → RBC synthesis, placental/fetal growth, ↓ risk of neural tube defects
- 1,000–1,300mg calcium/day supports pregnancy, lactation
- 60g protein daily supports tissue growth
- 27mg iron/day supports ↑ RBCs

LABOR

osms.it/labor

- **Labor (parturition)**: uterine contractions → cervical changes → delivery of baby, placenta
- Begins at term (37–42 weeks of gestation)
- Duration of three stages varies with gravidity (nulliparas typically longer than multiparas)

PREMONITORY SIGNS
- Cervical changes
  - Remodeling of cervix by enzymatic collagen dissolution, ↑ water content → softening, ↑ distensibility
- Cervical softening → expulsion of mucus plug → "bloody show" (pink-tinged mucus)

- Spontaneous rupture of amniotic membranes (ROM)

False labor
- AKA Braxton Hicks contractions
- *True labor*: regular, increase in frequency, duration, intensity; produce cervical changes (e.g. dilation/opening up, effacement/getting thinner); pain begins in lower back, radiates to abdomen, not relieved by ambulation
- *False labor*: irregular, intermittent contractions; no cervical changes; pain in abdomen; walking may decrease pain

FIRST STAGE OF LABOR

Early/latent
- 8–12 hours
- Mild contractions every 5–30 minutes
- Duration 30 seconds each
- Gradually increase in frequency, intensity, duration
- Cervical dilation 0–3cm/0–1.18in
- Effacement 0–30%
- Spontaneous ROM

Active phase
- 3–5 hours
- Contractions every 3–5 minutes
- Duration ≥ 1 minute
- Cervical dilation 3–7cm/1.18–2.76in
- Effacement 80%
- Progressive fetal descent

Transition phase
- 30 minutes–2 hours
- Intense contractions every 1.5–2 minutes
- Duration 60–90 seconds
- Cervical dilation 7–10cm/2.76–3.93in
- Effacement 100%

SECOND STAGE
- AKA pushing stage
- Begins with full dilation
- Navigation through maternal pelvis dictated by three Ps
  - Power, passenger, passage

Power
- Frequency, duration, intensity of uterine contractions
- Physiology of contractions
  - Stimulation of uterine myometrium
  - Alpha-receptors stimulate uterine contractions
  - Numerous oxytocin receptors, mostly on uterine fundus
- Contraction steps
  - Wave begins in fundus, proceeds downward to rest of uterus → muscle shortens in response to stimulus → increment (build up) → acme (peak) → decrement (gradual letting up) → relaxation → fetal descent, cervical effacement, dilation → amount of pressure exerted by uterine contractions (intrauterine pressure) measured in millimeters of mercury (mm Hg)

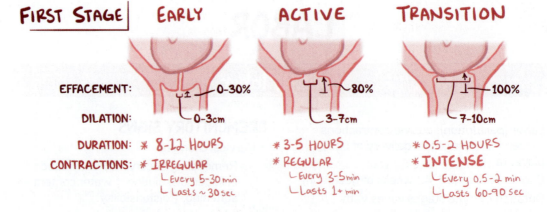

Figure 64.16 Features of the first stage of labor's phases.

Passenger
- Fetal size
  - Fetal head most critical; cephalopelvic disproportion → labor dystocia (difficult/obstructed)
  - Macrosomia (birth weight ≥ 90th percentile for gestational age/> 4500g) associated with shoulder dystocia (fetal shoulder unable to pass below maternal pubic symphysis), birth injuries
- *Fetal attitude*: relationship of fetal parts to one another
  - Full flexion (chin on chest; rounded back with flexed arms, legs); smallest diameter of head (suboccipitobregmatic diameter) presents at pelvic inlet
- *Fetal lie*: relationship of fetal cephalocaudal axis (spinal column) to maternal cephalocaudal axis
  - *Longitudinal (ideal)*: fetal spine lies along maternal
  - *Transverse*: fetal spine perpendicular to maternal
  - *Oblique*: fetus at slight angle
- *Fetal presentation*: fetal/presenting part enters pelvic inlet first
- *Cephalic*: head first
  - *Vertex (most common)*: optimal for easy delivery; head completely flexed onto chest → occiput (part of fetal skull covered by occipital bone) is presenting
  - *Brow*: fetal head partially extended; sinciput (part of fetal skull covered by frontal bone, anterior fontanelle to orbital ridge) presenting part
  - *Face*: fetal head hyperextended; fetal face from forehead to chin presenting part
- *Breech*: head up; bottom, feet, knees present first
  - *Frank breech*: hips flexed, knees extended; bottom presents
  - *Complete breech*: hips, knees flexed; bottom presents
  - *Incomplete breech*: one/both hips not completely flexed; feet present
  - *Shoulder*: transverse lie; shoulders present first

Passage
- Route through bony pelvis
- Size, type of pelvis
  - *Gynecoid*: rounded pelvic inlet, midpelvis, outlet capacity adequate; optimal for vaginal delivery
  - *Android*: heart-shaped pelvic inlet; ↓ midpelvis diameters, outlet capacity; associated with labor dystocia
  - *Anthropoid*: oval-shaped pelvic inlet; midpelvis diameters, outlet capacity adequate; favorable for vaginal delivery
  - *Platypelloid*: oval-shaped pelvic inlet, ↓ midpelvis diameters, outlet capacity adequate; not favorable for vaginal delivery
- Cardinal movements (mechanisms of labor)
  - *Descent*: presenting part reaches pelvic inlet (engagement) before onset of labor → degree of descent (fetal station), relationship of presenting part to maternal ischial spines → fetus moves from pelvic inlet (-5 station) down to ischial spines (0 station) to pelvic outlet (+4 station) to crowning at vaginal opening (+5 station)
  - *Flexion*: fetal chin presses against chest, head meets resistance from pelvic floor
  - *Internal rotation*: fetal shoulders internally rotate 45°; widest part of shoulders in line with widest part of pelvic inlet
  - *Extension*: fetal head passes under symphysis pubis (+4 station), moves (+5 station), emerges from vagina
  - *Restitution (external rotation)*: head externally rotates as shoulders pass through pelvic outlet, under symphysis pubis, turns to align with back
  - *Expulsion*: anterior shoulder slips under symphysis pubis, followed by posterior shoulder, rest of the body; marks end of second stage

THIRD STAGE
- Delivery of placenta, umbilical cord, fetal membranes; uterus contracts firmly, placenta begins to separate from uterine wall

FOURTH STAGE
- Physiological adaptation to blood loss, initiation of uterine involution

Second Stage

Fetal Attitude

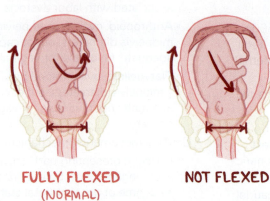

FULLY FLEXED (NORMAL)   NOT FLEXED

Fetal Lie

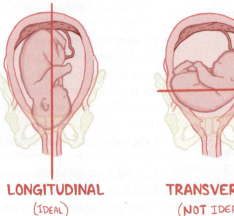
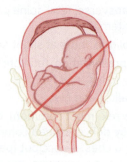

LONGITUDINAL (IDEAL)   TRANSVERSE (NOT IDEAL)   OBLIQUE (NOT IDEAL)

Fetal Presentation

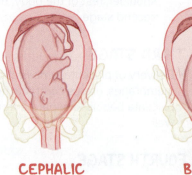
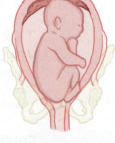
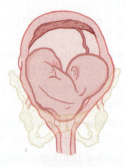

CEPHALIC (HEAD FIRST)   BREECH (BOTTOM FIRST)   BREECH (SHOULDER)

Figure 64.17 Fetal attitude, lie, and presentation are all critical factors in determining the fetus' ease of passage through the maternal pelvis.

Chapter 64 Reproductive Physiology: Female Reproductive System

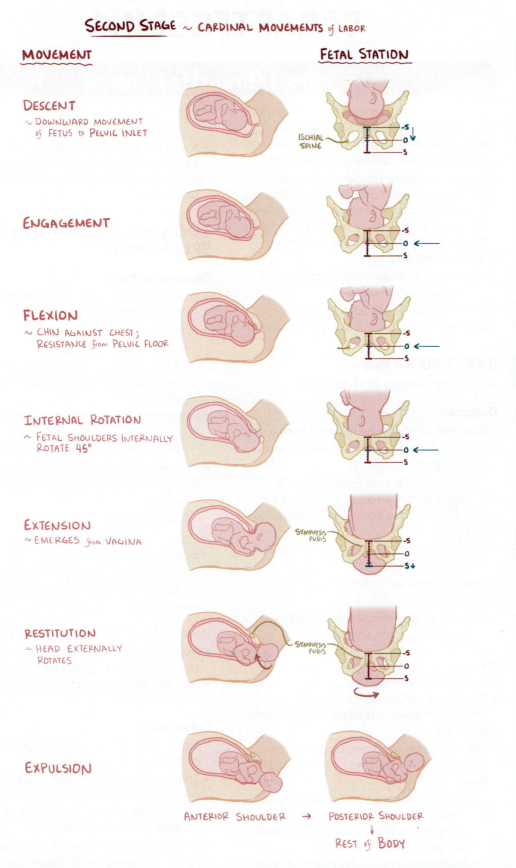

Figure 64.18 Second stage cardinal movements: the fetal position changes that occur during labor.

BREASTFEEDING

osms.it/breastfeeding

- Provision of breast milk from lactating breast; involves breast tissue development, initiation of milk secretion lactogenesis
- Pregnancy, human placental lactogen (hPL), progesterone released from placenta, + PL released from anterior pituitary gland → stimulates growth of breast glandular tissue → prepares epithelial cells lining alveoli to produce milk
    - Progesterone prevents lactation until after delivery of placenta
- Delivery of baby, placenta → ↓↓ progesterone → milk synthesized in alveoli

INFANT SUCKLING

- Stimulates release of oxytocin, PL

Oxytocin

- Required for milk to be released from alveoli
- Neuroendocrine reflex → let-down reflex (milk ejection)
    - Myoepithelial cells contract → milk ejection from alveolus → drained by milk-collecting ducts → transported to nipple
- Milk ejection continues as long as infant continues suckling
- Other triggers for oxytocin release, let-down reflex
    - Sounds/sights/smells connected to infant (e.g. infant crying)

PL

- Continues milk production
- Amount of milk produced depends on amount removed at feeding (supply meets demand)
- Milk extraction facilitated by good latch of baby onto nipple, frequent emptying of breast
    - Good latch: baby's mouth wide open, covering areola, lips flanged out, nipple up against roof of mouth, baby's tongue up against bottom of areola
    - Feedings every 1–2 hours at first, then every three hours
- If milk not removed, builds up → ↑ intramammary pressure → ↓ capillary blood flow → glandular tissue involutes → ↓ milk production

BIOCHEMICAL COMPOSITION OF BREAST MILK

Benefits for baby

- ↑ whey to casein ratio, enzymes, hormones → ↑ absorption, digestion of milk
- Immunoglobulins
    - ↓ risk of infection; esp. respiratory, gastrointestinal, otitis media; ↓ risk of necrotizing enterocolitis in premature infants
- Long-chain polyunsaturated fatty acids (PUFAs)
    - Aids neural. visual development
- ↑ beneficial bacteria (Lactobacillus, Bifidobacterium) in gut microflora
- Cytokines
    - Anti-inflammatory properties
- Ideal source of nutrition for newborns, including premature infants
- Milk composition transitions from early postpartum period to mature milk to meet infant needs

Benefits for mother

- Accelerated uterine involution, ↓ risk of chronic disease (e.g. diabetes Type II, arthritis, heart disease; cancers of breast, ovaries, uterus)

Colostrum

- Small amounts of milk produced during second half of pregnancy
- Thick, yellowish fluid (due to beta-carotene) rich in immune cells, antibodies, antioxidants, protein, fat-soluble vitamins, minerals; low in fat, lactose
- Protects newborn from infection; laxative effect → passage of first stool (meconium),

Chapter 64 Reproductive Physiology: Female Reproductive System

formed in fetal gastrointestinal tract
- Helps establish healthy gut microbiome

Transitional milk
- Produced 7–10 days postpartum; thinner than colostrum; light yellow color

Mature milk
- Produced two weeks postpartum
- Watery, slight bluish color; fat content increases during feeding
- Biologically complex
  - Protein, fat, sugars (e.g. lactose, oligosaccharides), vitamins, minerals, immunoglobulins, antibodies (esp. secretory IgA), immune cells (e.g. macrophages, neutrophils), immune-modulating factors (e.g. lactoferrin, lysozyme, lactoperoxidase)
- Low in vitamin D; supplementation often recommended
- Continues to be produced until lactation ceases
- Healthy maternal diet supports breast milk production

CONTRAINDICATIONS & CAUTIONS TO BREASTFEEDING

Contraindications
- Certain maternal medications (e.g. chemotherapy), illicit drugs (e.g. cannabis, heroin)
- HIV infection (in high-income settings)
- Herpes zoster, herpes simplex
  - If lesions on breast
- Tuberculosis
  - Until approx. two weeks of maternal pharmacotherapy

Cautions
- Smoking discouraged (↑ risk of SIDS, respiratory problems)
- Minimize alcohol; if consumed, wait two hours before breastfeeding
- Limit caffeine

BREASTFEEDING PROBLEMS

Engorgement
- *Cause*: milk accumulation in breast tissue, vascular congestion, resulting in pain
- *Presentation*: firm, tender breast; may have ↑ vascular markings
- *Treatment*: empty breasts (↑ breastfeeding, pumping); warm shower/compresses before feeding (enhances let-down), cool compresses after feeding; nonsteroidal anti-inflammatory drugs (NSAIDs); application of cool green cabbage leaves
- *Prevention*: frequent feedings, good latch to ensure emptying breast

Sore, cracked nipples
- *Cause*: improper latch, positioning
- *Presentation*: pain; blister/bleb on nipple if pores plugged
- *Treatment*: cool/warm compresses; apply expressed breast milk to nipple; mild analgesics (e.g. acetaminophen)
- *Prevention*: good breastfeeding technique

Mastitis
- *Cause*: bacterial infection
- *Presentation*: usually unilateral, localized warmth, tenderness/pain, edema, erythema, firmness; acute onset of flu-like symptoms (e.g. fever, fatigue)
- *Treatment*: continued breastfeeding, NSAIDs, antibiotics
- *Prevention*: good hygiene

Yeast infections
- *Cause*: Candida albicans; history of infant oral/diaper candidal infection/maternal vaginal candidal infection
- *Presentation*: infant may have white plaques in oral area; mother may experience pain, red/sore nipples
- *Treatment*: for mother, topical antifungal applied after feeding; infant, nystatin solution swabbed into oral mucosa after feeding
- *Prevention*: good hygiene; avoid excessive moisture by keeping breasts dry between feedings

MENOPAUSE

osms.it/menopause

- Diagnosed when menstrual cycles have stopped for entire year, no identified pathological cause
- Caused by natural effects of ovarian follicular depletion during aging process
- Usually begins age 50
- Preceded by perimenopause
  - Four years before final menstrual period; missed/irregular menstrual cycles, changes in bleeding patterns (heavy, prolonged, light)

HORMONAL CHANGES

- ↓ estrogen, progesterone → ↓ hypothalamic inhibition → ↑ bursts of GnRH → ↑ FSH, LH

PHYSIOLOGICAL EFFECTS OF ESTROGEN WITHDRAWAL

Hot flashes

- Caused by hypothalamus-associated thermoregulatory dysfunction → vasomotor instability
- Sensation of heat (centered on chest, face → generalized), diaphoresis, palpitations, anxiety
- Night sweats
  - Hot flashes occur at night → trouble sleeping
- Avoid triggers (e.g. hot drinks, spicy foods); maintain cool ambient temperature; dress in lighter clothing
- Stops within few years of onset

Vulvovaginal atrophy

- Vaginal dryness, loss of vaginal rugae → dyspareunia
- Vaginal estrogen creams, lubricants helpful

↓ protective effects from estrogen

- ↑ risk of cardiovascular disease
- ↓ bone marrow density → ↑ risk of osteoporosis, bone fractures
  - ↑ vitamin D, calcium (diet, supplements) helpful

Others

- Urinary tract dysfunction → dysuria, urinary urgency
- Mood instability → depression, anxiety
- Decline in cognitive function, difficulty concentrating
- ↓ collagen content in skin → ↑ skin wrinkling
- ↓ lean body mass
- Individualized approach for menopausal hormone therapy (MHT)
  - Estrogen/estrogen + progestin helpful in some cases

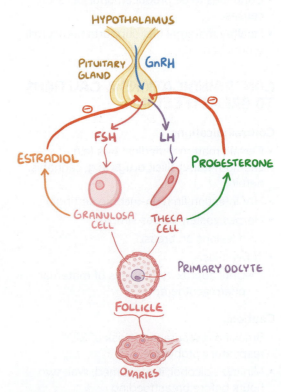

Figure 64.19 Hormone activity in a regular menstrual cycle. Estrogen and progesterone levels ↓ during menopause because the ovaries run out of functional follicles → no theca or granulosa cells to produce more hormones. So ↓ estrogen, progesterone → ↓ hypothalamic inhibition → ↑ bursts of GnRH → ↑ FSH, LH.

ESTROGEN & PROGESTERONE

osms.it/estrogen-progesterone

- Female steroid hormones, produced mainly by ovaries
  - Some estrogen produced in adrenal cortex, adipose tissue; secreted by placenta during pregnancy
  - Corpus luteum secretes estrogen, progesterone
- Three types
  - Estradiol (most biologically active), estrone, estriol

SYNTHESIS

- Cholesterol → theca cells → converted to pregnenolone via cholesterol desmolase → pregnenolone converted into progesterone via 3-beta-hydroxysteroid dehydrogenase (HSD) → released into blood → binds to plasma proteins (e.g. albumin) → transported to target tissues
- Remainder of pregnenolone converted to 17-hydroxypregnenolone → converted into dehydroepiandrosterone (DHEA) → finally converted into androstenedione (testosterone precursor) by 3-beta-HSD
- Androstenedione diffuses to nearby granulosa cells → androstenedione converted to testosterone by 17-beta-hydroxysteroid → testosterone converted to 17-beta-estradiol dehydrogenase aromatase (most biologically active type of estrogen during reproductive period)
- 17-beta-estradiol released into blood → binds to sex hormone-binding globulin (SHBG)
  - Plasma protein, carries 17-beta-estradiol to target tissues (e.g. uterus, vagina, bones)

SECRETION

- Regulated by hypothalamic-pituitary-ovarian axis through feedback loops
- At puberty, pulsatile release of GnRH from hypothalamus → anterior pituitary secretes FSH, LH → ovarian follicles differentiate into theca, granulosa cells → secrete estrogen, progesterone

EFFECTS OF ESTROGEN

- Maturation of female reproductive organs (e.g. uterus, fallopian tubes, vagina)
- Secondary sexual characteristics (e.g. breast growth, fat distribution)
- ↑ estrogen (pre-ovulation) → prepares uterine epithelium for implantation (endometrial proliferation); endometrial secretion in collaboration with progesterone
- Dominant hormone during the follicular phase of ovarian cycle; follicle maturation; initiates ovulation via FSH, LH surge

Pregnancy

- Secreted by placenta to support uterus; stimulates development of myometrium
- ↑ melanin-stimulating hormones → hyperpigmentation
- ↑ vascularity of upper respiratory tract; hypersecretion of mucus
- Preparation for labor
  - Stimulates development of myometrial gap junctions, promotes coordinated contractions
  - Promotes cervical ripening
  - ↑ uterine responsiveness to oxytocin (↑ oxytocin receptors), triggering parturition
- Breasts
  - Stimulates growth of duct cells

Systemic

- Required for closure of epiphyseal plates (both sexes)
- Anabolic effect on bones
- ↓ low-density lipoprotein (LDL), ↑ high-density lipoproteins (HDL)
- Maintains flexibility of blood vessels
- Promotes skin elasticity, fat deposition
- ↓ estrogen during perimenopausal/menopausal years → ↑ risk of cardiovascular morbidity, osteoporosis, sexual dysfunction

EFFECTS OF PROGESTERONE

- Dominant hormone during luteal phase of ovarian cycle
- ↑ progesterone (secretory phase of menstrual cycle) → forms decidual tissue for implantation

Pregnancy
- Maintains pregnancy: ↓ irritability of myometrium → ↓ risk of spontaneous abortion
- Cervis: forms mucus plug
- Breasts: ↑ alveolar-lobular development, prevents milk production during pregnancy (inhibits prolactin)
- Respiratory: ↑ sensitivity to CO_2, mild hyperventilation, ↓ airway resistance
- ↑ vasodilation

Systemic
- Works with estrogen to promote bone remodeling → ↑ bone density
- Promotes skin elasticity

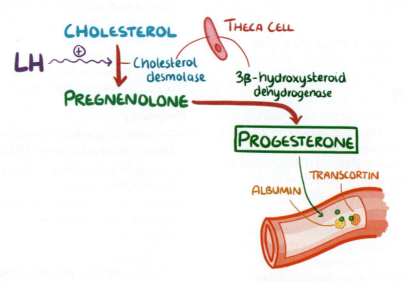

Figure 64.20 The steps of progesterone synthesis. LH stimulates proliferation of theca cells → cholesterol desmolase converts more cholesterol into pregnenolone.

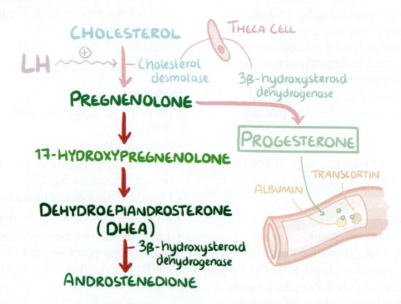

Figure 64.21 Synthesis of androstenedione from pregnenolone. Androstenedione will be used in the next steps to synthesize 17-beta-estradiol.

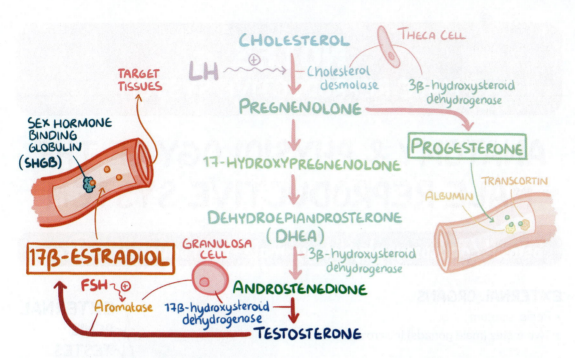

Figure 64.22 Synthesis of 17-beta-estradiol from androstenedione. FSH increases the activity of aromatase. Some target tissues for 17-beta-estradiol include the uterus and vagina, bones, and blood vessels.

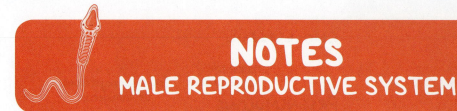

NOTES
MALE REPRODUCTIVE SYSTEM

ANATOMY & PHYSIOLOGY OF THE MALE REPRODUCTIVE SYSTEM

osms.it/anatomy-physiology-male-reproductive-system

EXTERNAL ORGANS
- Penis, scrotum
- Two testes (male gonads) in scrotum

Penis
- Smooth muscle cells
- Enlarged tip (glans penis), surrounded by loose skin (foreskin)
- Opens as external urethral orifice
- Three cylindrical bodies of erectile tissue (vascular spaces, surrounded by smooth muscle)
    - Corpus spongiosum, two corpora cavernosa
- Arousal → smooth muscle cells relax, blood flows into vascular spaces, corpora cavernosa distend → veins compress, blood doesn't drain → local engorgement → erection

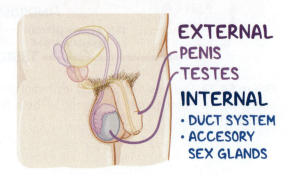

Figure 65.1 External and internal male reproductive system anatomy.

Testes
- **Functions:** produce sperm (in seminiferous tubules), testosterone (by Leydig cells)
    - Descend into scrotum from abdominal cavity (seventh month of gestation)
    - Scrotum provides cooler environment needed for spermatogenesis
- Contains epithelial, Sertoli, Leydig, sperm cells
- Separated by scrotal raphe
- Covered by tunica albuginea
    - Septa project towards center → 250 lobules (1–4 seminiferous tubules)
- Seminiferous tubules
    - Surrounded by epithelial lining,

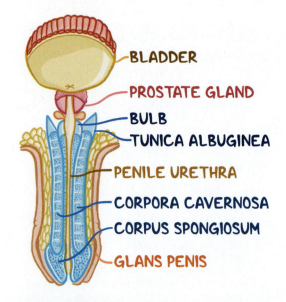

Figure 65.2 Penis anatomy.

Chapter 65 Reproductive Physiology: Male Reproductive System

capillaries, Leydig cells
- Spermatogonia (primordial sperm cells) → spermatocytes (towards lumen) → spermatids → sperm (most central); Sertoli cells (extend from margin to lumen; provide nutrients; establish blood-testis barrier)
- Tubules combine → rete testis (in mediastinum testis) → efferent ducts → epididymis

INTERNAL ORGANS
- Ducts for sperm, accessory glands (seminal vesicles, prostate gland, bulbourethral glands)

Sperm
- **Acrosome:** enzymes to penetrate oocyte (female gamete)
- **Neck (midpiece):** mitochondria for energy
- **Tail:** helps sperm swim
- Mature, swim in epididymis head; move through seminiferous tubules, rete testis by peristalsis

Spermatogenesis
- Begins at puberty
- Hypothalamus secretes gonadotropin-releasing hormone (GnRH) → pituitary secretes luteinizing hormone (LH), follicle-stimulating hormone (FSH)
  - LH binds to Leydig cells → stimulates testosterone production
  - FSH binds to Sertoli cells → produces androgen binding protein (ADP) → more testosterone crosses blood-testis barrier
- Spermatogonium (diploid cell) undergoes mitosis → two daughter cells (spermatogonia)
  - One spermatogonia cycled back to serve as spermatogonium
  - Second spermatogonia continues on to produce sperm
- Spermatogonia (diploid cell) undergoes mitosis → primary spermatocyte
- Primary spermatocyte undergoes meiosis I → secondary spermatocytes (haploid cells) emerge
- Secondary spermatocytes undergo meiosis II → spermatids (haploid)
- Spermatids enter lumen → cellular

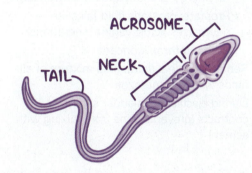

Figure 65.4 Sperm anatomy.

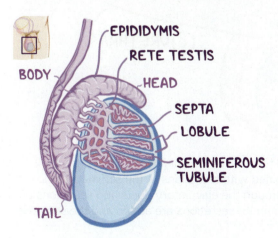

Figure 65.3 Testes anatomy.

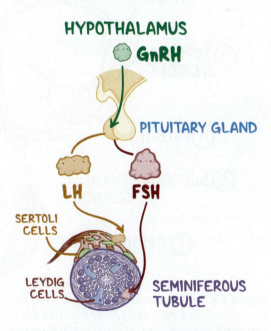

Figure 65.5 Hypothalamus secretes GnRH, stimulates pituitary release of FSH, LH (important to testosterone production).

differentiation → acquire tail → **mature sperm**
- Regulation via feedback loops
  - Sertoli cells secrete inhibin → negative feedback to pituitary → ↓ FSH
  - Leydig cells secrete testosterone → negative feedback to pituitary → ↓ LH

Ejaculation
- Mature sperm exit through tail of epididymis → vas deferens → secretions from seminal vesicle at ampulla → ejaculatory ducts → secretions from prostate gland → secretions from bulbourethral glands → empty into urethra
- Accessory glands secrete fluids into urethra
  - *Seminal:* seminal fluid (contains fructose for energy, prostaglandins for transport)
  - *Prostate:* prostatic fluid (alkaline → neutralizes acidic vaginal secretions)
  - *Bulbourethral:* lubricant
- Semen (seminal fluid): final mixture of all fluids with spermatozoa
- During ejaculation, bladder sphincter contracts (prevents urine from mixing with semen)

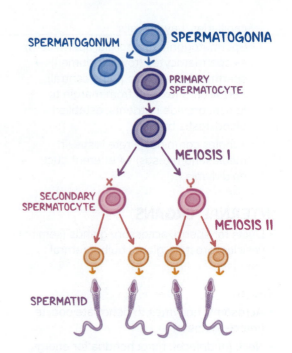

Figure 8.6 Spermatogenesis.

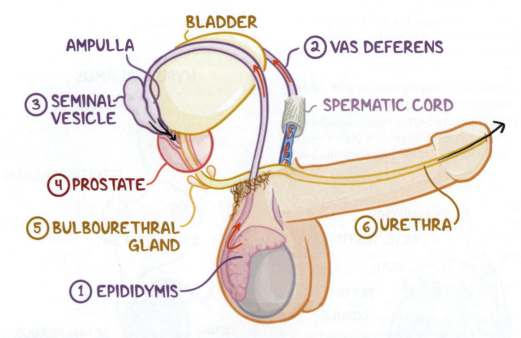

Figure 65.7 Once produced, the mature sperm exit the tail of the epididymis (1) and travel through the vas deferens (2) where they are combined with secretions of the seminal vesicles (3) at the ampulla. The mature sperm then pass through the ejaculatory ducts and secretions of the prostate gland (4). Finally, the bulbourethral gland (5) secretions are added and the semen is ejaculated through the urethra.

TESTOSTERONE

osms.it/testosterone

WHAT IS TESTOSTERONE?

- Main androgenic hormone
- Produced, released by Leydig cells of testes
- Synthesized from cholesterol in series of steps involving multiple enzymes
- Inactivated in liver → eliminated in urine, bile
- Active locally on Sertoli cells (paracrine action)
    - Sertoli cells produce androgen-binding protein (ABP) → keep testosterone levels high
    - Testosterone reinforces follicle-stimulating hormone (FSH) spermatogenesis stimulation
- Active in rest of body (endocrine action)

Circulation in bloodstream

- Approx. 98% bound to proteins (albumin, sex-hormone binding globulin)
    - Not biologically active when bound to protein
    - Functions as reservoir of free testosterone
    - Production regulated by androgens, estrogens
- Approximately 2% free, biologically active

PRODUCTION

Regulated by hypothalamic-pituitary axis

- Low testosterone → hypothalamic arcuate nuclei secrete GnRH into hypothalamic-hypophyseal portal blood → GnRH arrives to anterior lobe of pituitary gland → pituitary gland secretes FSH, LH (AKA gonadotropins)
    - LH → Leydig cells produce testosterone by increasing cholesterol conversion into pregnenolone (first step of testosterone production)
    - FSH → spermatogenesis, Sertoli cell function

NEGATIVE FEEDBACK REGULATION

- High testosterone levels → inhibits hypothalamus from secreting GnRH, pituitary gland from secreting LH
- Sertoli cells in testes secrete glycoprotein called inhibin → inhibits pituitary gland secreting FSH

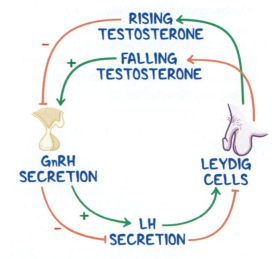

Figure 65.8 Testosterone production is regulated through a negative feedback loop by the hormones released by the hypothalamus and the Leydig cells.

MECHANISM OF ACTION

- Binding on androgen receptor in cell of target tissue → androgen-receptor complex moves into nucleus → gene transcription → generation of new proteins → physiological effects

EFFECTS OF ANDROGENIC HORMONES TESTOSTERONE & DIHYDROTESTOSTERONE

Testosterone

- Masculinizes internal genital tract in male fetus; promotes descent of testes before birth

- **Puberty:** muscle mass increases; epiphyseal plates close; penis, seminal vesicles grow; spermatogenesis; rise of libido; secondary sexual characteristics (thickens vocal cords, deepening voice, male pattern of hair growth)
- **Adulthood:** maintains reproductive tract; anabolic effect on proteins

Dihydrotestosterone (DHT)
- Produced from testosterone by 5 alpha-reductase in target tissues
- Determines
    - Fetal maturation of external male genitalia (penis, scrotum, prostate)
    - Hair distribution (baldness)
    - Sebaceous gland activity
- 5 alpha-reductase inhibitors block testosterone conversion in dihydrotestosterone → treats male pattern baldness, benign prostatic hypertrophy
    - Propecia (finasteride)

NOTES
SEXUAL DEVELOPMENT

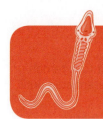

DEVELOPMENT OF THE REPRODUCTIVE SYSTEM

osms.it/reproductive-system-dev

SEXUAL DIFFERENTIATION

- Series of events begins at conception, ends with sexual characteristics acquisition (designated biologically male/female)
- During first five gestational weeks
  - Gonadal ridge develops, later becomes differentiated gonads
- Week 6
  - Primordial germ cells start migrating from yolk sac towards gonadal ridge
- Week 7
  - Primordial germ cells promote gene expression contained in sex chromosomes
- *Wolffian, Müllerian ducts*: structures that will develop into rest of reproductive tract; remain undifferentiated until week 8

MALE DEVELOPMENT

Male gonadal development

- Embryo genetically male → gene expression in Sex-determining Region in Y chromosome (SRY) promoted
  - SRY-region genes promote testis-determining factor production → testis-determining factor acts on undifferentiated gonads → gonadal transformation into testes
  - Gonadal ridge becomes seminiferous tubules, rete testis, straight tubules
- Testes contain three functional cell types
  - *Germ cells*: produce spermatogonia → produce male gametes in puberty
  - *Sertoli cells*: synthesize anti-Müllerian hormone
  - *Leydig cells*: synthesize testosterone

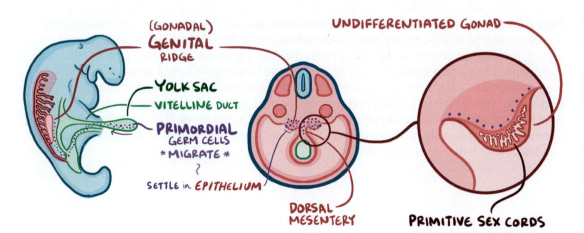

Figure 66.1 Illustration of the migration of primordial germ cells to the gonadal ridge in week 6. At this point, the gonad is undifferentiated, meaning that it can develop into ovaries or testes.

Male internal reproductive organ development

- Wolffian ducts give rise to male internal genitalia
  - AKA mesonephric duct/mesonephros
  - Meso = middle, in between; *nephros* = kidney
  - **Two functions**: connects primitive kidney to cloaca; develops into male genitalia
  - Growth, differentiation stimulated by testosterone
- Male internal reproductive organ development depends on Sertoli cells, Leydig cells, urogenital sinus
- *Sertoli cells*: synthesize, secrete anti-Müllerian hormone; AKA Müllerian inhibiting substance
  - Promotes Müllerian/paramesonephric-duct atrophy
- *Leydig cells*: synthesize, secrete testosterone → become internal male genitalia
  - Promotes Wolffian/mesonephric-duct growth, differentiation
- *Urogenital sinus*: develops into external reproductive organs; undifferentiated until gestational week 9
  - Urethral folds → urethra (both)
  - Labioscrotal swellings → scrotum
  - Primordial phallus → penis

Male external reproductive organ development

- Male external genitalia differentiation from urogenital sinus depends on testosterone presence
  - 5 alpha reductase in target tissues converts testosterone → more potent dihydrotestosterone
  - *Dihydrotestosterone*: responsible for masculinizing external genitalia

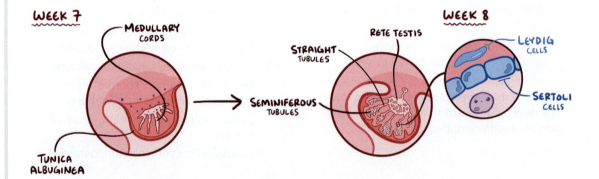

Figure 66.2 Biologically male sexual differentiation, week 7: genes in Sex-determining Region of Y chromosome (SRY) code for testis-determining factor (which initiates development of testes). Primitive sex cords → medullary cords that carry primitive germ cells deeper into mesoderm. The surface epithelial layer of each gonad thins out → tunica albuginea. Later, medullary cords → seminiferous tubules, straight tubules, rete testis. The primordial germ cells settle in seminiferous tubules mature into dormant spermatogonia. During puberty, spermatogonia start dividing → sperm (male gametes). During week 8, some cells in the seminiferous tubule walls differentiate into Sertoli cells, and cells between the seminiferous tubules differentiate into Leydig cells.

FEMALE DEVELOPMENT

Female gonadal development
- Without functional SRY gene
  - *Week 9*: ovaries begin developing
  - *Week 10*: ovarian cortex, inner medulla distinguishable
- Ovaries contain three functional cell types
  - *Germ cells*: produce oogonia; located in ovarian cortex (oogonia—haploid cells that remain arrested in prophase 1 of meiosis until ovulation)
  - *Granulosa cells*: synthesize estradiol
  - *Theca cells*: synthesize progesterone
- *Ovarian follicle*: oogonium surrounded by granulosa cells, connective tissue

Female internal reproductive organ development
- Müllerian duct → female genitalia
  - AKA paramesonephric duct/paramesonephros
  - *Para* = on the side of; *meso* = middle, in between; *nephros* = kidney
- Female internal reproductive organ development primarily depends on testes absence
- Lack of testosterone induces Wolffian duct degeneration
- Lack of anti-Müllerian hormone promotes Müllerian ducts persistence → develop into fallopian tubes, uterus, upper ⅓ of vaginal canal
- Rest of female reproductive organs arise from urogenital sinus

Female external reproductive organ development
- Urogenital sinus develops into external reproductive organs; undifferentiated until gestational week 9
  - Urethral folds → urethra (both ⚥), labia minora
  - Labioscrotal swellings → labia majora, mons pubis
  - Primordial phallus → clitoris
- Female external genitalia differentiation
  - Androgen absence-dependent (testosterone, dihydrotestosterone)
- Phenotypic differentiation complete at week 12 → earliest ultrasound-based sex-determination date

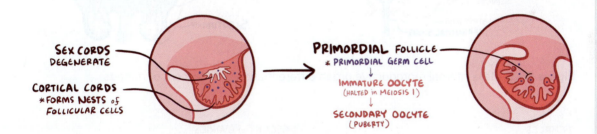

Figure 66.3 Biologically-female sexual differentiation. Since there is no Y chromosome to secrete Testis-determining factor, the undifferentiated gonads develop into ovaries. The rest of the reproductive tract acquires female characteristics in the absence of testosterone.

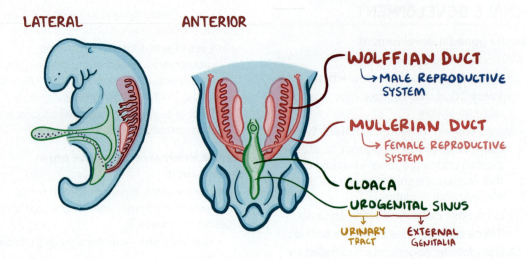

Figure 66.4 The genital ducts are initially undifferentiated, tubular structures that run down the embryo's back inside the two nephrogenic cords on either side of the embryo. The Wolffian and Müllerian ducts start in the thoracic and upper lumbar region and continue down the embryo's back until they open into the part of the cloaca called the urogenital sinus.

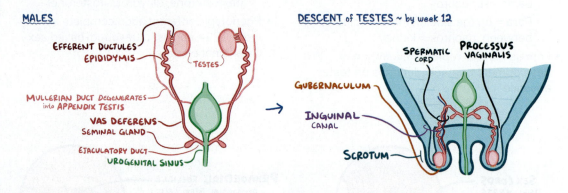

Figure 66.5 Male internal reproductive organ differentiation and descent of gonads.

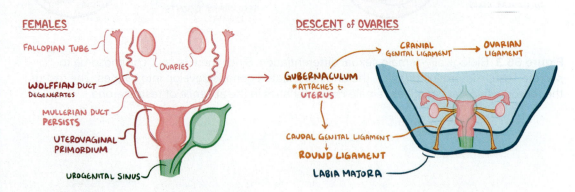

Figure 66.6 Female internal reproductive organ differentiation and descent of gonads.

Chapter 66 Reproductive Physiology: Sexual Development

SEX VS. GENDER

- Gender
  - Socially-constructed characteristics/behaviors associated with biologically male/female people
  - E.g. norms, roles, relationships between individuals
- Genetic sex
  - Individual's chromosomal composition
  - XY: males
  - XX: females
  - Established by oocyte, sperm cell fusion
- Gonadal sex
  - Individual's reproductive organs
  - *Male*: testes
  - *Female*: ovaries
- Phenotypic sex

Internal, external reproductive organ structure

- Male genitalia
  - *Internal*: prostate, seminal vesicles, vas deferens, epididymis
  - *External*: penis, scrotum
- Female genitalia
  - *Internal*: fallopian tubes, uterus, upper ⅓ vaginal canal
  - *External*: clitoris, labia majora, labia minora, lower ⅔ vaginal canal

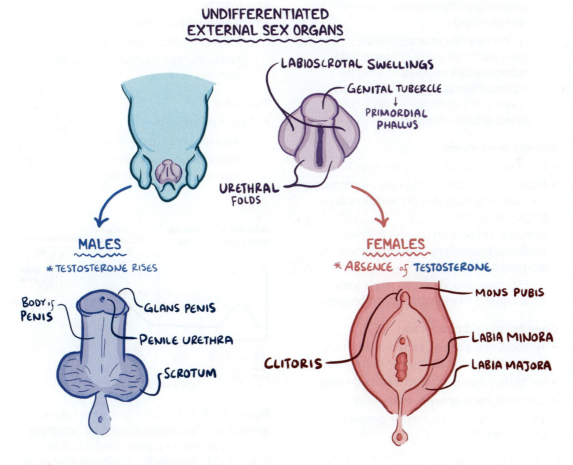

Figure 66.7 Male and female external sex organs. Phenotypical differentiation is complete at week 12.

PUBERTY & TANNER STAGING

osms.it/puberty-tanner-staging

PUBERTY
- Sexual maturation process involving endocrine, physical changes; controlled by hypothalamic-pituitary-gonadal axis
- Begins between ages 10–14 in females; between age 12–16 in males

GnRH secretion
- Pulses from hypothalamus regulate luteinizing hormone (LH), follicle-stimulating hormone (FSH) secretion from anterior pituitary → development of sexual characteristics
    - *Primary sex characteristics*: genitals (organs directly involved in sexual reproduction)
    - *Secondary sex characteristics*: sex-specific physical characteristic not necessary involved in sexual reproduction (e.g. pubic hair—both sexes, voice changes—males, breast development—females)

Gamete production
- Oocytes (females); sperm (males)
- *Males:* LH acts on Leydig cells → produces testosterone; FSH acts on Sertoli cells → produces sperm
- *Females:* LH acts on ovarian follicles → produces progesterone, androstenedione (converted into estrogen)
    - Estrogen, progesterone levels vary according to menstrual cycle phases

Gonadal steroid production
- Testosterone (males), estradiol (females) secretion → ↑ circulating sex hormones
- Secondary sexual characteristics develop
- Stimulate bone growth, ossification
- Involved in growth hormone production → growth spurt

EVENTS OF PUBERTY

Gonadarche
- Gonadal activation by FSH, LH

Adrenarche
- ↑ adrenal androgen production by adrenal cortex

Thelarche
- Breast tissue appears
    - Ovarian estradiol-guided

Menarche
- First menstruation occurs
    - Ovarian estradiol-guided
    - First menstrual cycles tend to be anovulatory

Spermarche
- First sperm production occurs
    - FSH, LH, testosterone-guided
    - Nocturnal sperm emissions, sperm appears in urine

Pubarche
- Pubic hair appears
    - Adrenal androgens-guided
    - *Association:* body hair; acne; apocrine sweat glands activation

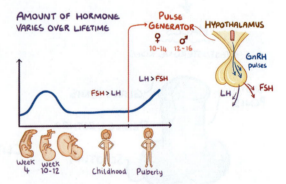

Figure 66.8 Puberty begins when pulse generator in hyothalamus begins secreting GnRH in pulses → pulsatile secretion of FSH and LH. In puberty, GnRH receptors in anterior pituitary become more sensitive to GnRH stimulation: small ↑ GnRH = large ↑ FSH, LH levels.

Chapter 66 Reproductive Physiology: Sexual Development

TANNER STAGING
- System for describing predictable steps during sexual maturation
- Centers on two, independent criteria
  - Appearance: pubic hair in males, females
  - Genital development: ↑ testicular volume, penile growth (males); breast development (females)

FIVE CATEGORIES OF TANNER STAGING

Stage 1: pre-pubertal
- ⚥ No pubic hair present in either sex
- ♂ Small penis, testes
- ♀ Have flat-chest

Stage 2
- ⚥ Soft pubic hair appears
- ♂ Measurable testes enlargement
- ♀ Breast buds appear

Stage 3
- ⚥ Pubic hair becomes coarser
- ♂ Penis begins to enlarge in size, length
- ♀ Breast mounds form

Stage 4
- ⚥ Pubic hair begins to cover pubic area
- ♂ Penis begins to widen
- ♀ Breast enlargement forms "mound-on-mound" breast contour

Stage 5: adult
- ⚥ Pubic hair extends to inner thigh
- ♂ Penis, testes enlarged to adult size
- ♀ Breast takes on adult contour

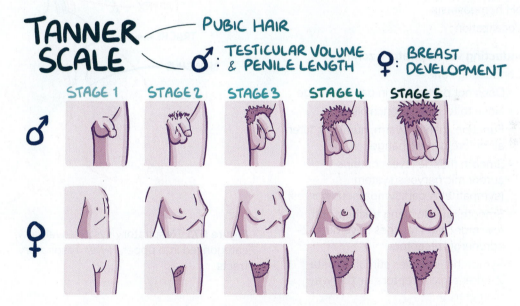

Figure 66.9 Illustration of the five stages of the Tanner scale in males and females.

NOTES

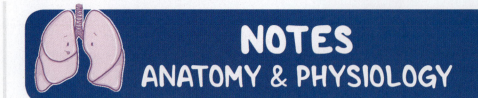

NOTES
ANATOMY & PHYSIOLOGY

RESPIRATORY SYSTEM

osms.it/respiratory-anatomy-physiology

RESPIRATORY SYSTEM
- Upper respiratory tract
  - Nose, pharynx, associated structures
- Lower respiratory tract
  - Larynx, trachea, bronchi, lungs

Respiratory system function
- Gas exchange between blood, atmosphere
- Protection against harmful particles, substances
- pH homeostasis
- Vocalization

Conducting vs. respiratory zone
- Conducting zone
  - Does not participate in gas exchange
  - Nose to terminal bronchioles
  - *Function*: inspire, warm, humidify, filter air before gas exchange
  - Smooth muscle layer contains autonomic nervous system (sympathetic, parasympathetic nerves)
  - Smooth muscle along trachea, first few bronchial branches have beta-2-adrenergic receptors
  - Sympathetic nerves stimulate beta-2-adrenergic receptors → ↑ airway diameter
  - Parasympathetic nerves stimulate muscarinic receptors → ↓ airway diameter
- Respiratory zone
  - Participates in gas exchange
  - Lined with alveoli
  - Terminal bronchioles–alveoli

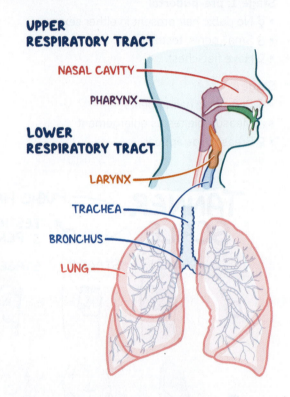

Figure 67.1 Respiratory system overview, categorized into upper, lower respiratory tracts.

Chapter 67 Respiratory Physiology: Anatomy & Physiology

RESPIRATORY SYSTEM ANATOMY

Nose
- *Function*: humidifies, warms, filters inspired air; voice resonance chamber; houses olfactory receptors
- Nasal vibrissae (hairs) coated with mucus → traps large particles (e.g. dust, pollen)

Nasal cavity
- Nasal cavity division
  - *Midline nasal septum*: composed of septal cartilage, anteriorly
  - *Vomer bone*: posteriorly
- Four paranasal sinuses (air-filled spaces inside bones) connected to nasal cavity
  - Ethmoid, frontal, sphenoid, maxillary sinuses
  - *Function*: warms, moistens inspired air; amplifies voice; lightens skull
- Roof formed by ethmoid, sphenoid bones
- Floor formed by palate
- Two mucous membrane types
  - *Olfactory mucosa*: olfactory epithelium containing smell receptors
  - *Respiratory mucosa*: pseudostratified ciliated columnar epithelium containing goblet cells; secretes mucus containing lysozyme, defensins
- Nasal conchae
  - Three mucosa-covered projections (superior, middle, inferior nasal conchae) of nasal cavity's lateral wall
  - *Meatus*: groove inferior to each conchae (superior, middle, inferior meatus)
  - *Function*: ↑ turbulence inside cavity to filter, humidify inspired air; reabsorb heat, moisture during nasal expiration

Palate
- Separates nasal cavity from oral cavity
  - *Hard palate*: anterior portion supported by palatine bones
  - *Soft palate*: posterior portion not supported by bones
  - Soft palate, uvula move together; forms valve that closes nasopharynx when swallowing (prevents food from entering nasopharynx)

Pharynx
- AKA throat
- Passageway connecting nasal cavity, larynx, oral cavity, esophagus
- *Nasopharynx*: region connecting nasal cavity to pharynx
  - Posterior to nasal cavity, inferior to sphenoid bone, superior to soft palate
  - Air-only passageway
  - Pharyngeal tonsils (adenoids); located on posterior wall; traps, kills pathogens
  - Pseudostratified ciliated epithelium (part of mucociliary escalator)
- *Oropharynx*: region connecting pharynx to oral cavity
  - Posterior to oral cavity, continuous with isthmus of fauces
  - Soft palate superior, epiglottis inferior
  - Food, air passageway
  - Pseudostratified columnar epithelium of nasopharynx → stratified squamous epithelium
  - Palatine tonsils located on lateral walls
  - Lingual tonsils cover posterior tongue
- *Laryngopharynx*: part of pharynx continuous with larynx (voice box)
  - Food, air passageway
  - Stratified squamous epithelium
  - Epiglottis anterior, esophagus posterior

Larynx
- Cartilage, connective tissue framework
  - Connects pharynx to trachea; houses vocal cords, epiglottis (cartilage flap atop larynx that seals airway off when swallowing—prevents food entering larynx)
- Location
  - Third to sixth cervical vertebra
  - *Superior*: hyoid bone
  - *Inferior*: trachea
- Function
  - Routes food, air into appropriate passageway; voice production
- Histology
  - *Superior portion*: contacts food; stratified squamous epithelium
  - *Inferior portion*: below vocal folds; pseudostratified ciliated columnar epithelium (part of mucociliary escalator)

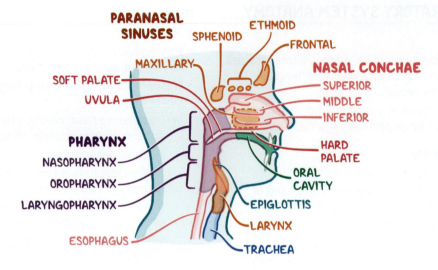

Figure 67.2 Anatomy of upper respiratory tract, surrounding structures.

- Contains nine cartilages
    - *Thyroid cartilage*: large shield-shaped midline cartilage, produces laryngeal prominence ("Adam's apple")
    - *Cricoid* cartilage: ring-shaped cartilage inferior to thyroid cartilage, superior to trachea
    - *Arytenoid, cuneiform, corniculate cartilages*: form posterior, lateral larynx walls (arytenoid cartilages anchor vocal cords)
    - *Epiglottis*: spoon-shaped cartilage is pulled superiorly to cover laryngeal inlet during swallowing (prevents food from passing through larynx)
- Vocal folds/ligaments
    - Attach arytenoid cartilages to thyroid cartilage
    - *True vocal cords*: sound production (function); composed of elastic fibers; core of mucosal folds; appears white (avascularity)
    - *False vocal cords*: superior to true vocal cords; does not participate in sound production; close glottis during swallowing (function)

Trachea
- AKA windpipe
- Mainstem bronchi, airways
- Trachea
    - Tube smooth muscle, connective tissue, C-shaped cartilage (provides support, maintains open passage for air)
    - Connected by trachealis muscle
    - Runs from larynx, divides into two main bronchi inferiorly at carina
- Layers (superficial to deep)
    - *Mucosa*: pseudostratified epithelium with goblet cells; mucociliary escalator
    - *Submucosa*: connective tissue layer (supported by 16–20 C-shaped cartilage rings)
    - *Adventitia*: connective tissue layer encasing cartilage rings

Right & left mainstem bronchus
- Right mainstem bronchus
    - Wider, more vertical
    - Something accidentally inhaled → goes into right lung (more likely)
- Inside lungs
    - Main bronchus subdivides into lobar bronchi → segmental bronchi → terminal bronchioles
- Trachea, first three bronchial generations
    - Wide, supported by cartilage rings
- Large airways lined by ciliated columnar cells, goblet cells (secrete mucus)
    - *Mucociliary escalator*: mucus traps particles → ciliated columnar cells beat rhythmically → moves mucus, trapped particles towards pharynx → spit out/swallowed

Chapter 67 Respiratory Physiology: Anatomy & Physiology

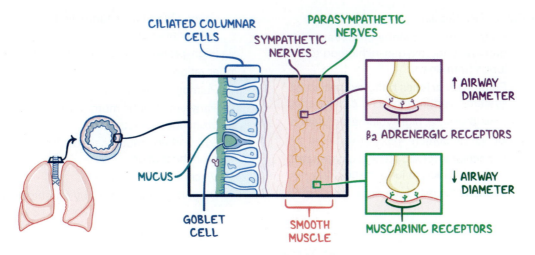

Figure 67.3 Section of tracheal wall showing its histology. Stimulation by sympathetic nerves dilates airways, stimulation by parasympathetic nerves constricts airways.

Histological changes as conducting tubes decrease
- Cartilage
  - Cartilage amount ↓ while elastic fibers ↑ (bronchioles contain no cartilage)
- Epithelium
  - Mucosal epithelium changes from pseudostratified columnar → columnar → cuboidal
  - Goblet cells, cilia ↓ (completely absent in bronchioles)
- Smooth muscle ↑

Bronchioles
- Narrow airways after first three bronchial generations
- *Terminal bronchioles*: last part of terminal bronchioles, end of conducting zone
- *Respiratory bronchioles*: distal to terminal bronchioles, first part of respiratory zone
- Terminal bronchiole → respiratory bronchiole → alveolar ducts → alveolar sac → alveoli

Alveoli
- Alveolar wall
  - Composed of a single simple squamous epithelium layer
- Elastic fibers surround alveoli → allow lung expansion during inspiration, recoil during expiration
  - *Type I pneumocytes*: primary gas exchange site; oxygen–carbon dioxide exchange occurs between alveolar gas, pulmonary capillary blood; thin walls, large alveoli surface-area maximizes gas exchange diffusion capabilities
  - *Type II pneumocytes*: secrete surfactant (↓ surface tension within alveoli → eases expansion, prevents collapsing
- Alveolar macrophages phagocytize particles inside lungs → conducting bronchioles → mucociliary escalator
- Respiratory membrane
  - Capillary, alveolar walls; basement membranes
- Alveolar pores connect adjacent alveoli
- Blood supply
  - Pulmonary capillary networks

Lungs
- Main respiration organs
- Right lung
  - *Three lobes*: upper, middle, lower lobe
- Left lung
  - *Two lobes*: upper, lower lobe
- Base of lungs rest on diaphragm
- *Pleura*: double-layered serosa covering lungs, pleural fluid lining pleural cavity between two layers
  - *Parietal pleura*: outer layer adherent to thoracic wall, superior surface of diaphragm
  - *Visceral pleura*: inner layer adherent to external lung surface

- Pulmonary circulation
  - Pulmonary veins (anterior to main bronchi) bring oxygen-rich blood to lungs from heart
  - Pulmonary arteries bring oxygen-poor systemic venous blood for oxygenation
  - Low-pressure, high-volume circulation
- Bronchial circulation
  - *Bronchial arteries*: provide oxygenated systemic blood to lung tissue
  - *Bronchial veins*: drain deoxygenated venous blood from lungs (with pulmonary veins)
  - High-pressure, low-volume circulation
- Innervation
  - Pulmonary plexus
  - Parasympathetic motor causes bronchoconstriction
  - Sympathetic motor causes bronchodilation
  - Visceral sensory
  - Diaphragm innervated by phrenic nerve

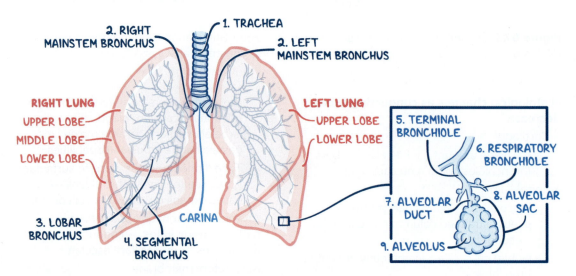

Figure 67.4 Trachea and lung anatomy. Numbered labels show sequence of airflow going into the airways from (trachea to alveoli).

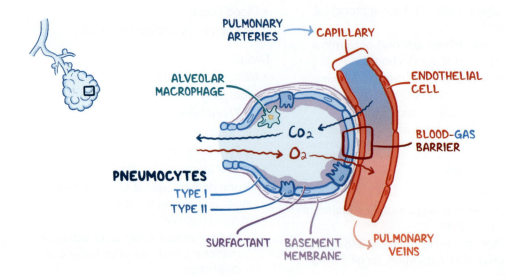

Figure 67.5 Alveolus structure. Gas exchange occurs at the blood-gas barrier. De-oxygenated blood from pulmonary arteries are oxygenated then sent to pulmonary veins.

VENTILATION

- **Ventilation (breathing)**: moving air in, out of lungs
- Oxygen pathway
    - Air inhaled through nostrils → nasal cavity → pharynx → larynx → trachea → mainstem bronchus → conducting bronchioles → terminal bronchioles → respiratory bronchioles → alveolar duct → alveoli → capillary → body
    - Carbon dioxide moves in reverse
- Airflow from atmosphere to lungs
    - Higher pressure → lower pressure
- Muscle movement creates pressure gradient
    - **Primary respiration muscles**: diaphragm, external intercostals, scalenes
    - **Forceful breathing**: other muscles recruited
- **Airflow resistance**: function of respiratory passage diameter
- **Passive inhalation**: negative pressure inside body generated → moves air into lungs
    - Diaphragm contracts downwards, chest muscles pull ribs outward → ↑ intrathoracic volume → ↓ intrathoracic pressure → air moved into lungs (air flows down pressure gradient)
- **Passive exhalation**: ↑ intrathoracic pressure generated → moves air out of lungs
    - Diaphragm relaxes (returns to resting position), external intercostal muscles relax, thoracic cage recoils → elastic lung recoil → ↓ intrathoracic volume → ↑ intrathoracic pressure → air pushed out of lungs

NOTES

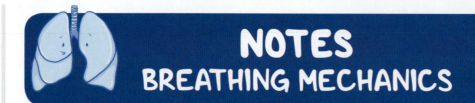

NOTES
BREATHING MECHANICS

LUNG VOLUMES & CAPACITIES

osms.it/lung-volumes-capacities

- **Spirometry:** spirometer used to measure air volume moving in, out of lungs
- **Static lung volumes:** volumes not involved in airflow rate
- **Capacities:** combination of > one lung volume

Volume variations
- Related to age, sex, body size, posture
- Tidal volume (V_T)
    - 500mL
    - Air volume inspired, expired during quiet breathing
- Inspiratory reserve volume
    - Maximum volume inhaled air above V_T = 3L
- Expiratory reserve volume
    - Maximum expired air volume below V_T = 1.2L
- Residual volume (RV)
    - Air remaining in lungs after forced expiration = 1.2L (not measured by spirometry)
- Functional residual capacity (FRC)
    - Expiratory reserve volume (ERV) + RV = 2.4L
- VT + inspiratory reserve volume = 3.5L
- Vital capacity (V_C)
    - V_T + inspiratory reserve volume (IRV) + ERV = 4.7L
- Total lung capacity (TLC)
    - Combination of all lung capacities = 5.9L

MEASURING FRC

Helium dilution method
- Helium placed in spirometer → inhaled
- Helium concentration in lungs equalizes with amount of helium placed in spirometer (helium insoluble in blood) after few breaths
- Total helium mass measured in spirometer = FRC

Body plethysmograph method
- Application of Boyle's law (P X V = k)
- Person sits inside plethysmograph (airtight box) → breathes in/out through mouthpiece → measures air pressure in mouth
- Mouthpiece closed after expiring V_T; as person attempts to breathe FRC calculated using measurements of alveolar pressure, lung volume, pressure changes within plethysmograph

Chapter 68 Respiratory Physiology: Breathing Mechanics

ANATOMIC & PHYSIOLOGIC DEAD SPACE

osms.it/anatomic-physiologic-dead-space

- **Dead space:** air volume enters airways, lungs; no gas exchange occurs

ANATOMIC DEAD SPACE
- Air inaccessible to body for gas exchange (due to anatomical structure)
- Air contained in conducting zone (nose → terminal bronchioles)
- Conduit for air movement in/out of lungs; warms, humidifies air; removes debris, pathogens
- Volume = 150mL (⅓ of tidal volume)

- Anatomic dead space = physiologic dead space
$$V_T = V_D + V_A$$
- V_T = tidal volume
- V_D = physiological dead space volume
- V_A = air volume present in functioning alveoli

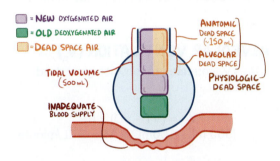

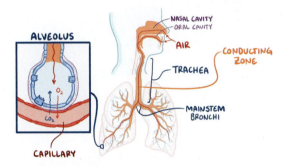

Figure 68.1 The volume of air contained in the conducting zone is called anatomic dead space because no gas exchange occurs here; therefore, no oxygen can be extracted from this air.

Figure 68.2 The green block represents residual air from the previous inhalation that participated in gas exchange. The purple blocks represent new oxygenated tidal volume inhaled during the current breath. Some of this new air also ends up being dead space air ("alveolar dead space") due to an inadequate blood supply to the alveolus.

PHYSIOLOGIC DEAD SPACE
- Air physiologically inaccessible to body for gas exchange
- **Composition:** anatomic dead space + dead space in respiratory zone (respiratory bronchioles, alveolar duct, alveolar sac, alveoli) that does not partake in gas exchange
  - **Ventilation/perfusion defect:** alveoli ventilated, not well perfused (alveolar dead space)
- Volume = approx. 0 (in healthy adult)

Physiological dead space volume (Bohr equation)
- Assumptions
  - Environmental air CO_2 = 0 (actual amount ≅ 0.04%)
  - Dead space CO_2 contribution = 0
  - All CO_2 in exhaled air comes from functioning alveoli
- $V_D = V_T \times$ arterial CO_2 partial pressure ($PaCO_2$) - expired CO_2 partial pressure ($PeCO_2$) ÷ $PaCO_2$

$$V_D = V_T \times \frac{Pa_{CO_2} - Pe_{CO_2}}{Pa_{CO_2}}$$

OSMOSIS.ORG 595

VENTILATION

osms.it/ventilation

- Air movement between environment, lungs
- **Ventilation rates:** measure air volume moving in/out of lungs over period of time

MINUTE VENTILATION (V_E)

- V_E = amount of air moved in/out of lungs in one minute; does not factor in physiological dead space

$$V_E = (VT) \times (\text{Respiratory Rate/RR})$$
$$V_E = 500\text{mL} \times 15/\text{minute} = 7.5\text{L/minute}$$

ALVEOLAR VENTILATION (V_A)

- $V_A = V_E$ corrected for physiological dead space

$$V_A = (VT - VD) \times RR$$
$$V_A = (500\text{ mL} - 150\text{mL}) \times 15 = 5.2\text{L/minute}$$

- V_A without measuring dead space
  - V_A = volume of CO_2 (V_{CO2}) ÷ fraction CO_2 (F_{CO2})

$$VA = (V_{CO2}) / (F_{CO2})$$

- **Partial pressure:** proportional to fractional concentration of that gas in mixture; based on constant **K**
  - Assumes gases are saturated with water vapor (normal body temperature, sea-level atmospheric pressure)
  - CO_2 partial pressure in alveolar air: $P_{CO2} = F_{CO2} \times K$
  - Alveolar ventilation equation: $V_A = [(V_{CO2}) / (P_{CO2})] \times K$
  - Replacing P_{CO2} with CO_2 pressure in arterial blood (Pa_{CO2}) in alveolar equation
  - Inverse relationship between alveolar ventilation, CO_2 partial pressure in alveolar air, pulmonary arteries (e.g. ↑ air ventilating the alveoli → ↓ CO_2 in blood, vice versa)

$$V_A = \frac{V_{CO_2} \times K}{P_{ACO_2}}$$

Chapter 68 Respiratory Physiology: Breathing Mechanics

ALVEOLAR GAS EQUATION

osms.it/alveolar-gas-equation

- Pressure in alveoli = atmospheric pressure (P_{atm}); air in alveoli contains water vapor
- Alveolar pressure (P_{atm}) = water vapor pressure (P_{vapor}) + gas mixture pressure → total alveolar pressure exerted from all gases minus water vapor = $P_{atm} - P_{vapor}$
- O_2 partial pressure dissolved in blood (P_{aO2}) = CO_2 partial pressure in alveoli (P_{ACO2}) ÷ by R (respiratory quotient)

$$P_{aO2} = (P_{ACO2}) / R$$

- Partial pressure of O_2 inside alveolus (P_{AO2}) = partial pressure of inspired oxygen (P_{iO2}) minus partial pressure of oxygen going into blood (P_{aO2})

Partial pressure: gas particle mixture

- Gas' partial pressure proportional to fractional gas concentration in mixture
- Fractional CO_2 concentration (F_{CO2}) = 0.3
  - Accounts for 30% of gas molecules (F_{CO2} × total pressure of gas mixture P_{gases})
- Fractional concentration of O_2 (F_{O2}) = 0.7
  - Accounts for remaining 70% (F_{O2} × total pressure of gas mixture P_{gases})

- Pressure exerted by O_2 > pressure exerted by CO_2 (proportional to fractional concentrations)
  - If P_{gases} = 20mmHg; partial pressure of O_2 = 14mmHg (0.7 × 20); partial pressure of CO_2 = 6mmHg (0.3 × 20)
  - Partial pressure of inspired air (P_{iO2}), fractional oxygen concentration in inspired air (F_{iO2}), accounting for water vapor

$$P_{iO2} = F_{iO2} \times (P_{atm} - P_{vapor})$$

Alveolar gas equation

- Relationship between O_2 partial pressure inside alveolus to CO_2 partial pressure in alveolus

$$P_{AO2} = [F_{iO2} \times (P_{atm} - P_{vapor})] - [(P_{ACO2}) / R]$$
$$P_{AO2} = 150 - (1.25 \times P_{ACO2})$$

- F_{iO2} = 0.21 (normal air = 21% O_2)
- Atmospheric pressure = 760mmHg
- Water vapor pressure i = 47mmHg
- R = 0.8

COMPLIANCE OF LUNGS & CHEST WALL

osms.it/compliance-lungs-chest-wall

- Compliance measures how changes in pressure → lung volume change
- **Lung, chest wall compliance:** inversely correlated with elastic, "snap back" properties (elastance)
  - Compliance = $\Delta V / \Delta P$
  - Elastance = $\Delta P / \Delta V$

- ↑ compliance → lungs easier to fill with air
  - *Forces promoting open alveoli:* compliance, transmural pressure gradient, surfactant
- ↓ compliance → lungs harder to fill with air
  - *Forces promoting collapse of alveoli:* elastic recoil/elastance, alveolar surface tension

COMBINED PRESSURE-VOLUME CURVES FOR THE LUNG & CHEST WALL

osms.it/pressure-vol_curves_lung_chest_wall

- Pressure-volume relationship is curvilinear
- Volume at FRC (zero airway pressure)
  - *Lung inward recoil:* balanced with chest wall's tendency to expand outward (e.g. at equilibrium with no tendency to collapse/expand)
- Volume > FRC
  - Positive transmural pressure
  - ↑ lung recoiling force
  - ↓ chest wall outward force
- Volume < FRC (forced expiration)
  - Negative transmural pressure
  - ↓ lung recoiling force
  - ↑ chest wall outward force
- Pressure-volume curves plotted on graph
  - X-axis: pressure
  - Y axis: volume
  - Slope of curve = compliance
- Curve flattens out when lung, chest wall compliance combined
- *Hysteresis:* compliance for inspiration, expiration are different → slopes will be different

ALVEOLAR SURFACE TENSION & SURFACTANT

osms.it/alveolar-surface-tension-surfactant

- Alveoli lined with fluid film; water tends to form spheres (e.g. drops)
  - Due to intrinsic surface tension (caused by attraction of water molecules to each other)
- Surface tension creates pressure → pulls alveoli closed → collapses into sphere → ↓ gas exchange
- *Law of Laplace:* pressure that promotes lungs' collapse is (1) directly proportional to surface tension, (2) inversely proportional to alveoli radius

  $$P = 2T/r$$

  - P = pressure on alveolus
  - T = surface tension
  - r = alveolar radius
- Smaller alveolus (r = 1) → ↑ pressure
  - P = 2 x 50/1 = 100
- Larger alveolus (r = 2) → ↓ pressure
  - P = 2 x 50/2 = 50
- Alveoli are small (allows ↑ surface area relative to volume), so have ↑ collapsing pressure

SURFACTANT

- ↓ collapsing pressure in alveoli → ↑ gas exchange, ↑ lung compliance, ↓ work of breathing
  - Lipoprotein mixture primarily containing dipalmitoyl phosphatidylcholine (DPPC)
  - Synthesized by type II pneumocytes, coats inside of alveoli

- Contains both hydrophilic, hydrophobic group (amphipathic nature)—intermolecular forces produced by repelling hydrophobic groups, attracting hydrophilic groups → ↓ surface tension, collapsing pressure

AIRFLOW, PRESSURE, & RESISTANCE

osms.it/airflow-pressure-resistance

AIR FLOW & PRESSURE
- Airflow in lungs determined by Ohm's law
  - Air flow directly proportional to pressure difference between alveoli, mouth/nose; inversely proportional to airway resistance

  $$Q = \Delta P/R$$

  - Q = air flow
  - ΔP = change in pressure
  - R = resistance
- Pressure gradient
  - Driving force for air flow
  - Diaphragm contracts during inspiration → creates pressure gradient (↑ lung volume, ↓ alveolar pressure) → air flows into lungs

RESISTANCE

Poiseuille's law
- Resistance in lungs determined by Poiseuille's law
  - Air flow directly proportional to resistance along airway

$$R = \frac{8nl}{\pi r^4}$$

  - R = resistance
  - n = gas viscosity
  - l = length of airway
  - πr^4 = flow is related exponentially to airway's radius
- Highlights critical importance of airway diameter on airflow
  - E.g. if airway radius ↓ by a factor of 2 → ↑ resistance by 24 (16-fold)

Resistance changes
- Parasympathetic muscarinic receptor stimulation → bronchial smooth muscle constriction → ↓ airway diameter → ↓ airflow; sympathetic stimulation of β2 receptors → bronchial smooth muscle relaxation → ↑ airway diameter → ↑ airflow
- ↓ lung volume → ↑ resistance; ↑ lung volume → ↓ resistance
- ↑ viscosity (e.g. deep sea diving) → ↑ resistance; ↓ viscosity (e.g. inhaling helium) → ↓ resistance

BREATHING CYCLE

osms.it/breathing-cycle

- Normal, quiet breathing phases
  - Rest (period between breaths), inspiration, expiration
- Involves changes in air volume, intrapleural pressure, alveolar pressure
- Affected by respiratory system's resistance, compliance

Rest

- Alveolar pressure (P_{alv}) = atmospheric pressure (P_{atm}) = 0
- No air movement in/out of lungs
  - Due to pressure gradient's absence
- Air volume in lungs = FRV
- Intrapleural pressure = -0.5cm0.2in H_2O
  - Transmural pressure gradient (intrapleural pressure always less than alveolar pressure) keeps lungs inflated
- Diaphragm relaxed

Inspiration

- Active process (requires muscle activity)
- Diaphragm (major inspiratory muscle; innervated by phrenic nerve) contracts, moves downward; external intercostal muscles contract (innervated by intercostal nerves) contract, elevate ribs outward, upward → enlarge thoracic cavity → ↑ lung volume → ↓ pressure in lungs (P_{alv} = -1cm/0.39in H_2O)
  - **Boyle's law ($P = k/V$):** gas pressure (P) in container (thorax, alveoli) at constant temperature (k) inversely proportional to volume (V)
- Pressure gradient causes air to flow into lungs until $P_{alv} = P_{atm}$ at inspiration's end
- Volume in lungs = FRC + VT
- Intrapleural pressure = -8cm/3.1in H_2O at expiration's end

Expiration

- Passive process
- Elastic forces of lungs compress alveolar air volume → ↑ pressure in lungs → $P_{alv} > P_{atm}$ → pressure gradient causes air to flow out of lungs until $P_{alv} = P_{atm}$ at inspiration's end
- Diaphragm, external intercostal muscles relax → ↓ thoracic cavity size → ↓ lung volume → ↑ pressure in lungs
- V_T expired → lung volume = FRC

NOTES
BREATHING REGULATION

BREATHING CONTROL

osms.it/breathing-control

WHAT IS BREATHING CONTROL?
- **Breathing (ventilation):** movement of gasses in, out of lungs
- Regulation maintains arterial partial pressures of O_2, CO_2 (PaO_2, $PaCO_2$)
- **Components:** brainstem respiratory centers; peripheral, central chemoreceptors; mechanoreceptors in lungs, muscles of respiration, joints

BRAINSTEM RESPIRATORY CENTERS

Dorsal respiratory group (DRG)
- Inspiratory center, located in dorsal medulla
- Sets basic rhythm of breathing
- Receives sensory input via cranial nerves (CN) IX, X from peripheral chemoreceptors, mechanoreceptors in lungs → sends motor output via phrenic nerve to stimulate contraction of diaphragm
    - DRG neurons generate repeating bursts of action potentials → period of quiescence
    - Bursts occur → action potential frequency "ramps up" → ↑ lung volume

Ventral respiratory group (VRG)
- Expiratory center, located in ventral medulla
- Inactive during basic, quiet breathing
- Provides high respiratory drive when ventilation needs to increase (e.g. exercise)

Pneumotaxic center
- Located in upper pons
- Limits inspiration by inhibiting DRG
- Limits tidal volume, increases respiratory rate
- Receives input from cerebral cortex

Apneustic center
- Located in lower pons
- Prolongs DRG inspiratory signal, diaphragm contraction → inspiratory gasps (apneusis)
- Associated with damage to pons/upper medulla

VOLUNTARY CONTROL

Cerebral cortex
- Sends commands to voluntarily override autonomic control of ventilation
- Hyperventilation
    - Voluntarily breathing at rate > that needed by metabolism
    - **Self-limiting:** hyperventilation → ↓ $PaCO_2$ (strongly inhibits autonomic respiratory centers, ventilation)
- Hypoventilation
    - Voluntarily breathing at rate insufficient for metabolism
    - **Self-limiting:** hypoventilation → ↓ PaO_2, ↑ $PaCO_2$

HYPOTHALAMIC CONTROL
- **Strong emotions, pain:** act via hypothalamus, limbic system → signal respiratory centers → modify respiratory rate, depth
- Rise in body temperature → ↑ respiratory rate
- Drop in body temperature → ↓ respiratory rate

PULMONARY CHEMORECEPTORS & MECHANORECEPTORS

osms.it/pulmonary-central-peripheral-chemoreceptors

CENTRAL CHEMORECEPTORS
- Located in ventral surface of medulla
- Sensitive to changes in H⁺ indirectly by sensing acute changes in $PaCO_2$ (unable to cross blood-brain barrier)
    - ↑ $PaCO_2$ → conversion to carbonic acid (H_2CO_3) by enzyme carbonic anhydrase → dissociation into H^+, HCO_3^- → ↓ CSF pH (↑ CSF [H^+]) → stimulates central chemoreceptors → stimulates DRG → ↑ ventilation → ↓ $PaCO_2$ (40mmHg)
- Crucial minute-to-minute control
    - Match ventilation with metabolism by monitoring $PaCO_2$

PERIPHERAL CHEMORECEPTORS
- Located in carotid bodies at bifurcation (near aortic arch)
- Responds directly to changes in PaO_2, $PaCO_2$
    - Strongly stimulated in linear fashion when PaO_2 < 60mmHg
    - Weakly stimulated by ↑ $PaCO_2$
    - Carotid bodies only: stimulated by ↑ arterial [H^+]
- Afferents send information to DRG via CN IX, X → directs ventilatory response to hypoxemia, acidemia, alkalemia

MECHANORECEPTORS

Lung stretch receptors
- Located in airway smooth muscle
- Respond to lung inflation → termination of inspiration (Hering–Breuer inspiratory-inhibitory reflex)

Joint and muscle receptors
- Respond to bodily movement → ↑ respiratory rate

Irritant receptors
- Respond to noxious gasses; particulates via CN X → coughing, bronchoconstriction

Juxtacapillary (J) receptors
- Located in alveoli, near capillaries
- Respond to capillary engorgement → ↑ respiratory rate

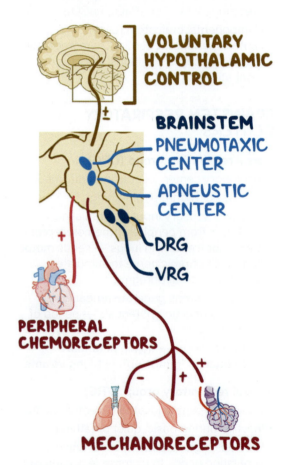

Figure 69.1 The brainstem is the respiratory center of the body. Many receptors throughout the body send signals to the brainstem so that it can regulate the breathing rate accordingly.

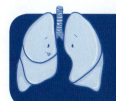

NOTES
GAS EXCHANGE

GAS EXCHANGE & LAWS
- Diffusion of oxygen (O_2), carbon dioxide (CO_2) in lungs, peripheral tissues
- Alveolar O_2 from inhaled gas → pulmonary capillary blood → circulation → tissue capillaries → cells
- CO_2 from cells → tissue capillaries → circulation → pulmonary capillary blood → CO_2 for exhalation from alveoli
- Gas exchange, gas behavior in solution is governed by fundamental physical gas properties → represented by gas laws

FORMS OF GAS IN SOLUTION

Dissolved gas
- All gas in solution are to some extent carried in a freely dissolved form
- For given partial pressure, the higher the solubility of a gas, the higher the concentration in solution
- In solution only dissolved gas molecules contribute to partial pressure
- Of the gases inspired as air, only nitrogen is exclusively carried in dissolved form

Bound gas
- O_2, CO_2, CO are bound to proteins in blood
- O_2, CO_2, CO can all bind to hemoglobin
- CO_2 also binds to plasma proteins

Chemically modified gas
- The ready back and forth conversion of CO_2 to bicarbonate (HCO_3^-) in presence of enzyme carbonic anhydrase allows CO_2 to contribute to gas equilibria despite chemical conversion
- Majority of CO_2 in blood carried as HCO_3^-

IDEAL (GENERAL) GAS LAW

osms.it/ideal-gas-law

- Relates multiple variables to describe state of a hypothetical "ideal gas" under various conditions
  - *Ideal gas:* theoretical gas composed of many randomly moving point particles whose only interactions are perfectly elastic collisions
  - All gas laws can be derived from general gas law
- $PV = nRT$
  - P = Pressure (millimeters of mercury (mmHg)
  - V = Volume (liters (L)
  - n = Moles (mol)
  - R = Gas constant (8.314 J/mol)
  - T = Temperature (Kelvin [K])
- *In gas phase:* body temperature, pressure (BTPS) used
  - T = 37°C/98.6°F/310K
  - P = Ambient pressure
  - Gas is saturated with water vapor (47mmHg)
- *In liquid phase/solution:* standard temperature, pressure (STPD) used
  - T = 0°C/32°F/273K
  - P = 760mmHg
  - Dry gas (no humidity)
- Ideal gas law can be used to interconvert between properties of same gas under BTPS, STPD conditions
  - E.g. gas volume (V_1) at BTPS → gas volume at STPD (V_2)

$$V_2 = V_1 \times \frac{T_1}{T_2} \times \frac{P_1 - P_{w1}}{P_2 - P_{w2}}$$

$$V_2 = V_1 \times \frac{273}{310} \times \frac{760 - 47}{760 - 0}$$

$$V_2 = V_1 \times 0.826$$

BOYLE'S LAW

osms.it/Boyles-law

- Describes how pressure of gas ↑ as container volume ↓
- $P_1V_1 = P_2V_2$
- For gas at given temperature, the product of pressure, volume is constant
- Inspiration → diaphragm contraction → ↑ lung volume
- If PV constant + lung volume ↑ → pressure ↓
- Pressure ↓ → disequilibrium between room, lung air pressures → air fills lungs to equalize pressure

DALTON'S LAW

osms.it/Daltons-law

- Total pressure exerted by gaseous mixture = sum of all partial pressures of gases in mixture → partial pressure of gas in gaseous mixture = pressure exerted by that gas if it occupied total volume of container
- $P_x = P_B \times F$
  - Px = partial pressure of gas (mmHg)
  - P_B = barometric pressure (mmHg)
  - F = fractional concentration of gas (no unit)
- Partial pressure = total pressure X fractional concentration of dry gas
- For humidified gases
  - $P_x = (P_B - P_{H2O}) \times F$
  - P_{H2O} = Water vapor pressure at 37°C/98.6°F (47mmHg)
  - If the sum of partial pressures in a mixture = total pressure of mixture → barometric pressure (P_B) is sum of the partial pressures of O_2, CO_2, N_2 (nitrogen), and H_2O
  - At barometric pressure (760 mmHg) composition of humidified air is O_2, 21%; N_2, 79%; CO_2, 0%
  - Within airways, air is humidified thus water vapor pressure is obligatory = to 47mmHg at 37°C/98.6°F

HENRY'S LAW

osms.it/Henrys-law

- For concentrations of dissolved gases
- When gas is in contact with liquid → gas dissolves in proportion to its partial pressure → greater concentration of a particular gas, in gas phase → more dissolves into solution at faster rate
    - $C_x = P_x \times$ Solubility
    - C_x = concentration of dissolved gas (mL gas / 100mL blood)
    - Concentration of gas in solution only applies to dissolved gas that is free in solution
    - Concentration of gas in solution does not include any gas that is presently bound to any other dissolved substances (e.g. plasma proteins/hemoglobin)
    - P_x = partial pressure of gas (mmHg)
    - Solubility = solubility of gas in blood (mL gas / 100mL blood per mmHg)
- Henry's law governs gases dissolved within solution (e.g. O_2, CO_2 dissolved in blood)

- To calculate gas concentration in liquid phase
    - Partial pressure of gas in gas phase → partial pressure in liquid phase → concentration in liquid
    - Partial pressure of gas in liquid phase (at equilibrium) = partial pressure of gas in gaseous phase
    - If alveolar air has PO_2 of 100mmHg → PO_2 of capillary blood that equilibrates with alveolar air = 100mmHg

HYPERBARIC CHAMBERS

- Hyperbaric chambers employ Henry's law
    - Contain O_2 gas pressurized to above 1 atm → greater than normal amounts of O_2 forced into the blood of the enclosed individual
    - Used to treat carbon monoxide poisoning, gas gangrene due to anaerobic organisms (cannot live in presence of high concentrations of O_2), improve oxygenation of skin grafts, etc.

FICK'S LAWS OF DIFFUSION

osms.it/Ficks-law-of-diffusion

- Describes diffusion of gases

$$V_x = \frac{DA\Delta P}{\Delta x}$$

- V_x = volume of gas transferred per unit time
- D = gas diffusion coefficient
- A = surface area
- ΔP = partial pressure difference of gas
- Δx = membrane thickness
- Driving force of gas diffusion is difference in partial pressures of gas (ΔP) across membrane (not the concentration difference)
    - If P_{O_2} of alveolar air = 100mmHg
    - P_{O_2} of mixed venous blood entering pulmonary capillary = 40mmHg
    - Driving force across membrane is 60mmHg (100mmHg - 40mmHg)
- Diffusion coefficient of gas (D) is a combination of usual diffusion coefficient (dependent on molecular weight) and gas solubility
- Diffusion coefficient dramatically affects

diffusion rate, e.g. diffusion coefficient for CO_2 is approximately 20x greater than that of O_2 → for a given partial pressure difference CO_2 would diffuse across the same membrane 20x faster than O_2

LUNG DIFFUSION CAPACITY (DL)

- A functional measurement which takes into account
    - Diffusion coefficient of gas used
    - Membrane surface area
    - Membrane thickness
    - Time required for gas to combine with proteins in pulmonary capillary blood (e.g. hemoglobin)
- Measured using carbon monoxide (CO) → CO transfer across alveolar-capillary barrier exclusively limited by diffusion process
- Lung diffusion capacity of carbon monoxide (DL_{CO}) is measured using a single breath
    - Individual breathes a mixture of gases with a low CO concentration → rate of CO disappearance is predictable in different disease states
    - Emphysema → destruction of alveoli → decreased surface area for gas exchange → decreased DL_{CO}
    - Fibrosis/pulmonary edema → increase in membrane thickness (via fluid accumulation in the case of edema) → decreased DL_{CO}
    - Anemia → reduced hemoglobin → reduced protein binding in a given time period → decreased DL_{CO}
    - Exercise → increased utilization of lung capacity, increased recruitment of pulmonary capillaries → increased DL_{CO}

GRAHAM'S LAW

osms.it/Grahams-law

- Diffusion rate of gas through porous membranes varies inversely with the square root of its density
- To compare rate of effusion (movement through porous membrane) of two gases → velocity of molecules determine the rate of spread
- Kinetic temperature in kelvin of a gas is directly proportional to average kinetic energy of gas molecules → at the same temperature, molecule of heavier gas will have a slower velocity than those of lighter gas

- Kinetic energy = $½mv^2$
- $½m_1v_1^2 = ½m_2v_2^2$
- $v_1^2 / v_2^2 = m_2 / m_1$
- $v_1 / v_2 = \sqrt{(m_2 / m_1)}$
- Which can be rewritten to give Graham's law

$$\frac{Rate_1}{Rate_2} = \sqrt{\frac{M_2}{M_1}}$$

GAS EXCHANGE IN THE LUNGS

osms.it/gas-exchange-in-lungs

PULMONARY GAS EXCHANGE

- AKA external respiration
- Pulmonary capillaries perfused with blood from right heart (deoxygenated)
- Gas exchange occurs between pulmonary capillary, alveolar gas
  - Room air → inspired air → humidified tracheal air → alveoli
  - O_2 diffuses from alveolar gas → pulmonary capillary blood
  - CO_2 diffuses from pulmonary capillary blood → alveolar gas
  - Blood exits the lungs → left heart → systemic circulation

Dry inspired air

- P_{O2} is approximately 160mmHg
  - Barometric pressure x fractional concentration of O_2 (21%)
  - P_{O2} = 760mmHg x 0.21
  - Assume no CO_2 in dry inspired air

Humidified tracheal air

- P_{O2} of humidified tracheal air is 150mmHg
  - Air is fully saturated with water vapor → "dilution" of partial pressures → calculations must correct for water vapor pressure (subtracted from barometric pressure)
  - At 37°C/98.6°F, P_{H2O} is 47mmHg
  - P_{O2} = (760mmHg − 47mmHg) x 0.21
  - Assume no CO_2 in humidified inspired air

Alveolar air

- Pressures of alveolar gas designated "PA"
- Alveolar gas exchange in lungs sees a drop in O_2 partial pressure, increase in CO_2 partial pressure
- PA_{O2} = 100mmHg
- PA_{CO2} = 40mmHg
- Amount of these gases entering/leaving alveoli correspond to physiological body needs (i.e. O_2 consumption, CO_2 production)

Pulmonary capillaries

- Blood entering pulmonary capillaries is mixed venous blood
- Tissues (metabolic activity alters composition of blood) → venous vasculature → right heart → pulmonary circulation
- P_{O2} = 40mmHg
- P_{CO2} = 46mmHg

Systemic arterial blood (oxygenated)

- Gas partial pressures of systemic arterial blood designated "Pa"
- In a healthy individual, diffusion of gas across alveolar, capillary membrane is so rapid that we can assume equilibrium is achieved between alveolar gases, pulmonary capillaries → P_{O2} and P_{CO2} of blood leaving pulmonary capillaries = alveolar air
- PA_{O2} = Pa_{O2} = 100mmHg
- PA_{CO2} = Pa_{CO2} = 40mmHg
- This blood enters systemic circulation to eventually return to lungs

Physiological shunt

- Small fraction of pulmonary blood flow bypasses alveoli → physiological shunt → blood not arterialized → systemic blood has slightly lower P_{O2} than alveolar air
- Shunting occurs due to
  - Coronary venous blood, drains directly into left ventricle
  - Bronchial blood flow
- Shunting may be increased in various pathologies → ventilation-perfusion defects/mismatches
- As shunt size increases → alveolar gas, pulmonary capillary blood do not equilibrate → blood is not fully arterialized
- **A-a difference**: difference in P_{O2} between alveolar gas (A), systemic arterial blood (a)
  - Physiological shunting → negligible/small differences
  - Pathology → notably increased difference

FACTORS AFFECTING EXTERNAL RESPIRATION

Thickness of respiratory membrane
- In healthy lungs, respiratory membrane → 0.5–1 micrometer thick
- Presence of small amounts of fluid (left heart failure, pneumonia) → significant loss of efficiency, equilibration time dramatically increases → the 0.75 seconds blood cells spend in transit through pulmonary circulation may not be sufficient

Surface area of respiratory membrane
- Greater surface area of respiratory membrane → greater amount of gas exchange
- Healthy adult male lungs have surface area of 90m²
- Pulmonary diseases (e.g. emphysema) → walls of alveoli break down → alveolar chambers enlarge → loss of surface area
- Tumors/pneumonia → prevent gas from occupying all available lung → loss of surface area

Partial pressure gradients and gas solubilities
- Partial pressures of O_2, CO_2 drive diffusion of these gases across respiratory membrane
- Steep O_2 partial pressure gradient exists
    - PO_2 of deoxygenated blood in pulmonary arteries = 40mmHg
    - PO_2 of 104mmHg in alveoli
    - O_2 diffuses rapidly from alveoli into pulmonary capillary blood
- O_2 equilibrium (PO_2 of 104mmHg on both sides of respiratory membrane) occurs in around 0.25 seconds of transit through lungs (about ⅓ of the time available)
- CO_2 has smaller gradient → 5mmHg (45mmHg vs 40mmHg), although pressure gradient for O_2 is much steeper than for CO_2, CO_2 is 20x more soluble in plasma, alveolar fluid than $O2$ → equal amounts of gas exchanged

Ventilation-perfusion coupling
- **Ventilation:** amount of gas reaching alveoli
- **Perfusion:** amount of blood flow in pulmonary capillaries
- These are regulated by local autoregulatory mechanisms → continuously respond to local conditions → some control in blood flow around lungs
- Arteriolar diameter controlled by P_{O2}
    - If alveolar ventilation is inadequate → blood taking O_2 away faster than ventilation can replenish it → low local P_{O2} → terminal arteriole restriction → blood redirected to respiratory areas with high P_{O2}, oxygen pickup more efficient
    - In alveoli where ventilation is maximal → high P_{O2} → pulmonary arteriole dilation → blood flow into pulmonary arterioles increases
    - Pulmonary vascular muscle autoregulation is opposite of that in systemic circulation
- Bronchiolar diameter controlled by P_{CO2}
    - Bronchioles connecting areas where PA_{CO2} high → dilation → allows CO_2 to be eliminated from body
    - Those with low CO_2 → constrict
- Independent autoregulation of arterioles, bronchioles → matched perfusion, ventilation
- Ventilation-perfusion matching is imperfect
    - Gravity → regional variation in blood, air flow (apices have greater ventilation but lesser perfusion, bases have greater perfusion, lesser ventilation)
    - Occasionally alveolar ducts may be plugged with mucus → unventilated areas

INTERNAL RESPIRATION
- Capillary gas exchange in body tissue
- Partial pressures, diffusion gradients are reversed from lungs however physical laws governing the exchanges remain identical
- Cells in body continuously use O_2, produce CO_2
    - PO_2 always lower in tissue than arterial blood (40mmHg vs 100mmHg) → O_2 moves rapidly from blood → tissues until equilibrated
    - CO_2 moves rapidly down its pressure gradient (P_{CO2} of 40mmHg in fresh blood arriving at capillary beds beds vs. P_{CO2} of 45mmHg in tissues) → venous blood → right heart

- Gas exchange at tissue level driven by partial pressures, occurs via simple diffusion

DIFFUSION-LIMITED & PERFUSION-LIMITED GAS EXCHANGE

osms.it/diffusion-limited-perfusion-limited-gas-exchange

Diffusion-limited gas exchange
- Diffusion is limiting factor determining total amount of gas transported across alveolar-capillary barrier
- As long as partial pressure gradient is maintained, diffusion continues
    - Gas readily diffuses across permeable membrane
    - Blood flow away from alveoli/chemical binding → partial pressure of gas on systemic end does not rise → partial pressure maintenance
    - Given a sufficiently long capillary bed diffusion will continue along entire length as equilibrium is not achieved
- Examples include
    - CO across alveolar-pulmonary capillary barrier
    - Oxygen during strenuous exercise/emphysema/fibrosis

Perfusion-limited gas exchange
- Perfusion (blood flow) is the limiting factor determining total amount of gas transported across alveolar-capillary barrier
- Increasing blood flow → increasing amount gas transported; examples include
    - **Nitrous oxide (N_2O):** not bound in blood → entirely free in solution; PA_{N2O} is constant, Pa_{N2O} = zero at start of capillary → initial large A-a difference → because no N_2O binds to any other components of blood, all of it remains free in solution → partial pressure builds rapidly → rapid equilibration, most of capillary length does not participate in gas exchange; new blood must be supplied to partake in further gas exchange with alveolar N_2O → "perfusion-limited gas exchange"
    - O_2 at rest
    - CO_2

Limitations of O_2 transport
- Under physiological conditions O_2 transport into pulmonary capillaries → perfusion-limited
- Diseased or abnormal conditions → diffusion-limited
- Perfusion-limited O_2 transport
    - PA_{O2} is constant = 100mmHg
    - At beginning of capillary Pa_{O2} = 40mmHg (mixed venous blood) → large partial pressure gradient → drives diffusion
    - As O_2 diffuses into pulmonary capillary blood → increase in Pa_{O2}
    - Hemoglobin binds O_2 → resists increase in Pa_{O2} → initially gradient is maintained; eventually equilibrium is achieved → perfusion-limitation
    - Therefore pulmonary blood flow determines net O_2 transfer (changes in pulmonary blood flow will affect net O_2 transfer)

Diffusion-limited O_2 transport
- Fibrosis → thickening of alveolar walls → increased diffusion distance for O_2 (decreases DL) → slowed rate of diffusion → prevents equilibration → partial pressure gradient maintained along length of capillary
- Increasing capillary length allows for more time for equilibrium to occur → diffusion-limitation

O₂ transport at high altitude
- High altitude reduces barometric pressure → reduced partial pressures
- Reductions in Pa_{O_2} → reduce oxygen amount available to diffuse into blood → reduced rate of equilibration at capillary → more time required for gas exchange, lower peak oxygen concentration reached once equilibrated

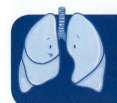

NOTES
GAS TRANSPORT

OXYGEN BINDING CAPACITY & OXYGEN CONTENT

osms.it/oxygen-binding-capacity-oxygen-content

MEASURES OF OXYGEN AVAILABILITY

O_2 binding capacity
- Maximum amount of O_2 bound to hemoglobin when 100% saturated (per blood volume)
  - More hemoglobin → more oxygen (per blood volume)
- Measurement
  - Expose blood to air with high P_{O_2} → complete hemoglobin saturation
  - Hemoglobin's oxygen affinity → 1g of hemoglobin A binds 1.34mL of O_2
  - Normal hemoglobin A concentration in blood → 15g/100mL
  - O_2 binding capacity = hemoglobin concentration × hemoglobin's affinity for oxygen
- *Example:* O_2 binding capacity = 15g/100mL × 1.34mL O_2/g hemoglobin = 20.1mL O_2/100mL blood

Oxygen content (CaO_2)
- Oxygen (mL) per 100mL of blood
- CaO_2 = O_2 binding capacity × % saturation + oxygen dissolved in solution
  - Correction for dissolved O_2 → solubility of O_2 in blood → 0.003mL O_2/100mL blood per mmHg
- CaO_2 = hemoglobin concentration (g/100mL blood) × hemoglobin oxygen affinity (mL O_2/g) × SaO_2 (arterial oxygen saturation) + partial pressure of oxygen (mmHg) × solubility of O_2 in blood (mL O_2/blood/mmHg)

- CaO_2 (ml O_2/100mL blood) = ([Hb] × 1.34 × SaO_2) + (PaO_2 × 0.003)

O_2 DELIVERY TO TISSUES
- Dependent on blood flow (determined by cardiac output), blood's oxygen content
- O_2 delivery = cardiac output × oxygen content

OXYGEN TRANSPORT
- Majority of oxygen in blood bound to hemoglobin, remainder dissolved in solution

Dissolved O_2
- Free in solution (1.5% of total blood O_2 content)
- Only free O_2 contributes to partial pressure → drives O_2 diffusion
- O_2 solubility in blood = 0.003mL O_2/100mL blood per mmHg → at normal PaO_2 of 100mmHg → concentration of dissolved O_2 is 0.3mL O_2/100mL blood
- Normal consumption of O_2 = 250mL O_2/minute
- Only dissolved O_2 delivered to tissues (cardiac output 5L/min) × dissolved O_2 concentration → 15mL O_2/min → incompatible with life
- Hemoglobin increases amount of O_2 carried by blood

Hemoglobin bound
- Hemoglobin → greater concentrations of O_2 carried to tissues by blood
- 98.5% of O_2 in blood bound to hemoglobin

- Four subunits of hemoglobin molecule
  - *Each subunit contains heme moiety:* iron-binding porphyrin, polypeptide chain (alpha/beta)
  - *Adult hemoglobin subunits ($\alpha_2\beta_2$)*: two alpha chains, two beta chains → each contains one iron molecule (Fe^{2+}) → binds one O_2 molecule → four molecules of O_2 per molecule of hemoglobin → oxyhemoglobin
  - Deoxygenated hemoglobin → deoxyhemoglobin

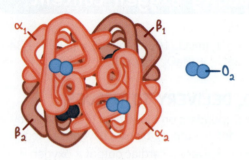

Figure 71.1 Each of the four hemoglobin subunits contains a heme group capable of binding one oxygen molecule.

- Heme binds oxygen in lungs → oxyhemoglobin
  - Oxygen diffuses from alveoli → across single cell thick alveolar walls → diffuses into blood → through red blood cell (RBC) membrane → interacts with heme → oxyhemoglobin (bright red blood)
- Oxygen binding to hemoglobin → conformational shift in heme structure → ↑ oxygen binding affinity → sigmoidal (S-shaped) oxygen-binding affinity/dissociation curve
- **At tissue level**: association process reversed
  - O_2 released → deoxyhemoglobin (dark red blood)
  - 20% of dissolved CO_2 → binds with globin amino acids (not heme group) of deoxyhemoglobin → carbaminohemoglobin

Fetal oxygen transport
- Fetal blood requires higher affinity for oxygen to facilitate movement of O_2 from maternal to fetal blood
- Fetal variant hemoglobin (hemoglobin F)
  - Contains two alpha chains, two gamma chains ($\alpha_2\gamma_2$) → greater affinity for oxygen

OXYGEN-HEMOGLOBIN DISSOCIATION CURVE

osms.it/oxygen-hemoglobin_dissociation_curve

- Proportion of saturated hemoglobin plotted against partial pressure of oxygen
- Illustrates how blood carries, releases oxygen as partial pressures vary
  - *Hemoglobin*: primary oxygen transporter in blood
  - Amount of oxygen bound to hemoglobin at any given time determined by environmental partial pressure of oxygen (high in lungs, lower in tissue capillary beds) → hemoglobin binds to oxygen in lungs, releases at tissue level
  - **Oxyhemoglobin dissociation curve**: determined by hemoglobin affinity for oxygen; rate hemoglobin acquires, releases oxygen into surrounding fluid; plots SO_2 against PO_2

Chapter 71 Respiratory Physiology: Gas Transport

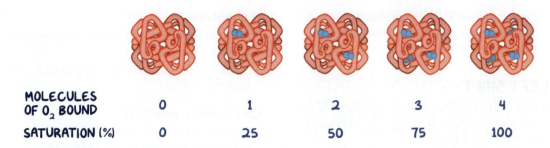

Figure 71.2 Each hemoglobin molecule can bind four O_2 molecules, but each hemoglobin isn't always 100% saturated, or bound, by O_2. A hemoglobin molecule with no O_2 bound (0% saturation) is called deoxyhemoglobin.

SIGMOIDAL SHAPE

- Oxyhemoglobin dissociation curve is sigmoidal
  - Positive cooperativity → each successive oxygen molecule binding to heme group → ↑ affinity
  - Approaches maximum saturation limit → few binding sites remain → little additional binding possible → curve levels off → large ↑ in oxygen partial pressure → no effect on hemoglobin saturation beyond saturation point
  - Partial pressures ↓ at tissue level → oxygen release → with each successive oxygen molecule release, subsequent release eases → rapid oxygen unloading at low partial pressures

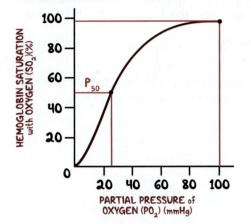

Figure 71.3 The oxygen-hemoglobin dissociation curve. O_2 saturation is influenced by the PO_2 of the blood. P_{50} indicates the partial pressure at which hemoglobin proteins are 50% saturated.

P_{50}

- P_{50}: partial pressure of oxygen in blood when hemoglobin 50% saturated (e.g. 26.6mmHg)
- Conventional measure of hemoglobin affinity for oxygen
- Physiological/disease processes may shift dissociation curve to left/right, alter P_{50}
  - Left shift → lower P_{50} → ↑ oxygen affinity
  - Right shift → raised P_{50} → ↓ oxygen affinity

RIGHT SHIFT

- Right shift → lower oxygen affinity → 50% saturation occurs at higher PO_2 → oxygen unloading

↑ PCO_2, ↓ pH

- ↑ metabolic activity of tissues → ↑ CO_2 → ↑ H^+ concentration → ↓ pH → ↓ hemoglobin oxygen affinity → oxygen unloading in metabolically active tissues
- Effect of PCO_2, pH on oxygen-hemoglobin dissociation curve → Bohr effect

↑ temperature

- Very metabolically active tissue (e.g. active muscle → ↑ heat production → ↓ hemoglobin oxygen affinity)

↑ 2,3-diphosphoglycerate (2,3-DPG) concentration

- 2,3-DPG (glycolysis byproduct) → binds deoxyhemoglobin beta chains → ↓ oxygen affinity → binds to hemoglobin beta chains → oxygen unloading
- 2,3-DPG production ↑ under hypoxic conditions (e.g. living at high altitude) →

hypoxemia → 2,3-DPG production in red blood cells → greater oxygen delivery to tissues

LEFT SHIFT
- Left shift → higher oxygen affinity → 50% saturation occurs at lower PO_2 → impairs oxygen unloading

↓ PCO_2, ↑ pH
- ↓ tissue metabolism → ↓ CO_2 production → ↓ H^+ concentration → ↑ pH → left shift → O_2 tightly bound to hemoglobin

↓ temperature
- ↓ tissue metabolism → ↓ heat production → ↓ O_2 unloading

↓ 2,3-DPG concentration
- ↓ tissue metabolism → ↓ 2,3-DPG concentration → ↓ O_2 unloading

Hemoglobin F
- Alternate molecular structure → ↑ oxygen affinity → left shift
- 2,3-DPG doesn't bind strongly to HbF gamma chains

Carbon monoxide (CO)
- Causes left shift, ↓ maximum saturation possible (curve levels off at lower PO_2)
- CO binds to hemoglobin with 250x affinity of O_2 (at partial pressure; 1/250 O_2, = O_2; CO bound to hemoglobin) → forms carboxyhemoglobin (longer-living molecule than oxyhemoglobin)
- CO binding to heme → confirmation shift → ↑ remaining heme molecules' affinity for oxygen (reducing oxygen release efficiency) → CO poisoning reduces blood's absolute oxygen-carrying capacity, impairs oxygen release → hypoxic injury

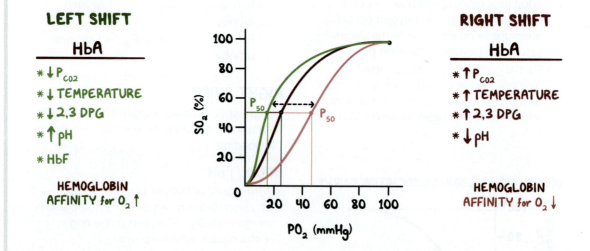

Figure 71.4 Summary of factors that can shift the oxygen-hemoglobin dissociation curve to the left (↑ hemoglobin's affinity for O_2) and to the right (↓ hemoglobin's affinity for O_2).

ERYTHROPOIETIN (EPO)

osms.it/erythropoietin

- Glycoprotein cytokine secreted by kidney (cellular hypoxia response) → stimulates erythropoiesis → RBCs

RENAL INDUCTION OF EPO SYNTHESIS

- ↓ O_2 delivery to kidneys (↓ hemoglobin concentration/PaO_2) → increased production of alpha subunit of hypoxia-inducible factor 1 (HIF1)
- Hypoxia-inducible factor 1-alpha (HIF1A) → acts on fibroblasts in renal cortex, medulla → upregulation of EPO messenger RNA (mRNA) → increased EPO synthesis
- EPO → promotes proerythroblast differentiation → mature to form erythrocytes (maturation not EPO-dependent)

RENAL SENSING OF HYPOXIA

- To effectively regulate EPO secretion, kidneys must distinguish between following:

Decreased blood flow

- → ↓ O_2 availability
  - ↓ renal blood flow → ↓ glomerular filtration → ↓ sodium (Na^+) filtration/reabsorption → ↓ O_2 consumption (Na^+ resorption closely linked to O_2 consumption in kidney)
  - O_2 delivery, consumption remain matched → EPO production not triggered

Decreased arterial blood O_2 content

- → ↓ O_2 availability
  - Renal blood flow remains normal → normal glomerular filtration → normal Na^+ filtration/reabsorption → reduced oxygen availability for given metabolic demand → stimulus for EPO secretion

CARBON DIOXIDE TRANSPORT IN BLOOD

osms.it/carbon-dioxide-transport-in-blood

- Carried as dissolved carbon dioxide (CO_2), carbaminohemoglobin (bound to hemoglobin), bicarbonate (HCO_3^-)

DISSOLVED CO_2

- Small fraction of CO_2 dissolved in blood (similar to oxygen)
- *Henry's law*: CO_2 concentration in blood = partial pressure x solubility of CO_2
- *Solubility*: 0.07mL CO_2/100mL blood per mmHg
- *Partial pressure*: 40mmHg

- Concentration = 2.8mL CO_2/100mL blood (5% of total CO_2 content of blood)

CARBAMINOHEMOGLOBIN

- CO_2 binds to terminal amino groups on proteins (e.g. albumin, hemoglobin)
- CO_2 bound to hemoglobin → carbaminohemoglobin (3% of total blood CO_2)
  - CO_2 binding to hemoglobin at different site than oxygen → conformational shift of protein structure → ↓ oxygen affinity

- → right shift in dissociation curve
- *Haldane effect*: less O_2 bound to hemoglobin → ↑ CO_2 affinity

BICARBONATE
- 90% of CO_2 in blood
- *Tissue level*: CO_2 produced by aerobic metabolism → driven by partial pressure gradient → CO_2 diffuses across cell membrane, capillary wall → enters RBCs

RBC blood pH regulation
- RBCs regulate blood pH via interaction with CO_2 in blood
- RBCs contain enzyme, carbonic anhydrase → catalyzes conversion of CO_2, water → carbonic acid (also catalyzes reverse reaction)
- Carbonic acid dissociates into bicarbonate, hydrogen ion in blood
  - $CO_2 + H_2O \rightleftharpoons H_2CO_3 \rightleftharpoons HCO_3^- + H^+$
  - Mass action drives reaction to right as tissues continuously supply CO_2
- H_2CO_3 dissociates → H^+, HCO_3^-
- H^+ remains in RBCs → buffered by deoxyhemoglobin
- If H^+ remains free in solution → acidifies RBCs, venous blood → H^+ must be buffered
- H^+ buffered by deoxyhemoglobin, carried in venous blood (deoxyhemoglobin more efficient buffer than oxyhemoglobin)
- H^+ production favors oxyhemoglobin conversion → deoxyhemoglobin (Bohr effect)
- HCO_3^- transported into plasma (exchanged for chloride)
  - Band 3 protein facilitates anion exchange of Cl^- for HCO_3^- (chloride shift)
  - HCO_3^- carried in plasma to lungs

Respiratory system blood pH regulation
- Respiratory system further regulates blood pH
  - Controls CO_2 elimination rate → CO_2 elimination ↑ pH by shifting equation to left
  - RBCs, carbonic anhydrase allow rapid reaction in lungs → reverse processes in blood at tissue level

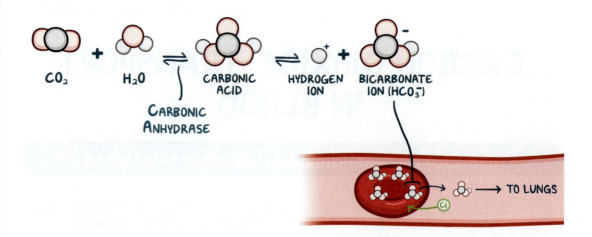

Figure 71.5 CO_2 transport in the form of bicarbonate. CO_2 undergoes a chemical reaction with H_2O to form carbonic acid, which then dissociates into hydrogen ions and bicarbonate ions. This reaction can occur in the plasma, but is sped up in red blood cells by the presence of carbonic anhydrase enzymes. Ionic exchange of bicarbonate ions and chloride occurs via facilitated diffusion to ensure charges stay balanced. Bicarbonate then travels to the lungs in the plasma.

REGULATION OF PULMONARY BLOOD FLOW

osms.it/pulmonary-blood-flow-regulation

- Regulated by altering arteriole resistance → controlled by arteriolar smooth muscle tone
- Regulatory changes mediated by local vasoactive substance concentrations

PULMONARY VASOACTIVE SUBSTANCES & STATES

Nitric oxide (NO)
- Retains similar function on pulmonary vascular beds (compared to systemic) → vasodilation
- Nitric oxide (NO) synthase inhibition → hypoxic vasoconstriction enhancement
- Inhaled NO → reduction in/prevention of hypoxic vasoconstriction

Thromboxane A_2
- Product of arachidonic acid metabolism via cyclooxygenase pathway (macrocytes, leukocytes, endothelial cells)
- Lung injury → potent vasoconstrictor of pulmonary arterioles, veins

Prostaglandin I_2 (prostacyclin)
- Product of arachidonic acid metabolism via cyclooxygenase pathway (endothelium)
- Potent local vasodilator

Leukotrienes
- Product of arachidonic acid metabolism via lipoxygenase pathway
- Potent airway constrictor

LUNG VOLUME
- Pulmonary blood vessels → alveolar capillaries that surround alveoli, extra-alveolar vessels which do not (arteries, veins)

Increased lung volume
- Crushes alveolar capillaries → ↑ resistance to blood flow
- Intrapleural pressure becomes more negative (↓ resistance) → pulls open extra alveolar vessels
- **Total pulmonary vascular resistance**: sum of alveolar, extra-alveolar resistance → increased lung volume effect dependent on larger effect
  - Low lung volumes (extra-alveolar vessels dominate) → ↑ volume → extra-alveolar vessels pulled open → ↓ resistance
  - High lung volume (alveolar capillaries dominate) → ↑ lung volume → alveolar vessels crushed, sharp ↑ resistance

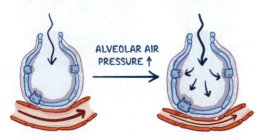
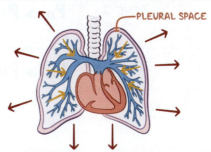

Figure 71.6 Blood vessel resistance associated with increased lung volume.

ZONES OF PULMONARY BLOOD FLOW

osms.it/zones-of-pulmonary-blood-flow

POSITIONAL EFFECT
- Supine gravitational effect largely uniform
- Upright distribution of blood flow (perfusion), ventilation throughout lungs not uniform
- Blood flow favors gravity-dependent lung regions → ↑ pulmonary arterial hydrostatic pressure moving inferiorly → blood flow in inferior (basal) regions > superior (apical) regions
- Ventilation favors apices → ventilation ↓ with move towards bases of lungs

LUNG ZONES
- Lungs divided into three vertical sections (based on pressure differences between compartments)

Zone I
- *Unobserved in healthy lung:* pulmonary arterial pressure (P_a) > alveolar pressure (P_A) in all parts of lung
- P_A generally = atmospheric pressure; can be overcome by low-pressure lung circulation
- Positive pressure ventilation → P_A > P_a in apices of lung → blood vessels collapse → physiological dead space (ventilated, not perfused)

Zone II
- P_a > P_A > pulmonary venous pressure (P_V)
- Capillary compression not problematic
- Perfusion driven by difference between P_a, P_A (not P_a, P_V; as in systemic vascular beds)

Zone III
- Majority of healthy lung volume
- No external resistance to blood flow
- Flow determined by P_a - P_V (both exceed P_A)

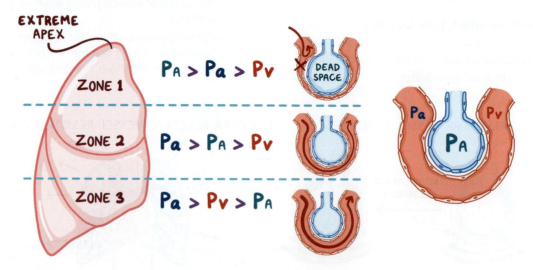

Figure 71.7 Relationships between P_A, P_a, and P_v in the three lung zones.

Chapter 71 Respiratory Physiology: Gas Transport

PULMONARY SHUNTS

osms.it/pulmonary-shunts

- Shunts occur when blood flow redirected from expected route, bypassing circulatory conduit

PHYSIOLOGICAL SHUNTS (ANATOMICALLY NORMAL)

- *Bronchial blood flow*: fraction of pulmonary blood which bypasses alveoli to supply bronchi
- *Coronary blood flow*: thebesian venous network allows for alternative myocardium drainage directly into left ventricle (not reoxygenated)

LEFT-TO-RIGHT SHUNTS

- More common
- Blood shunted from left to right heart
    - Due to septal defects (e.g. trauma, patent ductus arteriosus)
- Blood intended for systemic circulation directly circulated back to lungs → pulmonary blood flow exceeds systemic blood flow → fraction of blood does reach systemic circulation fully oxygenated → no hypoxia

BRONCHIAL BLOOD FLOW

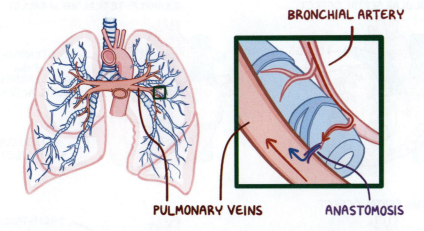

CORONARY BLOOD FLOW

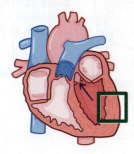
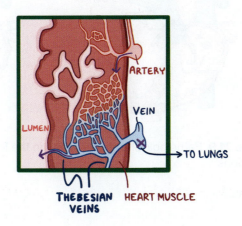

Figure 71.8 Physiologic shunts.

RIGHT-TO-LEFT SHUNTS

- Defect in wall between right, left sides of heart → blood shunted from right to left side of heart
- Allows for large cardiac output fraction to be shunted (approx. 50%) → bypasses lungs → oxygenated blood diluted with shunted deoxygenated blood → hypoxemia
- Not responsive to high P_{O_2} gas treatment → complete pulmonary blood saturation doesn't improve shunted blood oxygenation
- Causes minimal Pa_{CO_2} change → central chemoreceptors responsive to small Pa_{CO_2} increases (shunted blood not available for gas exchange) → ↑ ventilation rate → extra CO_2 expired
- Central O_2 receptors significantly less sensitive than CO_2 receptors → only ↑ ventilation once Pa_{O_2} < 60mmHg

Shunt fraction equation

- Oxygenation bypass of venous blood in lung capillaries
- $Q_S/Q_T = (C_{CO_2} - C_{AO_2})/(C_{CO_2} - C_{VO_2})$
- Q_S: blood flow through right-to-left shunt (L/min)
- Q_T: cardiac output (L/min)
- C_{CO_2}: oxygen content of nonshunted pulmonary capillary blood
- C_{aO_2}: oxygen content of systemic arterial blood
- C_{VO_2}: oxygen content of venous blood

LEFT-TO-RIGHT SHUNTS

VENTRICULAR SEPTAL DEFECT

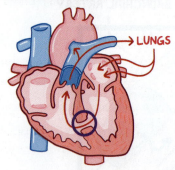

ATRIAL SEPTAL DEFECT

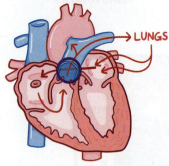

RIGHT-TO-LEFT SHUNTS

EXAMPLE: TETRALOGY of FALLOT

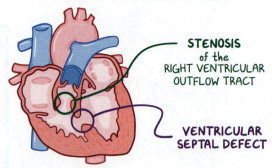

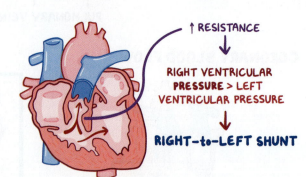

Figure 71.9 Pathologic shunts occurring in the left-to-right (more common) and right-to-left directions.

VENTILATION PERFUSION RATIOS & V Q MISMATCH

osms.it/ventilation-perfusion-ratios-V-Q-mismatch

- Ratio of amount of air to amount of blood reaching alveoli per minute ($\dot{V}/\dot{Q}$ ratio)

IDEAL SCENARIO
- Oxygen provided saturates blood fully → ratio of 1

NORMAL SCENARIO
- Average across entire lung → ratio of 0.8 (apex higher, bases lower)
- Normal breathing rate, tidal volume, cardiac output

DEFECTS
- Mismatching between ventilation, perfusion → abnormal gas exchange

Dead space
- Ventilation of lung regions not perfused
- No gas exchange (no blood to facilitate gas exchange)
- Alveolar gas same composition as humidified inspired air ($P_{A_{O_2}}$ = 150mmHg, $P_{A_{CO_2}}$ = 0)
- Pulmonary embolism

High $\dot{V}/\dot{Q}$
- High ventilation relative to perfusion (ventilation wasted)
- Usually due to ↓ blood flow (limited blood flow → limited gas exchange)
- Relatively high ventilation → pulmonary capillary blood with high P_{O_2}, low P_{CO_2}
- Emphysema

Low $\dot{V}/\dot{Q}$
- Low ventilation relative to perfusion (perfusion wasted)
- Usually due to ↓ ventilation → pulmonary capillary blood with low P_{O_2}, high P_{CO_2}
- Asthma, chronic bronchitis, pulmonary edema, etc.

Right-to-left shunt
- Perfusion of lung regions not ventilated
- No gas exchange occurs (no gas available to exchange)
- Same blood composition as mixed venous blood (Pa_{O_2} = 40mmHg, Pa_{CO_2} = 46mmHg)
- Airway obstruction, right-to-left cardiac shunts, etc.

	NORMAL SCENARIO	PULMONARY EMBOLISM	AIRWAY OBSTRUCTION
$\dot{V}/\dot{Q}$	NORMAL (0.8)	HIGH (can equal ∞)	LOW (can equal zero)
Pa_{O_2}	95 mmHg	N/A	↓ to 40 mmHg
Pa_{CO_2}	40 mmHg	N/A	↑ to 40 mmHg
$P_{A_{O_2}}$	100 mmHg	150 mmHg	N/A
$P_{A_{CO_2}}$	40 mmHg	0 mmHg	N/A

Figure 71.10 Normal $\dot{V}/\dot{Q}$, P_a, and P_A compared to pulmonary embolism and airway obstruction.

HYPOXEMIA & HYPOXIA

osms.it/hypoxemia-and-hypoxia

HYPOXEMIA
- Decrease in arterial Pa_{O_2}

High altitude
- Barometric pressure is decreased → decrease in P_{O_2} of inspired air → decreased PA_{O_2}
- Equilibration of alveolar air, pulmonary capillary blood (normal)
- Systemic arterial blood achieves same (lower) P_{O_2} of alveolar air
- Normal alveolar–arterial (A–a) gradient
- High altitude breathing supplemental O_2 → raised inspired P_{O_2} → raised PA_{O_2} → raised Pa_{O_2}

Hypoventilation
- Less inspired fresh air → decrease in PA_{O_2}
- Normal equilibration → pulmonary capillary blood achieves same (lower) PA_{O_2} as A–a gradient
- **Hyperventilation:** breathing supplemental O_2 → raised PA_{O_2} → raised Pa_{O_2}

Diffusion defects (fibrosis, pulmonary edema)
- Increased diffusion distance/decreased surface area → impaired equilibration
- Normal PA_{O_2}, decreased Pa_{O_2} → ↑ A–a gradient
- Breathing supplemental O_2 → raised PA_{O_2} → increased driving force for diffusion → raised Pa_{O_2}

Ventilation/perfusion mismatches
- Regions of well-ventilated (high PA_{O_2}), poorly-ventilated (low PA_{O_2}), well-perfused, poorly-perfused lung
- Poor perfusion to well-ventilated areas, adequate perfusion to areas poorly ventilated → low Pa_{O_2}
- Supplemental oxygen → raised PA_{O_2} in poorly-ventilated areas with adequate perfusion → increase in Pa_{O_2}
- ↑ A–a gradient

COMMON HYPOXEMIA CAUSES/THEIR EFFECT ON GAS EXCHANGE

CAUSE	PaO_2	A–a GRADIENT	SUPPLEMENTAL O_2 BENEFICIAL?
HIGH ALTITUDE	↓	Normal	Yes
HYPOVENTILATION	↓	Normal	Yes
DIFFUSION DEFECT	↓	↑	Yes
VENTILATION/PERFUSION MISMATCH	↓	↑	Yes
RIGHT-TO-LEFT-SHUNT	↓	↑	↑ shunt severity → ↓ effect

Right-to-left shunts (right-to-left cardiac shunts, intrapulmonary shunts)
- Shunted blood completely bypasses alveoli, cannot equilibrate
- Shunted blood mixes with, "dilutes" blood that did pass through alveoli → ↓ Pa_{O_2} (even if PA_{O_2} normal)
- ↑ A–a gradient
- Limited supplemental O_2 effect → raises PA_{O_2}, Pa_{O_2} of nonshunted blood, does not address underlying shunted blood/ oxygenated blood mixing → larger shunt, less effective supplemental O_2

HYPOXIA
- ↓ O_2 delivery to/utilization by tissues
- O_2 delivery → determined by cardiac output, O_2 content of blood
- ↓ cardiac output/localized blood flow → hypoxia
- Hypoxemia (any cause) → ↓ Pa_{O_2} → ↓ hemoglobin saturation → ↓ oxyhemoglobin concentration in blood → ↓ oxygen delivery to tissues → hypoxia
- Anemia (↓ hemoglobin concentration) → ↓ oxyhemoglobin concentration in blood → decreased oxygen delivery to tissues → hypoxia
- Carbon monoxide poisoning → irreversible binding with hemoglobin → ↓ oxyhemoglobin concentration in blood → ↓ oxygen delivery to tissues → hypoxia
- Cyanide poisoning → interferes with O_2 utilization on cellular level

HYPOXIC VASOCONSTRICTION
- Alveolar partial pressure of oxygen (PA_{O_2}) major factor controlling pulmonary blood flow
- ↓ PA_{O_2} → vasoconstriction (opposite to systemic vasculature where ↓ in Pa_{O_2} → vasodilation)
  - Vasoconstriction in response to poor oxygenation ensures blood flow coupled to areas of good ventilation → optimal gas exchange
  - In localized lung disease, areas of poorly-ventilated, diseased lung circumvented → blood directed towards healthy lung

COMMON HYPOXIA CAUSES/ARTERIAL OXYGENATION STATUS

CAUSE	MECHANISM	PaO2
↓ CARDIAC OUTPUT	↓ blood flow	Equilibrated
HYPOXEMIA	↓ PaO2 ↓ O2 saturation of hemoglobin ↓ O2 content of blood	↓
ANEMIA	↓ hemoglobin concentration ↓ O2 concentration of blood	Equilibrated
CARBON MONOXIDE POISONING	↓ O2 concentration of blood Left shift of O2-hemoglobin curve	Equilibrated
CYANIDE POISONING	↓ O2 utilization of blood	Equilibrated

Alveolar P$_{O_2}$ direct action on vascular smooth muscle → hypoxic vasoconstriction

- Pulmonary microcirculation surrounds alveoli
- O$_2$ highly lipid soluble → permeable across cell membranes
- Normal PA$_{O_2}$ (100mmHg), O$_2$ diffuses from alveoli → arteriolar smooth muscle → maintains relaxation, dilation of arterioles
- PA$_{O_2}$ decreases (70–100mmHg) → vascular smooth muscle sense change (hypoxia) → vasoconstriction → ↓ pulmonary blood flow to region
    - Vasoconstriction mechanism likely due to hypoxia → vascular smooth muscle depolarization → voltage-gated calcium channels open → calcium enters smooth muscle → contraction

HIGH ALTITUDE & HYPOXIC VASOCONSTRICTION

- Entire lung exposed to ↓ PA$_{O_2}$ (e.g. high altitudes) → global ↑ in pulmonary arteriolar resistance → ↑ pulmonary vascular resistance
- Chronic ↑ pulmonary vascular resistance → ↑ right heart afterload → right heart hypertrophy

FETAL HYPOXIC VASOCONSTRICTION

- Fetal circulation must acquire oxygen from maternal circulation via placenta → significantly lower Pa$_{O_2}$ → fetal lung vasoconstriction → reduction of blood flow to lungs (15% of cardiac output)
- At birth low pressure placenta circuit removed → ↑ systemic blood pressure → first breath after birth → ↑ PA$_{O_2}$ → 100mmHg → ↓ hypoxic vasoconstriction → ↓ pulmonary vascular resistance → pulmonary blood flow begins to normalize

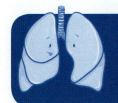

NOTES
NORMAL VARIATIONS

PULMONARY CHANGES DURING EXERCISE

osms.it/pulmonary_changes_during_exercise

RESPIRATORY RESPONSE TO EXERCISE

- Exercise → muscle workload increase → consumption of significant O_2 amounts, above baseline production of CO_2, lactic acid
- Increased O_2 demand → hyperpnea (ventilation increases 10–20x to compensate)
- Hyperpnea vs. hyperventilation
    - **Hyperpnea:** aims to maintain homeostasis → blood O_2, CO_2 levels remain relatively constant
    - **Hyperventilation:** excessive ventilation, blowing off too much CO_2 → low P_{CO2}, respiratory alkalosis
- Exercise-induced ventilation not initially prompted by alterations in blood gases (rising P_{CO2}, declining P_{O2}, pH)
- Ventilation increases abruptly as exercise begins due to neural factors
    - Psychological stimuli (conscious exercise anticipation)
    - Simultaneous cortical motor activation of skeletal muscle, respiratory centers
    - Proprioceptors moving muscles, tendons, joints → stimulate respiratory centers
    - Initial neural regulation → early compensation to exercise as opposed to waiting for change in blood values
- Initial abrupt increase in ventilation is followed by gradual increase (reflective of lung CO_2 delivery rate) → eventually, steady state of ventilation appropriate for intensity achieved
- Exercise cessation → initial small abrupt decline in ventilation (higher neurological stimulation ends) → followed by gradual decrease to pre-exercise respiratory rate (gradual decrease in CO_2 flow to lungs)

PULMONARY CIRCULATORY RESPONSE

- Cardiac output increases to meet tissue O_2 demand → increased right heart output → increased blood flow through pulmonary circulation → increased blood return to left heart → increased output to systemic circulation → increased O_2 tissue delivery
- Exercise → pulmonary resistance decrease → perfusion of more pulmonary capillary beds → more even distribution of pulmonary perfusion, ventilation → improved V/Q ratio (decreased physiological dead space) → increased gas exchange efficiency

HEMATOLOGICAL RESPONSE

Bohr effect
- Hemoglobin's oxygen binding affinity is inversely related to acidity, carbon dioxide concentration
    - Exercise → increased tissue P_{CO2}, decreased tissue pH, increased temperature → right shift of O_2-hemoglobin dissociation curve → decreased affinity of hemoglobin for O_2 → greater unloading of oxygen to exercising muscle

Regulation of blood gases during exercise
- Arterial P_{CO_2}, P_{O_2} remain nearly constant during exercise
- Venous P_{CO_2}, P_{O_2} may change significantly during exercise
    - Ventilation increases sufficiently to blow off all excess CO_2, maintain arterial homeostasis

Anaerobic respiration
- Leads to rise in lactic acid levels
- Not due to inadequate respiratory function
- Alveolar ventilation, pulmonary perfusion remain well matched during exercise → hemoglobin fully saturated
- Cardiac output limitation/limits of skeletal muscle to utilize oxygen → rising lactic acid

RESPIRATORY RESPONSE TO EXERCISE OVERVIEW

	RESPONSE
VENTILATION RATE	↑
PHYSIOLOGIC DEAD SPACE	↓
V/Q RATIO	More equal distribution throughout lungs
PULMONARY BLOOD FLOW, CARDIAC OUTPUT	↑
O_2 CONSUMPTION	↑
CO_2 CONSUMPTION	↑
ARTERIAL P_{O_2}, P_{CO_2}	No change
ARTERIAL pH	Light exercise: no change

PULMONARY CHANGES AT HIGH ALTITUDE & ALTITUDE SICKNESS

osms.it/pulmonary_changes_high_altitude_altitude_sickness

RESPIRATORY RESPONSE TO ALTITUDE

- Humans typically live at altitudes between sea level and 2400m/7800ft
- Altitudes > 2400m/7800ft → lower overall atmospheric pressure → lower P_{O_2} → hemoglobin less saturated at baseline
    - At rest at sea level hemoglobin typically unloads 20–25% O_2 content on a single trip through the circulatory system
    - Significant functional reserve allows for survival due to further hemoglobin unloading when poorly saturated

ACCLIMATIZATION

- Long-term, slow steady move from sea level to higher altitude → respiratory, hematopoietic adaptation
- Decrease in arterial P_{O_2} → peripheral chemoreceptors more responsive to increases in P_{CO_2} → chemoreceptors stimulate medullary inspiratory center → increased breathing rate

Initial (fast) adaptation

- Some changes occur immediately, others over course of days
- Pulmonary
    - Minute ventilation → 2–3L/min higher than sea level
    - Increased ventilation → decreased arterial CO_2 (<40mmHg) → respiratory alkalosis → increased blood pH → inhibition of central, peripheral chemoreceptors → offset increase in ventilation rate (initial effect)
    - As adaptation occurs → HCO_3^- excretion increases → HCO_3^- concentration in cerebrospinal fluid (CSF) decreases → CSF pH decreases toward normal → increased ventilation rate resumes
    - Respiratory alkalosis as result of rapid ascent to high altitude managed with carbonic anhydrase inhibitors → increased HCO_3^- excretion → mild compensatory metabolic acidosis
- Hematological
    - Increase in 2,3-bisphosphoglyceric acid (2,3-BPG) concentration → hemoglobin affinity for O_2 reduced → increased unloading of O_2 at tissue level (also decreases efficiency of oxygen loading in lungs)
- Cardiac
    - Increased heart rate
    - **Right heart hypertrophy:** low P_{O_2} alveolar gas → pulmonary vasculature vasoconstriction → increase in pulmonary vascular resistance → increased right heart strain → right ventricular hypertrophy
- Oxygen conservation
    - Non-essential body functions suppressed → reduction in food digestion efficiency (decreased circulation in favor of perfusing more important organs)

Late (slow) acclimatization

- Occurs over weeks to months
- **Hematological:** hypoxia → kidneys produce more erythropoietin → stimulates bone marrow production of red blood cells → total O_2 carrying capacity of blood increased
    - Essential compensation for living at altitude
    - Increases blood viscosity → greater blood flow resistance → greater heart workload
    - *Full acclimatization:* increase in red blood cell plateaus
- Effect on complete blood count parameters
    - *Total red cells:* ↑
    - *Hemoglobin:* ↑
    - *Hematocrit:* ↑

- Mean corpuscular volume: unchanged
- Mean corpuscular hemoglobin concentration: ↑

Exercise at altitude
- Adaptations normally serve to achieve homeostasis at rest → unless fully acclimatized intense physical activity → homeostasis loss → severe hypoxia
- This transient intentional hypoxia can be exploited by athletes → further adaptive changes to altitude → blood with greater oxygen carrying capacity → improved performance at lower altitude
- Late phase acclimatization of skeletal muscle includes: increased capillary concentration, increased myoglobin amount, increased mitochondria number, increased aerobic metabolism enzyme concentration

PHYSIOLOGICAL ACCLIMATIZATION TO HIGH ALTITUDE OVERVIEW

	RESPONSE
ALVEOLAR P_{O2}	↓ (lower barometric pressure → lower atmospheric P_{O2})
ARTERIAL P_{O2}	↓ (hypoxemia)
ARTERIAL pH	↑ (respiratory alkalosis due to hyperventilation)
HEMOGLOBIN CONCENTRATION	↑ red blood cell concentration
2,3-DPG CONCENTRATION	↑
MUSCLE METABOLISM	↑ efficiency of aerobic metabolism
O_2-HEMOGLOBIN DISSOCIATION CURVE	Right shift (more oxygen unloaded to tissues)
PULMONARY ARTERIAL PRESSURE	↑ (secondary to increased pulmonary vascular resistance)
PULMONARY VASCULAR RESISTANCE	↑ (vasoconstriction)
VENTILATION RATE	↑

ACUTE MOUNTAIN SICKNESS
- AKA altitude sickness
- Commonly associated with altitudes above 2400m/7800ft
  - Minor symptoms may occur at as low as 1500m/5000ft
  - **Death zone**: 5500m/18000ft, altitude considered incompatible with human life; acclimatization not possible
- Caused by sudden transition to altitude without sufficient acclimatization → low atmospheric pressure → low P_{O2} → hypoxia
- Contributing factors
  - Rate of ascent
  - Rate of water vapor loss from lungs
  - Activity level
- Sudden increase in altitude without taking time to acclimatize

Symptoms
- Headache, shortness of breath, nausea, dizziness, peripheral edema

Complications
- Severe complications of high altitude can be fatal
- High altitude pulmonary edema (HAPE)
  - Low atmospheric pressure → decreased oxygen partial pressures, poor oxygenation → increased pulmonary arterial, capillary pressures, idiopathic increase in permeability of vascular endothelium → fluid extravasation → pulmonary edema
- High altitude cerebral edema (HACE)
  - Hypoxia → increased cerebral microvascular permeability, failure of cellular ion pumps → vasogenic, cytotoxic edema

Treatment
- Supplemental oxygen/immediate descent

CREDITS

BIOCHEMISTRY

CARBOHYDRATE METABOLISM
Author: Thomas Bush

Editors: Andrea Day, MA; Lisa Miklush, PhD, RNC, CNS

FAT & CHOLESTEROL METABOLISM
Author: Thomas Bush

Editors: Damien Caissie; Tanner Harding; Ashley Thompson, BS, MD

NUCLEIC ACID METABOLISM
Author: Thomas Bush

Editors: Andrea Day, MA; Lisa Miklush, PhD, RNC, CNS

PROTEIN METABOLISM
Authors: Thomas Bush; Lisa Miklush, PhD, RNC, CNS

Editor: Andrea Day, MA

BIOSTATISTICS & EPIDEMIOLOGY

CAUSATION & VALIDITY
Author: Jorge Trevino-Calderon, MD

Editors: Fergus Baird, MA; Damien Caissie; Kyle Slinn, RN, MEd

COMMUNITY HEALTH
Author: Manuela Rizzo, MD

Editors: Fergus Baird, MA; Kyle Slinn, RN, MEd

EPIDEMIOLOGY MEASURES
Author: Lisa Miklush, PhD, RNC, CNS

Editor: Damien Caissie

INTRODUCTORY BIOSTATISTICS
Authors: Lisa Miklush, PhD, RNC, CNS; Manuela Rizzo, MD

Editors: Damien Caissie; Adleen Crapo, MA; Kyle Slinn, RN, MEd

NON-PARAMETRIC TESTS
Authors: Kaien Gu, BSc; Kath Quayle, PhD

Editors: Fergus Baird, MA; Damien Caissie

PARAMETRIC TESTS
Authors: Kaien Gu, BSc; Kath Quayle, PhD

Editors: Damien Caissie; Kyle Slinn, RN, MEd

STATISTICAL PROBABILITY DISTRIBUTIONS
Author: Kaien Gu, BSc

Editors: Fergus Baird, MA; Damien Caissie; Kyle Slinn, RN, MEd

STUDY DESIGN
Author: Kaien Gu, BSc

Editor: Kyle Slinn, RN, MEd

TESTING
Author: Jorge Treviño-Calderon, MD

Editors: Damien Caissie; Kyle Slinn, RN, MEd

CARDIOVASCULAR PHYSIOLOGY

BLOOD PRESSURE REGULATION
Author: Gordana Sendic

Editors: Fergus Baird, MA; Nahmi Lee; Kyle Slinn, RN, MEd; Ashley Thompson, MD Candidate

CARDIAC CYCLE
Authors: Sandra Hrncic; Lisa Miklush, PhD, RNC, CNS

Editors: Harry Delaney, MBChB; Jessica MacEachern, MA

CARDIAC ELECTROPHYSIOLOGY
Authors: Jorge Treviño-Calderon, MD; Sandra Hrncic

Editors: Andrea Day, MA; Harry Delaney, MBChB; Kyle Slinn, RN, MEd

CARDIOVASCULAR ANATOMY & PHYSIOLOGY
Authors: Jennifer Lee, BS, D.O. Candidate; Sandra Hrncic; Petrie Jansen van Vuuren, M.Sc.

Editors: Fergus Baird, MA; Damien Caissie; Harry Delaney, MBChB; Nahmi Lee; Kyle Slinn, RN, MEd

ELECTROCARDIOGRAPHY
Authors: Jennifer Lee, BS, D.O. Candidate; Kath Quayle, PhD

Editors: Peggy Hamilton; Elizabeth Krupa; Kyle Slinn, RN, MEd

HEMODYNAMICS
Author: Gordana Sendic

Editors: Elizabeth Krupa; Kyle Slinn, RN, MEd

NORMAL VARIATIONS OF THE CARDIOVASCULAR SYSTEM
Author: Kaien Gu, BSc.

Editors: Kyle Slinn, RN, MEd; Ashley Thompson

SPECIFIC CIRCULATIONS
Author: Ioana Tabarcea

Editors: Thomas Bush; Damien Caissie; Harry Delaney, MBChB; Gordana Sendic; Ashley Thompson

THERMOREGULATION

Authors: Pasquale Marra; Lisa Miklush, PhD, RNC, CNS

Editors: Fergus Baird, MA; Kyle Slinn, RN, MEd

CELLULAR PHYSIOLOGY
CELLULAR PATHOLOGY
Author: Thomas Bush

Editors: Andrea Day, MA; Lisa Miklush, PhD, RNC, CNS; Ashley Thompson BS, MD

CELLULAR STRUCTURES & PROCESSES
Authors: Thomas Bush; Nicole Findlay, D.O. Candidate; Lisa Miklush, PhD, RNC, CNS; Gordana Sendic; Petrie Jansen van Vuuren, M.Sc.

Editors: Thomas Bush; Damien Caissie; Paige Cooper, MLIS; Andrea Day, MA; Harry Delaney, MBChB; Lisa Miklush, PhD, RNC, CNS; Gordana Sendic; Kyle Slinn, RN, MEd; Ashley Thompson, MD

DERMATOLOGY
SKIN STRUCTURES
Author: Thomas Bush

Editors: Damien Caissie; Lisa Miklush, PhD, RNC, CNS

EMBRYOLOGY
EARLY WEEKS
Authors: Fergus Baird, MA; Gordana Sendic

Editors: Jessica MacEachern, MA; Kyle Slinn, RN, MEd

GERM LAYERS
Authors: Fergus Baird, MA; Gordana Sendic

Editors: Elizabeth Krupa; Kyle Slinn, RN, MEd

EARLY STRUCTURES
Authors: Fergus Baird, MA; Gordana Sendic

Editors: Elizabeth Krupa; Kyle Slinn, RN, MEd

BODY SYSTEM STRUCTURES
Author: Gordana Sendic

Editors: Andrea Day, MA; Lisa Miklush, PhD, RNC, CNS; Kyle Slinn, RN, MEd

HEAD & NECK STRUCTURE
Author: Gordana Sendic

Editors: Andrea Day, MA; Lisa Miklush, PhD, RNC, CNS; Kyle Slinn, RN, MEd

ENDOCRINE PHYSIOLOGY
ANATOMY & PHYSIOLOGY
Author: Thomas Bush

Editors: Elizabeth Krupa; Lisa Miklush, PhD

PITUITARY HORMONES
Author: Gordana Sendic

Editors: Elizabeth Krupa; Kyle Slinn, RN, MEd

ADRENAL HORMONES
Authors: Sandra Hrncic; Lisa Miklush, PhD, RNC, CNS

Editors: Elizabeth Krupa; Ashley Thompson

PANCREATIC HORMONES
Author: Gordana Sendic

Editors: Harry Delaney, MBChB; Elizabeth Krupa

CALCIUM & PHOSPHATE HORMONAL REGULATION
Author: Petrie Jansen van Vuuren, M.Sc.

Editors: Damien Caissie; Lisa Miklush, PhD, RNC, CNS

GASTROINTESTINAL PHYSIOLOGY
ANATOMY & PHYSIOLOGY
Authors: Jennifer Lee, BS, D.O. Candidate; Ashley Thompson

Editors: Andrea Day, MA; Elizabeth Krupa; Lisa Miklush, PhD, RNC, CNS; Ashley Thompson

GASTROINTESTINAL FUNCTION
Authors: Jennifer Lee, BS, D.O. Candidate; Ashley Thompson

Editors: Andrea Day, MA; Elizabeth Krupa; Lisa Miklush, PhD, RNC, CNS; Gordana Sendic

UPPER GASTROINTESTINAL TRACT
Author: Ashley Thompson

Editors: Elizabeth Krupa; Lisa Miklush, PhD, RNC, CNS

DIGESTION & ABSORPTION
Authors: Jennifer Lee, BS, D.O. Candidate; Ashley Thompson

Editors: Damien Caissie; Andrea Day, MA; Elizabeth Krupa; Lisa Miklush, PhD, RNC, CNS; Gordana Sendic

LIVER, GALL, BLADDER, & PANCREAS
Author: Jennifer Lee, BS, D.O. Candidate

Editors: Harry Delaney, MBChB; Jessica MacEachern, MA

GENETICS
POPULATION GENETICS
Author: Thomas Bush

Editors: Andrea Day, MA; Lisa Miklush, PhD, RNC, CNS; Ashley Thompson, BS, MD

TRANSCRIPTION, TRANSLATION, & REPLICATION
Author: Thomas Bush

Editors: Andrea Day, MA; Jessica MacEachern, MA; Lisa Miklush PhD; Ashley Thompson BS, MD

Credits

HEMATOLOGY

BLOOD COMPONENTS & FUNCTION
Author: Thomas Bush

Editors: Lyndsay Day, MA; Lisa Miklush, PhD, RNC, CNS

IMMUNOLOGY

B & T CELLS
Author: Thomas Bush

Editors: Jessica MacEachern, MA; Ashley Thompson, BS, MD

CONTRACTION OF THE IMMUNE RESPONSE
Author: Thomas Bush

Editors: Jessica MacEachern, MA; Lisa Miklush, PhD, RNC, CNS

IMMUNE SYSTEM
Author: Thomas Bush

Editors: Jessica MacEachern, MA; Lisa Miklush, PhD, RNC, CNS

INNATE IMMUNITY
Author: Thomas Bush

Editors: Damien Caissie; Lisa Miklush, PhD, RNC, CNS

MUSCULOSKELETAL PHYSIOLOGY

BONES, JOINTS, & CARTILAGE
Author: Thomas Bush

Editors: Andrea Day, MA; Lyndsay Day, MA; Jessica MacEachern, MA; Lisa Miklush, PhD, RNC, CNS; Ashley Thompson

MUSCLES
Author: Thomas Bush

Editors: Andrea Day, MA; Jessica MacEachern, MA; Lisa Miklush, PhD, RNC, CNS

NEUROLOGY

ANATOMY & PHYSIOLOGY
Authors: Thomas Bush; Jennifer Lee, BS, D.O. Candidate

Editors: Thomas Bush; Andrea Day, MA; Harry Delaney, MBChB; Jessica MacEachern, MA; Lisa Miklush, PhD, RNC, CNS; Gordana Sendic; Kyle Slinn, RN, MEd; Ashley Thompson, BS, MD

AUTONOMIC NERVOUS SYSTEM
Author: Gordana Sendic

Editors: Harry Delaney, MBChB; Paige Cooper, MLIS

BLOOD BRAIN BARRIER & CSF
Author: Pasquale Marra

Editors: Thomas Bush; Gordana Sendic

BRAIN FUNCTIONS
Author: Kaien Gu, BSc

Editors: Paige Cooper, MLIS; Lisa Miklush, PhD, RNC, CNS; Gordana Sendic

MOTOR NERVOUS SYSTEM
Author: Petrie Jansen van Vuuren, M.Sc.

Editor: Lyndsay Day, MA; Ashley Thompson

SENSORY NERVOUS SYSTEM
Authors: Thomas Bush; Lisa Miklush, PhD

Editors: Andrea Day, MA; Lisa Miklush, PhD, RNC, CNS

SPINAL CORD & NERVES
Author: Thomas Bush

Editors: Paige Cooper, MLIS; Lisa Miklush, PhD, RNC, CNS

RENAL PHYSIOLOGY

ACID-BASE PHYSIOLOGY
Author: Thomas Bush

Editors: Damien Caissie; Lisa Miklush, PhD, RNC, CNS

ANATOMY & PHYSIOLOGY
Author: Thomas Bush

Editors: Nahmi Lee; Lisa Miklush, PhD, RNC, CNS

FLUIDS IN THE BODY
Author: Thomas Bush

Editors: Nahmi Lee; Lisa Miklush, PhD, RNC, CNS

RENAL BLOOD FLOW REGULATION
Author: Thomas Bush

Editors: Jessica MacEachern, MA; Lisa Miklush, PhD, RNC, CNS

RENAL ELECTROLYTE REGULATION
Authors: Thomas Bush; Lisa Miklush, PhD, RNC, CNS

Editors: Damien Caissie; Andrea Day, MA

RENAL REABSORPTION & SECRETION
Authors: Thomas Bush; Lisa Miklush, PhD, RNC, CNS

Editor: Jessica MacEachern, MA

WATER REGULATION
Author: Thomas Bush

Editors: Nahmi Lee; Jessica MacEachern, MA; Lisa Miklush, PhD, RNC, CNS

REPRODUCTIVE PHYSIOLOGY

FEMALE REPRODUCTIVE SYSTEM
Authors: Thomas Bush; Lisa Miklush, PhD, RNC, CNS

Editors: Jessica MacEachern, MA; Ashley Thompson, BS, MD

MALE REPRODUCTIVE SYSTEM
Authors: Thomas Bush; Pasquale Marra

Editors: Harry Delaney, MBChB; Jessica MacEachern, MA; Lisa Miklush, PhD, RNC, CNS

SEXUAL DEVELOPMENT
Author: Jorge Trevino-Calderon, MD

Editors: Damien Caissie; Andrea Day, MA; Nahmi Lee; Lisa Miklush, PhD, RNC, CNS; Gordana Sendic

RESPIRATORY PHYSIOLOGY
ANATOMY & PHYSIOLOGY
Author: Jennifer Lee, BS, D.O. Candidate

Editors: Damien Caissie; Kyle Slinn, RN, MEd

BREATHING MECHANICS
Author: Lisa Miklush, PhD, RNC, CNS

Editor: Damien Caissie

BREATHING REGULATION
Author: Chris Brasel, PhD

Editors: Jessica MacEachern, MA; Lisa Miklush, PhD, RNC, CNS; Ashley Thompson

GAS EXCHANGE
Author: Petrie Jansen van Vuuren, M.Sc.

Editors: Ashley Thompson, Elizabeth Krupa

GAS TRANSPORT
Author: Petrie Jansen van Vuuren, M.Sc.

Editors: Damien Caissie; Jessica MacEachern, MA; Ashley Thompson

NORMAL VARIATIONS
Author: Petrie Jansen van Vuuren, M.Sc.

Editors: Elizabeth Krupa, Ashley Thompson

SOURCES

BIOCHEMISTRY

CARBOHYDRATE METABOLISM
Osmosis. Citric acid cycle.

Osmosis. Electron transport chain and oxidative phosphorylation.

Osmosis. Gluconeogenesis.

Osmosis. Glycogen metabolism.

Osmosis. Glycolysis.

Osmosis. Pentose phosphate pathway.

FAT & CHOLESTEROL METABOLISM
Osmosis. Cholesterol metabolism.

Osmosis. Fatty acid oxidation.

Osmosis. Fatty acid synthesis.

Osmosis. Ketone body metabolism.

NUCLEIC ACID METABOLISM
Osmosis. Nucleotide metabolism.

PROTEIN METABOLISM
Osmosis. Amino acids and protein folding.

Osmosis. Amino acid synthesis.

Osmosis. Enzyme function.

Osmosis. Nitrogen and urea cycle.

BIOSTATISTICS & EPIDEMIOLOGY

CAUSATION & VALIDITY
Gordis, L. (2014). *Epidemiology* (5 edition). Philadelphia, PA: Elsevier Saunders.

COMMUNITY HEALTH
Gordis, L. (2014). *Epidemiology* (5th ed.). Philadelphia, PA: Elsevier Saunders.

EPIDEMIOLOGY MEASURES
Gordis, L. (2014). *Epidemiology* (5 edition). Philadelphia, PA: Elsevier Saunders.

Osmosis. DALY and QALY.

Osmosis. Direct standardization.

Osmosis. Incidence and prevalence.

Osmosis. Indirect standardization.

Osmosis. Measures of risk.

Osmosis. Mortality rates.

Osmosis. Odds ratio.

The Global Burden of Disease concept. (n.d.). In WHO. Retrieved October 16, 2018, from http://www.who.int/quantifying_ehimpacts/publications/en/9241546204chap3.pdf

INTRODUCTORY BIOSTATISTICS
Osmosis. Descriptive statistics.

Osmosis. Introduction to biostatistics.

Osmosis. Mean, median, and mode

Osmosis. Probability

Osmosis. Range, variance, and standard deviation

Osmosis. Types of data

Weaver, A. & Goldberg, S. (2012). *Clinical Biostatistics and Epidemiology Made Ridiculously Simple*. Miami, FL: MedMaster, Inc.

NON-PARAMETRIC TESTS
Weaver, A. & Goldberg, S. (2012). *Clinical Biostatistics and Epidemiology Made Ridiculously Simple*. Miami, FL: MedMaster, Inc.

PARAMETRIC TESTS
Weaver, A. & Goldberg, S. (2012). *Clinical Biostatistics and Epidemiology Made Ridiculously Simple*. Miami, FL: MedMaster.

STATISTICAL PROBABILITY DISTRIBUTIONS
Gordis, L. (2014). *Epidemiology*. Philadelphia, PA: Elsevier/Saunders.

McClave, J. T. & Sincich, T. (2017). *Statistics*. Boston, MA: Pearson.

Weaver, A. & Goldberg, S. (2012). *Clinical Biostatistics and Epidemiology Made Ridiculously Simple*. Miami, FL: MedMaster, Inc.

STUDY DESIGN
Gordis, L. (2014). *Epidemiology*. Philadelphia, PA: Elsevier/Saunders.

LaMorte, W. W. (2016). Blinding (Masking), Placebos, and Shams. In *Boston University School of Public Health*. Retrieved September 24, 2017, from http://sphweb.bumc.bu.edu/otlt/MPH-Modules/EP/EP713_ClinicalTrials/EP713_ClinicalTrials5.html

LaMorte, W. W. (2017). Overview of Analytic Studies. In *Boston University School of Public Health*. Retrieved September 24, 2017, from http://sphweb.bumc.bu.edu/otlt/mph-modules/ep/ep713_analyticoverview/ep713_analyticoverview3.html

McClave, J. T. & Sincich, T. (2017). *Statistics*. Boston: Pearson.

STAT507: Epidemiological Research Methods: Lesson 6: Ecological Studies, Case-Control Studies. (n.d.). Retrieved September 24, 2017, from https://onlinecourses.science.psu.edu/stat507/06/intro

Weaver, A. & Goldberg, S. (2012). *Clinical Biostatistics and Epidemiology Made Ridiculously Simple*. Miami, FL: MedMaster, Inc.

TESTING
Gordis, L. (2015). *Epidemiology*. (5 edition). Philadelphia, PA: Elsevier Saunders.

Le, T., Bhushan, V., Sochat, M., & Chavda, Y. (2017). *First Aid for the USMLE Step 1 2017* (27 edition). New York, NY: McGraw-Hill Education / Medical.

Weaver, A. & Goldberg, S. (2012). *Clinical Biostatistics and Epidemiology Made Ridiculously Simple*. Miami, FL: MedMaster, Inc.

CARDIOVASCULAR PHYSIOLOGY
BLOOD PRESSURE REGULATION

Cardiovascular system: blood vessels. (n.d.). In *Lumen Learning*. Retrieved September 23, 2017, from https://courses.lumenlearning.com/boundless-ap/

Costanzo, L. S. (2017). *Physiology* (6 edition). Philadelphia, PA: Elsevier.

Marieb, E. N. & Hoehn, K. (2013). *Human Anatomy & Physiology* (9 edition). London, UK: Pearson.

CARDIAC CYCLE

Costanzo, L. S. (2017). *Physiology* (6 edition). Philadelphia, PA: Elsevier.

Hall, J. E. & Guyton, A. C. (2011). *Guyton and Hall Textbook of Medical Physiology* (12 edition). Philadelphia, PA: Saunders Elsevier.

Koeppen, B. M. & Stanton, B A. (2018). *Berne & Levy Physiology* (7 edition). Philadelphia, PA: Elsevier.

CARDIAC ELECTROPHYSIOLOGY

Costanzo, L. S. (2017). *Physiology* (6 edition). Philadelphia, PA: Elsevier.

Marieb, E. N. & Hoehn, K. (2013). *Human Anatomy & Physiology* (9 edition). London, UK: Pearson.

Hall, J. E. & Guyton, A. C. (2011). *Guyton and Hall Textbook of Medical Physiology*. Philadelphia, PA: Saunders Elsevier.

Osmosis. Action potentials in pacemaker cells.

Osmosis: Action potentials in myocytes.

Smith, T. W. & Morgan, J. P. (2015.). Excitation-contraction coupling in myocardium. In *UpToDate*. Retrieved August 2, 2018, from https://www.uptodate.com/contents/excitation-contraction-coupling-in-myocardium

CARDIOVASCULAR ANATOMY & PHYSIOLOGY

Agabegi, S. S. & Agabegi, E. D. (2016). *Step-Up to Medicine* (4 edition). Philadelphia, PA: Wolters Kluwer.

Aortic stenosis and aortic regurgitation. (2014). In *Khan Academy*. Retrieved July 18, 2018, from https://youtu.be/3t1n5szXriQ

Dennis, M., Bowen, W. T., & Cho, L. (2012). *Mechanisms of Clinical Signs* (1 edition). Chatswood, NSW: Elsevier Australia.

How to identify murmurs. (2014). In *Khan Academy*. Retrieved July 18, 2018, from https://youtu.be/sGHV5_ieDP4

Marieb, E. N. & Hoehn, K. (2013). *Human Anatomy & Physiology* (9 edition). London, UK: Pearson.

Mescher, A. L. (2013). *Junqueira's Basic Histology: Text & Atlas* (13 edition). New York, NY: McGraw Hill Medical.

Mitral valve regurgitation and mitral valve prolapse. (2014). In *Khan Academy*. Retrieved July 18, 2018, from https://youtu.be/Bjnw_jwDt1Q

Mitral stenosis. 2014). In *Khan Academy*. Retrieved October 21, 2014, from https://youtu.be/0k0iKKF2-Do

Osmosis. Anatomy & physiology of the circulatory system (heart).

Osmosis. Aortic valve disease (bicuspid, tricuspid) - stenosis, regurgitation, symptoms.

Osmosis. Mitral valve disease (regurgitation, stenosis) - causes, symptoms & pathology.

Osmosis. Pulmonic valve disease - causes, symptoms, diagnosis, treatment, pathology.

Osmosis. Tricuspid valve disease - causes, symptoms, diagnosis, treatment, pathology.

Strong, E. (2012). Heart Murmurs. [Course notes]

Strong, E. (2012). Heart Sounds. [Course notes]

Systolic murmurs, diastolic murmurs, and extra heart sounds - Part 1. (2014). In *Khan Academy*. Retrieved July 18, 2018, from https://youtu.be/6YY3OOPmUDA

Systolic murmurs, diastolic murmurs, and extra heart sounds - Part 2. (2014). In *Khan Academy*. Retrieved July 18, 2018, from https://youtu.be/ZUHpAaVpiY8

Valvular heart disease causes. (2014). In *Khan Academy*. Retrieved July 18, 2018, from https://youtu.be/R4qy9beFpHw

Valvular heart disease diagnosis and treatment. (2014). In *Khan Academy*. Retrieved July 18, 2018, from https://youtu.be/8HSeHRGihkY

What is Lymph? (n.d.). In *Khan Academy*. Retrieved November 24, 2017, from https://www.khanacademy.org/science/health-and-medicine/human-anatomy-and-physiology/lymphatics/v/what-is-lymph

What is valvular heart disease? (2014). In *Khan Academy*. Retrieved July 18, 2018, from https://www.youtube.com/watch?v=Wyxz0fgp6-A

ELECTROCARDIOGRAPHY

Dubin, D. (2000). *Rapid interpretation of EKG's: an interactive course*. Cover Publishing Company (6 edition). Tampa, FL: Cover Publishing.

O'Keefe, J. H., Hammill, S. C., Freed, M. S., & Pogwizd, S. M. (2009) *The Complete Guide to ECGs—A Comprehensive Study Guide to Improve ECG Interpretation Skills* (3 edition). Sudbury, MA: Jones and Bartlett Publishers.

HEMODYNAMICS

Boundless Anatomy and Physiology. (n.d.) In *Lumen Learning*. Retrieved January 29, 2019, from https://courses.lumenlearning.com/boundless-ap/

Costanzo, L. S. (2017). *Physiology* (6 edition). Philadelphia, PA: Elsevier.

Marieb, E. N. & Keller, S. M. (2013). *Human Anatomy & Physiology* (12 edition). NY, NY: Pearson

Osmosis. Blood flow, pressure and resistance.

Osmosis. Compliance of blood vessels.

Osmosis. Laminar flow and Reynold number.

Osmosis. Pressures in the cardiovascular system.

Osmosis. Resistance to blood flow.

NORMAL VARIATIONS OF THE CARDIOVASCULAR SYSTEM

Costanzo, L. S. (2014). *Physiology* (5 edition). Philadelphia, PA:

Saunders/Elsevier.

SPECIFIC CIRCULATIONS
Costanzo, L. S. (2017). *Physiology* (6 edition). Philadelphia, PA: Elsevier.

Marieb, E. N. & Hoehn, K. (2013). *Human Anatomy & Physiology* (9 edition). London, UK: Pearson.

THERMOREGULATION
Corneli, H. M. (2018). Hypothermia in children: Clinical manifestations and diagnosis. In *UpToDate*. Retrieved January 29, 2019, from https://www.uptodate.com/contents/hypothermia-in-children-clinical-manifestations-and-diagnosis

Costanzo, L. S. (2017). *Physiology* (6 edition). Philadelphia, PA: Elsevier.

Helman, R. S. (2017). Heat stroke. In *Medscape*. Retrieved September 29, 2017, from http://emedicine.medscape.com/article/166320-overview#a6

Marieb, E. N., & Hoehn, K. (2013). *Human Anatomy & Physiology* (9 edition). Boston, MA: Pearson.

Rosenberg, H., Pollock, N., Schiemann, A., Bulger, T., & Stowell, K. (2015). Malignant hyperthermia: a review. *Orphanet Journal of Rare Diseases 10(93)*. Retrieved October 31, 2017, from https://www.ncbi.nlm.nih.gov/pubmed/26238698

Zafren, K., & Mechem, C. C. (2018). Accidental hypothermia in adults. In *UpToDate*. Retrieved January 29, 2019, from https://www.uptodate.com/contents/accidental-hypothermia-in-adults

CELLULAR PHYSIOLOGY
CELLULAR PATHOLOGY
Osmosis. Atrophy, aplasia, and hypoplasia.

Osmosis. Free radicals and cellular injury.

Osmosis. Hyperplasia and hypertrophy.

Osmosis. Inflammation.

Osmosis. Ischemia.

Osmosis. Metaplasia and dysplasia.

Osmosis. Necrosis and apoptosis.

Osmosis. Oncogenes and tumor suppressor genes.

CELLULAR STRUCTURES & PROCESSES
Costanzo, L. S. (2017). *Physiology* (6 edition). Philadelphia, PA: Elsevier.

Marieb, E. N. & Hoehn, K. (2013). *Human Anatomy & Physiology* (9 edition). London, UK: Pearson.

Osmosis. Amino acids and protein folding.

Osmosis. Cell-cell junctions.

Osmosis. Cellular structures and functions.

Osmosis. Common cell signalling pathways.

Osmosis. Cytoskeleton and intracellular motility.

Osmosis. Endocytosis and exocytosis.

Osmosis. Nuclear structures.

Osmosis. Osmosis.

Osmosis. Resting membrane potential.

Osmosis. Selective permeability of the cell membrane.

Structure of a cell. (n.d.). In *Khan Academy*. Retrieved March 20, 2018, from https://www.khanacademy.org/science/biology/structure-of-a-cell

DERMATOLOGY
SKIN STRUCTURES
Osmosis. Hair, skin, and nails.

Osmosis. Skin anatomy and physiology.

Osmosis. Wound healing.

EMBRYOLOGY
EARLY WEEKS
Marieb, E. N. & Keller, S. M. (2013). *Essentials of Human Anatomy & Physiology* (9 edition). NY, NY: Pearson

Osmosis. Human development days 1-4.

Osmosis. Human development week 2.

Osmosis. Human development week 3.

Sadler, T. W. (2015). *Langman's Medical Embryology* (13 edition). Philadelphia: Wolters Kluwer Health/Lippincott Williams & Wilkins

GERM LAYERS
Marieb, E. N. & Keller, S. M. (2013). *Essentials of Human Anatomy & Physiology* (9 edition). NY, NY: Pearson

Osmosis. Ectoderm - derivatives of the germ layers.

Osmosis. Endoderm - derivatives of the germ layers.

Osmosis. Mesoderm - derivatives of the germ layers.

Sadler, T. W. (2015). *Langman's Medical Embryology* (13 edition). Philadelphia: Wolters Kluwer Health/Lippincott Williams & Wilkins

EARLY STRUCTURES
Marieb, E. N. & Keller, S. M. (2013). *Essentials of Human Anatomy & Physiology* (9 edition). NY, NY: Pearson

Osmosis. Development of the digestive system and body cavities.

Osmosis. Development of the fetal membranes.

Osmosis. Development of the placenta.

Osmosis. Development of the umbilical cord.

Osmosis. Development of twins.

Sadler, T. W. (2015). *Langman's Medical Embryology* (13 edition). Philadelphia: Wolters Kluwer Health/Lippincott Williams & Wilkins

BODY SYSTEM STRUCTURES
Dudek, R. W. (2014). *Embryology* (6 edition). Philadelphia: Wolters Kluwer Health.

Marieb, E. N. & Hoehn, K. (2013). *Human Anatomy & Physiology* (9 edition). London, UK: Pearson.

Osmosis. Development of the cardiovascular system.

Osmosis. Development of the gastrointestinal system.

Osmosis. Development of the muscular system.

Osmosis. Development of the renal system.

Osmosis. Development of the reproductive system.

Osmosis. Development of the respiratory system.

Osmosis. Development of the skeletal system.

Osmosis. Fetal circulation.

Sadler, T. W. (2014). *Langman's Medical Embryology* (13 edition). Philadelphia: Wolters Kluwer Health.

HEAD & NECK STRUCTURE
Dudek, R. W. (2014). *Embryology* (6 edition). Philadelphia: Wolters Kluwer Health.

Marieb, E. N. & Hoehn, K. (2013). *Human Anatomy & Physiology* (9 edition). London, UK: Pearson.

Osmosis. Tongue, pharyngeal arches, pouches and clefts

Sadler, T. W. (2014). *Langman's Medical Embryology* (13 edition). Philadelphia: Wolters Kluwer Health.

ENDOCRINE PHYSIOLOGY
ANATOMY & PHYSIOLOGY
Osmosis. Endocrine anatomy and physiology.

The pancreas. (n.d.). In *Lumen Learning*. Retrieved January 6, 2017, from https://courses.lumenlearning.com/boundless-ap/chapter/the-pancreas/

PITUITARY HORMONES
Costanzo, L. S. (2017). *Physiology* (6 edition). Philadelphia, PA: Elsevier

Growth hormone receptor signalling. (n.d.). In *Wikipathways*. Retrieved February 1, 2018, from https://www.wikipathways.org/index.php/Pathway:WP2657

Osmosis. Growth hormone and somatostatin.

ADRENAL HORMONES
Costanzo, L. S. (2017). *Physiology* (6 edition). Philadelphia, PA: Elsevier.

Hall, J. E., & Guyton, A. C. (2011). *Guyton and Hall Textbook of Medical Physiology*. (12 edition) Philadelphia, PA: Saunders Elsevier.

PANCREATIC HORMONES
Costanzo, L. S. (2017). *Physiology* (6 edition). Philadelphia, PA: Elsevier

CALCIUM & PHOSPHATE HORMONAL REGULATION
Costanzo, L. S. (2017). *Physiology* (6 edition). Philadelphia, PA: Elsevier.

Marieb, E. N. & Hoehn, K. (2013). *Human Anatomy & Physiology* (9 edition). London, UK: Pearson Education.

Osmosis. Calcitonin.

Osmosis. Parathyroid hormone.

Osmosis. Vitamin D.

GASTROINTESTINAL PHYSIOLOGY
ANATOMY & PHYSIOLOGY
Copstead, L.E. & Banasik, J. L. (2013). *Pathophysiology* (5 edition). St. Louis, MO: Elsevier.

Costanzo, L. S. (2017). *Physiology* (6 edition). Philadelphia, PA. Elsevier.

Hall, J. E. & Guyton, A. C. (2011). *Guyton and Hall Textbook of Medical Physiology.* (12 edition). Philadelphia, PA: Saunders Elsevier

Lieberman, M., Marks, A., Peet, A., & Chansky, M. (2013). *Marks' Basic Medical Biochemistry: A Clinical Approach.* (4 edition). Baltimore, MD: Wolters Kluwer Health/Lippincott Williams & Wilkins.

Marieb, E. N. & Hoehn, K. (2013). *Human Anatomy & Physiology* (9 edition). London: Pearson.

Osmosis. Small Intestinal Motility.

GASTROINTESTINAL FUNCTION
Copstead, L.E. & Banasik, J. L. (2013). *Pathophysiology* (5 edition). St. Louis, MO: Elsevier.

Costanzo, L. S. (2017). *Physiology* (6 edition). Philadelphia, PA: Elsevier.

Hall, J. E. & Guyton, A. C. (2011). *Guyton and Hall Textbook of Medical Physiology.* (12 edition). Philadelphia, PA: Saunders Elsevier.

Lieberman, M., Marks, A., Peet, A., Chansky, M.. (2013). *Marks' Basic Medical Biochemistry: A Clinical Approach.* (4 edition). Baltimore: Wolters Kluwer Health/Lippincott Williams & Wilkins,.

Marieb, E. N. & Hoehn, K. (2013). *Human Anatomy & Physiology* (9 edition). London: Pearson.

Osmosis. Small Intestinal Motility.

UPPER GASTROINTESTINAL TRACT
Costanzo, L. S. (2017). *Physiology* (6 edition). Philadelphia, PA: Elsevier.

Marieb, E. N. & Hoehn, K. (2013). *Human Anatomy & Physiology* (9 edition). London, UK: Pearson.

Osmosis. Chewing, Swallowing, and Salivary secretion.

Osmosis. Esophageal Motility.

Osmosis. Gastric Motility and Secretions.

DIGESTION & ABSORPTION
Copstead, L.E., & Banasik, J. L. (2013). *Pathophysiology* (5 edition). St. Louis, MO: Elsevier.

Costanzo, L. S. (2017). *Physiology* (6 edition). Philadelphia, PA: Elsevier.

Hall, J. E., & Guyton, A. C. (2011). *Guyton and Hall Textbook of Medical Physiology.* (12 edition). Philadelphia, PA: Saunders Elsevier.

Lieberman, M., Marks, A., Peet, A., & Chansky, M. (2013). *Marks' Basic Medical Biochemistry: A Clinical Approach.* (4 edition). Baltimore: Wolters Kluwer Health/Lippincott Williams & Wilkins.

Marieb, E. N. & Hoehn, K. (2013). *Human Anatomy & Physiology* (9 edition). London: Pearson.

Osmosis. Small Intestinal Motility.

LIVER, GALL, BLADDER, & PANCREAS
Copstead, L.E. & Banasik, J. L. (2013). *Pathophysiology* (5 edition.). St. Louis, MO: Elsevier.

Costanzo, L. S. (2017). *Physiology* (6 edition). Philadelphia, PA: Elsevier.

Hall, J. E. & Guyton, A. C. (2011). *Guyton and Hall Textbook of Medical Physiology* (12 edition). Philadelphia, PA: Saunders Elsevier.

Lieberman, M., Marks, A., Peet, A., & Chansky, M. (2013). *Marks' Basic Medical Biochemistry: A Clinical Approach*. Baltimore: Wolters Kluwer Health/Lippincott Williams & Wilkins.

Marieb, E. N. & Hoehn, K. (2013). *Human Anatomy & Physiology* (9 edition). London: Pearson.

GENETICS
POPULATION GENETICS
Osmosis. DNA mutations.

Osmosis. Evolution and natural selection.

Osmosis. Gel electrophoresis.

Osmosis. Gene regulation.

Osmosis. Hardy-Weinberg equilibrium.

Osmosis. Independent assortment of genes and linkage.

Osmosis. Inheritance patterns.

Osmosis. Lac operon.

Osmosis. Mendelian genetics and punnett squares.

Osmosis. Mitosis and meiosis.

Osmosis. Polymerase chain reaction.

TRANSCRIPTION, TRANSLATION, & REPLICATION
DNA cloning and recombinant DNA | Biomolecules | MCAT | Khan Academy. (2016). In *Khan Academy*. Retrieved July 24, 2018, from https://www.youtube.com/watch?v=5ffl-0OYVQU

Osmosis. DNA damage and repair.

Osmosis. DNA mutations.

Osmosis. DNA replication.

Osmosis. DNA structure.

Osmosis. Transcription.

Osmosis. Translation.

HEMATOLOGY
BLOOD COMPONENTS & FUNCTION
Osmosis. Blood components.

Osmosis. Blood groups and transfusions.

Osmosis. Clot retraction and fibrinolysis.

Osmosis. Coagulation (secondary hemostasis).

Osmosis. Platelet plug formation (primary hemostasis).

Osmosis. Role of Vitamin L in coagulation.

IMMUNOLOGY
B & T CELLS
Osmosis. B cell development.

Osmosis. T cell development.

CONTRACTION OF THE IMMUNE RESPONSE
Osmosis. B and T cell memory.

Osmosis. Contracting the immune response and peripheral tolerance.

IMMUNE SYSTEM
Osmosis. Introduction to the immune system.

Osmosis. Vaccines.

INNATE IMMUNITY
Osmosis. Innate immunity.

Osmosis. The complement system.

MUSCULOSKELETAL PHYSIOLOGY
BONES, JOINTS, & CARTILAGE
Osmosis. Bone remodeling and repair.

Osmosis. Cartilage.

Osmosis. Fibrous, cartilage, and synovial joints.

Osmosis. Skeletal system anatomy and physiology.

MUSCLES
Osmosis. ATP and muscle contraction.

Osmosis. Neuromuscular junction and motor unit.

Osmosis. Skeletal system anatomy and physiology.

Osmosis. Sliding filament model of muscle contraction.

Osmosis. Slow twitch and fast twitch muscle fibers.

NEUROLOGY
ANATOMY & PHYSIOLOGY
Copstead, L.E. & Banasik, J. L. (2013). *Pathophysiology* (5 edition). St. Louis, MO: Elsevier.

Costanzo, L. S. (2017). *Physiology* (6 edition). Philadelphia, PA: Elsevier.

Hall, J. E. & Guyton, A. C. (2011). *Guyton and Hall Textbook of Medical Physiology* (12 edition). Philadelphia, PA: Saunders Elsevier.

Hall, J. E. & Guyton, A. C. (2015). *Guyton and Hall Textbook of Medical Physiology* (13 edition). Philadelphia, PA: Saunders Elsevier.

Lieberman, M., Marks, A., Peet, A., & Chansky, M. (2013). *Marks' Basic Medical Biochemistry : A Clinical Approach*. Baltimore: Wolters Kluwer Health/Lippincott Williams & Wilkins,.

Marieb, E. N. & Hoehn, K. (2013). *Human Anatomy & Physiology* (9 edition). London, UK: Pearson.

AUTONOMIC NERVOUS SYSTEM
Autonomic nervous system. (n.d.) In *Lumen Learning*. Retrieved December 22, 2017 from https://courses.lumenlearning.com/boundless-ap/

Costanzo, L. S. (2017). *Physiology* (6 edition). Philadelphia, PA: Elsevier

Marieb, E. N. & Hoehn, K. (2013). *Human Anatomy & Physiology* (9 edition). London, UK: Pearson.

Osmosis. Sympathetic nervous system.

Osmosis. Parasympathetic nervous system.

BLOOD BRAIN BARRIER & CSF
Costanzo, L. S. (2017). *Physiology* (6 edition). Philadelphia, PA: Elsevier.

Marieb, E. N. & Hoehn, K. (2013). *Human Anatomy & Physiology* (9 edition). Boston, MA: Pearson.

BRAIN FUNCTIONS
Marieb, E. N. & Hoehn, K. (2018). *Human Anatomy & Physiology* (11 edition). London, UK: Pearson.

Stress. (2015). In *Cleveland Clinic*. Retrieved March 12, 2018, from https://my.clevelandclinic.org/health/articles/11874-stress

MOTOR NERVOUS SYSTEM
Costanzo, L. S. (2017). *Physiology* (6 edition). Philadelphia, PA: Elsevier.

Hacking, C., Palipana, D., et al. (n.d.). Anterior corticospinal tract. In *Radiopaedia*. Retrieved February 25, 2018, from https://radiopaedia.org/articles/anterior-corticospinal-tract

Hacking, C., Palipana, D., et al. (n.d.). Lateral corticospinal tract. In *Radiopaedia*. Retrieved February 25, 2018, from https://radiopaedia.org/articles/lateral-corticospinal-tract

Knierim, J. (n.d.) Spinal Reflexes and Descending Motor Pathways. In *Neuroscience Online*. Retrieved February 25, 2018, from http://nba.uth.tmc.edu/neuroscience/s3/chapter02.html

Marieb, E. N., & Hoehn, K. (2013). *Human Anatomy & Physiology* (9 edition). London, UK: Pearson.

Pandey, K. & Vanek, Z. F. (2018). Spasticity. In *Medscape*. Retrieved February 25, 2018, from https://emedicine.medscape.com/article/2207448-overview

Talley, N. J., & O'Connor, S. (2013). *Clinical Examination: A Systematic Guide to Physical Diagnosis* (7 edition). Chatswood, NSW: Elsevier Health Sciences

SENSORY NERVOUS SYSTEM
Osmosis. Auditory transduction and pathways.

Osmosis. Olfactory transduction.

Osmosis. Optic pathways.

Osmosis. Photoreception.

Osmosis. Somatosensory pathways.

Osmosis. Somatosensory receptors.

Osmosis. Taste and the tongue.

Osmosis. Vestibular transduction.

Osmosis. Vestibulo-ocular reflex and nystagmus.

SPINAL CORD & NERVES
Osmosis. Brachial plexus.

Osmosis. Cranial nerves.

Osmosis. Pyramidal and extrapyramidal tracts.

RENAL PHYSIOLOGY
ACID-BASE PHYSIOLOGY
Osmosis. Acid-base map and compensatory mechanisms.

Osmosis. Buffering and the Henderson-Hasselbalch equation

Osmosis. Metabolic acidosis.

Osmosis. Metabolic alkalosis.

Osmosis. Physiologic pH and buffers.

Osmosis. Plasma anion gap.

Osmosis. Respiratory acidosis.

Osmosis. Respiratory alkalosis.

Osmosis. The role of the kidney in acid-base balance.

ANATOMY & PHYSIOLOGY
Osmosis. Renal anatomy and physiology.

FLUIDS IN THE BODY
Osmosis. Body fluid compartments.

Osmosis. Renal clearance.

Osmosis. Water shifts between body fluid compartments.

RENAL BLOOD FLOW REGULATION
Osmosis. Measuring renal plasma flow and renal blood flow.

Osmosis. Regulation of renal blood flow.

RENAL ELECTROLYTE REGULATION
Costanzo, L. S. (2017). *Physiology* (6 edition). Philadelphia, PA: Elsevier.

Hall, J. E. & Guyton, A. C. (2011). *Guyton and Hall Textbook of Medical Physiology*. (12 edition). Philadelphia, PA: Saunders Elsevier.

Osmosis. Distal convoluted tubule.

Osmosis. Glomerular filtration.

Osmosis. Loop of Henle.

Osmosis. Proximal convoluted tubule.

RENAL REABSORPTION & SECRETION
Osmosis. Renal urea handling.

Osmosis. Tubular reabsorption of glucose.

Osmosis. Tubular secretion of PAH.

WATER REGULATION
Osmosis. Antidiuretic hormone.

Osmosis. Free water clearance.

Osmosis. Kidney countercurrent multiplication.

Osmosis. Osmoregulation.

REPRODUCTIVE PHYSIOLOGY
FEMALE REPRODUCTIVE SYSTEM
Blackburn, S. T. (2018). *Maternal, Fetal, and Neonatal Physiology: A Clinical Perspective*. St. Louis, MO: Elsevier.

Casper, R. F. (2018). Clinical manifestations and diagnosis of menopause. In *UpToDate*. Retrieved August 3, 2018, from https://www.uptodate.com/contents/clinical-manifestations-and-diagnosis-of-menopause

Costanzo, L. S. (2017). *Physiology*. Philadelphia, PA: Elsevier.

Ehsanipoor, R. M. & Satin, A. J. (2018). Normal and abnormal labor progression. In *UpToDate*. Retrieved August 3, 2018, from https://www.uptodate.com/contents/normal-and-abnormal-labor-progression

Hofmeyr, G. J. (2018). Overview of issues related to breech presentation. In *UpToDate*. Retrieved August 3, 2018, from https://www.uptodate.com/contents/overview-of-issues-related-to-breech-presentation

Kliegman, R. M., Stanton, B. F., St. Geme III, J. W., Schor, N. F., & Behrman, R. E. (2016). *Nelson Textbook of Pediatrics* (20 edition). Philadelphia, PA: Elsevier.

Lawrence, R. A. & Lawrence, R. M. (2016). *Breastfeeding: A Guide for the Medical Profession* (8 edition). Philadelphia, PA: Elsevier.

Martin, K. A., & Barbieri, R. L. (2018). Menopausal hormone therapy: Benefits and risks. In *UpToDate*. Retrieved August 3, 2018, from https://www.uptodate.com/contents/menopausal-hormone-therapy-benefits-and-risks

Osmosis. Anatomy and physiology of the female reproductive system.

Osmosis. Breastfeeding.

Osmosis. Estrogen and progesterone.

Osmosis. Menopause.

Osmosis. Oxytocin and prolactin.

Osmosis. Stages of labor.

Santen, R. J., Loprinzi, C. L. & Casper, R. (2018). Menopausal hot flashes. In *UpToDate*. Retrieved August 3, 2018, from https://www.uptodate.com/contents/menopausal-hot-flashes

Schanler, R. J. & Potak, D. C. (2018). Physiology of lactation. In *UpToDate*. Retrieved August 3, 2018, from https://www.uptodate.com/contents/physiology-of-lactation

Spencer, J. (2018). Common problems of breastfeeding and weaning. In *UpToDate*. Retrieved August 3, 2018, from https://www.uptodate.com/contents/common-problems-of-breastfeeding-and-weaning

Svena, J., & Galerneau, F. (2018). Face and brow presentations in labor. In *UpToDate*. Retrieved August 3, 2018, from https://www.uptodate.com/contents/face-and-brow-presentations-in-labor

MALE REPRODUCTIVE SYSTEM
Costanzo, L. S. (2017). *Physiology* (6 edition). Philadelphia, PA: Elsevier.

Osmosis. Anatomy and physiology of the male reproductive system.

SEXUAL DEVELOPMENT
Biro, F. M. & Chan, Y. (2017). Normal puberty. In *UpToDate*. Retrieved November 29, 2017, from https://www.uptodate.com/contents/normal-puberty

Gender, equity and human rights. (n.d.) World Health Organization. Retrieved July 20, 2018, from http://www.who.int/gender-equity-rights/en/

Osmosis. Sexual differentiation.

Osmosis. Puberty and Tanner staging.

RESPIRATORY PHYSIOLOGY
ANATOMY & PHYSIOLOGY
Costanzo, L. S. (2017). *Physiology* (6 edition). Philadelphia, PA: Elsevier.

Hall, J. E. & Guyton, A. C. (2011). *Guyton and Hall Textbook of Medical Physiology*. Philadelphia, PA: Saunders Elsevier.

Marieb, E. N. & Hoehn, K. (2013). *Human Anatomy & Physiology* (9 edition). London, UK: Pearson.

BREATHING MECHANICS
Costanzo, L. S. (2017). *Physiology* (6 edition). Philadelphia, PA. Elsevier.

Hall, J. E. & Guyton, A. C. (2015). *Guyton and Hall Textbook of Medical Physiology* (13 edition). Philadelphia, PA: Saunders Elsevier.

Le, T., Bhushan, V., Sochat, M., & Chavda, Y. (2017). *First Aid for the USMLE Step 1 2017* (27 edition). New York, NY: McGraw-Hill Education / Medical.

Marieb, E. N. & Hoehn, K. (2013). *Human Anatomy & Physiology* (9 edition). London, UK: Pearson.

Osmosis. Alveolar gas exchange.

Osmosis. Anatomic and physiologic dead spaces.

Osmosis. Lung volumes and lung capacities.

Osmosis. Ventilation.

BREATHING REGULATION
Costanzo, L. S. (2018). *Physiology* (6 edition). Philadelphia, PA: Elsevier.

Hall, J. E. (2016). *Guyton and Hall Textbook of Medical Physiology* (13 edition). Philadelphia, PA: Elsevier.

Marieb, E. N. & Hoehn, K.. (2013). *Human Anatomy & Physiology* (9 edition). Glenview, IL: Pearson Education, Inc.

GAS EXCHANGE
Costanzo, L. (2017). *Physiology*. (6 edition). Philadelphia: Elsevier.

Graham's law of diffusion | Respiratory system physiology | NCLEX-RN |. (2013). In *Khan Academy*. Retrieved January 30, 2019, from https://www.youtube.com/watch?v=g6QuuoTs2Oo

Marieb, E. N. & Hoehn, K. (2013). *Human Anatomy & Physiology*. (9 edition). London: Pearson

GAS TRANSPORT
Costanzo, L. S. (2017). *Physiology* (6 edition). Philadelphia, PA: Elsevier.

Bohr effect vs. Haldane effect | Human anatomy and physiology | Health & Medicine | Khan Academy. (2012). In *Khan Academy*. Retrieved July 20, 2018, from https://www.youtube.com/watch?v=dHi9ctwDUnc

Oxygen content | Human anatomy and physiology | Health & Medicine | Khan Academy. (2012). In *Khan Academy*. Retrieved July 20, 2018, from https://www.youtube.com/watch?v=a19T5CX2b-g

Marieb, E. N. & Hoehn, K. (2013). *Human Anatomy & Physiology* (9 edition). London, UK: Pearson.

Osmosis. Hypoxia and cellular injury - causes, symptoms, diagnosis, treatment & pathology.

Red blood cells. (n.d.). In *Lumen*. Retrieved November 20, 2017, from https://courses.lumenlearning.com/boundless-ap/chapter/red-blood-cells/

NORMAL VARIATIONS

Brothers, M. D., Doan, B. K., Zupan, M. F., Wile, A. L., Wilber, R. L., & Byrnes, W. C. (2010). Hematological and physiological adaptations following 46 weeks of moderate altitude residence. *High Altitude Medicine & Biology, 11*(3), 199-208.

Costanzo, L. S. (2017). *Physiology* (6 edition). Philadelphia, PA: Elsevier.

Hematy, Y., Setorki, M., Razavi, A., & Doudi, M. (2014). Effect of altitude on some blood factors and its stability after leaving the altitude. *Pakistan Journal of Biological Sciences: PJBS, 17*(9), 1052-1057.

Marieb, E. N. & Hoehn, K. (2013). *Human Anatomy & Physiology*. (9 edition). London, UK: Pearson.

INDEX

abaxial, 225
abdominal cavity, 206, 209, 216, 241, 295, 576
abducens nerve, 494, 504, 506
abduct, 412, 504
abembryonic, 200
ABO, 47, 370–371
ABP, 579
accessory nerve, 505, 508
ACE, 109, 530
acellular, 436
acetaminophen, 571
acetate, 16, 421
acetoacetate, 21
acetoacetyl, 13, 21
acetoacetylexercise, 21
acetone, 21
acetylation, 345–346
acetylcholine, 262, 280–281, 300, 302, 304, 313, 414, 421, 431–432, 445–446, 448, 452
acetylcholinesterase, 421
acetylglutamate, 36
acetyltransferase, 346, 452
ACH, 126, 313, 323, 331, 445–447, 452
acid, 518
acid, pantothenic, 330
acidemia, 517, 602
acidosis, 126, 158, 515–516, 518–521, 540–541, 627
acinar, 311, 313, 335
acini, 299, 311
acinus, 311
acne, 193, 586
aconitase, 1
ACP, 16
acromioclavicular, 500
acrosin, 196–197
acrosome, 196–197, 577
ACTH, 263, 268–270, 276, 278, 281
actin, 87, 119, 125, 166, 177, 225, 330, 370, 414–416, 419–420
acusticae, 259
acute mountain sickness, 628
acyl, 16, 18–19, 336–337
acyltransferase, 13, 18, 21
adam's apple, 590
ADAR, 346
ADCC, 384
adduction, 412
adenine, 18, 23–24, 38, 337, 349, 400
adenohypophysis, 254, 263, 268
adenoid, 93, 589
adenosine, 15, 23, 146, 153–154, 171, 174–175, 346, 399, 531
adenosine triphosphate, 163, 167, 171, 175, 285
adenylate, 171, 269, 272, 280, 283, 285, 305, 450, 452
adenylyl, 6, 126, 174–176, 313, 323–324, 331, 552
ADH, 106, 109, 148, 263, 268, 538, 542, 547–548, 552–554
adherens, 166
adipocytes, 18, 191, 269, 307–308, 330, 406
ADP, 3–4, 10, 153, 365, 420, 577
adrenal, 13, 157, 205, 256, 262–263, 265–266, 269–270, 276–279, 281, 446, 451–452, 520, 525, 542, 565, 573, 586
adrenal gland, 109, 204, 530
adrenal medulla, 268, 278, 431, 445, 451
adrenaline, 262, 265, 280–281, 286, 450, 530
adrenals, 265, 278, 432
adrenarche, 586
adrenergic, 127 262, 275, 283, 303, 313, 446–447, 450–451, 453–454, 530, 540–541, 588
adrenocortical, 265, 269–270, 276
adrenocorticotropic, 174, 263, 268–269, 276, 278
adrenodoxin, 276
adult hemoglobin, 612
adventitia, 238, 293–295, 317, 513, 590
AER, 227
afterbirth, 214
afterload, 86–87, 112, 115, 118, 120, 126, 624
agarose, 347
agella, 177
agglutination, 370
AID, 389
AIDS, 54
AIRE, 381, 391
airway obstruction, 521, 621
alanine, 4, 10, 33, 35, 280, 336
albuginea, 576, 582
albumin, 18, 32, 155, 274, 284, 289, 332–333, 336, 364, 518, 523, 573, 579, 615
alcohol, 324, 463, 571
alcoholism, 21, 287
aldolase, 5, 10
aldosterone, 13, 104, 109, 147, 175, 265, 276–277, 331, 513, 520, 525, 537, 541–542, 564
alimentary, 293, 325
alkalemia, 517, 602
alkalinization, 305
alkalosis, 515–516, 518, 520–522, 540–541, 564, 625, 627
allantois, 216, 218–219
allergens, 188
allergic, 385
allergy, 376–377, 385, 499
allocortex, 255
allosteric, 16, 31, 36
alothane, 158
alpha, 32, 330, 432
alphastores, 432
ALT, 33
alternans, 96
altitude, 627
altitude sickness, 627–628
alveoli, 85, 163, 232, 236–237, 248, 521, 560, 563, 570, 574, 588, 591–600, 602–603, 605–609, 612, 617–619, 621–624, 626–627
alveolus, 560, 570, 592, 595, 597–598
ambulation, 566
ameloblasts, 252
amenorrhea, 562
amino acid, 16, 29–30, 32–33, 36, 38–39, 262, 272, 281–282, 284, 286, 323, 328, 331, 336, 355–356, 360, 373, 547
aminoacyl, 355
aminobutyric, 478
aminohippuric, 532, 545
aminopeptidase, 328
aminotransferase, 32
amitotic, 424
ammonia, 32–37, 336, 519
amnion, 200, 210, 214, 216, 218–219, 565–566
amphipathic, 599
amplitude, 99, 129–131, 133–134, 458–459, 476
ampulla, 196, 297, 443–444, 493, 555, 578
ampulla of vater, 297, 334–335
ampullae, 259
ampullare, 259
ampullaris, 259, 493
ampullary, 196
amygdala, 477
amygdaloid, 253–255
amylase, 31, 295, 309, 312, 326, 335
amylin, 265
anabolic, 265, 272, 282, 306, 573, 580
anaemia, 98
anaerobic, 418, 605, 626
anal, 201, 207, 241–242, 246, 298, 301, 316
analgesics, 571
analysis, 63
anamnestic, 396
anaphase, 358–359
anaphylatoxins, 404
anastomoses, 90, 152
androgen, 193, 265, 277–278, 577, 579, 583, 586
androgenic, 277, 579
androstenedione, 277, 557, 573–575, 586
anemia, 143, 564, 606, 623
anergy, 395, 399
anesthesia, 458
anesthetic, 158
aneuploidy, 360–361
anger, 428
angina, 134
angiogenesis, 194
angiomas, 565
angiotensin, 104, 109–110, 147, 265, 277, 513, 520, 530, 542, 552, 564
angiotensinogen, 109, 542
anhydrase, 322, 331, 517, 519, 602–603, 616, 627
anion, 123, 169, 518–520, 523, 541, 546, 616
anisocytosis, 186
ankles, 405, 564
annealing, 348
annular, 438
annulus, 224
anova, 65–67
anovulatory, 586
ANP, 106, 542
anses, 241
antacid, 520
anterior pituitary, 154, 263, 268–269, 271,

276, 278, 560–561, 564, 570, 573, 586
anteriorly, 239, 435, 437, 589
anterograde, 316
anterolateral, 482
anteroposterior, 564
anthrax, 53
anthropoid, 567
antiapoptotic, 378, 390
antibacterial, 295
antibiotic resistance, 353
antibiotics, 351, 571
anticoagulation, 369
anticodon, 39
antidiuretic, 174, 552
antidiuretic hormone, 109, 175, 263, 268, 525, 537–538, 547, 552, 554
antifreeze, 519
antifungal, 571
antigen, 91, 183, 189, 370, 372–375, 377–381, 383–391, 393, 395–397, 399, 402
antigenic, 387
antigravity, 471
antimuscarinics, 323
antioxidants, 187, 570
antiport, 3
antithrombin, 369
antitrypsin, 336
antral, 322, 324
antrum, 259, 296, 319, 321, 440, 557
anvil, 440
anxiety, 193, 462, 522, 572
aorta, 85–86, 88, 93–94, 96, 98, 100, 103, 107, 113, 115–118, 126, 136–139, 141, 144–145, 147, 153, 226, 228–229, 231–232, 234, 245, 505, 510
aortic arch, 105, 231, 505, 602
aortic regurgitation, 98–101
aortic stenosis, 98–101, 117
aortic valve, 85, 94, 96, 100–101, 103, 113, 116
aorticopulmonary, 231
aorticorenal, 445
AP, 126, 315, 320
APAF, 181
aperture, 430, 456
aphasia, 461
apically, 321
aplasia, 186–187
apnea, 159
apneusis, 601
apocrine, 192–193, 247, 586
apoferritin, 330
apolar, 257
apoproteins, 329, 336
apoptosis, 166, 174, 176, 181–184, 186, 227, 271, 357, 362, 373, 381, 384–385, 391, 395–396, 410, 562
apoptosome, 181
appendix, 93, 221, 241, 298, 405–406
appetite, 265, 278, 308
aPTT, 367
aquaporin, 536–537, 547, 552–554
aqueduct, 430, 456
aqueduct of sylvius, 430
aqueous, 155, 261, 311, 335, 435–436, 439, 523
arachidonic, 278, 617
arachnoid, 261, 430, 456–457

archicortex, 255
archipallium, 255
arcuate, 461, 510–511, 579
areola, 294, 560, 563, 565, 570
arginase, 36
arginine, 36, 176, 280, 305–306
argininosuccinate, 36
arium, 101
armpits, 193
aromatase, 573, 575
arousal, 428, 445, 460, 462, 576
ARR, 58
arrector pili, 192–193, 247
arrhythmia, 129, 158–159
artemis, 362, 393
arterial, 87, 90, 99, 104, 106–107, 111–112, 116, 118, 138–139, 147, 149, 152–156, 188, 231, 238, 297, 334, 365, 510, 541–542, 595–596, 601–602, 607–608, 611, 615, 618, 620, 622, 626–628
arterial pressure, 86, 104, 112, 137–139, 147, 158, 525, 618
arterializedo, 607
arteriole, 85, 88–89, 105, 109, 112, 138–139, 141, 147–148, 152, 154–155, 157, 232, 268, 334, 431, 510–512, 530–531, 533–534, 541, 608, 617, 624
arteriosclerosis, 144
arteriosum, 232
arteriosus, 98–99, 231–232, 234, 619
arteriovenous, 159
arthritis, 570
articular, 227, 406, 408–409, 412
arytenoid, 236, 590
aspartate, 2, 33, 36
aspirin, 158
AST, 36
asthma, 621
astrocyte, 254, 257, 425, 455
asystole, 159
ataxia, 476–477
atherosclerosis, 105, 143, 188, 195
athletes, 628
atkins, 21
ATP, 2–4, 6, 9–10, 13, 15–16, 18–21, 36–37, 125, 161, 163, 167, 169, 171, 175, 181, 272, 285, 327, 418, 420, 517, 523, 535–537, 539–540, 552
atpase, 125–127, 162–163, 275, 291, 312, 322, 327, 331, 415, 418, 420, 523, 535–537, 540–541, 549
atria, 85–87, 94–98, 103, 106, 111, 116–117, 123, 126, 128, 131–133, 147–148, 176, 229–230, 432, 530, 542
atrial myxoma, 103
atrioventricular, 85, 94–96, 116, 123, 229–231, 450
atrioventricular node, 123, 231
atrium, 85–86, 95–96, 100–101, 103, 121, 139, 141, 153, 229–234, 564
atropine, 323
auditory tube, 259
auerbach, 256, 302, 315, 432
auricle, 259, 440
auscultate, 94–97, 98–101, 103–104, 562–563

autocatalyzes, 327
autocrine, 170, 383–384, 390
autoimmune, 93, 370, 381, 391, 399
autologous, 370
automaticity, 121, 129, 131, 415
autonomic, 256, 300, 313, 423, 431–432, 445, 452, 456, 459, 471, 478, 480, 504, 601
autonomic nervous system, 88, 126, 146, 256–257, 294, 319, 423, 431, 445, 447, 449, 451, 453, 458, 514, 588
autonomous, 300, 432
autophosphorylation, 282
autopod, 227
autoreceptors, 450
autoregulation, 152, 154, 531, 608
autosomal, 49, 341–342
AV, 116–117, 121, 123, 128, 131–132, 450
AV node, 121, 123, 131–132
avascular, 435–436, 590
AVPR, 552
axial, 221, 258, 405–406, 471, 493
axolemma, 424
axon, 257–258, 260, 263, 421–422, 424–425, 428, 431–434, 437, 440, 443–444, 465, 475–476, 481–482, 487, 495, 498, 504, 552, 559
azurophilic, 400–401

b cell, 92, 373, 377–383, 389, 391, 397, 399
bacteria, 93, 166, 193, 297–298, 322, 330, 332, 345, 351, 353, 383, 400, 570
bacterial infections, 383, 563
bainbridge, 106
balance, 518
baldness, 192, 342, 580
barometric, 604, 607, 610, 622
baroreceptor, 104–107, 147, 149, 505, 541, 548, 552
barrier, 455
basal, 194, 214, 247, 252–254, 256–257, 274, 285, 296, 430, 455, 470, 477–478, 498, 618
basal ganglia, 254, 430, 452, 464, 477–478
basal metabolic rate, 264, 274–275, 564
basale, 190–191, 247, 289
basalis, 199–200, 214
base, 515, 518
base sequence, 38–39
basement membrane, 88, 164, 237, 336, 511, 533
basilar, 152, 258, 442–443, 489–490
basolateral, 273, 291, 312, 322, 325–327, 330–331, 519, 535–537, 541, 543–546, 549, 552
basophil, 372, 377, 383, 404
bayesian, 69–70
BBB, 402, 404
beer, 502
belly, 249–250, 414
Bergmann, 254
beta blockers, 119, 158
bias, 41, 49–50, 71, 77
bicep, 421, 500
biconcave, 364
bicuspid, 85
bifurcate, 107, 236, 476, 602
bilaminar, 200–202, 206

642 OSMOSIS.ORG

Index

bilayer, 155, 162, 179
bile, 13, 239, 289, 297, 299–300, 303, 305–306, 328–329, 332–335, 337, 579
biliary, 239, 306, 331
bilirubin, 332, 334
biliverdin, 332
billows, 101
bilobed, 372
bimodal, 43
binocular, 439
biochemical, 31, 570
biochemistry, 3, 5, 7, 9, 11, 15, 17, 19, 21, 25, 27, 31, 33, 35, 37, 39
biopharmaceuticals, 351
biostatistics, 41, 43, 45, 47, 49, 51, 53, 57, 59, 61, 63, 67, 69, 73, 81
biosynthesis, 336
biotin, 15, 18, 330
biotransformation, 336
biphasic, 133
bipolar, 129, 257, 425, 437, 439, 443–444, 494, 496
birth, 75–76, 216, 223, 230, 232, 234–235, 237, 248, 259, 460, 562, 567, 579, 624
bisphosphatase, 5
bisphosphate, 5, 9–10, 171, 286
bisphosphoglyceric, 627
bladder, 58–60, 207, 216, 218, 235, 246, 332–333, 335, 337, 416, 432, 446–447, 450, 513–514, 556, 564, 578
bladder cancer, 58–60
blastema, 243
blastocoel, 197, 218
blastocyst, 197, 199–200
blastomeres, 197
bleb, 181, 571
blind, 74, 311, 437
blister, 571
blockage, 134, 188, 534
blocker, 112, 323, 415
blood, 603, 608, 611
blood cell, 91, 143, 168, 533, 564, 612, 627
blood clot, 194
blood coagulation, 284, 367
blood transfusion, 112, 370
blood urea nitrogen, 548
blood-brain barrier, 152, 425, 602
bloodborne, 373
bloodstream, 13, 18, 21, 90, 261–262, 265, 281, 321, 326, 535, 554, 560, 579
bloody show, 565
BMI, 41
BMR, 274–275, 564
BNP, 542
Bohr, 595, 613, 616, 625
bolus, 304, 309–310, 318, 320, 325
bone density, 574
bone marrow, 93, 222, 372–373, 378, 391, 406–407, 572
bordetella pertussis, 375
bowditch, 127
bowel, 93
BPM, 87, 121, 129–131
brachial, 104, 258, 500
brachial artery, 104, 137
brachial plexus, 500–502
brachialis, 500

brachii, 500–501
brachioradialis, 501
bradycardia, 105, 131, 159
bradykinin, 312
brain, 455
brain death, 458
brainstem, 105, 108, 152, 256, 309, 314, 325, 426–428, 443, 447, 459, 464, 468, 474–475, 482, 503, 521–522, 601–602
breast, 83, 185, 263, 560, 562, 565, 570–571, 573, 586–587
breast milk, 570–571
breastfeeding, 263–264, 559, 561, 570–571
breath, 232, 515, 519, 521–522, 594–595, 600, 606, 624, 628
breech, 567
Breuer, 602
Broca, 428, 461–462
Brodmann, 490
bromocriptine, 478
bronchi, 236, 265, 432, 588, 590–592, 599, 607, 619
bronchiolar, 608
bronchiole, 236–237, 450, 588, 590–591, 593, 595, 608
bronchitis, 621
bronchoconstriction, 447, 592, 602
bronchodilation, 446, 592
bronchomediastinal, 90
bronchus, 590, 593
brosis, 194, 342, 351, 609, 622
brow, 567
Brunner, 297
buccal, 295, 311, 325, 505
buccopharyngeal, 238
Budd–Chiari syndrome, 188
buffered, 616
buffering, 516
buffy, 364
bula, 227, 405
bulbar conjunctiva, 434
bulbourethral, 577–578
bulbourethral gland, 578
bulboventricular, 229
bulbus, 229
BUN, 548
bundle branch block, 96, 132
Burk, 32
Burkitt lymphoma, 184
burn, 49, 156, 194
bursa, 239
bypass, 159, 620

cabbage, 571
cadherins, 164–166
caffeine, 324, 571
cajal, 299, 315
calbindin, 291–292, 330
calcidiol, 287
calcifediol, 289
calcitonin, 174, 264, 284–285, 411
calcitriol, 286, 288–289
callosum, 255, 428
calmodulin, 176
calor, 188
calsequestrin, 125
calyces, 244, 511–513
canalicular, 236
canaliculi, 334, 434

canalized, 248
cancer, 48, 50, 54, 58–60, 76–78, 90, 93, 185, 187, 190, 364, 373, 570
candida, 571
candida albicans, 571
candidal, 571
cannabis, 571
CaO, 611, 620
capacitance, 144
capacitation, 196
capillaries, 602
capsularis, 214
carbaminohemoglobin, 612, 615
carbamoyl, 36–37
carbon monoxide poisoning, 623
carbonate, 364, 443
carbonic, 322, 331, 517, 519, 602–603, 616, 627
carboxyhemoglobin, 614
carboxyl, 13, 15, 18, 29, 33, 327, 517
carboxylase, 4, 15–16, 18, 367
carboxylation, 367
carboxypeptidase, 327–328, 337
carcinogenic, 48
cardiac, 125
cardiac muscle, 83, 119, 121, 126, 225, 415, 480
cardiac output, 86–87, 99, 104–107, 111, 120, 136–137, 139, 141, 143, 146–147, 149, 265, 275, 432, 510, 563, 611, 620, 623–626
cardinal, 231, 372, 556, 567, 569
cardio, 83
cardiomyocyte, 125, 415
cardiomyopathy, 97, 99–100
cardiopulmonary, 106–107, 159
cardiopulmonary bypass, 159
caregivers, 326
carina, 590
carnitine, 18, 336
carotene, 570
carotid, 98, 100, 105, 107, 147, 149, 152, 231, 505, 602
carpal, 227, 405, 412
carpometacarpal, 412
cartilage, 164, 194, 205, 221–223, 227, 236, 258–259, 272, 405, 407–409, 411–413, 440, 589–591
cartilaginous, 221–224, 258, 411–412
casein, 570
caseosa, 247
caseous, 181
caspase, 181, 183, 384, 395–396
catabolic, 275
catabolism, 32–33, 278
catabolite, 345
catalase, 187
catalysis, 31
catalytic, 171
catalyze, 6, 160, 175, 273, 287, 451–452, 517, 616
catechol, 451
catecholamine, 157, 265, 275, 278, 446, 450–451
cauda equina, 427
caudad, 303–304, 319–320
caudal, 201, 204–207, 210, 213, 224, 241, 243, 257, 445
caudate, 253–255, 333, 430, 477
cava, 85, 106, 136, 139, 141, 232–233, 334, 511, 563–564

cavae, 86
cavas, 231
caveolae, 155, 416
caverns, 161
cavity, 83, 93, 197, 200, 206, 209–211, 214–216, 218, 228, 239, 241, 252–254, 256, 259, 293, 295, 309, 311, 313, 318, 406, 425, 434, 440, 494, 498, 504, 555–557, 576, 589, 591, 593, 600
cavity, abdominal, 210
CCK, 299–300, 305–306, 321–322, 328, 337
CD, 373, 378–380, 383–387, 389–391, 395–398
ceca, 260
cecum, 241, 298, 300, 316
celiac, 238, 294, 297, 303, 319, 445
cell / cellular, 83, 160–161, 163, 165–169, 171, 173–175, 177, 179, 181, 183, 185–187, 189, 200, 278, 284, 323, 325, 331, 357, 375, 387, 426, 478, 540, 577, 615, 623, 628
cell cycle, 184, 351, 357–358
cellulose, 298
Celsius, 47
cementoblasts, 252
cementum, 252
central nervous system, 146, 158, 275, 305, 313, 423, 444–445, 455, 480
centralis, 437
centrifuge, 364
centrioles, 358
centromere, 180
centrosomes, 358
cephalic, 201, 204, 224, 323, 567
cephalocaudal, 257, 567
cephalopelvic, 567
cerebellar, 254, 474–476
cerebelli, 430
cerebellum, 152, 253–254, 427, 429–430, 444, 464, 470–471, 474–475, 477
cerebral, 141, 146–147, 152, 154, 253–255, 427–428, 430, 452, 456, 458, 460, 464, 468, 470, 474, 478–479, 601, 628
cerebral edema, 152, 628
cerebri, 254, 430, 468
cerebrospinal, 254, 425, 442, 456, 627
cerebrospinal fluid, 456
cerebrum, 254, 428–429
ceruloplasmin, 187, 336
cerumen, 193, 440
ceruminous, 193, 440
cervical, 50, 92, 98, 313, 316, 318, 427, 445, 470–471, 500, 505, 556, 562, 565–566, 573, 589
cervical cancer, 50
cervis, 574
cervix, 196, 263, 556, 561, 563, 565
cessation, 175, 421–422, 625
cGMP, 174, 176, 439
Chadwick, 562
Chaikoff, 274
Chatelier, 516
cheese, 181
chemical reaction, 616
chemoattractants, 196
chemokines, 188, 194
chemoreceptor, 104, 107–108, 110, 147, 300, 313, 494, 505, 519–522, 601–602, 620, 627
chemotactic, 386
chemotaxins, 404
chemotherapy, 571
chenodeoxycholic, 13, 334
chest, 598
chiasm, 253, 437, 440, 487, 504
chiasmata, 359
childbirth, 263, 556
childhood, 99, 556
chiral, 30
chloasma, 564
chloride, 171, 364, 456, 495, 519, 531, 549, 616
cholecalciferol, 287, 289, 330
cholecystokinin, 280, 283, 299, 305–306, 321, 335, 337
cholelithias, 564
cholera, 53, 331
cholestasis, 564
cholesterol, 13–15, 17, 19, 21, 42, 46, 77, 167, 190, 262, 276, 289, 328–329, 334, 336, 573–574, 579
cholic, 13, 334
choline, 421, 452
cholinergic, 157, 302–303, 445–447, 452–454, 478
cholinesterase, 452
chondroblasts, 407–409
chondrocranium, 222
chondrocyte, 221–222, 227, 272, 407–409
chondrogenesis, 227
chorda tympani, 504
chordae, 85, 97, 101, 103
chordal, 222
chorea, 478
chorion, 214, 216, 218–219
chorionic, 174, 200, 214–216, 218, 562
choroid, 253–255, 260–261, 430, 436, 456–457
choroidal, 438
choroidea, 253–254
chromaffin, 204, 256, 445, 451
chromatid, 180, 357–358, 362
chromatin, 161, 179–180, 350, 354, 358
chromatophilic, 424
chromosomal, 585
chromosome, 179–180, 184, 197, 213, 338–341, 342, 351, 358–361, 381, 391, 557, 581–583
chronic bronchitis, 621
chronic myeloid leukemia, 184
chronotropic, 275, 450
chyle, 90
chyli, 91
chylomicrons, 289, 329
chyme, 295, 297, 300, 303–304, 306–307, 319–320, 324, 335, 337
chymotrypsin, 327, 337
chymotrypsinogen, 327, 335, 337
CI, 67–68
cigarette, 48, 50–51
cilia, 177, 372, 400, 425, 442–443, 456, 491, 494, 496, 555, 591
ciliaris, 260, 504
ciliary, 253–254, 256, 260–261, 432, 435–437, 439, 447, 504
ciliated, 589–590
cimetidine, 323
cingulate, 468
cinulin, 528
circle of Willis, 152
circulation, 13, 85–86, 88, 94, 107, 112, 116, 137, 139–140, 152–154, 200, 214–215, 230, 232, 274, 276, 289, 294, 321–322, 329, 332–334, 336, 425, 430, 456–457, 552, 554, 579, 592, 603, 607–608, 618–619, 624–625, 627
circulatory, 86, 104, 152, 205, 209, 229, 232, 234–235, 619, 625, 627
circulatory system, 205, 209, 229, 234, 627
circumvallate, 497
circumventricular, 455–456
cirrhosis, 334
cistern, 160, 456
cisterna, 91, 160
citrate, 1, 15–17
citric, 1–2, 10, 15–16, 18–19, 21, 161, 313
citrulline, 36, 176
clathrin, 167
claudin, 166, 535
claustrum, 253–255
clavicle, 221–222, 405
Cl-coupled, 331
cleft, 89, 155, 249–251, 259, 421, 426
clitoris, 193, 246, 514, 555, 583, 585
cloaca, 201, 206–207, 238, 241, 243, 246, 582, 584
clonal, 372, 383–384, 389–390, 395–396, 399
cloning, 348, 351, 353
clot, 188, 364, 369–370
clotting, 333, 367, 539, 564
cloverleaf, 39
CMP, 23–25
CMR, 55
CN, 495
coagulation, 158, 284, 336, 367–368, 370
coagulative, 181, 369
coarctation, 98
coarctation of aorta, 98
cobalamin, 330
coccygeal, 427
coccyx, 406
cochlea, 204, 253, 258, 442–443, 489–490, 505
cochlear, 253, 258, 442–443, 489, 505, 507
codon, 38–40, 355–356, 360
coefficient, 64
coelom, 209, 218
coenzyme, 2, 336
cognition, 460
cognitive, 459–460, 462, 477, 572
coherence, 48, 67
cohort, 60, 76
coitus, 196
Coli, 297, 351
colic, 298
colipase, 328
collagen, 84, 88, 164–165, 191, 194–195, 365, 367, 406–408, 410, 436, 565, 572
collagenase, 410, 412
colliculi, 254, 440
colliculospinal, 471
colliculus, 443, 471
colloid, 89, 155, 273–274
colon, 241, 297–298, 300, 302–303, 331
colonic, 300
colony, 385–386

Index

colony-stimulating factor, 287, 386
colostrum, 563, 570–571
coma, 158–159, 458–460
combat, 322
commissure, 254–255
commissures, 255
common bile duct, 335
communicable disease, 52
compacta, 478
compaction, 197
compensatory, 515
complement, 402
complete blood count, 627
concentration, 312
conception, 581
conchae, 589
condensation, 30, 227
conductance, 156
conduction, 49, 121, 123–124, 132, 153, 425, 433–434, 443, 450, 465–466
conduit, 595, 619
condylar, 309
condyle, 406
condyloid, 412
cone, 83, 260, 437, 486–487
conformational, 9, 171, 175, 271, 402–403, 612, 615
confounding, 48, 50, 55, 75–76
congenital heart disease, 98
congestive, 127
conjugation, 13, 336
conjunctiva, 434
connective tissue, 84, 91, 191, 194, 227, 236, 259–260, 265, 278, 293, 317, 334, 407, 414, 440, 465, 485, 494, 510, 563, 565, 583, 589–590
connexins, 166
connexons, 426
consanguineous, 342
consciousness, 427, 458, 460–461
constipation, 307, 564
constrictive pericarditis, 96
consumption, 615
contagiousness, 54
contamination, 52, 194
contractile, 105, 112, 115, 119, 123, 126–127, 146–147, 194, 275, 316, 334, 432, 450, 560, 562
contraction, 125
convertase, 402–404
COPD, 96
coracobrachialis, 500
cordis, 229
cornea, 204, 260, 434–436, 439
corneum, 191
corniculate, 590
corona, 128, 197–198, 425, 468, 477, 514
coronary, 84–85, 134, 141, 146, 153–154, 231, 607, 619
coronary artery, 134, 153
corpora cavernosa, 576
corpus, 199–200, 254–255, 428, 557, 559, 562, 565, 573, 576
corpuscle, 93, 191, 247, 484–485, 511, 533, 535, 628
correlation, 48, 64, 67–69
cortex, 92–93, 146, 205, 254–255, 265–266, 269–270, 276, 278, 427–428, 438, 443–444, 452, 458, 460, 464, 468, 470, 475–479, 482–483, 487–488, 490, 495, 504, 510–511, 542, 549, 555–556, 573, 583, 586, 601, 615
Corti, 258–259, 442–443, 489–491
cortical, 197, 378–379, 406–407, 458–459, 468, 478, 482, 510–511, 547, 625
cortices, 464
corticobulbar, 254, 468, 470
corticopapillary, 547, 549, 551–552
corticopontine, 254
corticospinal, 254, 258, 427, 468–470
corticosteroid, 13, 276
corticosterone, 277
corticotropic, 269, 281
corticotropin, 174, 263, 268–269, 278
cortisol, 13, 263, 265, 269, 276–279, 463, 565
cortisone, 277
costal, 224, 407–408
costimulation, 383–384, 390, 395
costochondral, 412
cotransport, 326, 328, 330
cotransporter, 292, 327, 331, 519, 535, 537, 540–542, 549
cottage, 181
cotyledon, 214, 216
countercurrent, 536, 549, 552
coupling, 125
covalent, 194
covalently, 176, 350
covariates, 63
CPB, 159
CPS, 36–37
CR, 378, 380
cranial, 201, 204–207, 210, 213, 222, 241, 249, 253, 256–257, 259, 325, 423, 427, 430, 442, 447–448, 468, 470, 487, 503, 601
cranial nerves, 253, 256, 325, 423, 427, 448, 468, 470, 503, 601
cranio, 243
craniocaudal, 205, 213, 225, 229, 249
craniosacral, 432
creamy, 181
creatinine, 543
crenation, 168
crescendo, 98, 100
crescendovalvular, 98
crescent, 193, 230, 265
crest, 204, 222, 226, 247, 252, 256, 258, 406, 436
CRH, 263, 268–269, 278
cri du chat syndrome, 361
cribriform, 504
cricoid, 236, 590
cricothyroid, 250
crista, 259, 493
cristae, 161, 259
crossbred, 338–339
crossing over, 340–341, 487
crosstabs, 62
crura, 212
crus, 254, 259, 468
crypt, 93, 297–298, 331
crystalloid, 159
crystals, 443
CSF, 287, 386, 425–426, 430, 442, 455–457, 602, 627
CTP, 25
cuboidal, 200, 236–237, 536, 591
cult, 53, 76, 567
culty, 572
cumulus, 196
cuneate, 482
cuneiform, 590
cupula, 443, 493
curve, 598, 612
curvilinear, 598
cutaneous, 427, 500, 565
cuticle, 193
CV, 46
CVD, 58
CVP, 137
cyanide poisoning, 623
cyclase, 6, 13, 126, 171, 174–176, 269, 272, 280, 283, 285, 305, 313, 323–324, 331, 450, 452, 552
cycleas, 33
cyclins, 184
cyclization, 13
cyclooxygenase, 617
cysteine, 16, 38
cystic, 334–335, 342, 351
cytidine, 23, 378, 389
cytochrome, 2–3, 181, 276, 289, 291, 336
cytokine, 166, 188, 194, 271, 287, 334, 372–373, 378, 380, 383, 385, 389–390, 395, 397–400, 570, 615
cytokinesis, 359
cytolysis, 372
cytoplasm, 2–4, 9–10, 15, 17, 36, 39, 158, 160–162, 171, 179, 286, 374, 414, 424, 426
cytoplasmic, 276, 374
cytosine, 23–24, 38, 345–346, 349
cytoskeleton, 167, 177–178, 181, 384
cytosol, 160, 167
cytosolic, 175–176, 183
cytotoxic, 183, 373, 384, 386–387, 390, 395, 398, 628
cytotrophoblast, 200, 202, 214, 218

DAG, 174–175, 286, 323, 450, 452
Dalton, 604
DALY, 61
dAMP, 24, 188–189
dandruff, 191
dantrolene, 158
dataset, 43
dCMP, 24
DCT, 245
deacetylases, 346
deactivates, 6, 410
deafness, 259, 343
deaminase, 32, 378–379, 389
deaminated, 32
deamination, 32–33, 451
debranching, 6
debrided, 194
debris, 167, 194, 425, 595
debt, 153–154
decamethonium, 158
decarboxylase, 13, 451
deceleration, 494
decerebration, 471
decidua, 199–200, 202, 214
decidual, 200, 214, 216, 574
deciduous teeth, 252
decoy, 287
decrement, 566
decrescendo, 98, 100–101, 103
decubitus, 97

decussate, 427, 468–470, 482–483
decussation, 468, 504
defecation, 297, 300–301, 326
defect, 96, 565, 595, 607, 619, 620–622
defensin, 191, 297, 312, 589
deferens, 585
deformation, 486
degeneration, 218, 244–245, 478, 583
deglutition, 310, 325
degradation, 24, 153, 160, 174–175, 181, 194, 200, 330, 370, 385, 387, 421, 426, 451–452, 532, 561
degranulation, 404
dehelicization, 354
dehydration, 190, 313, 326, 520, 548
dehydrocholesterol, 13, 289
dehydroepiandrosterone, 277, 573
dehydrogenase, 1–2, 4–5, 10, 15, 18, 21, 33, 36, 277, 337, 573
deiodinase, 274
Deiters, 471
deltoid, 406, 501
dementia, 478
demineralization, 291
denaturation, 348
dendrite, 92, 189–190, 257, 372–374, 397, 424–425, 428, 465, 475–476, 481, 494
dendrocytes, 91
denervation, 186
denominator, 53
densa, 109–110, 512–513, 531
density, 70, 143, 310, 336, 364, 408, 437, 572–573, 606
dental, 252
dentin, 252
deoxyadenosine, 24
deoxycytidine, 24
deoxygenated, 85–86, 153, 214, 231–232, 234, 592, 607–608, 612, 620
deoxyguanosine, 24
deoxyhemoglobin, 612–613, 616
deoxynucleotide, 393
deoxyribonucleases, 328
deoxyribonucleic acid, 349
deoxyribose, 23–24, 349
deoxythymidine, 24
depletion, 4, 540, 572
depolarization, 105, 116, 121–124, 125, 128, 131, 158, 171, 315, 421, 426, 433, 439, 443, 452, 481, 490–491, 493, 495, 499, 624
deposition, 195, 222, 280, 282, 573
depression, 132, 134, 158, 201, 247, 572
deprivation, 424
derangement, 158
dermal, 194, 247
dermatology, 191, 193, 195
dermatome, 205, 225, 427
dermcidin, 193
dermis, 190–194, 205, 247, 484–485
dermomyotome, 225
Descemet, 436
desensitization, 174
desmin, 177
desmolase, 276, 573–574
desmosomes, 123, 415
desquamated, 247
detrusor, 432, 446–447, 450, 513–514
deviation, 41–42, 46–47, 65, 69, 71–72, 131–133

dextrinase, 326
dextrins, 326
dGMP, 24
DHAP, 4–5, 10
DHEA, 277, 573
DHP, 420
diabetes, 21, 61, 78, 195, 343, 544, 570
diabetes mellitus, 21, 78, 343, 544
diabetic, 58, 519
diabetogenic, 278, 565
diacylglycerol, 171, 174, 286, 323
diakinesis, 359
diamniotic, 219
diapedesis, 177
diaper, 571
diaphoresis, 572
diaphysis, 412
diarrhea, 326, 331, 518–520, 525
diastasis, 116, 565
diastole, 86, 88, 94, 96, 98, 101, 103, 113, 116–117, 119, 127, 137, 144–145, 153
DIC, 158
dichorionic, 219
dichotomous, 47, 69
dicrotic, 116, 138
diencephalon, 253–254, 428–429, 477
dietary, 32, 78, 288–289, 328, 330, 336, 367, 541
differential, 49, 344
differential diagnosis, 95–96
diffusion, 9, 18, 21, 88–89, 91, 155, 162–163, 170, 175–176, 212–213, 232, 262, 281, 284, 286, 289, 291, 323, 327–329, 331, 334, 421, 426, 435, 452, 455, 519, 531, 535, 540–541, 544, 547, 549, 573, 591, 603, 605–609, 610–612, 616, 622, 624
digastric, 249–250
digest, 167, 181, 194, 294–295, 297, 299, 305, 320–321, 322, 326–328, 330, 410, 432, 447
digestive, 209, 226, 235, 238, 293–294, 296, 299–300, 305, 313, 325, 335, 505
digitoxin, 127
diglycerides, 328
digoxin, 112, 119, 127
dihydroacetone, 4, 10
dihydrogen, 517
dihydropyridine, 420
dihydrotestosterone, 579–580, 582–583
dihydroxycholecalciferol, 175, 288–289, 291, 330
dihydroxymandelic, 451
dihydroxyphenylacetic, 451
diiodotyrosine, 273
dilated, 118, 259, 443
dilator, 226, 260, 436, 450
dilution, 312, 523, 542, 594, 607, 620, 623
dimensional, 213
dimer, 176, 377
dimerization, 175–176, 271
dinucleotide, 18, 337, 400
dioxide, 15, 18, 37, 83, 85, 88–89, 214, 455, 505, 516, 591, 593, 603, 615, 625
dioxygenase, 399
dipalmitoyl, 598
dipeptidase, 328

dipeptides, 327–328
diphosphate, 24, 26, 170, 174–175
diphosphoglycerate, 10, 613
diphtheria, 376
diploid, 197–198, 359, 557, 577
diplotene, 359
dipstick, 42
disability, 61
disaccharidases, 297
disaccharides, 326
discoloration, 562
discontinued, 436
discrete, 47, 64, 428
diseased, 79–80, 94, 609, 623
disequilibrium, 604
disintegrate, 181, 201, 358
disjoint, 44
dismutase, 187, 400–401
disorder, 478, 515
dispersion, 42
displaced, 112, 130, 360, 443, 563
disseminated intravascular, 158
dissipation, 157, 565
dissociation, 18, 96, 132, 174, 402, 404, 516, 602, 612–614, 616, 625
distal, 227, 331, 541
distend, 113, 144, 300–301, 310, 513, 576
distensibility, 144, 293, 562–563, 565
distensible, 88
distension, 144, 300, 305, 318, 320, 322–324
distress, 462
DIT, 273–274
diuresis, 158
diuretic, 158, 326, 520, 539, 541, 542
diurnal, 269, 278
diverticulum, 207, 216, 239, 254
dizygotic, 219
dizziness, 628
DN, 391
DNA, 23–24, 26, 38–39, 161, 175, 179–180, 187, 219, 275, 341, 345–357, 360, 362, 389, 393, 540
DNA cloning, 351, 353
DNA polymerase, 348, 351, 362
DNA replication, 348, 351–352, 362
DNA sequence, 346
dobutamine, 127
dolor, 188
dominance, 338, 547, 617
Donnan, 523
dopa, 451
dopamine, 127, 264, 268, 450–451, 478, 530, 559
dopaminergic, 478, 530
dormant, 252, 582
dorsally, 259
dorsolateral, 227
dorsomedial, 225
dose, 48, 67, 375
double helix, 349, 351
downregulation, 174, 391
downsloping, 133
DPG, 613–614
DPPC, 598
DR, 387
drainage, 156, 188, 298, 435, 619
DRG, 601–602
dromotropic, 450
dry mouth, 326
DS, 500

Index

dTMP, 24
ductal, 311–313, 335
ductus, 98–99, 231–234, 258, 619
ductus arteriosus, 98–99, 231–232, 234, 619
duodenal, 297, 305–307, 320–321
duodenum, 238–239, 241, 293, 296–297, 300, 303, 305, 315–316, 320–321, 325, 330, 335, 337
dura, 261
dura mater, 260, 430, 436
DW, 61
dysarthria, 477
dysdiadochokinesia, 476–477
dysfunction, 90, 96, 158, 477–478, 572
dyskinesias, 470
dysmetria, 477
dyspareunia, 572
dysphagia, 468
dysplasia, 185–186
dystocia, 567
dystrophic, 181
dysuria, 572

e. Coli, 345, 353
EABF, 541
EABV, 541–542
ear, 193, 204–205, 207, 249–251, 258–259, 312, 406, 408, 440–441, 443, 489, 491–492, 504
eardrum, 193, 259, 440, 489
eccrine, 193, 247
ECF, 109, 525, 539–542
ECG, 116, 128–131, 133–134
ECMO, 159
ecologic, 78
EcoRI, 347, 353
ecosystem, 298
ectoderm, 200–202, 204–207, 209–210, 221, 225–227, 241, 247, 249–254, 256, 258–259, 260, 298
ectopic, 131
EDD, 562
EDHF, 153
Edinger, 254
EDV, 111, 113, 115–117, 119–120
EEG, 458–459
EF, 87, 115, 120
effacement, 566
effector, 174, 383–384, 398–399, 423, 431–432, 446–447, 450, 452, 480
efferent nerve, 468
eicosanoids, 188
Eisenmenger, 96
ejaculation, 196, 446, 514, 578
ejaculatory, 578
ejection click, 100–101
ejection fraction, 87, 115, 120, 126
EKG, 128
elastance, 144–145, 597
elasticity, 293, 416, 573–574
elastin, 88, 164, 191, 407–408
elbow, 104
electrocardiography, 128–129, 131, 133, 135
electrochemical, 163, 291, 322, 327, 539
electrode, 128–129, 458
electroencephalogram, 458
electrolyte, 158, 193, 297, 311–312, 331, 364, 455–456, 533, 535, 537, 539, 541, 543

electron, 2–4, 10, 15, 18, 30, 123, 161, 187, 367
electronegativity, 541
electroneutrality, 523
electrophoresis, 347
electrophysiology, 121, 123, 125, 127
electrostatic, 169
ellipsoid, 412
emboli, 369
embolism, 96, 158, 522, 621
embryo, 197, 200–202, 204–207, 210, 212–214, 216, 218–291, 221, 226, 228–229, 240–241, 243, 251, 563, 581, 584
embryoblast, 197, 200, 218
embryogenesis, 187
embryological, 268, 275, 293, 298
embryology, 197, 199, 201, 203, 205, 207, 211, 213, 215, 217, 219, 223, 225, 227, 229, 231, 233, 235, 237, 239, 241, 243, 245, 247, 251, 253, 255, 257, 259, 261
embryonic, 176, 201–202, 212–213, 408, 562
emotion, 428, 460, 462, 601
emotional, 428, 461–463
emphasis, 50, 464
emphysema, 606, 608–609, 621
empyema, 430
emulsify, 328, 334
enamel, 252
enantiomers, 30
endocardial, 228, 230–231
endocardium, 84, 228
endocervical, 563
endochondral, 221–222, 224
endochromaffin, 322
endocrinocytes, 303
endocytose, 274, 334
endocytosis, 163–164, 167, 274, 276
endoderm, 200–201, 206–207, 209–210, 221, 235–236, 238–239, 249, 251–252, 259, 298
endodermal, 259
endolymph, 258, 442–444, 489, 493
endometrial, 77, 185, 200, 214, 561, 573
endometrial cancer, 77
endometrium, 199, 214, 218, 556, 561–562
endomysium, 414, 416
endonucleases, 362
endopeptidases, 327
endoplasmic, 4, 13, 160, 171, 175, 273, 286, 334, 387, 414, 424, 499
endorphin, 269
endosome, 167, 387
endothelial, 88–90, 153, 155, 176, 188–189, 226, 228, 334, 336, 365, 367, 455, 523, 530, 533, 617
endothelin, 153–154, 365
endothelium, 153, 237, 436, 511, 533, 617, 628
engagement, 567
engorgement, 571, 576, 602
enkephalin, 303, 307
enolase, 10
enoyl, 18
enterochromaffin, 304
enterocolitis, 570
enterocyte, 288–289, 326–330
enteroendocrine, 296–297, 305–306, 321

enterohepatic, 13, 332–334
enterokinase, 327
enteropeptidase, 337
entropy, 168
enzymatic, 171, 284, 299, 306, 539, 565
eosin, 372
eosinophils, 372, 377, 383, 404
ependymal, 253, 255, 257, 425, 430, 456
epiblast, 200–201, 218
epicardium, 83–84, 228–229
epicondyle, 406
epidemiology, 43, 45, 47, 49, 51, 53, 55, 57, 59, 61, 63, 67, 69, 73, 75, 77, 81
epidermal, 176, 190, 192, 194, 247
epidermis, 190–191, 194, 204, 227, 247–248, 287, 484
epididymis, 577–578, 585
epigenetics, 345–346
epiglottis, 236, 253, 295, 310, 325, 408, 498, 505, 589–590
epimerase, 10
epimysium, 414
epinephrine, 6, 119, 127, 157, 262, 426, 431–432, 446, 450–451, 463, 530
epiphyseal, 272, 573, 580
epiphysis, 412
epiploic, 297
epistaxis, 564
epithalamus, 253–254
epithelia, 166
epithelial, 4, 84, 93, 155, 164, 166, 186, 196, 199, 207, 225, 236–237, 247–248, 252, 258–261, 273–274, 293–294, 317, 321–322, 325, 327–329, 331, 369, 436–437, 494, 536, 555, 560, 570, 576, 582
epithelialization, 225
epithelium, 84, 161, 186, 190, 204, 207, 209, 236, 238–239, 252, 257, 259, 293–298, 321, 400, 424, 434, 436, 486, 494, 511, 513, 533, 536, 556, 573, 589–591
epithelization, 194
epitrichium, 247
EPO, 615
eponychium, 193
epoxide, 367
EPSPs, 433, 439
equilibrium, 122, 127, 168–169, 259, 344, 427, 491, 493, 505, 516–517, 534, 598, 605, 607–609
equimolar, 281
Erb, 94
erectile, 555, 576
erection, 447, 576
ergocalciferol, 289
ERV, 594
erythema, 565, 571
erythrocyte, 91, 161, 334, 364, 615
erythropoiesis, 615
erythropoietin, 278, 615, 627
esophageal, 238–239, 295, 310, 316–318, 320, 325, 564
esophagus, 212, 236, 238–240, 293–295, 302–303, 310, 312, 316–318, 320, 325, 498, 589
ester, 328–329
estradiol, 13, 277, 557, 573–575, 583, 586
estriol, 573
estrogen, 174–175, 200, 248, 263, 268,

OSMOSIS.ORG **647**

271, 276, 330, 555, 557, 561–565, 572–574, 579, 586
estrone, 573
ESV, 113, 115, 120
ethanol, 306
ethmoid, 504, 589
euchromatin, 180, 350
Eustachian tube, 93, 251, 259, 440
eustress, 462
evagination, 254
evolution, 213, 344
excision, 362, 389
excitability, 124
excitable, 414, 424, 540
excitation, 125–126, 426, 439, 443, 476, 478
excitatory, 300, 304, 433, 439, 471, 475–476, 478–479
exclusion, 381, 391
excretion, 24, 32, 36, 106, 265, 287–288, 300, 331–332, 334, 336, 515, 519–522, 532, 539–542, 544, 546–547, 554, 564, 627
executing, 427
exercise, 625
exhalation, 24, 99, 593, 603
exhaled, 21, 595
exhaustion, 158, 395, 399, 463
exibility, 13, 191, 407, 412, 573
exible, 216, 407–408, 430
exion, 567
exive, 325, 365
exocoelomic, 200
exocrine, 262, 265–266, 283, 294, 299, 305, 335, 434, 452
exocytic, 387
exocytosis, 163–164, 167, 426
exogenous, 362, 387–388
exons, 354
exonucleases, 346, 362
exopeptidases, 327
exor, 227, 467, 470–471, 500
expel, 167
experimental, 48, 67, 70, 78
experimentally, 72
expiration, 94, 96, 99, 589, 591, 594, 598, 600
expiratory, 594, 601
expire, 301
expired, 594–595, 600, 620
expiring, 594
exploited, 628
expression, 43, 213, 282, 345, 365, 378, 385, 395, 427, 462, 468, 504, 561, 581
expulsion, 167, 565, 567
extensible, 414
extensive, 134, 255
extensor, 227, 467, 470–471, 501
externa, 88, 295, 313–319
external ear, 440, 443
extracellular, 164–165, 167, 170–171, 174, 176, 265, 282, 284, 286–289, 326, 334, 386, 407–408, 421, 428, 433, 442, 499, 517, 523–525, 539–540
extracorporeal, 159
extracranial, 507
extrafusal, 465–467
extraglomerular, 512
extranitric, 617
extraocular, 438, 444

extrapyramidal, 468, 470
extrasystole, 127
extravasation, 188–189, 628
extrinsic, 119, 154–155, 183, 253, 300, 302, 316, 318–319, 367–368, 436, 438–439, 497
extrudes, 326–327
exure, 298
eye, 205, 219, 253, 260, 421, 432, 434–439, 459, 465, 474, 487, 494, 504, 506
eyelid, 434, 438, 504

facets, 224
facial, 204, 223, 313, 406, 427, 448, 462, 468, 503–504
facial nerve, 250, 259, 434, 498, 504, 507
FADH, 1–2, 18–19, 337
failure, 96–97, 156, 187, 274, 381, 391, 519, 521, 628
fainting, 149
falciform, 333
fallopian, 555–556, 573, 583, 585
fallopian tube, 557, 559, 562
false negative, 70, 79
false positive, 79
falx, 430
family tree, 373
farnesyl, 13
FAS, 183, 395–396
fascia, 265, 510
fascicle, 132, 414, 482
fascicular, 132
fasciculata, 265, 269–270, 276–277
fasciculi, 254
fasciculus, 444, 461
fatality, 60–61
fatty, 4, 15–20, 162, 181, 280–281, 305–306, 321, 328–329, 336–337, 510
fatty acids, 15, 18, 161, 181, 271, 280, 282–283, 306, 321, 328–329, 334, 336–337, 570
fauces, 589
Fe, 3, 330, 612
fecal, 300, 316
feces, 13, 297, 299–301, 331–332, 334
female external genitalia, 583
femora, 405
femur, 227, 405–406, 409
fenestration, 89, 155–156, 334, 336, 533–534
ferment, 298
ferrous, 330
fertilization, 196–198, 219, 555, 557, 559, 561–562
fetal, 91, 93, 202–204, 207, 210, 214–215, 218–219, 223, 232–235, 259, 261, 333, 561–563, 565–569, 571, 580, 612, 624
fetal circulation, 232, 624
fetal development, 557
fetal movement, 562
feto, 214–215
fetus, 201, 204, 214, 216, 565, 567–568, 579
feverishly, 372
fiber, 421
fibrin, 181
fibrinogen, 364
fibrinoid, 181

fibrinolysis, 369–370
fibroblasts, 191, 194
fibrocartilage, 408
fibroplasia, 194
fibrosis, 606, 609
fibrous, 84, 411, 436, 513
Fick, 111, 163, 532, 546, 605
filament, 419
filiform, 497
filtrate, 512, 534, 536–537
filtration, 89, 155, 533–534, 539–543, 545
fimbriae, 555
first stage of labor, 566
Fisher's exact test, 62
fissure, 261
flexibility, 117
flexion, 567
flora, 298
foci, 131
foliate, 497
folic acid, 330, 565
follicle, 91–93, 174, 191–193, 219, 247–248, 263–264, 268, 272–273, 378–379, 555–557, 559–562, 572–573, 583, 586
follicle-stimulating hormone, 174, 219, 557
follicular, 264, 272–274, 383, 396–397, 555, 557, 559, 561, 572–573
folliculitis, 193
fontanelle, 223, 567
footplate, 440
foramen, 152, 230, 232, 234, 239, 406, 430, 504–505, 508
foramen magnum, 152, 406, 505, 508
foramen ovale, 230, 232, 234
foramina, 430, 456, 495
forearm, 500–501
forebrain, 253, 260, 478
foregut, 207–208, 235–236, 238–241
forehead, 152, 504–505, 567
forelimb, 248
foreskin, 576
formalin, 375–376
formic, 518–519
fornix, 255, 556
fortel, 254
fossa, 232, 406, 474
fourth ventricle, 430, 456
fovea, 437
fragile x syndrome, 343
Frank–Starling, 87, 111–112, 119, 126
fraternal, 219
FRC, 594, 598, 600
free radical, 187
frondosum, 214
fructose, 5, 9–10, 326–327, 334, 578
frustration, 463
FRV, 600
FSH, 219, 263, 268, 557, 560–561, 565, 572–573, 575, 577–579, 586
fumarase, 1
fumarate, 1, 36
functio laesa, 188
fundal, 562–563
fundus, 296, 300, 319, 556, 563, 566
fungal, 181, 383
fungi, 383, 400
fungiform, 497
fungiform papillae, 497
funiculus, 482–483
fusiform, 416

Index

fusion, 161, 184, 197–198, 230, 334, 585

g protein, 170–171, 174–176, 305
GABA, 426, 478
GABAergic, 475, 478
galactose, 326, 331, 334, 345
galactosidase, 345
gall, 332–333, 335, 337
gallbladder, 13, 207, 238–239, 241, 299, 305–306, 332, 334–335, 337, 564
gamete, 263, 339–341, 360, 577, 581–582, 586
gamma, 170, 174, 265, 269, 378, 385, 396, 398, 467, 612, 614
ganglia, 204, 256–258, 302–303, 307, 313–314, 423, 430, 432, 442, 445–447, 452, 470, 477, 481
ganglion, 256, 258, 260, 313, 319, 423, 431, 437, 439, 443–445, 447, 486–487, 504
ganglionic, 446, 448
gangrene, 181, 605
gangrenous, 181
garments, 157
gas, 50, 158, 232, 236, 364, 521, 588, 591–592, 595–600, 603–611, 613, 615, 617, 619–621, 623, 625, 627
gas gangrene, 605
gastric, 283, 295–296, 300, 303, 305–308, 318–324, 327–328, 330, 432, 520, 564
gastrin, 283, 296, 300, 305–306, 320–324
gastrocolic, 300
gastroenteritis, 52
gastroesophageal, 295, 318, 325
gastrointestinal, 207, 238, 283, 288, 293, 295, 297, 299–303, 305, 307, 311, 313–315, 317, 319, 321, 323, 325, 327, 329, 331, 333, 335, 337, 446–447, 450, 459, 564, 570
gastrointestinal tract, 166, 207, 253, 294, 302, 309, 311, 313–315, 317, 319, 321, 323, 450, 571
gastrulation, 201, 221
GATA, 383
Gaussian, 42, 46
GDP, 1, 170, 174–175
gel, 347, 407–408, 434, 533
gelatinous, 216, 443
gender, 585
gene expression, 13, 179, 213, 262, 345–346, 390, 581
gene therapy, 351
generation, 157, 338–339, 342, 344, 421–422, 424, 426, 428, 579, 590–591
generator, 586
genetic mutations, 360
genetically, 192, 246, 581
geniculate, 254, 437, 440, 443–444, 487, 504
genital, 193, 243, 246, 579, 584, 586–587
genitalia, 580, 582–583, 585
genitourinary, 201, 206, 446–447
genotype, 338–339, 342–343
geranyl, 13
germ, 200–201, 204–205, 207, 581–583
germinal, 91–92, 254, 378–379, 389
germinative, 247
germline, 360
gestation, 562, 565, 576

gestational, 275, 563, 567, 581–583
GFR, 530–531, 534, 539, 542, 564
GH, 268, 271, 281
GHIH, 263
GHR, 271
ghrelin, 265, 296, 307–308
GHRH, 263, 268, 271
GI, 86, 171–172, 174, 283, 288, 294, 299–300, 302–303, 313, 315–316, 321, 324–325, 432, 450, 452, 454
GI tract, 275, 293–296, 299–300, 302–304, 307, 313, 315–316, 318, 320, 322, 331, 432, 450
Gibbs, 523
GIP, 306, 320
girdle, 221, 405
glandular, 236, 263, 570
glans, 193, 576
glenohumeral, 500
glial, 257, 425–426
glioblasts, 257
globin, 612
globular, 415
globules, 299, 329
globulin, 364, 573, 579
globus, 253, 255, 430, 477–479
globus pallidus, 253, 430, 477–479
glomerular, 106, 512, 530, 533–534, 540–543, 547, 564, 615
glomeruli, 475–476, 534
glomerulosa, 109, 265, 276–277
glomerulus, 243–244, 511, 518, 530, 533–534, 543
glossopharyngeal, 105, 310, 313, 448, 503
glossopharyngeal nerve, 105, 250, 498, 505, 508
glottis, 99, 301, 590
GLP, 306, 308
glucagon, 6, 9–10, 16, 18, 174, 262, 265, 275, 280–281, 283, 299, 305–306, 335–336
glucoamylase, 326
glucocorticoid, 175, 265, 269, 276–278, 565
glucokinase, 9
gluconeogenesis, 4–5, 265, 271, 275, 280, 282, 306, 336, 432, 446, 450
glucose, 4–6, 8–10, 15, 18, 21, 33, 35, 46–47, 49, 155, 161–163, 214, 265, 269, 271, 275, 278, 280–283, 299, 305–306, 326–327, 330–331, 334–336, 345, 418, 424, 455–456, 535, 538, 543–545, 548, 564–565
glucose-6-phosphate, 5–6, 9–10, 330
glucose-6-phosphate dehydrogenase, 10
glucosidase, 6
glucuronidation, 336
glut, 9, 163, 281–282, 326–327, 544–545
glutamate, 32–33, 36, 426, 439, 478, 490–491
glutamic, 367
glutaminase, 33
glutamine, 33–34, 336, 535
glutamyl, 367
glutathione, 187
glyceraldehyde, 10
glycerol, 2, 4–5, 18, 328–329
glycine, 13, 426
glycochenodeoxycholic, 13
glycocholic, 13
glycogen, 6–9, 32, 158, 160, 265,

282–283, 299, 306, 330, 333, 336, 418, 562
glycogenesis, 447
glycogenin, 6
glycogenolysis, 4, 6, 265, 271, 278, 280, 282, 306, 336, 432, 450
glycolipids, 190–191
glycolysis, 4, 6, 9, 11, 15–16, 161, 280, 336, 613
glycolytic, 418
glycoprotein, 194, 196–197, 272–273, 311, 336, 370, 579, 615
glycosaminoglycan, 407
glycosides, 127
glycosidic, 6, 326
glycosuria, 544, 564
glycosylase, 389
glycosylation, 161
GMP, 23–24, 28, 174, 439
GNRH, 263, 268, 560–561, 572–573, 577, 579, 586
goblet, 297–298, 589–591
Golgi, 160, 167, 254, 286, 334, 424, 475–476, 485
gomphoses, 411
gonad, 13, 243, 262–263, 275, 555, 576, 581–584
gonadal, 581, 583, 585–586
gonadarche, 586
gonadotropin, 174–175, 200, 263, 268, 561–562, 577, 579
gonorrhea, 53
Goodell, 563
goosebumps, 157, 193
GP, 365
Graafian follicles, 557, 559
gracilis, 482
gradient, 2–4, 89, 96, 98–99, 112, 136, 138, 155, 162–163, 169, 188–189, 213, 291, 318, 322, 327, 530, 535–537, 539–540, 544, 547, 549, 551–552, 593, 597, 599–600, 608–609, 616, 622–623
grafts, 605
granular, 247, 475, 512
granulation, 194, 456–457
granule, 188, 190, 197, 254, 284, 286, 335, 372–374, 377, 384, 400–401, 475–476
granulocyte, 372, 374, 386
granulosa, 555, 557, 559, 561, 572–573, 583
granulosum, 190
granzymes, 384
gravid, 563–564
gravida, 562
gravidarum, 565
gravidity, 565
gravitational, 618
gravity, 88, 318, 443, 565, 608, 618
gray matter, 257, 425, 427–428, 430
GRFs, 174
growth, 271
growth factor, 176, 184, 228, 383
growth hormone, 175–176, 263, 268, 271, 275, 281, 586
GRP, 323
GTP, 1, 170, 174–176
GTPAL, 562
GTPase, 174–175, 184
guanine, 23–24, 38, 170, 345–346, 349

OSMOSIS.ORG 649

guanosine, 23, 170, 174, 354
guanylyl, 176
Guillain-Barré syndrome, 376
gunshot, 49, 440
gustation, 497
gustatory, 498–499
gut, 204–207, 209–210, 226, 238, 241–242, 294, 298, 300, 305, 313, 332–334, 400, 570–571
GVA, 445
GVE, 445
gynecoid, 567
gyri, 255, 428–429
gyrus, 443, 464, 468

habenular, 254
HACE, 628
haemophilus, 375
hairless, 484–485
hairpin, 39, 354
haldane, 616
handgrip, 99
HAPE, 628
haploid, 358–359, 557, 577, 583
haptocorrin, 330
hard palate, 309–310, 325, 589
harmonics, 99
Hasselbalch, 515–517
Hauser, 200
haustra, 297, 300
Haversian, 406
Hayflick limit, 351
hCG, 200, 562–563, 565
Hct, 546
HDL, 573
headache, 628
healthcare, 61
heart failure, 127, 156, 608
heart murmur, 98
heart valve, 99
heartburn, 564
hegar, 562
height, 47, 133–134, 405, 562–563
helical, 179
helicase, 351
helicotrema, 443, 489
helix, 30, 38
helper, 373, 378, 383–385, 387, 390, 396–398
helpless, 463
hematocrit, 158, 364, 525, 532, 546, 564, 627
hematologic, 564
hematological, 625, 627
hematology, 365, 367, 369, 371
hematopoiesis, 372
hematopoietic, 239, 372, 385, 391, 406, 627
hematoxylin, 372
heme, 2, 18, 612–614
hemisphere, 253–255, 427–428, 430, 461, 474
hemispheric, 477
hemizygotes, 342
hemizygous, 342
hemodialysis, 159
hemodilution, 564
hemodynamics, 99, 136–137, 139, 141, 143, 145
hemoglobin, 30, 76, 332, 334, 364, 517, 521–522, 603, 605–606, 609, 611–616, 623, 625–628
hemoglobin a, 611
hemoglobin f, 612, 614
hemolytic, 370
hemophilia, 342–343
hemorrhage, 112, 146–147, 149, 565
hemorrhoids, 563
hemostasis, 194, 365, 367, 369–370
Henderson, 516
Henderson–Hasselbalch, 516
Henle, 244–245, 331, 512, 518, 535–537, 539, 547, 549, 551
Henrys, 605
heparin, 372
hepatic, 188, 232, 239, 265, 278, 280, 282, 289, 297–298, 327–329, 332–334, 336, 540
hepatic duct, 334
hepatitis, 375
hepatitis A, 375
hepatitis B, 375
hepatocytes, 161, 239, 289, 299, 330, 332–334, 336
hepatomegaly, 188
hepatopancreatic, 297
heptamer, 393
herd, 54
hereditary, 478
Hering, 602
herniates, 216, 241
herniation, 216, 241–242
heroin, 571
herpes, 571
herpes zoster, 571
Herring, 263, 554, 559
Hertz, 458
Heschl, 443
heterochromatin, 180, 350
heteroreceptors, 450
heterotrimer, 280
heterotrimeric, 174
heterozygotes, 341–342
heterozygous, 338, 342
hexagonal, 333
hexokinase, 6, 9
hiatus, 295, 317
Hicks, 566
HIF, 615
high blood pressure, 531
highsecretion, 573
hillock, 259, 424, 433
hilum, 93, 510
hindbrain, 253, 256
hindgut, 207–208, 216, 218, 238, 241–242
hindlimb, 248
hinge, 412
hippocampal, 255
hippocampus, 253–255, 424, 452
hippuric, 518–519
histamine, 154, 170, 188, 286, 296, 306, 321–324, 372, 426
histocompatibility, 373, 378, 386
histological, 264, 408, 591
histone, 179–180, 345–346, 350
HIV, 54, 571
HIV infection, 571
HIV/AIDS, 54
HLA, 386–387
holistic, 460
holosystolic, 98
homeobox, 213

homeobox gene, 213
homeostasis, 157, 262, 265, 284, 320, 335, 445, 455, 539–541, 588, 625–626, 628
homeostatic, 104, 149, 428
homogeneity, 65
homologous chromosomes, 359
homologues, 358
homovanillic, 451
homozygotes, 341–342
homozygous, 338–339, 342
homunculus, 428, 464
hormonal, 16, 154, 174–175, 185–186, 284–285, 287, 289, 291, 299, 315, 320, 411, 544, 572
hormonally, 104, 109, 313, 320
hormone, 269, 271–273
hormone secretion, 163, 262, 272, 274–275
hormone therapy, 572
hormone, follicle-stimulating, 174
hormone, thyrotropin, 175
horseshoe, 228
housekeeping, 432
howship, 410
Hox, 213
HOXA, 213
HOXB, 213
HOXC, 213
HOXD, 213
HPA, 265, 278
hPL, 570
HPV, 375
HRT, 77
HSD, 573
HT, 304
human, 196, 199
human chorionic gonadotropin, 200
human leukocyte antigen, 386
humeri, 405
humerus, 227, 405–406, 412
humidify, 588–589
humidity, 603
humor, 261, 434–436, 439
humoral, 154, 373, 375, 377
hunger, 307–308, 499
Huntington's disease, 341, 478
HVA, 451
hyaline, 197, 221, 227, 408, 412
hyaloid, 260–261
hyaluronan, 407
hyaluronic, 298, 407, 412
hyaluronidase, 196
hydratase, 18
hydrate, 164–165
hydration, 326, 548
hydraulic, 156
hydrochloric, 410
hydrolase, 328–329, 400
hydrolysis, 174, 274, 336
hydrolytic, 181, 197
hydrolyze, 326–327–329
hydronephrosis, 564
hydrophilic, 29, 162, 170, 174, 262, 386, 599
hydrophobic, 29–30, 162, 170, 176, 262, 329, 386, 599
hydroquinone, 367
hydrostatic, 89, 147, 149, 155–156, 534, 618
hydroxy, 13, 21

Index

hydroxyacyl, 18
hydroxyapatite, 406, 410
hydroxybutyrate, 21
hydroxycholecalciferol, 287, 289, 330
hydroxyl, 18, 187, 289
hydroxylase, 277, 287, 289, 291, 330, 451
hydroxylation, 289, 291, 336
hydroxymandelic, 451
hydroxypregnenolone, 573
hydroxysteroid, 277, 573
hymen, 556
hyoid, 250, 589
hyothalamus, 586
hyperactivation, 158
hyperalbuminemia, 518
hyperaldosteronism, 541
hyperbaric, 605
hypercalcemia, 518
hyperchloremic, 518–519
hypercholesterolemia, 78
hyperchromatism, 186
hypercoagulable state, 564
hypercortisolism, 565
hyperdynamic, 95–96, 98
hyperemia, 152–154, 564
hyperextended, 567
hyperkalemia, 518–519, 540
hypermagnesemia, 518
hypermutation, 389, 396
hyperosmotic, 525, 554
hyperovulation, 219
hyperphosphatemia, 518
hyperpigmentation, 564, 573
hyperplasia, 185, 194, 562–563, 565
hyperpnea, 625
hyperpolarization, 107, 121, 433, 439, 443, 493
hyperpolarize, 439
hyperpolarizing, 105, 153, 439
hypersecretion, 573
hypertension, 41, 80, 96–97, 104–105, 117, 181, 185
hyperthermia, 158
hyperthyroid, 98
hypertonic, 168, 549
hypertonic solution, 168
hypertrophic, 99–100
hypertrophy, 97, 117, 130–131, 133, 185, 265, 562–563, 565, 580, 624, 627
hypervariable, 393
hyperventilation, 152, 564, 574, 601, 622, 625
hypnosis, 460
hypo, 540
hypoalbuminemia, 518
hypoaldosteronism, 541
hypoblast, 200–201, 218
hypocalciuric, 539
hypodermis, 190–191
hypogastric, 298, 303
hypoglossal, 503, 505
hypoglossal nerve, 505, 509
hypoglycemia, 265, 271, 305
hypokalemia, 520
hypomagnesemia, 287
hypongram, 459
hypoosmotic, 554
hypophyseal, 263, 268, 406, 579
hypophysis, 254, 268
hypoplasia, 186–187
hyposmotic, 525

hypotension, 104, 149, 564
hypotensive, 563
hypothalamic, 157–158, 254, 263, 265, 269, 274, 278, 308, 426, 572–573, 579, 586, 601
hypothalamus, 109, 157, 253–255, 263–264, 268–269, 271–272, 274, 278, 307–308, 428–430, 446–447, 455, 459, 504, 548, 552, 554, 559–561, 572–573, 577, 579, 586, 601
hypothermia, 158–159
hypotonia, 477
hypotonic, 168, 193, 312, 320
hypotonic solution, 168
hypoventilation, 159, 601, 622
hypoxanthine, 24
hypoxemia, 147, 602, 614, 620, 622–623
hypoxia, 153, 522, 615, 619, 622–624, 627–628
hypoxic, 181, 232, 613–614, 617, 623–624
hysteresis, 598
Hz, 458

iatrogenic, 158
ICF, 525, 539–541
idiopathic, 628
idioventricular, 96
IFN, 378, 383, 385
IFNs, 385
IFNα, 383
IFNβ, 383
Ig, 378–379
IgA, 297, 375, 377, 397, 571
Igβ, 379
IgD, 377–378, 381, 396–397
IgE, 377–378, 397
IgF, 271
IgG, 375, 377–378, 384, 396–399
IgM, 377–378, 381, 396–398
IL, 377–378, 383–386, 390, 397–400
ileal, 241, 297
ileocecal, 297–298, 300, 316
ileum, 297, 303, 316, 321, 325, 330–332
iliac, 232, 234, 244–245, 298, 406
ilium, 241, 406
illicit, 571
immature, 93, 186, 284, 381, 391
immersion, 158
immobile, 166
immobility, 156
immune, 400
immune response, 188, 372–373, 389, 395–399
immune system, 92, 189, 370, 372–373, 375–376, 385, 400
immunization, 54
immunize, 53
immunizing, 54
immunogenic, 375
immunoglobulin, 32, 214, 373, 375, 377, 570–571
immunoglobulin A, 312, 377
immunoglobulin D, 377
immunoglobulin E, 377
immunoglobulin G, 377
immunoglobulin M, 377
immunologic, 372, 396
immunological, 53
immunology, 373, 375, 379, 381, 383, 385, 387, 389, 391, 393, 397, 399, 401, 403

immunoreceptor, 378, 390
immunosuppressive, 265, 278, 386
IMP, 26
impaired, 156, 158, 521, 622
impermeable, 166, 312, 537, 541–542, 549
impermeant, 455
implantation, 197, 199, 573–574
inactivate, 149, 174, 197, 305, 326, 328, 369, 375–376, 395, 433, 579
incerta, 254
incidence, 60
incisura, 138
incontinence, 564
incretins, 306
incus, 223, 249, 259, 440, 489
indigestible, 298–299
indoleamine, 399
inducible, 615
induction, 243, 271, 615
inert, 538
inertia, 493
inexpensive, 53
inexpensively, 76
infancy, 557
infant, 54, 158, 459, 560, 562, 570–570
infarction, 134, 158, 188, 415, 565
infected, 52, 54, 166, 373, 383–385
infections, 54, 93, 156, 181, 383, 499, 563, 571
infectious, 52, 90, 166
infective, 52
inference, 41, 69
inferiorly, 590, 618
inflammation, 188
infrahyoid, 225
infraspinatus, 500
infundibulum, 254, 263, 268, 552, 555
infusion, 370, 525
ingested, 309, 312, 322, 326
ingestible, 519
ingestion, 283, 295, 299, 305–306, 330, 520
ingests, 325, 387
inguinal, 92, 298, 565
inhalation, 139, 593, 595
inheritance, 338, 341–343
inherited, 339, 341
inhibin, 557, 565, 578–579
inhibit, 126–127, 158, 181, 263–264, 271–272, 287, 305–308, 310, 312, 318, 324, 346, 385, 399, 444, 459, 475–476, 478–479, 541, 559, 582, 601
inhibition, 31, 50, 126, 157, 174, 286–287, 305–307, 324, 336, 415, 426, 439, 443, 450, 459, 478, 481, 561, 572, 617, 627
inhibitor, 184, 212, 286, 322, 336, 402, 404, 478, 580, 627
inhibitory, 31, 174, 263, 283, 300, 303–306, 320, 384, 399, 415, 439, 450, 452, 475–476, 478–479, 481
inhibits, 15–16, 143, 171, 212, 262, 265, 268–269, 271–272, 274, 280, 282–283, 287, 300, 303, 305–306, 320, 324, 335, 345, 395, 411, 415, 439, 467, 470–471, 478–479, 540, 560, 563, 574, 579, 601
initiation, 38, 278, 299, 310, 346, 351–352, 355, 474, 567, 570

injected, 320
injuries, 567
injury, 90, 181, 187, 365, 614, 617
inlet, 567, 590
innate, 54, 372–373, 384–385, 400–401, 403
inner ear, 204, 440–441, 489, 491–492
innervate, 157, 227, 249–250, 253, 256, 258–259, 293, 300, 302–304, 309, 313, 323, 421, 427, 431–432, 434, 445, 465–468, 470, 489–490, 498, 500–501, 504–505, 508–509, 592, 600
innervation, 253, 294, 297–298, 300, 302–303, 311, 313, 318–319, 414, 431, 465–466, 504–505, 592
inorganic, 160
inosine, 346
inositol, 171, 174, 286
inotropes, 126
inotropic, 119, 126–127, 275, 450
inotropic agents, 112, 119
inotropism, 126–127
inotropy, 112, 119–120
INSIG, 13
insoluble, 13, 594
inspiration, 94, 96, 99, 591, 598–602, 604
inspiratory, 594, 600–601, 627
instability, 121, 572
insula, 255
insulated, 424
insulates, 191, 218
insulin, 6, 9–10, 15–16, 175–176, 239, 265, 271, 278, 280–283, 299, 306, 308, 320, 330, 335–336, 351, 450, 540–541, 544, 565
insulinotropic, 306
intake, 109, 274, 326, 541–542
integrin, 164–165, 197, 199, 370
integumentary, 190, 247, 564
intention tremor, 476–477
interaction, 50–51, 53, 174, 187, 196–197, 227, 252, 263, 287, 397, 603, 616
intercalary, 555
intercalated, 83, 123, 226, 311, 415, 519, 537, 541
intercellular, 155, 416
interconversion, 333
interconvert, 603
intercorrelations, 69
intercostal, 94, 100–101, 103, 225, 593, 600
intercourse, 52
interferon, 278, 378, 385, 400
interleukin, 170, 278, 377, 385
interlobar, 510–511
intermediolateral, 256
intermembrane, 161
intermolecular, 599
interna, 87–88
interneuron, 300, 321, 425, 459, 467, 475–476, 480–484, 486, 494
internodal, 123
interobserver, 63
interosseous, 411
interpersonal, 52
interphase, 357, 359
intersection, 436
interstitium, 89, 155, 326, 535–537, 547, 549–550, 552
interval, 47, 61, 64–65, 67–68, 95–96, 116, 128–130, 132, 179, 316, 320
interventricular, 153, 430, 456
interventricular foramen, 430
interventricular septum, 153, 231
intervertebral, 224, 408
intervertebral disc, 202, 224
intestinal, 90, 93, 216, 241, 289, 291, 297, 300, 302–305, 307–308, 318, 320, 324–328, 330–332, 337
intestine, 4, 13, 32, 90, 155, 216, 241, 288–289, 291–292, 294–300, 302–307, 316, 319–320, 324–331, 335
intraabdominal, 318
intracellular, 125, 127, 160, 170–171, 174–177, 181, 262, 271, 282, 286, 313, 323, 326, 331, 379, 383, 400, 443, 499, 517, 523–524, 539–541
intracranial, 456, 507
intracytoplasmic, 177
intradermally, 375
intraembryonic, 209
intraepithelial, 297
intraesophageal, 318
intrafusal, 465–467
intrahepatic, 564
intraluminal, 305
intramammary, 570
intramembranous, 221–223
intramuscular, 375
intramuscularly, 375
intranasally, 375
intraocular, 435
intraocular pressure, 435
intraperitoneal, 293, 297
intrapleural, 600, 617
intrapulmonary, 623
intraretinal, 260
intrasellar, 565
intrathoracic, 94, 99, 318, 593
intrauterine, 248, 261, 566
intravascular, 149, 158
introns, 38, 346, 354
inulin, 523, 528, 538
invade, 247, 252
invaders, 400
invaginate, 163, 167, 201, 247, 258, 260, 415
invagination, 93, 167, 201, 252–253, 416
invasive, 80
inversion, 132–134, 361
inverted, 134
investigation, 52–53, 72
investigators, 74
involuntary, 293, 298, 309–310, 325, 415–416, 423, 431, 445, 470, 480, 494, 514
involutes, 570
involution, 559–561, 567, 570
iodide, 274
iodinated, 274
iodinates, 273
iodine, 273–274
ion, 89, 123–124, 155, 160, 162, 166, 168–169, 171, 173, 179, 181, 284, 291, 311, 320, 326, 328, 331, 335, 400–401, 414, 419–422, 424–425, 433, 481, 495, 499, 516–522, 531, 547–550, 616, 628
ionization, 187, 284, 362, 547
ionotropic, 439, 452
iosine, 26
IP, 126, 174–175, 286, 313, 322–323, 450, 452
ipsilateral, 444, 470–471, 495
IPSPs, 439
iridica, 260
iridocorneal, 261
iridopupillary, 260
iris, 253–254, 260–261, 435–436, 439, 450
iron, 91, 167, 187, 330, 564–565, 612
irradiated, 156
irradiation, 455
irregularly, 435
irritant, 188, 602
IRS, 282
IRSs, 271
IRV, 594
ischaemic, 97
ischemia, 134, 147, 154, 181, 186, 188, 456
ischemic, 188
ischial, 567
islet, 265–266, 299, 305–306, 335
isocitrate, 1
isocortex, 255
isoelectric, 29, 130, 347
isohydric, 515
isomerase, 5, 10
isometric, 99, 420
isopentenyl, 13
isoproterenol, 127
isosmotic, 331, 525, 541–542
isotonic, 168, 311–312, 320, 420, 525
isotonic solution, 168
isovolumetric, 115–116
isovolumic, 113, 116
isthmus, 555–556, 562, 589
ITAM, 378, 390

JAGS, 69
JAK, 271
Janus, 176
jaw, 226, 252, 468
jejunal, 241
jejunum, 241, 297, 331
jelly, 197
jet, 101
jugular, 90, 505, 508
junction, 123–124, 131, 166, 193, 197, 295, 298–299, 315–316, 322, 325, 331, 411, 415, 421, 425–426, 452, 455, 513, 535, 573
junctional, 131, 201, 214–215
juxtacapillary, 602
juxtaglomerular, 109–110, 147, 512–513, 530–531, 533, 542
juxtamedullary, 511

kallikrein, 312
Kaplan, 63
kappa, 63, 378, 381, 391, 393
kB, 378, 390
kegel exercises, 514
Kelvin, 603, 606
keratin, 164, 177, 190, 192
keratinization, 190, 192–193
keratinized, 247
keratinocyte, 190–191, 247, 287, 289
keratohyalin, 190
Kerckring, 325

Index

keto, 32, 280, 282
ketoacid, 33, 518–519
ketoacidosis, 519
ketoacyl, 16, 18
ketogenesis, 306
ketogenic diet, 21
ketoglutarate, 1, 32–33, 36
ketone, 21–22, 336
ketone bodies, 21, 330, 336
ketothiolase, 18, 21
Kf, 156, 534
kidney, 4, 89, 92, 106, 109, 147, 155, 166, 194, 244, 265, 268, 280, 287, 291, 330, 337, 450, 510–512, 518, 520, 530, 542–543, 545–546, 549, 582–583, 615
kinase, 4, 6, 9–10, 13, 171, 175–176, 184, 269, 271–272, 280, 282, 305, 323, 362, 390
kinetic, 31, 137, 143–145, 168, 606
kinetochores, 358
kininogen, 312
kinocilia, 492
kinocilium, 443, 491
knee, 408
Korotkoff, 104
Krebs, 1–2, 161
ku, 393
Kupffer, 239, 333–334
kurtosis, 42
kurtotic, 42

L-dopa, 451, 478
labia, 514, 555, 583, 585
labia majora, 555, 583, 585
labia minora, 514, 555
labioscrotal, 582–583
labor, 214, 559, 561, 565–567, 569, 573
lacrimal, 434, 504
lacrimal gland, 434
lactase, 326, 345
lactate, 4, 146, 154, 570
lactation, 560, 565, 570–571
lacteal, 90, 329
lactic, 158, 519, 625
lactic acid, 518–519, 626
lactiferous, 248, 563
lactobacillus, 570
lactoferrin, 571
lactogen, 570
lactogenesis, 268, 570
lactoperoxidase, 571
lactose, 326, 330, 345, 570–571
lactotroph, 559, 565
lacunae, 200–201, 214–215, 407, 410
lacunar, 200, 214
laesa, 188
laeve, 214
lagging, 351
lamellar, 190, 485
lamellipodia, 370
lamentous, 179, 192, 415
laminal, 253
laminar, 98, 143
langerhans, 265–266, 335
lanosterol, 13
lanugo, 247
Laplace, 117–118, 154, 598
large intestine, 241, 297–298, 300, 331
lariasis, 156
laryngeal, 236, 250, 310, 590

laryngopharynx, 295, 589
larynx, 235–236, 250, 295, 310, 325, 408, 498, 505, 588–590, 593
lateral ventricle, 430
laterally, 227, 406, 435, 444
laterial, 310–311
laxative, 570
LBBB, 132
LCK, 390
LDL, 573
leakage, 322
leaked, 90, 200
leaky, 166, 331, 334, 535
lectin, 402, 404
left bundle branch block, 132
left heart, 85, 99, 111, 607, 625
left ventricle, 85–86, 95–96, 99–101, 103, 111, 113, 118, 131–132, 153, 229, 607, 619
lemniscal, 482–483
lemniscus, 443, 482
lens, 204–205, 260–261, 434–436, 439
lenticular, 254
leptin, 307–308
leptokurtic, 42
leptotene, 358
lesion, 468, 476
leucine, 4, 305–306
leukemia, 184
leukocyte, 161, 188–189, 364, 372, 385–386, 400, 617
leukorrhea, 563
leukotrienes, 278, 617
levator, 250, 438, 504
levelo, 623
levo, 30
Leydig, 576–579, 581–582, 586
LH, 174, 263, 268, 557, 560–561, 565, 572–574, 577–579, 586
lial, 338
libido, 265, 580
life, 611
lifestyle, 50
lifetime, 63, 77, 345, 424, 459
ligament, 216, 227, 232, 252, 258, 260, 333, 406, 411, 436, 490, 555–556, 590
ligamentum, 232, 333
ligand, 170–171, 174, 176, 183, 197, 286–287, 334, 378, 395–396, 398–399, 410, 421
ligase, 351, 353, 362
lightheadedness, 149, 326
limbic, 428, 495, 601
limbus, 258–259, 436
limitans, 253, 257
limpid, 456
linea, 564
linear, 30, 64, 67–68, 97, 272, 443–444, 517, 602
linearly, 544, 546
Lineweaver, 32
lingual, 93, 295, 312, 328, 589
linkage, 338–339, 378
lip, 225, 504
lipase, 18, 295, 312, 321, 328, 335
lipid, 2, 15, 42, 89, 155, 160–161, 167, 187, 193, 295, 299, 312, 328–330, 336–337, 377, 396, 455, 547, 624
lipofuscin, 424
lipoic, 1

lipolysis, 265, 271, 275, 278, 280, 282, 321, 450
lipoprotein, 13, 289, 336, 573, 598
lipotropin, 269
lipoxygenase, 617
liquefactive, 181
liver, 4, 6, 8, 13, 15, 18, 21, 32–36, 156, 160, 188, 194, 207, 216, 232–233, 238–241, 271, 274, 280–283, 287, 289, 293–294, 297, 299, 305–306, 327–330, 332–337, 402, 432, 450, 510, 579
LMP, 562
lobar, 236, 590
lobe, 109, 254, 263–264, 333–334, 438, 443–444, 468, 474, 477, 482–483, 487–488, 504, 579, 591
lobular, 563, 574
lobulated, 161
localization, 443
localized, 227, 296, 571, 623
locally, 579
location, 71, 78, 83, 91–94, 98, 106–108, 121, 134, 208, 212, 216, 230, 244, 249, 263–264, 266, 286, 302, 308, 310, 316, 322, 330, 333–335, 347, 393, 411, 414, 443, 452, 460, 462, 464, 474, 477, 498, 500–501, 556, 589
locomotion, 470–471
lodged, 534
logarithmic, 517
logically, 47
logistic, 69
logit, 69
longevity, 424
loop diuretics, 539, 542
looping, 229–230, 346
loops, 113, 115
loosening, 563
lordosis, 565
loudness, 99
low blood pressure, 104, 277, 530
LT, 500
LTM, 461
lubricates, 296, 321, 412
lubricating, 312, 331
lubrication, 295, 309, 311
lubricin, 412
lucidum, 190–191
lumbar, 90, 212, 243, 314, 426–427, 431, 445, 456, 584
lumbar puncture, 456
lumbar vertebrae, 456
lumberjack, 185
lumbosacral, 258
lumen, 88, 238–239, 260, 273, 289, 291, 299–300, 317, 321–322, 331, 519, 535–537, 541, 549, 552, 577
luminal, 312, 325, 540–541
lung, 48–50, 76, 232, 235–239, 590–594, 597–602, 604, 606, 608, 617–618, 620–625
lung cancer, 48, 50, 76
lunula, 193
Luschka, 430
lutea, 437
luteal, 557, 559, 562, 574
luteinized, 557
luteinizing, 174
luteinizing hormone, 174, 263, 268, 557,

577, 586
luteum, 199–200, 557, 559, 562, 565, 573
lyase, 15, 21, 36, 277
lymph, 90–93, 156, 293, 298–299, 329, 372–373, 378–379, 396
lymph node, 90, 92, 373, 379
lymphatic, 90–93, 155–156, 191, 289, 293–294, 297, 317, 378, 434, 436, 510
lymphatic system, 90–91, 289, 378
lymphedema, 90
lymphocyte, 91, 93, 189, 297, 334, 381, 390, 395
lymphoid, 91–93, 294, 298, 372–373, 378–379, 381, 391, 398
lymphoid tissue, 91, 93, 294, 298
lymphoma, 184, 383
lymphopoiesis, 381, 391
lyses, 168
lysine, 4
lysis, 189, 540
lysolecithin, 328–329
lysosomal, 160–161, 181, 197, 275, 410
lysosome, 167, 274, 387, 400–401, 434
lysozyme, 295, 297, 312, 372, 400, 571, 589

MAC, 402, 404
macrocytes, 617
macromolecule, 160, 179, 275, 347
macrophage, 91, 93, 167, 183, 188–189, 191, 194, 287, 332, 334, 372–373, 377, 383, 385–386, 404, 571, 591
macroscopic, 523
macrosomia, 567
macula, 109–110, 437, 443–444, 491–492, 512–513, 531
macula lutea, 437
Magendie, 430
magnesium, 286–287, 330, 456, 539
magnitude, 43, 347
magnum, 152, 406, 505, 508
mainstem, 590, 593
majora, 555, 583, 585
malate, 1–2, 4, 36
male external genitalia, 582
malic, 15
malleus, 223, 249, 259, 440, 489
malnourishment, 156
malonate, 16
malonyl, 15–17
MALT, 93, 294, 298
maltase, 326
maltose, 326
maltotriose, 326
mammary, 193, 204, 226, 248
mammillary, 253–255
mandible, 221–223, 249, 309, 312, 406
mandibular, 223, 249, 259, 406, 504–505, 507
Mann, 63
mannitol, 523–524
mannose, 402, 404
mantle, 255, 257, 260
manubrium, 224
MAO, 451, 478
MAP, 94, 137–138, 443, 515–516
MAPKs, 176
margin, 94, 100–101, 103, 577
MARMU, 502
marrow, 90, 93, 222, 372–373, 378, 391, 406–407, 572, 627
masculinizes, 579
masculinizing, 582
mask of pregnancy, 564
masking, 74
masseter, 249, 309–311
mast, 188–189, 372, 374, 377, 383, 404
mast cell, 404
masticate, 309
mastication, 295, 309–311, 325, 468
mastitis, 571
mastoid, 259, 440
mater, 430, 456
mathematics, 70
maturation, 93, 194, 275, 377, 389, 573, 580, 586–587, 615
maxilla, 221, 223, 249, 504
maxillary, 231, 504, 507, 589
maximal, 126, 174, 608
maximally, 331
maximized, 325
meal, 13, 265, 280, 308, 320–322, 334
measles, 54, 375
measures, 65
meatal, 259
meatus, 250–251, 259, 406, 434, 440, 504–505, 507, 589
mechanical, 103, 177, 295, 299, 325, 411, 456, 486, 562
mechanically, 310
mechanics, 594–595, 597, 599
mechanism, 48, 87, 104, 109, 125, 131, 136, 146, 149, 152, 154, 157–158, 171, 173–176, 187, 262, 284, 291, 303–304, 315, 321–324, 330–331, 345, 362–363, 393, 399, 419, 450, 452–454, 462, 515, 519–522, 531, 541, 567, 579, 608, 624
mechanoreceptors, 105, 309, 313, 318, 320, 442, 484, 560, 601–602
mechanosensors, 484–485
mechanosensory, 489
Meckel, 207, 216, 223
Meckel's diverticulum, 207, 216
meconium, 570
medialis, 489
medially, 227, 439, 444
mediastinum, 83–84, 93, 577
mediate, 104–105, 109, 147, 154, 167, 175–176, 197, 212, 286, 300, 318, 320, 324, 373, 375, 383–384, 439, 470–471, 486, 617
mediation, 300
mediators, 188–189, 334
meditation, 460
medulla, 93, 105, 107–108, 147, 149, 253, 256, 265–266, 268, 278, 310, 313, 427–428, 431, 444–446, 451–452, 468–470, 475–476, 478, 482, 505, 511, 549, 555–556, 583, 601–602, 615
medulla oblongata, 253, 468, 478
medullary, 93, 149, 406, 468, 471–472, 547, 582, 627
Meier, 63
meiosis, 197, 339–340, 358–359, 557, 559, 577, 583
meiotic, 197, 557
Meissner, 191, 247, 256, 293, 300, 302, 317, 432, 484
melanin, 177, 190, 192–193, 424, 573
melanocyte, 174, 190, 192, 194, 204, 247, 269–270, 436, 563–564
melanosomes, 190, 192
melasma, 564
melatonin, 264, 428, 459
mellitus, 21, 78, 343, 544
membrane, 2–4, 6, 13, 15, 18, 88, 121–122, 124–125, 155, 159–164, 166–169, 171, 174–177, 179, 181, 183, 187–188, 200–201, 206–207, 209–210, 212, 216, 218, 227, 237–238, 241–242, 258–260, 262, 272, 274, 286, 289, 291, 294, 299, 312, 315, 320, 322–323, 325–331, 336, 358, 367, 387, 402–403, 411–412, 414, 421–422, 424, 426, 433–434, 436, 439–440, 442–443, 455, 481, 486, 489–491, 495, 499, 510–511, 519, 533, 539–541, 544, 546, 552, 556, 589, 591, 605–609, 612, 616
membrane attack complex, 402–403
membranous, 160, 222, 230, 246, 258, 440
memory, 275, 372, 375, 383, 396–400, 427, 459, 461, 463
memory B cells, 375, 383, 396–398
menarche, 586
Mendel, 338
Mendelian, 338
meninges, 426, 430–431
meningitidis, 375
menisci, 227
meniscus, 408
menopausal, 572–573
menopause, 572
menses, 561
menstrual, 219, 560–562, 572, 586
menstrual cycle, 557, 559, 561, 572, 574, 586
menstruation, 561, 586
Menten, 31–32
Merkel, 484
merocrine, 193
mesangial, 512
mesencephalon, 253–254, 427
mesenchymal, 221–222, 224, 227–228, 252, 259
mesenchyme, 227, 247–248, 252–253, 258–261
mesenteric, 238, 241, 294, 297–298, 303, 445
mesentery, 206, 209, 212, 259, 293, 297, 333
mesh, 91, 194, 367, 370
meshwork, 435
meso, 582–583
mesocardium, 228
mesocolon, 297
mesoderm, 200–207, 209–210, 212, 214, 216, 218, 221–222, 224–226, 228, 230, 235–236, 238–239, 243–245, 247, 249, 259, 582
mesodermal, 202, 212, 225, 265
mesogastria, 238
mesogastrium, 238–240
mesometrium, 556
mesonephric, 243, 246, 582
mesonephros, 243–244, 582
mesosalpinx, 555
mesothelial, 555

Index

mesothelium, 293
messenger, 174–175, 322, 354, 450, 452, 615
messenger rna, 38, 174–175, 321, 385
metabolic, 32, 88, 154, 157–159, 257, 265, 278, 334, 424–425, 435, 446–447, 455, 515–516, 518–521, 540, 563, 607, 613, 615, 627
metabolic acidosis, 515–516, 518–520, 627
metabolic alkalosis, 515, 518, 520–521
metabolically, 613
metabolises, 126
metabolism, 1, 3, 5–7, 9, 11, 13, 15, 17, 19, 21, 23, 25, 27, 29, 31–33, 35, 37, 39, 154, 160, 264, 271–272, 275, 298, 336, 543, 601–602, 614, 616–617, 628
metabolite, 146, 152–154, 174, 278, 291, 336, 435, 456
metabolize, 193, 345, 418
metabolizer, 336
metabotropic, 439, 450, 452
metacarpals, 227, 405
metacarpophalangeal, 412
metal, 2, 187, 336
metallic, 103
metanephric, 243–245
metanephrine, 451
metanephros, 243–244
metaphase, 358–359, 559
metaplasia, 186
metarhodopsin, 439
metarteriole, 89, 155
metatarsals, 227, 405
metatarsophalangeal, 412
metencephalon, 253–254
methanol, 519
methoxy, 451
methoxytyramine, 451
methyl, 345–346, 354
methylation, 336, 345–346, 451
methylglutaryl, 13, 21
methylmalonyl, 18
methyltransferase, 451
mevalonate, 13–14
MHC, 373, 378, 383–388, 390–391
MHT, 572
micelles, 289, 329–330
Michaelis, 31–32
microbial, 188
microbiome, 400, 571
microcirculation, 89, 155, 624
microcracks, 410
microglia, 257
microglial, 425
microglobulin, 386
micrometer, 608
microorganisms, 372, 400
microtubules, 177, 424
microvascular, 628
microvilli, 163, 177, 296–298, 325, 498, 535, 537, 543, 545
micturition, 514
midbrain, 253–254, 256, 427–428, 440, 443, 468, 470, 477–478, 482, 504
midclavicular, 94, 100–101
middle ear, 249–251, 440, 489, 504
middlevalues, 43
midgut, 207–208, 216, 238–239, 241
midpelvis, 567

midpiece, 577
migrated, 255, 257
migrating, 303, 320, 581
milk teeth, 252
mimic, 100, 459, 478
mineralization, 289, 291
mineralocorticoids, 265, 276–277
minivalves, 90
minora, 514, 555, 583, 585
miosis, 447
miscalculation, 79
mismatch, 362, 389, 607, 621
missense mutation, 360
MIT, 273–274
mitochondria, 1, 3–4, 15–18, 21, 32–33, 36, 83, 161, 181, 197, 289, 334, 415, 418, 424, 562, 577, 628
mitochondrial, 2–4, 15, 18–20, 161, 181–182, 336–337, 341, 343
mitochondrial dna, 161, 341
mitochondrial inheritance, 341, 343
mitogen, 176
mitosis, 177, 186, 225, 357–359, 577
mitotic, 177, 186, 197, 557
mitral, 86, 94, 96–101, 103, 113, 117, 230
mitral regurgitation, 98–101
mitral stenosis, 95–96, 99, 101, 103
mitral valve, 85, 94, 96, 100–101, 103, 113, 116
mitral valve prolapse, 101
MLF, 444
MMFAE, 337
MMRV, 375
mobility, 565
mobilization, 282
mobilize, 300
modalities, 53
modiolus, 258, 489
modulate, 315, 468, 470–471, 476, 571
modulation, 322
modulators, 303
modulatory, 468
moiety, 176, 612
moist, 313
moisten, 434, 589
moisture, 193, 571, 589
monoamine, 451
monoamniotic, 219
monochorionic, 219
monocyte, 91, 170, 372, 404, 410
monoglyceride, 328–329
monohydrogen, 517
monoiodotyrosine, 273
monomer, 176–177, 325, 377
monomeric, 175
mononucleated, 200
mononucleotide, 2
monophasic, 132
monophosphate, 23–24, 26, 171, 174–175
monosaccharide, 327, 331
monosynaptic, 480
monotone, 64
monotonic, 64
monoxide, 605–606, 614
monozygotic, 219
mons, 555, 583
mood, 462, 572
morbid, 318
morning sickness, 562, 564
mortality, 60
morula, 197

mossy, 475–476
motilin, 283, 303, 305, 320
motility, 177, 283, 299–300, 305, 313, 316, 318–321, 432, 446–447
motivation, 462
mound, 587
mountain sickness, 628
mouthpiece, 594
movement, 2–3, 89, 94, 123, 155–157, 163, 168, 177, 179, 294–295, 299–300, 302, 304, 310, 312, 325, 331, 361, 411–412, 427–428, 430, 438, 440, 444, 455, 459–460, 464–465, 468, 470–471, 474–478, 491–494, 497, 504–506, 519, 525, 534–535, 537, 540, 562, 567, 569, 593, 595–596, 600–602, 606, 612
movement disorders, 470
mRNA, 38–39, 160, 175, 346, 354–356, 385, 615
MSH, 389
MSP, 112
mucin, 295, 298, 311
mucociliary, 589–591
mucosa, 91, 93, 294–298, 300, 304, 306–307, 311, 317, 319–321, 323, 332, 334, 425, 497, 555, 561, 571, 589–590
mucosae, 294, 298
mucosal, 93, 299, 318, 322, 377, 556, 590–591
mucous, 295–296, 311, 321, 434, 440, 556, 589
mucus, 294–298, 311–312, 317, 321–322, 331, 434, 494, 563, 565, 573–574, 589–590, 608
mulberry, 197
Müller, 100
Müllerian, 581–584
multinucleated, 200, 225, 410
multiparas, 565
multipolar, 257, 425, 465
multipotent, 201, 372
multisystem, 158
mumps, 375
Munro, 430
murmur, 47, 98–101, 103
muscarinic, 126, 313, 431–432, 447–448, 452–454, 588, 599
muscle relaxants, 158
muscularis, 293–296, 298, 300, 313–319
musculature, 258, 468
musculocutaneous, 500
musculoskeletal, 407, 409, 411, 413, 415, 417, 419, 421, 565
mushy, 310
mutagens, 360
mutase, 10, 18
mutate, 185
mutation, 49, 184, 187, 213, 341, 344, 347, 360–361, 389
myasthenia gravis, 521
MYC, 184
mycobacterial, 181
mydriasis, 446
myelencephalon, 253
myelin, 258, 424–425
myelinate, 258, 424–425, 433–434, 465, 482–483
myelinates, 258
myelination, 257–258

myeloid, 184, 372
myeloid leukemia, 184
myenteric, 293, 296, 300–303, 313–315, 317–319, 321, 432
mylohyoid, 249, 309
myoblasts, 225–226, 228
myocardial, 87, 111, 116, 118, 123–124, 126, 134, 158, 228, 231, 415
myocardial infarction, 134, 158
myocardium, 83–84, 87, 123, 153, 228, 231, 540, 619
myocyte, 83, 106, 118, 122–123, 125, 166, 185, 231, 330, 414–415
myoelectric, 303, 320
myoepithelial, 311, 560, 570
myogenic, 154, 225, 531
myoglobin, 418, 628
myometrial, 561, 573
myometrium, 556, 560–561, 566, 573–574
myopathy, 100
myosin, 87, 119, 125, 225, 330, 370, 414–416, 419–420
myotome, 205, 224, 226–227
myotubes, 225
myxoma, 103

nachos, 1
NAD, 1–2, 10, 18
nadh, 1–2, 10, 18–19
NADP, 10, 15
NADPH, 10, 15–16, 21, 276, 289, 291, 400–401
Naegele, 562
nares, 100
nasal septum, 589
nasolacrimal, 434
nasopharynx, 310, 325, 440, 589
nasteride, 580
natriuresis, 542
natriuretic, 106, 176, 530, 542
navigation, 566
necrotizing, 570
necrotizing enterocolitis, 570
negative, false, 79
negatively, 42, 162, 168, 284, 367, 518
negligible, 94, 532, 607
neisseria meningitidis, 375
neocortex, 255, 478
neocortical, 255
neonatal, 61, 93
neonatal mortality rate, 61
neonate, 232
neopallium, 255
nephrogenic, 243, 584
nephron, 109, 244–245, 510–512, 518, 533, 538–539, 543, 545, 549, 552, 554
nephros, 582–583
nephrotic syndrome, 156
nephrotomes, 243
Nernst, 169
nerve cell, 257, 260
nerve growth factor, 176
neurally, 104, 311, 313
neurilemma, 258
neuroblast, 253–255, 257
neurochemicals, 302
neurocranium, 222–223
neurocrines, 302–303
neuroectoderm, 254
neuroectodermal, 254, 265

neuroendocrine, 560, 570
neuroepithelial, 255, 257
neuroepithelium, 256–257
neuroglia, 261, 425
neurohormones, 268
neurohypophysis, 253–254, 263, 268
neurolemmocytes, 425
neuromodulators, 302
neuromuscular, 421, 452, 521, 539
neuron, 105, 107, 149, 194, 204, 255–257, 260, 263, 300, 302–304, 307, 313, 320, 414, 421, 423–426, 431–433, 437, 445–448, 450–452, 458–460, 464–471, 475, 478, 480–484, 486, 491, 493–495, 504, 552, 554, 601
neuronal, 284, 458
neuropeptide, 304, 445, 447
neuropore, 204–205, 257
neurotransmitter, 167, 174, 302, 304, 323, 331, 424–426, 431–432, 439, 445, 450, 452, 478, 499
neurulation, 202–204
neutralization, 320
neutralize, 196, 297, 321, 335, 364, 520, 578
neutrophil, 167, 177, 188–189, 194, 278, 372, 377, 404, 571
newborn, 54, 570
NF, 378, 390, 400
NFAT, 378, 390
nicotinamide, 18, 400
nicotinic, 330, 421, 431–432, 446, 448, 452
nicotinic acid, 330
nifedipine, 127
night sweats, 572
nigra, 254, 451, 477–478, 564
nigrostriatal, 470
nipple, 248, 511, 560, 563, 565, 570–571
Nissl, 424
nitric, 153–154, 176, 188–189, 300, 304, 365, 369, 617
nitrogenous base, 23, 349
nitrous oxide, 609
NK cell, 372–373, 383–384, 387, 395–396
nmethyltransferase, 451
nn, 452
nociceptors, 484, 486
nocturia, 564
nocturnal, 586
nodal, 128
nodularity, 563
noise, 99, 440, 462
nominal, 47, 62
nonamer, 393
nonampullare, 259
noncausal, 48
noncellular, 372
noncompliant, 117
nonconcurrent, 76
noncovalently, 176
nonfenestrated, 156
nonframeshift, 360
nonfunctional, 360
nonionic, 547
nonkeratinized, 295, 434
nonleukocytes, 385
nonlinear, 67–68, 544
nonparametric, 42, 63
nonpathogenic, 375, 377
nonphagocytes, 372

nonpolar, 163
nonsense, 360
nonshunted, 620, 623
nonsteroidal, 571
nonverbal, 461
noradrenaline, 262, 265, 450
norepinephrine, 127, 157, 262, 303, 313, 431–432, 445–446, 450–451
normetanephrine, 451
norms, 585
norovirus, 52
nostrils, 593
notch, 116, 138
notochord, 202, 204–205, 212–213, 224–225
nourish, 86, 244–245, 557, 561
nourishment, 218
novo, 24–26, 276
noxious, 427, 602
NPV, 81
NREM sleep, 459
NSAIDs, 571
NSTEMIs, 134
nuclease, 335, 389
nucleated, 386
nuclei, 253–254, 256, 263, 414–415, 430, 443–444, 446–447, 465–466, 470–471, 474–477, 494, 504, 548, 552, 554, 579
nucleic, 328, 374
nucleic acid, 23, 25, 27, 328
nucleobase, 23, 38, 349
nucleolus, 179–180, 358
nucleoplasm, 179–180
nucleoporin, 179
nucleosidases, 328
nucleoside, 23–24
nucleosome, 180, 350
nucleotide, 23–24, 26, 38, 170, 174, 336, 345–351, 354–356, 360, 362, 389, 393
nucleus, 38–39, 105, 161, 175, 179–181, 197, 202, 224, 253–255, 269, 275, 278, 307–308, 313, 346, 355, 372, 390, 416, 424, 430, 437, 443, 470–471, 477–479, 487, 494, 504, 579
nulliparas, 565
nutrient, 32, 83, 88–89, 155, 163, 186, 195, 218, 222, 294, 296–297, 299–300, 305–306, 320, 330–331, 333–334, 430, 455–456, 555, 563, 577
nutritional, 543, 565
nystagmus, 477, 494
nystatin, 571

obesity, 77, 96, 318, 521
oblique, 231, 296, 319, 504, 567
obliterated, 260
oblongata, 253, 468, 478
obstetric, 562
obstructed, 567
obstruction, 96, 98, 156
obtention, 76
occipital, 152, 221, 255, 428, 438, 474, 487–488, 504
occipital bone, 406, 567
occiput, 567
occludins, 166
occulonodular, 444, 474, 477

Index

octanoyl, 337
ocular, 159, 494–495
oculi, 438
oculomotor, 254, 448, 494, 503
oculomotor nerve, 254, 439, 504, 506
odontoblasts, 252
odontogenesis, 252
odor, 193
odorants, 494–495
Okazaki, 351
olfaction, 428, 494
olfactory, 253–256, 424–425, 478, 494–497, 503–504, 589
olfactory nerve, 494, 504–505
oligodendrocyte, 254, 258, 424–425
oligodendroglial, 257
oligosaccharides, 326, 571
oliguria, 158
olivary, 253, 443
omental, 239
omentum, 239, 293
omeprazole, 322
omphalomesenteric, 231
oncogene, 184
oncosis, 181
oncotic, 155–156, 364, 534, 542
oocyte, 196–198, 263, 555, 557, 559, 561, 577, 585–586
oogenesis, 557
oogonia, 557, 583
oogonium, 583
openbugs, 69
operating room, 158
operon, 345
ophthalmic, 152, 504, 507
opiates, 307
opiomelanocortin, 269
opsonin, 377, 404
opsonization, 189
opsonizes, 404
opthalmic, 504
optic nerve, 253, 260–261, 436–437, 439, 487, 506
optica, 260
orad, 303, 318–320
orally, 375
orbicularis, 438
orbital ridge, 567
organelle, 160–161, 177, 181, 187, 357, 364, 489
organism, 52, 54, 160, 351
organisms, 53, 344, 605
orgasm, 263
orifice, 98, 236, 295, 513–514, 576
ornithine transcarbamylase, 36
oropharyngeal, 201, 206–207
oropharynx, 310, 325, 589
orthopedic, 186
orthostatic hypotension, 104, 149
oscillating, 315
oscillatory, 309
osmolality, 510, 540
osmole, 548
osmoreceptors, 548, 552
osmoregulation, 548, 564
osmotic, 155, 168, 428, 536, 540
ossicles, 259, 440, 443
osteoblast, 222, 272, 275, 287, 406, 409–410
osteoclast, 161, 222, 275, 284–285, 287–288, 291, 406, 410

osteocyte, 285, 406, 410
osteoid, 222, 410
osteon, 406
osteoporosis, 572–573
osteoprotegerin, 287, 410
ostium, 230
otic, 204–205, 258–259, 447
otitis media, 440, 570
otocysts, 258
otolith, 443–444, 491
otolithic, 491
ouabain, 127
outbreak, 52–53
outcome, 36, 42, 44, 50, 58–59, 65, 68–69, 77–78, 188, 246
outer ear, 258, 489
outgrowth, 258
outlier, 43, 69
outpocketing, 216, 254
oval, 440, 442–443, 489, 567
ovale, 230, 232, 234, 504
ovalis, 232
ovarian, 555–556, 560, 572–574, 583, 586
ovary, 555–556
overabundance, 219
overdose, 521–522
overdrive, 131
overexpression, 184
overhydration, 548
overlie, 255
override, 309, 601
overshoot, 476
overwhelmed, 158
overwinding, 351
oviduct, 196
ovulation, 196, 557, 559–562, 573, 583
ovum, 557
oxalate, 284, 370
oxalic, 330, 518–519
oxaloacetate, 1, 4, 15, 17, 33, 36
oxidase, 3, 400–401, 451
oxidation, 4, 18–20, 161, 187, 280, 282, 336–337
oxidative, 2, 4, 10, 15, 33, 187, 374, 400, 418
oxidatively, 32
oxide, 153–154, 176, 188–189, 300, 304, 365, 369, 617
oxidosqualene, 13
oximeter, 82
oxygenated, 85, 153, 214–215, 232, 592, 595, 607, 619–620, 623
oxyhemoglobin, 612–614, 616, 623
oxyntic, 321
oxytocin, 175, 263, 268, 559–561, 565–566, 570, 573
oxytocinase, 561

pacemaker, 121–122, 131, 231, 278, 299–300, 315, 415
pachytene, 359
Pacinian, 191, 485
$PaCO_2$, 595–597, 601–602, 607–608, 620–621
pah, 532, 545–546
painful, 93
palate, 253, 309–310, 325, 498, 504, 589
palatine, 93, 504, 589
palatini, 249–250
paleocortex, 255
paleopallium, 255

pallidum, 255
pallidus, 253, 430, 477–479
palmar, 565
palmitoyl, 15, 17
palms, 190, 192
palpebrae, 438, 504
palpebral, 434
palpitations, 572
palsy, 468
PAMP, 188–189, 400–401
pancreas, 181, 207, 238–239, 241, 265–266, 293, 297, 299, 305, 307, 332–333, 335–337, 450, 520
pancreatic, 239, 265, 280–281, 283, 297, 299–300, 303, 305–306, 321, 326–328, 330–331, 335, 337, 565
pancreatic juice, 299, 303, 337
pancreatitis, 181
paneth, 297
panic, 522
pansystolic, 100–101
PaO, 597, 601–602, 609–611, 620–624
papilla, 192, 247, 252, 297, 511
papillae, 191, 247, 497–499
papillary, 85, 191, 247
papillary muscle, 85
parabolic, 143
paracellular, 325, 331, 535, 539
paracortical, 378
paracrine, 170, 262, 265, 321, 323, 542, 579
parafollicular, 204, 251, 264, 284
paralysis, 459
paramesonephric, 582–583
paramesonephros, 583
parameter, 41, 53, 112, 115, 627
parametric, 42, 62–65, 67, 69, 72
paranasal, 406, 589
parasite, 372, 383, 385
parasitic, 156
parasternal, 101
parasympathetic, 105, 107, 121, 126, 146–147, 149, 253, 256, 294, 297, 300, 302–303, 307, 311, 313–314, 319–320, 337, 423, 431–432, 434, 436, 439, 445, 447–448, 450, 452, 505, 588, 591–592, 599
parasympathetic nervous system, 256, 262, 280–281, 300, 447
parasympathomimetic, 452
parathyroid, 207, 251–252, 264–265, 286–287
parathyroid gland, 251, 286
parathyroid hormone, 174, 264–265, 284, 286, 291, 411, 537, 539, 565
paraventricular, 263, 552, 554
paravertebral, 445–446
paraxial, 202–203, 205–206, 221–222, 225–226, 247
parietal, 84, 152, 204, 206–207, 209–210, 221–225, 255, 293, 296, 306, 321–324, 330, 428, 468, 482–483, 591
parietal lobes, 152, 430
parietal pericardium, 84
Parkinson's disease, 478
parotid, 311, 505
particle, 90–91, 166, 309, 320, 499, 588–591, 597, 603
particulates, 602
partitioned, 237

partitioning, 230
parturition, 565, 573
passageway, 406, 589
passenger, 566–567
passive immunity, 375
passively, 100, 117, 331, 539, 547
patella, 406
patent ductus arteriosus, 98–99, 619
pathologic, 134, 187, 620
pathological, 21, 94, 97, 134, 185–186, 572
pathway, 6, 10, 12–16, 24, 28, 50, 106–107, 123, 170, 170–173, 174, 181–183, 186, 196, 212, 221, 253–254, 257, 260, 269, 271–272, 275, 280, 282–283, 291, 304, 324–326, 328–330, 332, 334, 336, 367–368, 377, 387–388, 402–404, 418, 425, 434–435, 443–444, 469–470, 477–479, 482–484, 487–489, 494–496, 499, 514, 552–554, 593, 617
Pavlov, 313, 323
pCO_2, 107, 147, 152, 515–516, 596, 607–608, 613–614, 621, 625–626
PCT, 245
PD, 395, 399
pea, 286, 338
peanuts, 377
Pearson, 64, 67
$PeCO_2$, 595
pectinate, 207, 298
pectoral, 405, 500
peduncle, 468, 474
peg, 411
pellucida, 196
pendrin, 273
penetrance, 49
penetration, 197–198
penicillin, 535
penile, 587
penis, 193, 246, 514, 576, 580, 582, 585, 587
pentamer, 377
pentose, 10, 12, 328
penumbra, 188
PEP, 4, 10
PEPCK, 4
pepsin, 321–322, 324, 327
pepsinogen, 296, 321–322, 324
peptidase, 286, 297
peptide, 30, 106, 160, 176, 262, 271, 280–281, 283, 302–303, 305–308, 318, 320, 322–324, 327–328, 356, 386–387, 390, 396, 530, 542, 552, 559
peptidergic, 302–303, 318, 320
peptidic, 262
peptidyl, 355
percentile, 567
perception, 158, 427, 438, 460, 499
perforin, 384
perfused, 595, 607, 618, 621–622
perfuses, 541
perfusing, 627
perfusion, 106, 109, 147, 188, 542, 563, 595, 607–609, 618, 621–622, 625–626
pericardial, 84, 96, 103, 209–210, 228
pericardial effusion, 96
pericarditis, 96, 103

pericardium, 83–84, 229
perichondrium, 407–408
periderm, 247
perilymph, 442–443, 489
perilymphatic, 258
perimenopausal, 573
perimenopause, 572
perimetrium, 556
perimysium, 414, 485
perineal, 514
periodic, 316, 320
periodically, 320
periodontal, 252, 411
periosteum, 406
peripheral nervous system, 204, 423, 445
peristalsis, 293, 295–296, 300, 304, 316, 319, 325, 432, 564, 577
peristaltic, 300–301, 304, 310, 316, 318
peritoneal, 159, 209–210, 239, 293, 510, 557
peritoneum, 293, 297, 333, 514, 555
peritubular, 511–512, 519, 533, 535–537, 542–546, 549, 552
permeability, 156, 163, 169, 188–189, 385, 425, 455, 534–535, 539, 565, 628
permeable, 168–169, 179, 425, 549, 609, 624
permeant, 455
permease, 345
peroxidase, 187, 273
peroxidation, 187
peroxide, 187, 337, 400–401
peroxisomal, 18
peroxisome, 18, 161, 334, 337
pertussis, 375–376
petrosal, 504
Peyer, 93, 297
phagocyte, 372–374, 400–401
phagocytic, 257, 400
phagocytize, 425, 591
phagocytose, 189, 401
phagocytosis, 91, 163, 167, 181, 278, 333, 373, 404
phagolysosome, 374, 387, 400–401
phagosome, 167, 374, 400–401
phalanges, 405
phallus, 582–583
pharmaceuticals, 336
pharmacologically, 74
pharmacotherapy, 571
pharyngeal, 93, 223, 225, 236, 238, 249–253, 259, 310, 325, 504, 589
pharyngeal pouch, 251, 259
pharyngotympanic, 440
pharynx, 93, 207, 238–239, 253, 295, 310, 316, 318, 325, 498, 505, 588–590, 593
phasic, 315–316, 481
phenotype, 338–339, 344
phenotypical, 583, 585
phenylethanolamine, 451
Philadelphia chromosome, 184
phonology, 461
phosphatase, 5–6, 8, 328
phosphate, 1–2, 4–6, 9–10, 12–13, 16, 23–25, 36–37, 162, 171, 222, 264, 284–289, 291–292, 328, 330, 345, 367, 349–350, 400, 406, 410, 420, 517, 519, 523, 540
phosphatidylcholine, 598
phosphatidylinositol, 171, 174–175

phosphaturia, 540
phosphodiesterase, 126, 175, 439
phosphoenolpyruvate, 4, 10
phosphofructokinase, 9–10
phosphoglucoisomerase, 9
phosphoglucomutase, 6
phosphogluconate, 10
phosphoglycerate, 10
phospholamban, 126–127
phospholipase, 171, 175–176, 286, 323, 328–329, 450, 452
phospholipid, 13, 162, 179, 262, 323, 329, 334, 373
phosphomevalonate, 13
phosphoproteins, 175
phosphorus, 330
phosphorylase, 6
phosphorylate, 4, 9, 13, 171, 176, 378
phosphorylated, 127
phosphorylates, 171, 175–176, 390
phosphorylation, 2, 4, 15, 126, 161, 175–176, 187, 269, 271–272, 280, 282, 291
photoreception, 439, 486
photoreceptor, 437, 439, 486
phototransduction, 439, 487
phrenic, 500, 592, 600–601
phytates, 330
pia, 261
pia mater, 253, 260, 430
pigmented, 177, 260, 435–437, 439
piloerection, 157
pineal, 254
pineal gland, 253, 264, 428, 455, 459
pinealocytes, 264
pinna, 440, 489
pinnae, 408
pinocytic, 155
pinocytosis, 167
pinulin, 538
PIP, 175, 286
piriform, 495
pisiform, 406
pituitary gland, 109, 170, 204, 263, 268, 428–429, 455, 552, 554, 565, 570, 579
pKA, 126
PL, 268, 559–560, 570
placebo, 65, 74
placenta, 197, 202–203, 214–216, 218–219, 232, 234, 557, 559, 561, 563, 565, 567, 570, 573, 624
placental, 214–215, 230, 561, 564–565, 570
placode, 204–205, 256, 258, 260
plaque, 143, 166, 188, 571
plasma cell, 92, 377
plasmid, 348, 351, 353
plasmin, 370
plasminogen, 370
plateau, 31, 64, 121–122, 125–126, 315, 545, 627
platykurtic, 42
platypelloid, 567
pleated, 30
plethysmograph, 594
pleura, 591
pleural, 159, 209–210, 591
pleuropericardial, 210
pleuroperitoneal, 210, 212
plexiform, 437, 486

Index

plexus, 253–255, 258, 293–294, 296–298, 300–303, 313–315, 317–319, 321, 423, 430, 432, 456–457 500, 555, 592
plop, 103
pluripotent, 197
pneumatization, 259
pneumocytes, 237, 591, 598
pneumonia, 521–522, 608
pneumoniae, 375
pneumotaxic, 427, 601
PNMT, 451
PNS, 258, 423–426, 431, 445
pO_2, 82, 107, 147, 517, 605, 607–608, 611–614, 620–622, 624, 626–628
podocytes, 511, 533
poikilocytosis, 186
Poiseuille, 141, 599
poisoning, 605, 614, 623
polar, 29, 162–163, 197, 262
polarity, 336
polarization, 122–123, 315
pole, 200, 359
polio, 375
polyadenine, 354
polyadenylate, 354
polymer, 6, 16–17
polymerase, 38–39, 345–346, 348, 351, 354–356, 362, 389
polymerase chain reaction, 348
polymerize, 177, 415
polymers, 377
polymodal, 486
polymorphonuclear, 161, 372, 374
polynucleotide, 349
polypeptide, 39, 106, 265, 284, 286, 299, 327–328, 355–356, 612
polyploidy, 360–361
polysaccharide, 375
polyspermy, 197
polysynaptic, 480
polyubiquitinated, 186
polyunsaturated, 570
POMC, 269
pons, 152, 253–254, 256, 313, 427–428, 430, 443–444, 468, 470–471, 482, 494, 504–505, 514, 601
pontine, 254, 471–472, 474–475, 478, 514
pontocerebellar, 254, 475–476
pontocerebellum, 474
popula, 53
porous, 606
porphyrin, 612
portal, 13, 263, 268, 297–298, 332–334, 579
portal vein, 32, 232, 289, 327–329, 334
positive, false, 79
positively, 42, 168, 433
postadaptive, 400
postcapillary, 89
postdiagnosis, 61
posterior pituitary, 263, 268, 455, 552–554, 559–561
posteriorly, 239, 430, 435–436, 589
posterolateral, 231
posteromedial, 308
postextrasystolic, 127
postganglionic, 256, 302–303, 313, 320, 431–432, 445–447, 450–452
postmeal, 320
postmitotic, 225

postnatal, 258
postpartum, 559–560, 565, 570–571
postrema, 455
postsynaptic, 421, 426, 433, 439, 445, 478
posture, 254, 414, 427, 443, 470–471, 474, 476, 594
potassium, 121–122, 146, 169, 171, 265, 282, 327, 364, 425, 433, 443, 455–456, 490–491, 540, 549
potatoes, 312
pouch, 204, 249–251, 254, 259, 297–298
PPV, 81
PPY, 305
PR, 95–96, 116, 128, 130, 132, 286
prealbumin, 274
preaortic, 256
precancerous, 186
precapillary, 89, 155
prechordal, 222
precision, 82
precordial, 129, 132
precursor, 15, 26, 187, 190, 265, 287, 289, 478, 557, 573
preexcitation, 96
preexisting, 76
preformed, 282
preganglionic, 256, 302–303, 313–314, 431–432, 445–448, 452
pregnenolone, 573–574, 579
pregnolone, 276
preload, 86, 94, 111, 115, 117, 120, 126
premature, 61, 76, 570
premature birth, 76
premonitory, 565
premotor, 428, 464, 468
prenatal, 247
preprocalcitonin, 284
preproglucagon, 280
preproinsulin, 281
preproparathyroid, 286
prepropth, 286
pressure, 115, 603
pressure ulcers, 194
pressurized, 605
presynaptic, 421, 426, 445, 450
presystolic, 103
pretectal, 504
preterm, 562
preterminal, 500
prevalence, 53, 58, 77, 81
prevention, 53, 195, 365, 402, 571, 617
preventive, 58
prevertebral, 256, 445
primase, 351
primaxial, 225
primer, 348, 351
primordial, 557, 559, 561, 577, 581–583
primordium, 260
primum, 230
principle, 6, 111, 465, 516, 523, 532, 546
prioritization, 61
probability, 41, 44–45, 48, 58, 62, 69–73, 81, 342, 344
probit, 69
problematic, 618
procalcitonin, 284
procarboxypeptidase, 327, 335, 337
process, 9
procolipase, 328
procollagen, 164
proctodeum, 207, 241

proenzyme, 329, 335
proepicardial, 226, 228
proerythroblast, 615
progenitor, 372, 381, 391
progesterone, 13, 174–175, 199–200, 248, 263, 268, 555, 557, 559, 561–565, 570, 572–574, 583, 586
progestin, 572
proglucagon, 280
prognenolone, 276
proinsulin, 281
projection, 91, 239, 406, 424, 455, 476, 479, 488, 497, 589
prolactin, 175, 264, 268, 559–560, 563, 574
prolapse, 99, 101
proliferate, 194, 200, 225, 227–228, 230, 238–239, 247–248, 254–255, 259, 297, 381, 389, 391, 561
proliferation, 174, 176, 199, 247, 259, 278, 385, 561, 565, 573–574
proliferative, 561
prometaphase, 358
promoter, 38, 184, 345–346, 354
prompted, 625
pronator, 227
pronephric, 243
pronephros, 243–244
pronuclei, 197–198
pronucleus, 197
proopiomelanocortin, 269
propecia, 580
prophase, 339, 358–359, 583
propionyl, 18
propria, 260–261, 293–294, 296–297, 317, 321, 494
proprioception, 442, 474, 482–483, 485, 504
proprioceptive, 505
proprioceptors, 484–485, 625
proPTH, 286
propulsion, 295, 297, 299, 325
propulsive, 304
prosencephalon, 253–254
prostacyclin, 153, 369, 617
prostaglandin, 157–158, 278, 324, 365, 530, 578, 617
prostate, 514, 577–578, 580, 585
prostate gland, 577–578
prostatic, 246, 514, 578, 580
protease, 312, 327, 330, 335–337, 370, 400, 402
proteasome, 186, 387
proteinases, 412
proteins, 289
proteinuria, 42
proteoglycan, 164–165, 336, 407–408
proteolysis, 275, 282
proteolytic, 275
prothrombin, 367
prothrombin time, 367
prothrombinase, 367
protid, 312
proton, 2–4, 322, 328
protoplasmic, 179, 257
protrusions, 201, 214
proximally, 193
PRRs, 188, 400–401
pseudobulbar, 468
pseudoglandular, 236
pseudopodia, 177

pseudopods, 167
pseudounipolar, 481
pSMAC, 384
PT, 367
pterygoid, 249, 309–311
pterygopalatine, 256
PTH, 286–289, 291, 539–540
ptyalism, 564
pubarche, 586
pubertal, 587
puberty, 192–193, 247–248, 271, 557, 573, 577, 580–582, 586
pubic, 265, 586–587
pubic symphysis, 567
pubis, 412, 555, 563, 565, 567, 583
public health, 53
pulmonary, 625, 627
pulmonary artery, 111, 231–232, 234
pulmonary edema, 158, 521, 606, 628
pulmonary embolism, 96, 158, 522, 621
pulmonary hypertension, 96
pulmonary valve, 85, 94, 100
pulmonary vein, 111, 139
pulmonic, 86, 94, 98, 100–101, 103, 116–118
pulmonic regurgitation, 98, 101
pulp, 91, 252
pulposus, 202, 224
pulsatile, 271, 278, 573, 586
pulsation, 90, 113
pulse, 86, 103, 113, 116, 137–139, 144–146, 586
pulsus, 96
puncta, 434
Punnett, 338–339, 342–343
pupil, 226, 260–261, 432, 435–436, 439, 446–447, 504
pupillae, 253, 260, 436, 439, 504
pupillary, 159, 260, 439
purine, 23–24, 26–27, 349
Purkinje, 121, 123, 128, 231, 254, 475–476
purplish, 562–563
putamen, 253–255, 430, 477
PV, 603–604, 618
PW, 604
Px, 538, 604–605
pyloric, 296, 300, 316, 320–321
pylorus, 239, 296, 320
pyramid, 265, 427, 468, 470, 510–511
pyramidal, 468
pyrimidine, 23–25, 349
pyrogens, 157
pyrophosphate, 13
pyrophosphorylase, 6
pyrosis, 564
pyruvate, 4, 9–10, 15–16, 33, 161
PYY, 308

QALY, 61
QRS, 129–132
QRS complex, 116, 128, 131–132
QTc, 130
quadrate, 333
quaternary, 30
quickening, 562
quiescence, 601
quinone, 367
quotient, 597

RA, 111–112, 117

RAAS, 110, 147, 265, 513, 542, 564
rabies, 375
radially, 143
radiata, 197–198, 468
radiolabeled, 523
radius, 118, 141, 154, 227, 405, 411–412, 598–599
RAG, 381, 391, 393
rami, 258
ramps, 601
ramus, 406
randomization, 41, 78
randomized, 76, 78
randomly, 65, 78, 351, 393, 603
rank, 64
RANKL, 287, 410
Ranvier, 424
raphe, 576
rate, 60, 602, 606
rater, 63
Rathke, 254
ratio, 47–48, 55, 57–59, 62, 64–65, 67, 69, 158, 339, 476, 528, 534, 538, 570, 621, 625
RBBB, 132
RBC, 370, 546, 564–565, 612, 615–616
RBF, 546
RCT, 78
rDNA, 179
reabsorb, 13, 89, 109, 332, 457, 518–522, 528, 535, 538–543, 547–548, 552, 554, 589
reabsorbable, 541
reabsorptive, 539
reactants, 516
reaction, 4, 30–33, 74, 175–176, 196–197, 200, 273, 276, 336, 348, 370, 463, 480, 517, 539, 616
reactivated, 396
reading frame, 360
rearrange, 18, 136, 381, 391, 393
rearrangement, 384, 391, 393
reattach, 170, 361, 393
recanalization, 238–239
reception, 170, 442
receptive, 318, 320, 481, 484–485
reciprocal, 243, 304
recoil, 88, 137–139, 144–145, 591, 593, 597–598
recolonize, 298
recombinant, 339, 341, 351, 353
recombinase, 381, 391, 393
recombination, 363, 381, 393
recombinational, 393
recombine, 393, 519
recruitment, 606
recta, 536
rectal, 298, 301
rectum, 297–298, 300–301, 303, 513, 556
recumbent, 563
recycle, 274, 332, 547
red blood cell, 91, 143, 168, 533, 564, 612
reddish, 372
redness, 188, 372
reductase, 13, 24, 276, 367, 580, 582
reduction, 58–59, 105, 186, 188, 276, 336, 519, 610, 617, 624, 627
reflex, 105, 107, 480, 494
reform, 354
refractive, 436, 439
regeneration, 425

regenerative, 194
regional, 608
regressed, 214
regression, 68–69
regularity, 458
regulator, 88, 284, 286, 381
regulatory, 13, 171, 274, 284, 345–346, 386, 395, 399, 419–420, 519–522, 617
regurgitant, 101, 103
regurgitation, 96, 98–101
rehearsal, 461, 464
rejuvenated, 194
relationship, 119
relaxant, 158
relaxation, 86, 94, 113, 116, 125–126, 154, 176, 303, 315–316, 318, 320, 432, 439, 450, 458, 514, 564, 566, 599, 624
relaxin, 563, 565
relay, 147, 171, 253, 321, 427–428, 482
relayed, 297
release, 337
REM sleep, 459
remainder, 252, 539, 573, 611
remnant, 202, 216, 218, 232, 333, 235
remodel, 411
remodeling, 194, 410–411, 565, 574
renal, 32, 106–107, 109, 111, 141, 147–148, 158, 243–245, 265, 278, 287, 289, 331, 510–513, 516–521, 525, 527–535, 537, 539, 541–547, 549, 551, 553, 564, 615
renal capsule, 510
renal failure, 519
renal pelvis, 244, 511, 513
renal tubular acidosis, 519
renal tubule, 511–512, 518, 535, 547
renin, 104, 109–110, 147, 265, 450, 513, 520, 530, 533, 542, 564
renina, 253
reoxygenated, 619
repeatability, 42, 82
repeatable, 82
repeatedly, 48, 236, 381, 391
reperfusion, 188
repetition, 339, 461, 480
repigmentation, 194
replicate, 160, 192, 348, 351, 353, 357, 372, 375, 389
replication, dna, 351
repolarization, 116, 121–122, 128, 132, 315, 433
reportable, 53
reposition, 239, 310
repressor, 345–346
reproduce, 82, 342
reproductive, 360, 480, 555, 557, 559, 561–563, 565, 567, 569, 571, 573, 575–577, 579–585, 587
RER, 160, 179, 273
resegmentation, 224
reservoir, 54, 91, 579
residual, 594–595
residue, 6, 16, 171, 175, 271, 273–274, 345, 367, 378, 386, 390
resistant, 53, 330, 408
resonance, 30, 589
resonant, 94
resorbed, 410
respiratory acidosis, 515, 521

Index

respiratory alkalosis, 515, 522, 564, 625, 627
respiratory rate, 459, 519–522, 596, 601–602, 625
restitution, 567
restorative, 459
restraint, 101
restriction, 347, 351, 353, 608
resultant, 103
rete, 577, 581–582
retention, 519–520, 543, 552, 564
reticular, 91, 191, 427, 444, 471
reticularis, 265, 276–278
reticulata, 478
reticulin, 164
reticulospinal, 471–472
reticulum, 4, 13, 125–126, 158, 160, 171, 175, 252, 273, 286, 334, 387, 414–415, 419–420, 424, 499
retina, 254, 260–261, 425, 435, 437, 439–440, 443, 459, 486–488, 504
retinae, 260
retinal, 435, 437–439
retraction, 369–370
retrograde, 316
retroperitoneal, 293, 297, 335, 510–511
retroperitoneally, 265
retropulsion, 320
reuniens, 258
rewarming, 159
RF, 427
Rh, 370–371
rho, 64
rhombencephalon, 253–254, 258
rhomboid, 500
rhombomeres, 256
rhythmic, 123, 228, 458
rhythmically, 590
rib, 221, 224, 333, 412
ribonuclease, 328
ribonucleotide, 24
ribose, 10, 23–24, 349
ribosomal, 39, 160, 179
ribosome, 30, 39–40, 160–161, 346, 354–356
ribozyme, 160
ribulose, 10
richly, 260, 293, 436
ridge, 227, 230, 236, 243, 248, 258, 406, 474, 581
right bundle branch block, 96, 132
right heart, 99, 111, 607–608, 619, 624–625, 627
right ventricle, 85, 96, 99–101, 117, 132, 139, 229, 232, 234
right ventricular hypertrophy, 130–131, 133
rigidity, 159
ripening, 573
RNA, 23–26, 38–39, 175, 180, 345–347, 349–351, 354–356, 385, 615
RNA polymerase, 38–39, 345–346, 354–356
rods, 260, 406, 437, 486–487
rootlets, 505
rope, 177
rostral, 253–254, 445
rostrally, 210
rotate, 227, 439, 567
rotation, 112, 131, 238, 240, 412, 443, 493–494, 567
rotational, 440, 443–444

rotavirus, 375
rotundum, 504
RPF, 534, 546
RR, 58, 129–130, 341, 596
rRNA, 39, 160, 179
RSV, 76
RTKs, 176
rubella, 375
rubor, 188
rubrospinal, 470–471
Ruffini corpuscles, 484–485
rumble, 103
rumbling, 99, 103
rupture, 167, 181, 241–242, 557, 559, 566, 561
RV, 117–118, 594
ryanodine, 125, 127, 158, 420
RYR, 158

SA, 450
SA node, 121, 123, 129, 131
saccular, 492
saccule, 258–259, 443–444, 491–492
sacral, 224, 314, 427, 447
sacrum, 406, 556
saddle, 412
safeguard, 378
sagittal, 428–430, 513
sagittal sinus, 430
salicylates, 522
saline, 159
saliva, 31, 295, 309–313, 499, 504, 564
salivary, 253, 295, 311–313, 326, 330, 450, 505
salivating, 313
salivation, 325, 445–447, 450
salivatory, 313
salt, 332, 337
saltatory, 425, 433–434
salvage, 24, 28, 336
sanitation, 53
SaO_2, 611
sarcolemma, 414–415, 420
sarcolemmal, 125–126
sarcomere, 117–119, 414–416, 419
sarcoplasm, 125–126, 158, 175, 414–415, 419–420
satellite, 425
satiety, 307–308
savory, 497
scab, 194
scala, 258, 442–443, 489
scalae, 442
scalenes, 593
scap, 13
scapulae, 405–406
scapular, 500
scar, 194
scarpa, 444
scarring, 194
scatterplots, 68
Schlemm, 261, 435
Schwann, 204, 258, 424–425
Schwann cell, 258
sclera, 260–261, 436
scleral, 261, 435
sclerotome, 205, 224–225
scores, 71
scrotal, 576
scrotum, 576, 580, 582, 585
SD, 41, 46, 65, 68–70

sea, 596, 599, 627
sebaceous, 192–193, 563
sebaceous gland, 247, 265, 580
sebum, 193, 247
second, 322
secrete, 84, 92, 106, 109, 147, 161, 170, 190–191, 193–194, 190, 199–200, 202, 212–213, 218, 222, 239, 243, 247, 262–266, 268–269, 271–274, 276, 278, 280–281, 283–284, 293–297, 299, 303–308, 311–313, 317, 319–322, 324–325, 327–331, 334–336, 373, 377–378, 385, 398, 400, 406–407, 409–410, 426, 436, 440, 455, 478, 480, 513, 520, 528, 530, 533, 538, 541–543, 546–547, 555, 557, 559, 562–563, 573, 577–579, 582–583, 586, 589–591, 615
secretin, 283, 299, 306, 320, 335, 337
secretion, 106, 109, 147–148, 160, 190–191, 193, 262, 265, 269, 271–272, 274, 278–281, 283–284, 286–287, 295–300, 302–303, 305–307, 311–313, 319–324, 326, 331–332, 335–337, 365, 432, 434, 446–447, 450, 505, 518–520, 528, 535–539, 541, 543, 545–548, 559–560, 563–564, 570, 573, 586, 615
secretory, 161, 199, 247–248, 256, 268, 281–282, 284, 286, 300, 305–307, 313, 321–322, 455–456, 555, 562, 571, 574
sectional, 77
secundum, 230
seeping, 190
segmental, 236, 300, 303, 510, 590
segmentation, 152, 213, 296, 300
segregate, 338
segregation, 338
selectin, 199
SEM, 72
semen, 514, 578
semicircular, 253, 258–259, 440, 443–444, 491, 493–494
semiconservative, 351
semilunar, 85, 94, 116, 231
seminal, 196, 514, 577–578, 580, 585
seminal vesicle, 578
seminiferous, 576–577, 581–582
semipermeable, 162, 168
senescence, 362
sensation, 190, 326, 427, 443, 486, 497, 572
sensitive, 18, 79–80, 105, 107–108, 437, 466–467, 484–485, 487, 497, 513, 530, 586, 602, 620
sensitivity, 79–80, 105, 126, 174, 278, 467, 481, 499, 561, 574
sensors, 326
sepsis, 98, 522
septa, 214, 216, 576
septae, 237
septal, 96, 129, 589, 619
septum, 83, 121, 153, 210, 212, 230–231, 236, 238–239, 241, 246, 589
sequential, 80, 123, 141, 318
sequentially, 162
SER, 160
serine, 171, 176, 402
serosa, 293–295, 319, 591

serotonin, 154, 188, 296, 304, 307, 321, 365, 426
serous, 84, 205–206, 209, 311, 434
serous membrane, 209
serratus, 500
sertoli, 576–579, 581–582, 586
sesame, 406
sesamoid, 406
setpoint, 105
sex chromosome, 341
sexual dysfunction, 573
SF, 79
SGLT, 163, 327
SH, 1, 13
shaft, 192–193, 247
shallow, 247
shallower, 515
sharpey, 411
SHBG, 573
sheath, 222, 247, 252, 258, 424–425, 465
sheehan, 565
SHH, 202, 213
shield, 590
shock, 104, 158, 351, 412
shock, spinal, 158
short-term memory, 461
shoulder, 221, 225, 412, 500, 505, 567
shoulder joint, 412
shrimp, 229
shunt, 89, 231–232, 234, 607, 619–621, 623
shuttle, 2, 17–18
sickle cell disease, 360
sickness, 627
sigmoid, 241, 297–298, 300, 303
sigmoidal, 612–613
silence, 345–346
silencer, 346
silent, 98, 360
silver, 349
simplex, 571
simulate, 69, 99
simultaneous, 80, 96, 141, 460, 493, 625
simultaneously, 99, 104, 304
sinciput, 567
sinoatrial, 450
sinoatrial node, 123, 231
sinus, 85, 92–93, 105, 128–129, 131, 147, 149, 228–229, 231, 241, 246, 261, 406, 430, 435, 505, 582–584, 589
sinus arrhythmia, 129
sinus bradycardia, 131
sinus node, 128–129
sinus rhythm, 129
sinus tachycardia, 131
sinusoidal, 334, 336
sinusoids, 91, 200, 214, 334
skeletal, 6, 8, 18, 86, 107, 126, 146, 154, 157–158, 161, 194, 221, 225–226, 293, 295, 298, 301, 311, 315, 405, 414–416, 418, 421, 427, 432, 440, 450, 459, 465, 467, 480, 539, 625–626, 628
skeletal muscle, 6, 107, 146, 154, 157–158, 161, 194, 226, 293, 295, 298, 301, 311, 315, 414–415, 418, 421, 432, 450, 459, 465, 467, 480, 539, 625–626
skeleton, 83, 221, 276, 405, 408, 565
skin cancer, 190
skull, 152, 221–223, 405–406, 411, 474, 505, 508, 567, 589
sleep, 157, 271, 278, 313, 427, 458–460, 478, 504
sleep disturbances, 478
slick, 88
slippery, 293
slowness, 470, 478
SLP, 390
slurred, 132
SMAC, 384
small intestine, 32, 90, 241, 288, 292, 294, 296–300, 303–307, 316, 319–320, 324, 326–331, 335
smallpox, 375
smokers, 58, 72, 76
smooth muscle, 88, 139, 153–155, 176, 225–226, 256, 278, 293–295, 297–303, 307, 315–316, 320–321, 334, 365, 416, 432, 436, 452, 480, 505, 530–531, 555–556, 564, 576, 588, 590–591, 599, 602, 617, 624
SMR, 55
SN, 79
SO_2, 612
sodium, 121–122, 163, 169, 171, 181, 265, 287, 292, 326–328, 330, 335, 364, 421–422, 433, 436, 439, 443, 456, 494, 511, 513, 519, 525, 531, 538, 541, 543–544, 548–549, 564, 615
soft palate, 310, 325, 498, 589
solitarius, 105
solitary, 253
solubilities, 608
solubility, 603, 605, 611, 615
solubilized, 329
soluble, 89, 155, 176, 289, 330, 332, 410, 455, 547, 570, 608, 624
solute, 163, 168, 312, 331, 511–512, 523, 525, 529, 533, 535–537, 549, 554
solution, 159, 311, 525, 548, 571, 603, 605, 609, 611, 616
solutions, 168, 516
soma, 424
somatic, 202, 207, 209, 228, 253–254, 341, 357, 360, 389, 396, 423, 445, 480, 482, 484, 505, 565
somatomedin, 271
somatosensory, 310, 428, 468, 481–482, 484
somatostatin, 170, 263, 265, 271, 280, 283, 296, 299, 305–306, 321, 324, 335
somatotropic, 271
somatotropin, 268, 271
somite, 205–206, 212, 224–227
somitic, 225
somitomeres, 225
sonic, 202, 212–213
sore, 571
span, memory, 275
sparking, 188
spasm, 365
spastic, 468
spatial, 427, 491
Spearman, 64
species, 54, 187, 344
specificity, 79
specimens, 41
sperm, 196–198, 219, 263, 576–578, 582, 585–586
spermarche, 586
spermatids, 577
spermatocyte, 577
spermatogenesis, 576–580
spermatogonia, 577, 581–582
spermatogonium, 577
spermatozoa, 196–197, 578
sphenoid, 406, 589
sphenoid bone, 406, 589
sphere, 117–118, 598
spherical, 161, 439
sphincter, 89, 155, 226, 239, 253, 260, 293, 295–298, 300–301, 303, 310, 316–318, 320, 325, 432, 436, 439, 450, 504, 514, 578
sphygmomanometer, 104
spicy, 572
spider nevi, 565
spikes, 300, 476
spinal, 224, 227, 253, 257–258, 408, 423, 427, 432, 456, 466, 468, 470, 480, 482, 502, 505, 514
spinal column, 243, 427, 456, 567
spinal cord, 158, 224, 254, 256–257, 301, 313–314, 423, 425–428, 430–431, 444–447, 456, 459, 464, 468, 470–471, 474, 480, 482–483, 500–501, 503, 505, 507, 509, 560–561
spinal nerve, 227, 427
spindle, 177, 358–359, 465–467, 485
spine, 567
spinocerebellar, 475–476
spinocerebellum, 474
spinosum, 190, 289
spinothalamic, 482–484
spinous, 247
spiral, 199, 214, 258–259, 442–443, 465, 490
spiraling, 231
spirometer, 100, 594
spirometry, 594
splanchnic, 107, 207, 209, 225–226, 228, 294, 297, 432
splay, 544
spleen, 91–92, 240, 275, 294, 335, 389
splenic, 91, 298
splenic artery, 91
splice, 346, 354, 378, 381, 391
spliceosomes, 38, 346, 354
spongiosum, 576
spongy, 406–407, 514
spontaneous, 21, 121, 123, 315, 360, 402, 404, 458, 562, 566, 574
spurt, 586
squalene, 13
squamous, 84, 186, 190, 293–295, 298, 434, 436, 536, 556, 589, 591
squared, 62
squat, 100
squatting, 100
squeezed, 13
squeezing, 146
SR, 126
Src, 271
SREBP, 13
SRY, 581–583
stability, 177, 351
stabilizes, 31, 414, 494
stabilizing, 367
staircase, 127

Index

stalk, 216, 218, 243–244, 246, 254, 260–261, 263, 268
standardization, 55–57
standardize, 55, 57, 71
stapedial, 231
stapedius, 250, 259, 440, 504
stapes, 223, 250, 259, 440, 443, 489
starch, 312, 326
Starling, 119, 155–156, 533–534, 542
starvation, 186, 274, 308, 336, 346
STAT, 271, 383
static, 177, 466, 491, 594
stationary, 414
statistic, 41, 65
statistical, 41–42, 62, 68–69, 71–73
statistician, 68
statoacoustic, 258
stellate, 252, 254, 334, 475–476
stem cell, 190, 391
stemi, 134
stenosis, 95–96, 98–101, 103, 117
stenotic, 96, 100, 103, 117–118
stercobilin, 332, 334
stereocilia, 443, 489, 491, 493
sternal, 94, 100–101, 103
sternocleidomastoid, 505, 508
sternum, 83, 93, 221, 224, 405–407, 412
steroid, 13, 160, 175, 262, 265, 276, 278, 289, 455, 565, 573, 586
sterol, 13
stethoscope, 98–99, 104
stiffness, 490
stimulant, 300, 305–307, 324, 561
stimulation, 119, 185, 265, 269, 271–272, 274, 280–282, 286, 289, 291, 305–307, 313, 320, 322–324, 330, 335, 337, 383–384, 390, 419–420, 530, 566, 579, 586, 591, 599, 625
stimulatory, 174, 263, 324, 397, 450, 452
stimulus, 124, 174, 186, 286–287, 299, 307, 313, 323, 337, 423, 427, 433, 455, 459–460, 462, 471, 480–482, 566, 615, 625
stirrup, 440
STM, 461
stomodeum, 207, 254
stool, 570
STPD, 603
strain, 133, 627
strand, 38–39, 180, 192, 346, 348, 350–352, 354–356, 362, 415
stranded, 351, 362–363
stratum, 190–191, 247, 289
strength, 30, 41, 48, 64, 67, 69, 87, 94, 115, 119, 164, 166, 194, 315–316, 320, 389, 407–408, 412, 481, 562, 565
strenuous, 117, 609
streptococcus, 375
streptococcus pneumoniae, 375
stress incontinence, 564
stressful, 431
stressor, 186, 278, 353, 462
stretchy, 88, 117
striae, 565
striatal, 478
striated, 83, 253, 301, 310–311, 415
striations, 226
striatum, 254, 477–479
stringy, 311
striola, 491–492

stroke, 87, 99, 104, 112–113, 115, 119–120, 146, 158, 419–420, 521, 563
stroke volume, 87, 99, 104, 112–113, 115, 119–120, 146, 563
stroma, 200, 436
structural, 160, 164–165, 176–177, 181, 252, 275, 345, 361, 425
structurally, 361
study, 75, 77
stylohyoid, 250
styloid, 250
stylomastoid, 505
stylopharyngeus, 250, 505
stylopod, 227
subarachnoid, 430, 456
subcapsular, 92–93
subclavian, 90, 156, 231
subcortical, 477
subcostal, 564
subcutaneous, 191, 485
subcutaneously, 375
subendocardial, 134
subendothelial, 88, 367
subfornical, 455
sublingual, 311–312
submandibular, 256, 311–312, 447
submucosa, 293–297, 302, 313–314, 317, 319, 590
submucosal, 300, 302–303, 313–314, 317, 319
suboccipitobregmatic, 567
subphases, 357
subpial, 255
subscapular, 500
subset, 41, 460
substantia, 254, 260–261, 451, 477–478
substituting, 136
substitutions, 360
substrate, 4, 31, 271, 282, 289, 336
subthalamic, 254, 477–479
subthalamus, 253–255
subthreshold, 315
subunit, 160, 170–171, 174–175, 179, 269, 272, 280, 282, 375–376, 415, 420, 612, 615
succinate, 1–2, 21
succinyl, 1, 18, 21
succinylcholine, 158
sucking, 318
suckling, 560, 570
sucrase, 326
sucrose, 326
sudoriferous, 192–193
suicidal, 463
sulci, 255, 428–429
sulcus, 153, 229, 253, 257, 464, 497
sulfate, 541
sulfation, 336
sulfonation, 161
sunlight, 78
sunscreen, 190
superfamily, 175, 305
superimposed, 460
superimposition, 98
superioris, 438, 504
superiorly, 590
superoxide, 187, 400–401
supinator, 227
supplemental, 622–623, 628
supplementation, 564, 571
supplements, 572

suppress, 481
suppression, 131, 306
suppressor, 184
suprachiasmatic, 269, 278, 504
supramolecular, 384
supranormal, 124
supraoptic, 263, 548, 552, 554
suprascapular, 500
supraspinatus, 500
suprasternal notch, 317
surface, 519
surfactant, 237, 591, 597–598
surge, 278, 561, 573
surgical, 194
surrogate, 68, 76, 381
surveillance, 53, 434
survival, 58, 63, 174, 344, 627
survivors, 63
susceptible, 53–54, 154, 158
suspensory, 260, 436, 555–556
sustain, 200, 418
SV, 87, 112–113, 115–116, 119–120
SVR, 118, 137, 563
SW, 113
swabbed, 571
sweat, 157, 190–193, 204, 226, 247–248, 431, 452, 525, 586
sweating, 157–158, 326, 446, 525
SWS, 459
Sylvius, 430
symmetrical, 42
symmetry, 43, 201
sympathetic, 99, 105, 107, 109, 119, 121, 126, 139, 146–147, 149, 157, 204, 256–257, 269, 278, 294, 297, 300, 302–303, 311, 313–314, 319–320, 423, 427, 431–432, 436, 439, 445–446, 450–452, 530, 542, 588, 591–592, 599
sympathetic nervous system, 153–154, 157, 193, 256, 262, 280–281, 283, 445–446, 463, 541
sympathomimetic, 450
symphysis, 412, 562–563, 565, 567
symphysis pubis, 412, 563, 565, 567
symport, 273
symporter, 273
symptomatic, 52
synapse, 105, 303, 313–314, 424, 426, 431, 437, 440, 445–447, 466–470, 475–476, 480, 482–484, 487, 504
synapsis, 358
synaptic, 421–422, 426, 486, 490–491
synarthrosis, 411
synchondrosis, 412
synchronicity, 458
synchronize, 231, 415, 426
syncope, 149
syncytial, 202, 214
syncytiotrophoblast, 199–201, 214, 218
syncytium, 123, 200, 299, 415
syndesmoses, 411
synergism, 50
synergistic, 51
synergistically, 291
synergy, 474–475
synovial, 227, 411–413, 440
synthase, 1, 4, 6, 13, 16, 21, 176, 277, 617
synthesis, 4, 6–7, 10, 13–18, 21–22, 24–26, 32, 37–39, 109, 160, 174–175, 269, 272–278, 280–282,

291–292, 306, 331–333, 336, 357, 385, 424, 451–452, 537, 540, 559, 565, 573–575, 615
synthesize, 15, 32, 38, 161, 181, 225, 264, 268, 273, 276–277, 284, 286–287, 298, 330, 336, 348, 362, 385, 445, 450, 452, 530, 542, 559, 570, 574, 579, 581–583, 598
synthetase, 18, 24, 33–34, 36, 336
syringe, 100
system, 109, 400, 402, 517
systole, 86, 88, 94–96, 98, 100–101, 103, 113, 116–119, 126–127, 137, 144–145, 153
systolic, 47, 66, 86, 97–104, 113, 115, 137–139, 144–145, 149, 291, 531

T cell, 91, 183, 278, 374–375, 378, 380, 383–384, 389–392, 394–396
tachyarrhythmias, 117
tachycardia, 98, 103, 131, 159
tachypnea, 159
Tanner scale, 586–587
tannins, 330
tapasin, 387
tapered, 335
Taq, 348
tarsal, 405, 412
tarsus, 434
tastants, 498–499
taste bud, 498
TATA, 354
taurine, 13
taurochenodeoxycholic, 13
taurocholic, 13
taut, 85, 439
TBP, 274
TCRs, 393
TDaP, 376
TdT, 393
tectorial, 258–259, 442–443, 489–490
tectospinal, 471
teenagers, 409
teeth, 90, 252, 295, 299, 309–310, 411, 504, 539
tegmental, 451
tegmentum, 478
tela, 253–254
telencephalon, 253–255
telomere, 351
telophase, 358–359
temporal bone, 223, 250, 309, 504
temporal lobe, 443, 504
temporalis, 249, 309–311
temporality, 48
tender, 571
tenderness, 562, 571
tendinae, 85
tendineae, 85, 97, 101, 103
tendinous, 212, 438
tenia, 297
tensile, 164, 194, 408
tension, 86, 117–119, 125–127, 154, 164, 315, 419–420, 465, 591, 597–599
tensor, 249, 259, 440
tentorium, 430
teres, 333, 501
terminalis, 253–255, 455, 497
terminalization, 359
termination, 38–39, 351–352, 354–355, 399, 602

terminator, 39
terminus, 175, 424
tertiary, 30, 194, 202, 214, 236, 557, 559
test, 62–63
testes, 13, 205, 262–263, 268, 277, 576–577, 579, 581–583, 585, 587
testicular, 587
testis, 577, 581–583
testosterone, 13, 175, 263, 271, 276–277, 573, 576–583, 586
tetanus, 376
tether, 85
tetrads, 358–359
tetraiodothyronine, 273
tetramer, 282
TF, 367, 538, 542
Tfh, 383
TG, 273–274
TGF, 383, 385–386, 399
Th, 383
thalamic, 254, 430, 504
thalamus, 253–254, 428–429, 437, 443, 477–479, 482–483, 487, 504
thebesian, 619
theca, 555, 557, 561, 572–574, 583
thelarche, 586
thermal, 348, 486
thermogenesis, 157–158, 450
thermoreceptors, 157, 484, 486
thermoregulation, 88, 157–159, 326
thermoregulatory, 157, 572
thermostat, 157
thermostatic, 428
theta, 458–459
thiamine, 1
thiazide, 520, 539, 541–542
thiazide diuretics, 539, 542
thiokinase, 1
thiophorase, 21
third stage of labor, 214
third ventricle, 254, 430, 456
thirst, 109, 326, 428
thoracic duct, 91, 156
thoracic vertebrae, 224
thoracolumbar, 445
threonine, 171, 176
threshold, 95, 121, 124, 299, 315–316, 320, 465, 544
thrill, 99
thrombin, 367, 369
thrombomodulin, 369
thromboplastin, 367
thrombosis, 156
thromboxane, 278, 365, 369, 617
thrombus, 143
thymic, 93
thymidylate, 24
thymine, 23–24, 38, 349
thymus, 93, 207, 251, 373
thyroglobulin, 273
thyroid, 157, 175, 204, 207, 236, 251–252, 262–265, 268, 272–275, 286, 590
thyroid gland, 170, 264, 272, 274, 284–285, 565
thyroid hormone, 272–275
thyroid-stimulating hormone, 174, 263, 268, 272, 274, 565
thyrotropic, 272, 274
thyrotropin, 175, 263, 268, 272, 274, 560
thyroxine, 264, 274
tibia, 227, 405

tidal, 564, 594–595, 601, 621
tide, 322, 331
tilting, 444
timbre, 99
TLC, 594
TLRs, 400
TNF, 183, 385
TNFα, 400
tobacco, 186
toenails, 247
tolerance, 381, 391, 399
tolerate, 88
toll, 400
toluene, 519
tongue, 93, 226, 251–253, 295, 309–310, 312, 325, 468, 497–498, 504–505, 509, 570, 589
tonic, 315–316, 443, 481
tonically, 301, 315
tonicity, 312
tonotopic, 443
tonsils, 93, 207, 251, 589
tooth, 194, 252, 312
topographically, 464, 475, 478
topoisomerase, 351
towels, 99
toxoid, 375–376
TPR, 104–105, 109, 112, 136, 146–147
trabeculae, 91–92, 406
trabecular, 406, 435
trachea, 207, 235–236, 310, 316, 588–590, 592–593
tracheal, 408, 591, 607
trachealis, 590
tracheoesophageal, 236, 238–239
tract, 98, 201, 206–207, 228–229, 235, 253–255, 258, 288, 299, 313, 315, 325, 424, 427, 437, 444, 450, 468–472, 475, 480, 483, 487, 495, 497, 504, 579–581, 583, 588
tractus, 105
transacetylase, 345
transacylase, 16
transaminase, 4, 33, 36
transamination, 32–33
transcriptional, 346
transcytosis, 328
transducer, 383
transducin, 439
transduction, 170, 174–175, 184, 282, 442, 486, 489, 491, 494
transection, 158
transfer RNA, 39, 355
transferase, 13, 393, 421
transferrin, 187, 330, 336
transform, 186, 224, 248, 252, 261, 383, 385, 440
transformation, 581
transfusion, 76, 112, 370
transient, 99, 134, 202, 486, 628
transiently, 316
transit, 608
transitional, 253, 513, 571
translation, 39–40, 160, 275, 346, 349, 351, 353–357, 359–361, 363
translocates, 282, 331
translocation, 184, 361
transmembrane, 170–171, 176, 386
transmission, 52–54, 123, 424, 426, 451–452
transmit, 105–106, 108, 440, 444, 464

Index

transmural, 597–598, 600
transportation, 162, 274, 387, 456
transporter, 9, 163, 273, 281–282, 287, 312, 322, 326–328, 331, 336, 387, 537, 544–545, 612
transportn, 609
transversal, 207
transverse, 128, 207, 241, 297–298, 300, 302–303, 414–415, 443, 511, 567
transversum, 210, 212, 239
trapezius, 505, 508
tremor, 476–478
Treppe, 127
TRH, 263, 268, 272, 274, 560
triacylglyceride, 4
triacylglycerol, 306, 336
triad, 333–334
triangular, 513
triceps, 501
tricuspid regurgitation, 98, 101
tricuspid stenosis, 98, 103
tricuspid valve, 85, 94, 96, 100–101, 103
trigeminal, 253, 309, 503–504
trigeminal nerve, 249, 259, 504, 507
triglyceride, 18, 328–329, 334
trigone, 246, 513
triiodothyronine, 264, 273
trilaminar, 201–202
trimester, 562–565
trimodal, 43
tripeptides, 327–328
triphosphate, 15, 170, 174, 286
triplet, 38
triploidy, 360
trisphosphate, 171, 174
tRNA, 39–40, 160, 355–356
trochlear, 254, 503
trochlear nerve, 504, 506
trophic, 272, 274
trophoblast, 197, 199–200, 202, 214
tropic, 268
tropocollagen, 164
tropomyosin, 125, 225, 415, 420
troponin, 125–126, 225, 415, 419–420
troughs, 458
TRPM, 486
TRPV, 486
truncal, 477
truncus arteriosus, 229, 231
trunk, 85, 90, 225, 238, 294, 464, 468, 471, 482, 500
trypsin, 286, 327–329, 337
trypsinogen, 327, 335, 337
TSH, 170, 263, 272, 274, 565
tubal, 93
tubercle, 246, 406, 563
tuberculosis, 571
tuberosity, 406
tubes, 228, 243, 555–556, 573, 583, 585, 591
tubular, 166, 258, 287, 426, 518–519, 538, 542–543, 545, 547, 584
tubule, 109–110, 166, 194, 243–245, 268, 285, 287, 289, 331, 414–416, 420, 511–513, 518–520, 531, 534–547, 549, 553–554, 564, 576–577, 581–582
tubulins, 177
tubuloacinar, 434
tubuloglomerular, 531
tuft, 511, 533

tumor necrosis factor, 183, 278
tumour, 103
tunica albuginea, 576, 582
tunica intima, 87
tunica media, 88
tunics, 87–88
turbulence, 589
turbulent, 98, 143
twin, 219–220
twitch, 315, 418, 465
tympani, 249, 258–259, 440, 442–443, 489
tympanic, 259, 440, 443
tympanic membrane, 440, 443
type i, 69–70, 164, 171, 237, 383, 385, 406, 408, 418, 591
type i error, 69–70
type ii, 69–70, 164, 171, 237, 378, 383, 385, 408, 467, 475, 570, 591, 598
type ii error, 69–70
type iii, 164
type iv, 164
tyrosine, 6, 171, 175–176, 184, 262, 271, 282, 378, 390, 451
tyrosyl, 273

ubiquinone, 2
ubiquitin, 186
UFR, 546
UGA, 355
UGC, 38
ulna, 227, 405, 411–412
ulnar, 501
ulnar nerve, 501
ultimo, 251
ultrasonic, 562
umami, 497, 499
umbilical, 207, 216, 231–232, 234–235, 333
umbilical cord, 214, 216–218, 232, 235, 241, 567
umbilicus, 562
UMP, 23–24
unabsorbed, 300
unbound, 274, 539, 545
uncharged, 547
uncoil, 359
unconjugated, 332
unconscious, 99, 423, 459–460
unconsciousness, 458
underpowered, 68
underreporting, 53
undifferentiated, 227, 322, 581–584
unexposed, 58–60
unidirectional, 156, 426
unidirectionally, 88, 426
unipolar, 129, 425
unlearned, 480
unloading, 613–614, 625, 627
unmineralized, 222
unmyelinated, 313, 425
unpackaging, 354
unpacked, 354
unpaired, 63, 187
unpleasant, 99
unpredictability, 463
unpredictably, 129
unresponsiveness, 395
unstressed, 105
untreated, 58
unventilated, 608

unzipped, 38
upmediated, 384
upper respiratory tract, 573, 588, 590
upregulate, 174, 287–289, 537
upregulation, 174, 287, 378, 390, 615
uptake, 32, 272, 282, 330, 336, 351, 426, 540, 564
urachus, 216, 218
uracil, 23, 38, 346, 349, 389
urea, 32–33, 36–37, 336, 535, 538, 543, 547–548
ureter, 244, 246, 510–511, 513, 534
ureteric, 243–244, 246
ureterovesical, 513
urethra, 207, 218, 246, 514, 578, 582–583
urethral, 513–514, 555, 576, 582–583
uric, 519
uric acid, 24, 27
uridine, 23, 389
urinalysis, 564
urinary bladder, 218
urinary sphincter, 432
urinary tract, 49, 572
urinary tract infection, 49
urinating, 326
urine pH, 519, 547
urobilin, 332
urobilinogen, 332
urodilatin, 542
urogenital, 205, 241, 243, 246, 514, 582–584
urorectal, 241, 246
uterine, 196, 199–200, 214, 216, 263, 555–556, 560–567, 570, 573
uterine tube, 196
uteroplacental, 200
uterosacral, 556
uterus, 174, 196, 199, 218–219, 268, 416, 513, 555–557, 559–567, 570, 573, 575, 583, 585
utility, 61
utilize, 626
UTP, 6
utricle, 258–259, 443–444, 491
utricular, 492
UUU, 38
UV, 287, 289
uvea, 436
uvula, 310, 589

Va, 367, 595–596
vaccinated, 54
vaccination, 53–54, 58, 375
vaccine, 375–376
vacuoles, 160, 186, 200, 214, 258
vacuolization, 260
vagal, 149, 305, 320, 323–324, 335
vagina, 513, 556, 563, 567, 573, 575
vaginal, 196, 555, 562, 567, 571–572, 578, 583, 585
vaginal opening, 514
vagotomy, 320
vagovagal, 302
vagus, 297, 305, 310, 325, 337, 503
vagus nerve, 105, 236, 250, 294–295, 302–303, 314, 318–320, 322–323, 335, 498, 505, 508
valence, 377
Valsalva, 99–100
Valsalva maneuver, 99, 301
valve, 84–86, 88–90, 94–96, 98–101, 103,

116–118, 137–138, 144, 156, 230–231, 297–298, 300, 316, 589
valvular, 98
vapor, 596–597, 603–604, 607, 628
variability, 67, 393
varicella, 375
varicose veins, 563–564
varicosities, 445
vas, 585
vas deferens, 578
vasa, 536
vascular endothelial growth factor, 228
vascularity, 563, 573
vascularization, 298
vascularized, 260, 265, 293, 436, 562
vasculature, 112, 116, 136, 607, 623, 627
vasculitis, 181
vasculogenesis, 202
vaso, 88
vasoactive, 152, 154, 302–303, 305, 307, 318, 617
vasoconstriction, 88, 107, 109, 139, 146–148, 152, 154, 157, 232, 446, 450, 534, 541–542, 617, 623–624, 627
vasoconstrictive, 278
vasoconstrictor, 153, 617
vasodilatation, 106
vasodilate, 88, 154
vasodilation, 105–106, 146, 152–154, 188–189, 312, 400, 450, 534, 563, 574, 617, 623
vasodilator, 153, 617
vasogenic, 628
vasomotor, 89, 149, 427, 572
vasopressin, 154, 263, 268, 552, 564
vasopressors, 159
vasorum, 88
vasovagal, 320
vault, 222
VC, 594
V_{CO_2}, 596
VD, 595–596
VDJ, 393
VEGF, 228
vehicle, 52
veli, 249
vellus, 192
velocity, 31, 98–99, 116, 118, 123, 136, 143, 419, 465–466, 606
vena, 85–86, 106, 136, 139, 141, 231–233, 334, 511, 563–564
venereal, 52
venial, 512
venoconstriction, 144
venosum, 232
venosus, 228–229, 231–233
venous, 89, 91, 98–100, 106, 111–112, 116–117, 119, 137, 139, 149, 155–156, 188, 231, 261, 322, 430, 435, 456, 592, 605, 607–609, 616, 618–621, 626
venous return, 87, 99–100, 111–112, 117, 139, 146–147, 149, 230, 563
venovenous, 159
ventilated, 595–596, 618, 621–623
ventilation, 107, 519–522, 593, 595–596, 601–602, 607–608, 618, 620–623, 625–627
ventilator, 522
ventilatory, 564, 602

ventral, 201, 223, 225, 227, 231, 238–240, 251, 253, 257–258, 261, 308, 427, 443, 451, 468, 477, 504, 601–602
ventrally, 201, 206, 210
ventricle, fourth, 456
ventricular, 86–87, 94–100, 113, 115–118, 123, 126, 128, 130–131, 133–134, 137, 159, 230–231, 254, 257, 431, 450, 456–457, 627
ventricular hypertrophy, 97, 130–131, 133, 627
ventricular septal defect, 98–99
ventrolateral, 225, 227
ventromedial, 307, 471
venule, 85, 88–89, 91, 141, 155, 334
vermis, 444, 474, 477
vernix, 247
vertebra, 589
vertebrae, 221, 224, 405–406, 456, 510
vertebral, 152, 224, 258, 427, 446, 483
vertebral column, 83, 426
vesical, 235, 246
vesicle, 155, 160–161, 163, 167, 177, 204, 244–245, 253–254, 258–260, 274, 276, 281–282, 286, 374, 387, 421–422, 426, 490–491, 514, 577–578, 580, 585
vesicular, 155, 163, 387
vessels, 83–85, 88–90, 92–93, 105, 118, 137, 139, 141–144, 147, 149, 153, 155–157, 164, 188, 191, 194, 200, 202–203, 214, 216, 222, 228, 232, 235, 247, 252, 261, 263, 268, 293–294, 317, 319, 364, 369, 406–407, 416–418, 430, 436, 438, 450, 452, 480, 513, 555–556, 573, 575, 617–618
vestibular, 253, 258–259, 443–444, 470–471, 474–475, 491, 494, 505, 507
vestibular apparatus, 491, 494
vestibular system, 443–444
vestibule, 442, 489, 505, 555
vestibuli, 258, 442–443, 489
vestibulo, 494–495
vestibulocerebellar, 476
vestibulocerebellum, 474
vestibulocochlear, 258, 503, 505
vestibulocochlear nerve, 491, 494, 507
vestibulospinal, 444, 471
viability, 200
vibrate, 440, 443, 489
vibration, 99, 191, 440, 442, 482, 485, 489–490
vibratory, 443
vibrissae, 589
vice, 596
villi, 90, 200–203, 214–215, 218, 296, 298, 325, 327–329, 331, 430
villous, 203
villus, 202, 297
vimentin, 177
vinegar, 313
VIP, 300, 303–307, 318, 320, 331
virally, 384–385
viruses, 400
viscera, 253, 293
visceral, 83–84, 206–207, 209–210, 225–226, 229, 236, 253–254, 293, 305, 313–314, 333, 427, 445, 447, 480, 591–592

visceral pericardium, 83–84, 229
viscerocranium, 222–223
viscosity, 98, 141, 143, 599, 627
viscous, 311, 407–408
vision, 423, 427, 432, 436–437, 439, 504
visual acuity, 437
vitamin A, 334, 437
vitamin B, 32, 330
vitamin C, 330
vitamin D, 190, 284, 288–292, 330, 411, 571–572
vitamin K, 297–298, 330, 367, 369
vitelline, 218, 228, 231
vitelline duct, 207, 210, 216, 218, 238, 241
vitreous, 261, 434–435, 439
vitreous humor, 434–435, 439
VLDL, 336
VMA, 451
V_{max}, 31–32
vocal, 236, 580, 589–590
vocalization, 588
voice box, 589
Volkmann, 406
voltage, 125, 127, 129–130, 132, 163, 421–422, 426, 433, 452, 458, 481, 490–491, 499, 624
volume, 113, 115
vomer, 589
von Willebrand, 365, 367
VPN, 308
VpreB, 381
vQ, 134
VRG, 601
VT, 594–596, 600
vulva, 556, 565
vulvar, 555
V_x, 605

waddling, 565
wakefulness, 458–459
Wald, 69
wall, 598
warmth, 571
watery, 321, 434, 571
waveforms, 459
wavefront, 131
wavelengths, 289
way, 65
WBC, 564
weakly, 306, 385, 602
weather, 193
Weinberg, 344
Wernicke, 428, 461–462
Westphal, 254
Wharton's jelly, 216, 235
whey, 570
white blood cell, 564
white matter, 254, 257, 425, 427–428, 468
Whitney, 63
whoosh, 103
Windkessel, 144–145
windpipe, 590
withdrawal, 572
wither, 235
Wolff, 274, 411
Wolffian, 581–584
womb, 220
workbench, 39
working memory, 461
workload, 185, 530, 625, 627
workup, 98

worldwide, 219
wrinkled, 339
wrinkling, 572
wrinkly, 339
writhing, 478

X-linked dominant, 342–343
X-linked recessive, 342–343
Xa, 367
xenobiotic, 336
xiphoid process, 224, 406
xylulose, 10

Y chromosome, 581–583
Y-linked, 341–342
Y-linked inheritance, 342
yeast, 571
yeast infections, 571
yellow fever, 375
yield, 42, 54, 117
yielding, 326
YLD, 61
YLL, 61
yolk, 207
yolk sac, 200, 204, 207, 210, 214, 216, 218–219, 228, 238, 581
yolk stalk, 207
yr, 339
yy, 308
yyrr, 339

ZAP, 390
zeta, 390
zeugopod, 227
zinc, 175
zona, 196–197, 254, 265, 269–270, 276–278
zona pellucida, 196–198
zonula, 260
zonule, 436, 439
zoster, 375, 571
ZP, 197
zwitterion, 29
zygomatic, 223, 249, 505
zygomatic arch, 309
zygote, 196–199, 219–220, 555
zygotene, 358
zymogen, 335

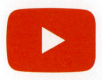

Watch our new videos every week:
www.youtube.com/osmosis

Follow us on Facebook:
@osmoseit

Follow us on Twitter:
@osmoseit

Follow us on Instagram:
@osmosismed